THE LUNG AT DEPTH

LUNG BIOLOGY IN HEALTH AND DISEASE

1. Immunologic and Infectious Reactions in the Lung, *edited by Charles H. Kirkpatrick and Herbert Y. Reynolds*
2. The Biochemical Basis of Pulmonary Function, *edited by Ronald G. Crystal*
3. Bioengineering Aspects of the Lung, *edited by John B. West*
4. Metabolic Functions of the Lung, *edited by Y. S. Bakhle and John R. Vane*
5. Respiratory Defense Mechanisms (in two parts), *edited by Joseph D. Brain, Donald F. Proctor, and Lynne M. Reid*
6. Development of the Lung, *edited by W. Alan Hodson*
7. Lung Water and Solute Exchange, *edited by Norman C. Staub*
8. Extrapulmonary Manifestations of Respiratory Disease, *edited by Eugene Debs Robin*
9. Chronic Obstructive Pulmonary Disease, *edited by Thomas L. Petty*
10. Pathogenesis and Therapy of Lung Cancer, *edited by Curtis C. Harris*
11. Genetic Determinants of Pulmonary Disease, *edited by Stephen D. Litwin*
12. The Lung in the Transition Between Health and Disease, *edited by Peter T. Macklem and Solbert Permutt*
13. Evolution of Respiratory Processes: A Comparative Approach, *edited by Stephen C. Wood and Claude Lenfant*
14. Pulmonary Vascular Diseases, *edited by Kenneth M. Moser*
15. Physiology and Pharmacology of the Airways, *edited by Jay A. Nadel*
16. Diagnostic Techniques in Pulmonary Disease (in two parts), *edited by Marvin A. Sackner*
17. Regulation of Breathing (in two parts), *edited by Thomas F. Hornbein*
18. Occupational Lung Diseases: Research Approaches and Methods, *edited by Hans Weill and Margaret Turner-Warwick*
19. Immunopharmacology of the Lung, *edited by Harold H. Newball*
20. Sarcoidosis and Other Granulomatous Diseases of the Lung, *edited by Barry L. Fanburg*

21. Sleep and Breathing, *edited by Nicholas A. Saunders and Colin E. Sullivan*
22. *Pneumocystis carinii* Pneumonia: Pathogenesis, Diagnosis, and Treatment, *edited by Lowell S. Young*
23. Pulmonary Nuclear Medicine: Techniques in Diagnosis of Lung Disease, *edited by Harold L. Atkins*
24. Acute Respiratory Failure, *edited by Warren M. Zapol and Konrad J. Falke*
25. Gas Mixing and Distribution in the Lung, *edited by Ludwig A. Engel and Manuel Paiva*
26. High-Frequency Ventilation in Intensive Care and During Surgery, *edited by Graziano Carlon and William S. Howland*
27. Pulmonary Development: Transition from Intrauterine to Extrauterine Life, *edited by George H. Nelson*
28. Chronic Obstructive Pulmonary Disease: Second Edition, Revised and Expanded, *edited by Thomas L. Petty*
29. The Thorax (in two parts), *edited by Charis Roussos and Peter T. Macklem*
30. The Pleura in Health and Disease, *edited by Jacques Chrétien, Jean Bignon, and Albert Hirsch*
31. Drug Therapy for Asthma: Research and Clinical Practice, *edited by John W. Jenne and Shirley Murphy*
32. Pulmonary Endothelium in Health and Disease, *edited by Una S. Ryan*
33. The Airways: Neural Control in Health and Disease, *edited by Michael A. Kaliner and Peter J. Barnes*
34. Pathophysiology and Treatment of Inhalation Injuries, *edited by Jacob Loke*
35. Respiratory Function of the Upper Airway, *edited by Oommen P. Mathew and Giuseppe Sant'Ambrogio*
36. Chronic Obstructive Pulmonary Disease: A Behavioral Perspective, *edited by A. John McSweeny and Igor Grant*
37. Biology of Lung Cancer: Diagnosis and Treatment, *edited by Steven T. Rosen, James L. Mulshine, Frank Cuttitta, and Paul G. Abrams*
38. Pulmonary Vascular Physiology and Pathophysiology, *edited by E. Kenneth Weir and John T. Reeves*
39. Comparative Pulmonary Physiology: Current Concepts, *edited by Stephen C. Wood*
40. Respiratory Physiology: an Analytical Approach, *edited by H. K. Chang and Manuel Paiva*
41. Lung Cell Biology, *edited by Donald Massaro*
42. Heart–Lung Interactions in Health and Disease, *edited by Steven M. Scharf and Sharon S. Cassidy*
43. Clinical Epidemiology of Chronic Obstructive Pulmonary Disease, *edited by Michael J. Hensley and Nicholas A. Saunders*
44. Surgical Pathology of Lung Neoplasms, *edited by Alberto M. Marchevsky*
45. The Lung in Rheumatic Diseases, *edited by Grant W. Cannon and Guy A. Zimmerman*

46. Diagnostic Imaging of the Lung, *edited by Charles E. Putman*
47. Models of Lung Disease: Microscopy and Structural Methods, *edited by Joan Gil*
48. Electron Microscopy of the Lung, *edited by Dean E. Schraufnagel*
49. Asthma: Its Pathology and Treatment, *edited by Michael A. Kaliner, Peter J. Barnes, and Carl G. A. Persson*
50. Acute Respiratory Failure: Second Edition, *edited by Warren M. Zapol and Francois Lemaire*
51. Lung Disease in the Tropics, *edited by Om P. Sharma*
52. Exercise: Pulmonary Physiology and Pathophysiology, *edited by Brian J. Whipp and Karlman Wasserman*
53. Developmental Neurobiology of Breathing, *edited by Gabriel G. Haddad and Jay P. Farber*
54. Mediators of Pulmonary Inflammation, *edited by Michael A. Bray and Wayne H. Anderson*
55. The Airway Epithelium, *edited by Stephen G. Farmer and Douglas Hay*
56. Physiological Adaptations in Vertebrates: Respiration, Circulation, and Metabolism, *edited by Stephen C. Wood, Roy E. Weber, Alan R. Hargens, and Ronald W. Millard*
57. The Bronchial Circulation, *edited by John Butler*
58. Lung Cancer Differentiation: Implications for Diagnosis and Treatment, *edited by Samuel D. Bernal and Paul J. Hesketh*
59. Pulmonary Complications of Systemic Disease, *edited by John F. Murray*
60. Lung Vascular Injury: Molecular and Cellular Response, *edited by Arnold Johnson and Thomas J. Ferro*
61. Cytokines of the Lung, *edited by Jason Kelley*
62. The Mast Cell in Health and Disease, *edited by Michael A. Kaliner and Dean D. Metcalfe*
63. Pulmonary Disease in the Elderly Patient, *edited by Donald A. Mahler*
64. Cystic Fibrosis, *edited by Pamela B. Davis*
65. Signal Transduction in Lung Cells, *edited by Jerome S. Brody, David M. Center, and Vsevolod A. Tkachuk*
66. Tuberculosis: A Comprehensive International Approach, *edited by Lee B. Reichman and Earl S. Hershfield*
67. Pharmacology of the Respiratory Tract: Experimental and Clinical Research, *edited by K. Fan Chung and Peter J. Barnes*
68. Prevention of Respiratory Diseases, *edited by Albert Hirsch, Marcel Goldberg, Jean-Pierre Martin, and Roland Masse*
69. *Pneumocystis carinii* Pneumonia: Second Edition, Revised and Expanded, *edited by Peter D. Walzer*
70. Fluid and Solute Transport in the Airspaces of the Lungs, *edited by Richard M. Effros and H. K. Chang*
71. Sleep and Breathing: Second Edition, Revised and Expanded, *edited by Nicholas A. Saunders and Colin E. Sullivan*
72. Airway Secretion: Physiological Bases for the Control of Mucous Hypersecretion, *edited by Tamotsu Takishima and Sanae Shimura*

73. Sarcoidosis and Other Granulomatous Disorders, *edited by D. Geraint James*
74. Epidemiology of Lung Cancer, *edited by Jonathan M. Samet*
75. Pulmonary Embolism, *edited by Mario Morpurgo*
76. Sports and Exercise Medicine, *edited by Stephen C. Wood and Robert C. Roach*
77. Endotoxin and the Lungs, *edited by Kenneth L. Brigham*
78. The Mesothelial Cell and Mesothelioma, *edited by Marie-Claude Jaurand and Jean Bignon*
79. Regulation of Breathing: Second Edition, Revised and Expanded, *edited by Jerome A. Dempsey and Allan I. Pack*
80. Pulmonary Fibrosis, *edited by Sem Hin Phan and Roger S. Thrall*
81. Long-Term Oxygen Therapy: Scientific Basis and Clinical Application, *edited by Walter J. O'Donohue, Jr.*
82. Ventral Brainstem Mechanisms and Control of Respiration and Blood Pressure, *edited by C. Ovid Trouth, Richard M. Millis, Heidrun F. Kiwull-Schöne, and Marianne E. Schläfke*
83. A History of Breathing Physiology, *edited by Donald F. Proctor*
84. Surfactant Therapy for Lung Disease, *edited by Bengt Robertson and H. William Taeusch*
85. The Thorax: Second Edition, Revised and Expanded (in three parts), *edited by Charis Roussos*
86. Severe Asthma: Pathogenesis and Clinical Management, *edited by Stanley J. Szefler and Donald Y. M. Leung*
87. *Mycobacterium avium*–Complex Infection: Progress in Research and Treatment, *edited by Joyce A. Korvick and Constance A. Benson*
88. Alpha 1–Antitrypsin Deficiency: Biology • Pathogenesis • Clinical Manifestations • Therapy, *edited by Ronald G. Crystal*
89. Adhesion Molecules and the Lung, *edited by Peter A. Ward and Joseph C. Fantone*
90. Respiratory Sensation, *edited by Lewis Adams and Abraham Guz*
91. Pulmonary Rehabilitation, *edited by Alfred P. Fishman*
92. Acute Respiratory Failure in Chronic Obstructive Pulmonary Disease, *edited by Jean-Philippe Derenne, William A. Whitelaw, and Thomas Similowski*
93. Environmental Impact on the Airways: From Injury to Repair, *edited by Jacques Chrétien and Daniel Dusser*
94. Inhalation Aerosols: Physical and Biological Basis for Therapy, *edited by Anthony J. Hickey*
95. Tissue Oxygen Deprivation: From Molecular to Integrated Function, *edited by Gabriel G. Haddad and George Lister*
96. The Genetics of Asthma, *edited by Stephen B. Liggett and Deborah A. Meyers*
97. Inhaled Glucocorticoids in Asthma: Mechanisms and Clinical Actions, *edited by Robert P. Schleimer, William W. Busse, and Paul M. O'Byrne*
98. Nitric Oxide and the Lung, *edited by Warren M. Zapol and Kenneth D. Bloch*

99. Primary Pulmonary Hypertension, *edited by Lewis J. Rubin and Stuart Rich*
100. Lung Growth and Development, *edited by John A. McDonald*
101. Parasitic Lung Diseases, *edited by Adel A. F. Mahmoud*
102. Lung Macrophages and Dendritic Cells in Health and Disease, *edited by Mary F. Lipscomb and Stephen W. Russell*
103. Pulmonary and Cardiac Imaging, *edited by Caroline Chiles and Charles E. Putman*
104. Gene Therapy for Diseases of the Lung, *edited by Kenneth L. Brigham*
105. Oxygen, Gene Expression, and Cellular Function, *edited by Linda Biadasz Clerch and Donald J. Massaro*
106. Beta$_2$-Agonists in Asthma Treatment, *edited by Romain Pauwels and Paul M. O'Byrne*
107. Inhalation Delivery of Therapeutic Peptides and Proteins, *edited by Akwete Lex Adjei and Pramod K. Gupta*
108. Asthma in the Elderly, *edited by Robert A. Barbee and John W. Bloom*
109. Treatment of the Hospitalized Cystic Fibrosis Patient, *edited by David M. Orenstein and Robert C. Stern*
110. Asthma and Immunological Diseases in Pregnancy and Early Infancy, *edited by Michael Schatz, Robert S. Zeiger, and Henry N. Claman*
111. Dyspnea, *edited by Donald A. Mahler*
112. Proinflammatory and Antiinflammatory Peptides, *edited by Sami I. Said*
113. Self-Management of Asthma, *edited by Harry Kotses and Andrew Harver*
114. Eicosanoids, Aspirin, and Asthma, *edited by Andrew Szczeklik, Ryszard J. Gryglewski, and John R. Vane*
115. Fatal Asthma, *edited by Albert L. Sheffer*
116. Pulmonary Edema, *edited by Michael A. Matthay and David H. Ingbar*
117. Inflammatory Mechanisms in Asthma, *edited by Stephen T. Holgate and William W. Busse*
118. Physiological Basis of Ventilatory Support, *edited by John J. Marini and Arthur S. Slutsky*
119. Human Immunodeficiency Virus and the Lung, *edited by Mark J. Rosen and James M. Beck*
120. Five-Lipoxygenase Products in Asthma, *edited by Jeffrey M. Drazen, Sven-Erik Dahlén, and Tak H. Lee*
121. Complexity in Structure and Function of the Lung, *edited by Michael P. Hlastala and H. Thomas Robertson*
122. Biology of Lung Cancer, *edited by Madeleine A. Kane and Paul A. Bunn, Jr.*
123. Rhinitis: Mechanisms and Management, *edited by Robert M. Naclerio, Stephen R. Durham, and Niels Mygind*
124. Lung Tumors: Fundamental Biology and Clinical Management, *edited by Christian Brambilla and Elisabeth Brambilla*
125. Interleukin-5: From Molecule to Drug Target for Asthma, *edited by Colin J. Sanderson*
126. Pediatric Asthma, *edited by Shirley Murphy and H. William Kelly*

127. Viral Infections of the Respiratory Tract, *edited by Raphael Dolin and Peter F. Wright*
128. Air Pollutants and the Respiratory Tract, *edited by David L. Swift and W. Michael Foster*
129. Gastroesophageal Reflux Disease and Airway Disease, *edited by Mark R. Stein*
130. Exercise-Induced Asthma, *edited by E. R. McFadden, Jr.*
131. LAM and Other Diseases Characterized by Smooth Muscle Proliferation, *edited by Joel Moss*
132. The Lung at Depth, *edited by Claes E. G. Lundgren and John N. Miller*
133. Regulation of Sleep and Circadian Rhythms, *edited by Fred W. Turek and Phyllis C. Zee*

ADDITIONAL VOLUMES IN PREPARATION

Anticholinergic Agents in the Upper and Lower Airways, *edited by Sheldon L. Spector*

Control of Breathing in Health and Disease, *edited by Murray D. Altose and Yoshikazu Kawakami*

Immunotherapy of Asthma, *edited by Jean Bousquet and Hans Yssel*

Chronic Lung Disease of Early Infancy, *edited by Richard D. Bland and Jacqueline J. Coalson*

Diagnostic Pulmonary Pathology, *edited by Philip T. Cagle*

Multimodality Treatment of Lung Cancer, *edited by Arthur T. Skarin*

Cytokines in Pulmonary Infectious Disease, *edited by Steven Nelson and Thomas Martin*

Asthma's Impact on Society: the Social and Economic Burden, *edited by Kevin B. Weiss, A. Sonia Buist, and Sean D. Sullivan*

Asthma and Respiratory Infections, *edited by David P. Skoner*

New and Exploratory Therapeutic Agents for Asthma, *edited by Michael Yeadon and Zuzana Diamant*

Particle–Lung Interactions, *edited by Peter Gehr and Joachim Heyder*

Tuberculosis: A Comprehensive International Approach, *edited by Lee B. Reichman and Earl S. Hershfield*

The opinions expressed in these volumes do not necessarily represent the views of the National Institutes of Health.

THE LUNG AT DEPTH

Edited by

Claes E. G. Lundgren
State University of New York at Buffalo
Buffalo, New York

John N. Miller
University of South Alabama
Mobile, Alabama

MARCEL DEKKER, INC. NEW YORK • BASEL

ISBN: 0-8247-0158-5

This book is printed on acid-free paper.

Headquarters
Marcel Dekker, Inc.
270 Madison Avenue, New York, NY 10016
tel: 212-696-9000; fax: 212-685-4540

Eastern Hemisphere Distribution
Marcel Dekker AG
Hutgasse 4, Postfach 812, CH-4001 Basel, Switzerland
tel: 41-61-261-8482; fax: 41-61-261-8896

World Wide Web
http://www.dekker.com

The publisher offers discounts on this book when ordered in bulk quantities. For more information, write to Special Sales/Professional Marketing at the headquarters address above.

Current printing (last digit):
10 9 8 7 6 5 4 3 2 1

PRINTED IN THE UNITED STATES OF AMERICA

To our wives

INTRODUCTION

Undoubtedly, when Jules Verne first introduced underwater adventures in his popular novels, the reaction was one of both astonishment and dreams! ''Why not?'' wondered the free spirits of the time. That was in the mid-nineteenth century.

It was truly the second World War that defined the possibilities—and then the risks—of diving. Since then, those interested in the physiology of the underwater environment have opened a world of biological exploration that has been extraordinarily productive. This productivity has been felt in many areas. First and foremost, we have learned about the response and adaptation of the body to increased environmental barometric pressure. With this knowledge, the field enlarged remarkably to encompass industrial projects as well as recreational possibilities. Many events of the last few years have illustrated all the possibilities that arise from being able to manage in the undersea world.

Futuristic though his vision may have been, even Jules Verne would never have dreamed of diving to 700 meters underwater and coming back safely to continue a more mundane life at sea level. To put it simply, this has been a result of the hard work and imagination of a great number of engineers and life scientists.

Soon, this series of monographs will introduce a volume describing adaptations to low barometric pressure, that is, high altitude. It will be followed by another volume showing the effect of microgravity, that is, space. It seemed appropriate that these two forthcoming volumes should be preceded by a monograph on the lung at depth. Claes Lundgren was an ideal choice to edit such a volume, as he brought to this task decades of extensive and novel research in the field of deep-sea adaptation. He developed a roster of contributors that is quite remarkable; indeed, anyone who has read in this field will recognize the names of the research pioneers who have made possible deep-sea diving as we know it today.

Jules Verne made us dream. The authors of this monograph contributed immensely to making this dream a reality. I am grateful to the opportunity to present them and to introduce their work to the readers of the *Lung Biology in Health and Disease* series.

Claude Lenfant, M.D.
Bethesda, Maryland

PREFACE

The underwater world severely challenges human physiology and especially respiratory function. It does so because water is not respirable by humans under normal circumstances, because it exerts pressure on the body, and because it is likely to disturb human thermal balance. The most critical of functions—namely the supply of adequate amounts of oxygen at an appropriate pressure—can be compromised in the diving environment at two extremes, i.e., by hypoxia in the breath-hold diver and the drowning victim, and by oxygen toxicity in the diver using breathing gear. Another kind of dualism pertains to the cooling effects of water. By facilitating the diving response, it may conserve oxygen and enhance the breath-hold diver's endurance and chance of survival in near-drowning accidents; however, cooling the breathing gas may endanger divers using breathing gear.

Current deep-sea diving has penetrated beyond 700 meters of depth; at 700 meters, divers will experience a 71-fold increase in pressure. The respiratory impediment caused by gas density—even with optimal mixtures of hydrogen, helium, and oxygen—may limit physical performance and compromise carbon dioxide elimination. Moreover, lung function in divers may undergo long-term changes, even in the absence of obvious injury mechanisms. By contrast, the abnormal condition of intravascular gas embolization, which forces the lung to act as a bubble filter, is often endured without any apparent unfavorable effects. Notwithstanding the tolerance of the respiratory system to various stresses, having healthy lungs is considered a prerequisite for divers. Nevertheless, the permissibility of a history of asthma in diver candidates is under debate. However, even in the absence of any pre-dive abnormalities, severe lung injury, known as pulmonary barotrauma, may be sustained in diving due to inadequate technique and/or technology. Yet modern breathing gear built to the best design standards is able to keep a working diver at a relatively adequate physiological steady state at great depths.

By contrast, the breath-hold diver is in a profoundly unsteady state, the operational limits of which are currently being explored in record-setting attempts around the world. Although it pales in comparison to the performance of the natural divers of the animal kingdom, the current human depth record for breath-hold diving, at 133 meters, is impressive. This performance relies on adaptability of respiratory functions to the stresses of apneic immersion, which only a few decades ago was considered improbable by respiratory physiologists. Paradoxically, the recent observations of potentially life-threatening pulmonary edema from as commonplace an activity as swimming at the surface were equally surprising to our profession.

This book attempts to offer a comprehensive view of the many-faceted aspects of lung function in the water environment. To the extent that it succeeds, it is due in large measure to the wisdom and good work of my coeditor, John N. Miller, M.D., whose involvement with the project was cut short by his untimely death in 1997.

I would like to take this opportunity to convey the editors' thanks to the authors of this volume for both their professional contributions and their good-spirited indulgence when circumstances beyond our control caused delays in the project. Thanks are also due to the colleagues who provided peer reviews of the manuscripts, and to Ms. Jeanne M. Catalano for excellent technical support in preparing the material for publication. It is also important to recognize that this book was inspired by Dr. Claude Lenfant, Executive Editor of this series, who has been a much appreciated source of inspiration and encouragement throughout the project.

Claes E. G. Lundgren

CONTRIBUTORS

Jolie Bookspan, Ph.D. Former Research Associate, Institute for Environmental Medicine, University of Pennsylvania, Philadelphia, Pennsylvania

Alf O. Brubakk, M.D., Ph.D. Professor, Department of Physiology and Biomedical Engineering, Medical Faculty, Norwegian University of Science and Technology, Trondheim, Norway

John R. Clarke, Ph.D. Scientific Director, Navy Experimental Diving Unit, Panama City, Florida

David M. Denison, Ph.D., F.R.C.P. Emeritus Professor of Clinical Physiology, Royal Brompton Hospital and National Heart and Lung Institute, London, England

Massimo Ferrigno, M.D., F.C.C.M. Staff Anesthesiologist, Brigham and Women's Hospital and Harvard Medical School, Boston, Massachusetts

Valerie Flook, Ph.D., C.Phys., M.Inst.P. Department of Biomedical Sciences, University of Aberdeen, and Unimed Scientific Ltd., Aberdeen, Scotland

Edward T. Flynn, Jr., M.D. Research Associate Professor of Anesthesia, Institute for Environmental Medicine, University of Pennsylvania, Philadelphia, Pennsylvania

T. James R. Francis, Ph.D., M.F.O.M. Biomedical Department, Naval Submarine Medical Research Laboratory, Groton, Connecticut

Robert S. Howard, M.D., Ph.D., L.D. Center for Marine Biotechnology and Biomedicine, Scripps Institution of Oceanography, University of California, San Diego, La Jolla, California

Gerald L. Kooyman, Ph.D. Professor in Residence, Center for Marine Biotechnology and Biomedicine, Scripps Institution of Oceanography, University of California, San Diego, La Jolla, California

Johannes A. Kylstra, M.D., Ph.D. Professor Emeritus, Department of Medicine, Duke University Medical Center, Durham, North Carolina

Edward H. Lanphier, M.D. Senior Scientist Emeritus, Department of Preventive Medicine, University of Wisconsin Medical School, Madison, Wisconsin

A. Joseph Layon, M.D. Professor, Departments of Anesthesiology, Surgery, and Medicine, and Chief, Division of Emergency Medicine, University of Florida and Shands Hospital, Gainesville, Florida

Claes E. G. Lundgren, M.D., Ph.D. Director, Center for Research and Education in Special Environments, and Professor, Department of Physiology, State University of New York at Buffalo, Buffalo, New York

Jerome H. Modell, M.D. Associate Vice-President for Health Affairs and Professor of Anesthesiology, University of Florida College of Medicine, Gainesville, Florida

Tom S. Neuman, M.D. Professor of Medicine and Surgery, Department of Medicine, University of California, San Diego, Medical Center, San Diego, California

James C. Parker, Ph.D. Professor, Department of Physiology, College of Medicine, University of South Alabama, Mobile, Alabama

Paul J. Ponganis, M.D., Ph.D. Associate Research Physiologist, Center for Marine Biotechnology and Biomedicine, Scripps Institution of Oceanography, University of California, San Diego, La Jolla, California

James W. Reed, Ph.D. Senior Lecturer in Physiology, Department of Physiological Sciences, Medical School, University of Newcastle, Newcastle upon Tyne, England

Aubrey E. Taylor, Ph.D. Louise Lenoir Locke Eminent Scholar, Professor, and Chairman, Department of Physiology, College of Medicine, University of South Alabama, Mobile, Alabama

Einar Thorsen, M.D., Ph.D. Norwegian Underwater Technology Centre A/S, Laksevåg, Norway

Anne Vik, M.D., Ph.D. Department of Neurosurgery, Norwegian University of Science and Technology, Trondheim, Norway

CONTENTS

1

Respiratory Function at Depth

JOHN R. CLARKE

Navy Experimental Diving Unit
Panama City, Florida

VALERIE FLOOK

University of Aberdeen
and Unimed Scientific Ltd.
Aberdeen, Scotland

I. Introduction: Physics and Physiology

A. Relative Changes

The evolution of humans from their land-dwelling mammalian forebears presumably occurred under conditions of stable environmental pressure. Today, ''standard'' physical conditions are based upon the assumption that the mean barometric pressure at sea level is 760 mmHg. [We analyzed over 200,000 mean monthly sea level pressures stored on the National Oceanic and Atmospheric Administration's Global Historical Climatology Network (GHCN) (1) and found that the average pressure was 759.4 mmHg, reassuringly close to standard pressure.] Since much of the earth's inhabited land masses are above sea level, the average meteorological reporting station's pressure should be somewhat less than 760 mmHg. Indeed, the GHCN database yields an average station pressure of 724.7 mmHg.

The scales on household barometers provide a handy estimate of the expected meteorological variation in barometric pressure; it varies roughly between 700 and 800 mmHg (933 and 1066 mbar). Consequently, transient weather phenomena affect barometric pressure by roughly $\pm$ 7% of the mean. [The lowest pressure ever recorded was 653 mmHg (870 mbar) in a hurricane.] Not surprisingly, altitude can have a greater impact on barometric pressure than does weather. Atmospheric pressure in barely inhabited 6000-m altitude regions of the Andes Mountains of Chile (2,3) drops to 372 mmHg. However, humans generally inhabit regions of higher atmospheric pressure, so it is safe to assume that their exposure to varying pressure on dry land ranges between 50 and 100% of the absolute pressure at sea level and more typically ranges within 10% of standard pressure. On an absolute scale, that is not a large variation.

In the face of relatively constant barometric pressure, there is no reason for humans to have evolved the biochemical and physiological ability to deal with very high ambient pressure. However, in diving, one is being thrust into an underwater environment where the atmospheric pressure increases tens of times over that of the normal environment, with 1 atm of pressure being added for every 10 m increase in depth.* Just as in flight, we have learned to use technology to equip us in ways that evolution did not. In recent years, humans have spent prolonged periods at depths greater than 2000 fsw (613 msw), at an ambient pressure of 45,960 mmHg (889 psi, 61.3 bar, $6.13 \cdot 10^6$ Pa). There is no place on earth where the human body can experience such dramatic environmental changes, on an absolute scale, and then return relatively unscathed.

The body surface area of a man 177 cm tall, weighing 70 kg, is approximately 1.86 m^2. When multiplied by the pressure (force per unit area) acting on that body surface at a depth of 2000 fsw, we find an astonishing force of $1.15 \cdot 10^8$ newtons applied to the outside of the diver's body. Were it not for the incompressibility of the majority of the diver's body and the use of modern underwater breathing apparatus, the diver would be crushed. Crushing does not occur because of Pascal's principle: pressure exerted on an enclosed fluid is transmitted equally to every part of the fluid and to the walls of the fluid's container. In other words, for the above example, there is a force pressing out on the body that exactly matches the force pressing in.

Unfortunately, there is a catch. Gas is compressible. If a diver were to hold his breath and make an unplanned descent to 2000 fsw, his lungs would be filled with gas trapped at a pressure of 1 atm absolute (101 kPa). The increasing pressure across his chest would not be counterbalanced, and his chest would be crushed long before 2000 fsw was reached. An underwater breathing apparatus (UBA; Chap. 12) keeps this from happening by maintaining an airway pressure that is very nearly identical to the pressure of the surrounding water column (see Fig. 1).

---

*Pressure is related to depth through the law of hydrostatics: $P = h \cdot \rho \cdot g$, where h is the height of the water column at the point of interest, ρ is water density, and g is the acceleration due to gravity. The hydrostatic pressure at a depth of 1m of seawater (msw) is defined as 10 kPa, assuming a ρ of 1.01972 g/mL at 4°C. The primary definition (3) of 1 ft of seawater (fsw) is 1 bar/32.646, assuming a seawater density (ρ) of 1.02480 g/mL at 4°C. From the above primary definitions, we obtain 10 msw = 1 bar.

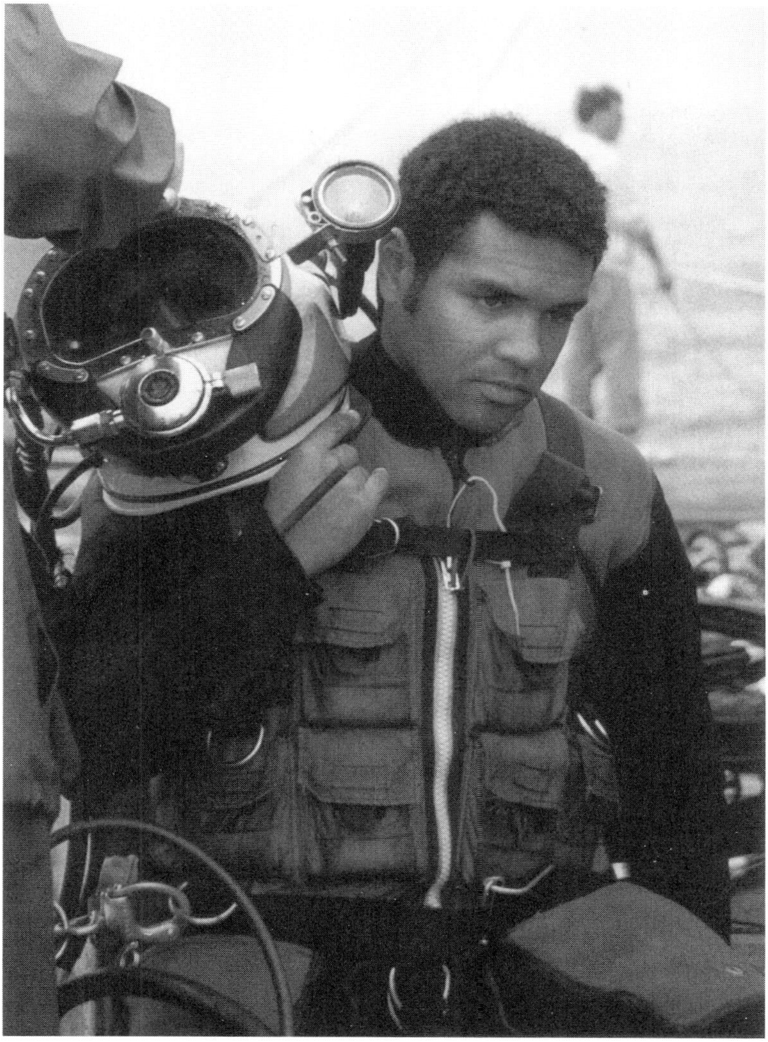

Figure 1 A Navy diver prepares for his next dive during search and recovery operations at the TWA 800 crash site at Moriches Inlet, Long Island, N.Y. (*Official U.S. Navy photo by Journalist Second Class Ligia I. Manning.*)

While technology allows us to deal with large changes in environmental pressure by artificially minimizing pressure gradients across the chest, there is a physiological price to be paid: that is, the mass and density of the breathing medium inevitably increases as environmental pressure increases. It is astonishing, however, that this price is not prohibitive. An individual can tolerate prolonged periods under enormous ambient pressures with little more than mild exercise limitation. Indeed, a deep-sea diver is akin to a patient with pulmonary disease who endures a constraint on physical activity but is essentially normal otherwise. The diver's quality of life may suffer, but the environment is tolerable.

B. The Approach

In this chapter we explore the effects of these unavoidable physical changes on the physiology of the human respiratory apparatus. To this end, we will describe the respiratory system as two distinct yet largely interrelated entities—one being a complex network of conducting tubes that could function inanimately almost as well as in life. The other is the biological function that modulates the basic mechanical function of the airways and is vastly more complex than a mere assemblage of air passages.

We treat the mechanics of gas flow at depth in a quantitative manner through the methods of fluid dynamics. However, we will not attempt to present the fluid dynamics portion of this chapter with anything like the detail and authority of those who have gone before us. Rather, we will interject into the subject those teachings that are best illustrated by—and in some cases are peculiar to—diving and hyperbaria.

II. Introduction to Flow in Airways

The pressure required to drive gas through respiratory airways is dependent on the physical properties of the gas and the flow rate. The physical property most affected by depth is gas density; it increases in direct proportion to an increase in atmospheric pressure. Since hydrostatic pressures increase approximately 1 atm for each 10 m of depth (1 atm=1.013 bar), the pressure at 100 msw is 10 atm plus the atmosphere above sea level, for a total of 11 atm absolute. Consequently, air with a gas density of 1.1 $g \cdot L^{-1}$ BTPS at the surface would turn into a 12.1 $g \cdot L^{-1}$ gas at 100 msw. Not surprisingly, the respiratory pressures required to force such a dense gas through human airways is considerably greater than that required for normal air. At the surface, an expired ventilation ($\dot{V}_E$) of 75 $L \cdot min^{-1}$ causes 83 g of air to pass on a round trip through the airways each minute. At 60 msw, that same expired ventilation sends 466 g of compressed air through the respiratory tree each minute.

The respiratory airways are composed of both pulmonary and extrapulmonary passages. We will see that as gas density increases, the maximal flow rate that can be achieved becomes limited. However, the site of that limitation varies between pulmonary and extrapulmonary regions, depending on the phase of ventilation. Furthermore, the mechanism of flow limitation seems to vary as well.

To understand the effect of increased gas density on respiratory mechanics, we have to understand the physical basis of the different types of flow in the airway. Respiratory flow is complex, in part because the flow is cyclic; it changes direction on the change from inspiration to expiration and vice versa. The characteristics of inspiratory flow (Fig. 2) are different from those for expiratory flow (Fig. 3) because airway bifurcations present a completely different shape to the flow profile depending on flow phase. The two flow streams merge during expiratory flow but split during inspiratory flow.

The vocal cords also contribute to phasic differences; they change shape and the aperture through them changes size as flow reverses. The aperture is open as inspiration starts and continues to increase with lung volume (4,5); during expiration the aperture size decreases. During inspiration, the pressure gradients across the airways all tend to expand the airway lumen. It is generally believed that dynamic compression of the airways, which can occur during expiration (Sec. V), should not be possible. However, we will show in Sec. VI that this assertion is not valid in diving.

Phase-related differences in airway geometry occur at localized regions within the airways. However, we gain further insight into respiratory flow by first considering the airways in toto and by envisioning them very simplistically as assemblages of pipes. Consequently, the engineering principles gleaned from nineteenth-century studies of pipe flow can illustrate basic concepts in respiratory flow.

A. Flow Regimes

Flow regimes in pipes can be characterized by a "Reynolds number." Osborne Reynolds was a British engineering professor who, in 1883, showed that the pressure drop along the length of a pipe was proportional to a dimensionless ratio of pipe and fluid parameters describing the relative importance of a flow's inertial forces to its viscous forces. This ratio, named the Reynolds number (Re) in his honor, is defined as:

$$\mathrm{Re} = \frac{v \cdot D \cdot \rho}{\mu} \tag{1}$$

where D is the tube diameter in centimeters, ρ is gas density in grams per liter, v is mean fluid velocity in centimeters per second, and μ is gas viscosity in micropoise.

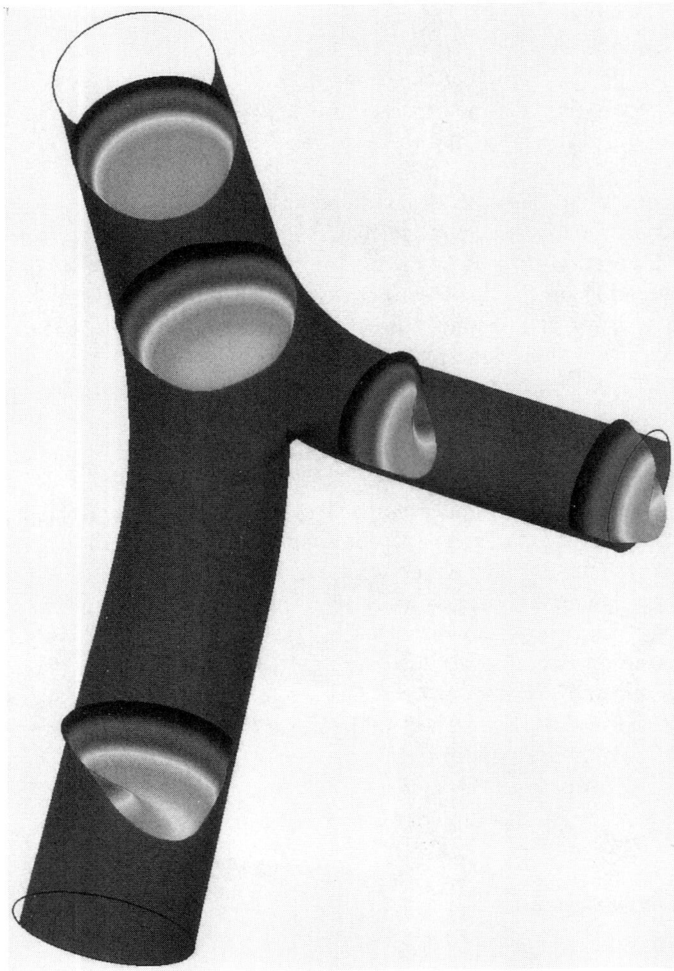

Figure 2 Velocity profiles for a computational fluid dynamic (CFD) simulation of laminar flow through a model bifurcation during quasi-steady flow typical of inspiration. The geometry of the model, such as the 70° branching angle and the diameter ratios of parent and daughter tubes, is characteristic of the small airways of the lung. The flow is for a Reynolds number of 500. The highly distorted profiles are caused by strong secondary cross flows, which are generated primarily by the axial curvature of the tubes. (*Courtesy of NSF Engineering Research Center, Mississippi State University.*)

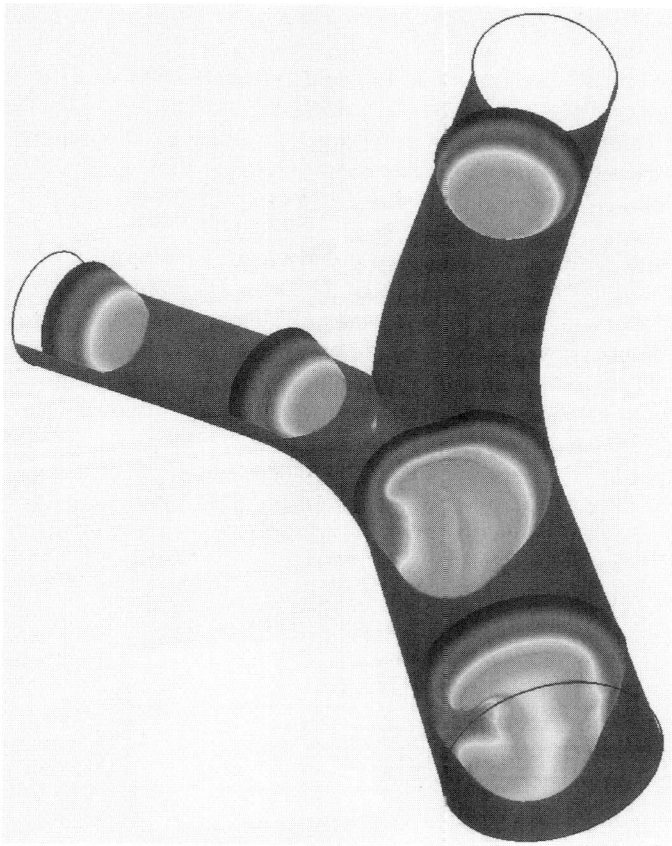

Figure 3 Velocity profiles for CFD simulation of laminar flow through a model bifurcation during quasi-steady flow typical of expiration. (*Courtesy of NSF Engineering Research Center, Mississippi State University.*)

When inertial forces based on fluid density and velocity are large relative to viscous forces, turbulence is favored. When viscosity is high relative to fluid inertia, Reynolds number is low and laminar flow is favored. The continuum of possible ratios of inertial and viscous forces is usually subdivided into flow regimes based on Reynolds numbers as follows:

1. Laminar flow, where the Reynolds number is below 2000. For this type of flow, the resistance to flow (R), defined as the ratio of

driving pressure to volumetric flow ($\Delta P/\dot{V}$), is independent of fluid velocity.

2. Critical, changing flow, Reynolds numbers 2000 to 4000. Resistance becomes dependent on fluid velocity.
3. Transitional turbulent flow, Reynolds numbers 4000 to 10,000.
4. Turbulent flow, Reynolds numbers greater than 10,000. Resistance to flow is proportional to flow$^{0.75}$ ($R \propto \dot{V}^{0.75}$).

Laminar flow is characterized by an orderly forward movement of fluid molecules (Fig. 4). For conditions in which the Reynolds number is less than 2000, any flow disturbances that occur are damped quickly by the fluid viscosity, and laminar flow is restored. For Reynolds numbers increasing from 2000 to 10,000, the effect of viscous damping is gradually reduced until, at Reynolds numbers of 10,000 or above, even the smallest flow disturbance is undamped and fully developed turbulence occurs.

To put these ranges of Reynolds numbers into perspective (6), the Reynolds number for blood flowing in a medium sized artery is about 1000, air flowing past a fast baseball has a Reynolds number of roughly 200,000, and air

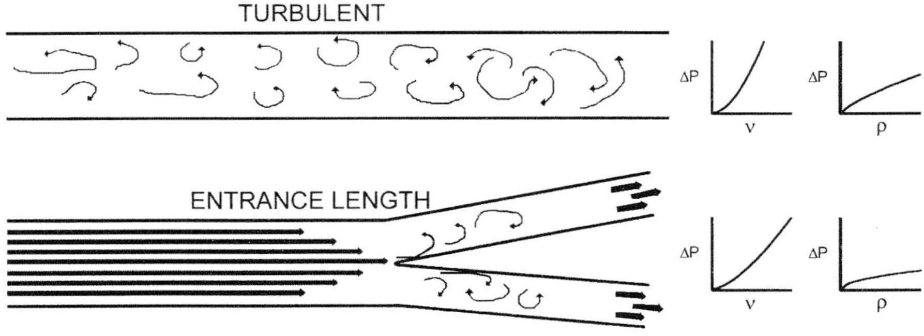

Figure 4 Highly simplified depiction of laminar, turbulent, and entrance length flow, along with plots of the respective relationships between ΔP and both flow velocity and gas density.

flowing over the fuselage of a cruising jetliner has a Reynolds number on the order of 100 million.

B. The Fifth Flow Regime: Orifice Flow

The upper airway includes a constriction at the larynx (Fig. 5). A sudden reduction in the diameter of a pipe through which a fluid is flowing may result in a type of flow called *orifice flow*. With fully developed orifice flow, the resistance to flow is linearly proportional to flow rate ($R \propto \dot{V}^{1.0}$). As will become clear in the course of this chapter, the presence of the larynx and the resultant flow patterns through it strongly influence pressure–flow relationships in the pulmonary airway tree. This influence applies to both inspiration and expiration, but the mechanisms are different in the two cases.

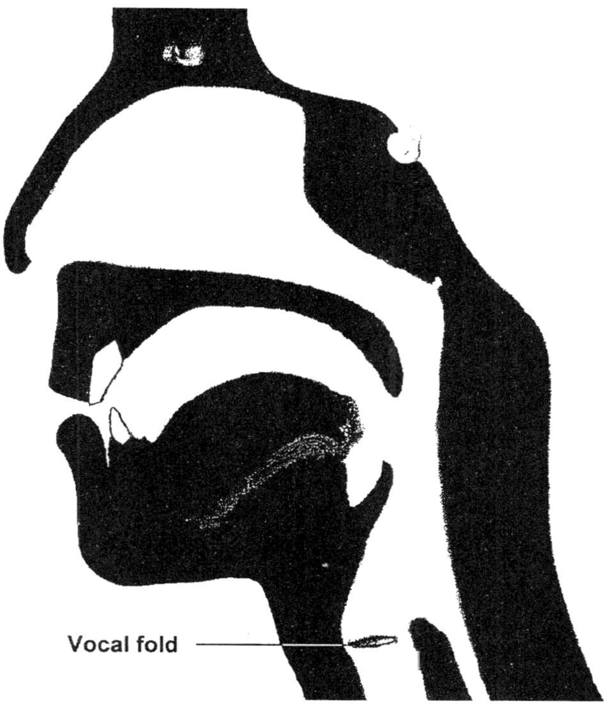

Figure 5 Silhouetted section of the upper airways, including oral cavity and pharynx.

Much of the following discussion is concerned with ways in which airway flow can be described within these five flow types.

C. Reynolds Number

The Reynolds number is very helpful for analyzing flow relationships. Table 1 lists values reproduced from Olson et al. (7) for Reynolds numbers calculated for each airway generation for an inspiratory flow of 60 $L \cdot min^{-1}$, calculated using two mathematical models of the airway tree. Weibel's model (8) assumes symmetrical bifurcations at the end of every airway down to the terminal bronchioles; the model of Olson et al. (7) allows for asymmetrical branching, has fewer bifurcations, and uses hydraulic diameter in place of geometric diameter. Hydraulic diameter is defined as twice the ratio of the cross-sectional area to

Table 1 Reynolds Number and Cumulative Pressure Drop Down Airways for Two Models of the Airway Tree

	Weibel		Olson	
Order	Reynolds number	Cumulative pressure	Reynolds number	Cumulative pressure
Mouth	2986	9.6	2986	15.4
Trachea	3500	23.2	3513	36.0
1	3114	35.6	2930	47.5
2	2295	45.8	2019	59.1
3	1698	57.7	1509	72.6
4	1058	67.2	672	78.0
5	679	75.1	512	83.9
6	424	82.6	239	86.4
7	259	87.5	177	89.3
8	160	91.4	137	92.3
9	96.4	93.3	57.3	93.5
10	57.1	96.0	47.2	95.0
11	34.1	97.4	22.2	95.8
12	19.6	98.4	16.5	96.7
13	11.3	99.0	12.4	97.6
14	6.3	99.5	5.8	98.4
15	3.6	99.7	4.4	99.0
16	1.9	99.8	3.2	99.8
17	1.1	99.9	1.2	99.9
18	0.6	100	0.6	100
19			0.2	100

Source: Data from Ref. 7.

the perimeter, thereby allowing definition of a characteristic diameter for noncircular pipes. Despite the differences in the models of Weibel and Olson, both show that the Reynolds number is below 2000 and never exceeds 10,000 for much of the airway tree, so that we may expect a successful fluid dynamic model of the airway tree to be one dealing with laminar, critical and transition flows (flow regimes 1, 2, and 3). For a lower flow rate of 30 $L \cdot min^{-1}$ (not shown), the Olson model predicts Reynolds numbers below 2000 for all generations. Reynolds numbers approach 10,000 in the upper airways only for flows in excess of 120 $L \cdot min^{-1}$.

It is axiomatic that no mathematical representation of the airway tree simple enough to be useful can be anatomically accurate, not least because not all respiratory bronchioles are at the ends of identical branching pathways. Thus Olson et al. define what they refer to as an ''effective'' pathway and Weibel defines an ''average'' pathway; both are intended to give a reasonable approximation to the anatomy that will allow a good simulation of the behavior.

Also included in Table 1 are the values for the cumulative pressure drop at each generation, expressed as a percentage of the total pressure drop down the airway. These are drawn from Olson (7) and are discussed in more detail later. They are presented here to show that most of the pressure drop occurs in the upper airways.

The conclusions to be drawn from Table 1 are that in the majority of airways, flow is more laminar than turbulent, but that most of the pressure losses are in the upper airways, where the flow is either critical or transitional. For all flows except those during quiet breathing, the dominant flow in the airway tree has Reynolds numbers in the region of 2000 to 10000, where the exact nature of the flow velocity profiles is difficult to describe.

D. Reynolds Number in Heliox

Because of its low density relative to nitrogen, helium is used as an inert gas instead of nitrogen in dives to depths in excess of 61 msw. Its low density yields reduced breathing resistance (9,10). Helium is also nonnarcotic at pressures relevant to diving (see Secs. VI.D and IX.A). Although helium has a density approximately one-seventh that of air, this difference is reduced in practice, because when helium is used in deep saturation diving, it is usual to add 40 to 45 kPa (0.4 to 0.45 atm) of oxygen. The density of this heliox mixture at sea level is more than half that of air at similar pressure and temperature.

The general statement that most airways have Reynolds numbers within the range for laminar flow and that most of the pressure losses occur in the upper airways is also true for heliox breathing except at normal pressure (1 atm absolute or 101 kPa). Table 2 gives the airway generation number at which the Reynolds number is first less than 2000 for air and heliox for a range of pres-

Table 2 Airways That Have Reynolds Numbers Less Than 2000

Air				Heliox, 40 kPa oxygen			
1 atm	2 atm	4 atm	8 atm	1 atm	10 atm	20 atm	40 atm
3	4	6	6	0	4	5	6

sures. The calculations from which this was derived were based on the numbers for the Olson model in Table 1.

E. Entrance Length and Density-Dependent Flow

Fully developed laminar flow is the only type of flow that is independent of changes in gas density. Its properties are described by the Hagen-Poiseuille equation for flow through smooth circular tubes of diameter D and length l:

$$\Delta P = 32\mu v \frac{l}{D^2}$$

where ΔP is the pressure drop down the length l, v is average linear velocity in $\text{cm} \cdot \text{sec}^{-1}$, and, as before, μ is the viscosity of the fluid. When flow is expressed as a volumetric rate, then the above equation becomes:

$$\Delta P = 128\mu \dot{V} \frac{l}{\pi D^4} \tag{2}$$

Dividing Eq. (2) by $\dot{V}$ gives flow resistance, with units of $Pa{\cdot}L^{-1}{\cdot}sec$.

$$R = \frac{\Delta P}{\dot{V}} = 128\mu \frac{l}{\pi D^4}$$

Thus, in laminar flow, flow resistance R is dependent on viscosity (μ) and not on fluid density (ρ).

However, these equations apply for only a very special type of laminar flow; that which is fully developed and has a parabolic velocity profile (Fig. 4). Fluid entering a tube or dividing at an airway bifurcation takes time and distance to build up a parabolic profile by accelerating the more central layers of the fluid relative to the layers closer to the walls. Thus there is an inertial (i.e., acceleration-dependent) component to flow, dependent on density, until the parabolic velocity profile is fully developed (11).

At each airway bifurcation, the parabolic flow profile is altered. The faster central layers end up close to the walls of the daughter tubes and decelerate, while the new central layers are accelerated (Fig. 3). Thus gas must flow some distance to generate a parabolic velocity profile in the next generation.

The distance required to develop laminar flow independent of fluid density is termed the *entrance length* (L), which, for smooth, round tubes has been found empirically (12) as

$$L = 0.0288\ \mathrm{Re}\cdot D \tag{3}$$

Thus the length of tube required to develop density-independent laminar flow depends on density [from the Reynolds number, Eq. (1)], and therefore will be different for different breathing gases and at different depths.

Within the entrance length for laminar flow, the energy dissipation per unit length of airway is higher than further into the airway, where parabolic laminar flow exists, because it takes energy to accelerate some of the fluid within the entrance length. Since flow within the entrance length of a tube depends on both density and viscosity, laminar flow is also in a sense dependent on these physical properties of the breathing gas.

Distance is also required for the development of turbulent flow, and an entrance length for that type of flow can also be defined. In general the entrance length for turbulent flow is about one-third of that for laminar flow. However, for most of the airway, fully developed turbulent flow plays a role only at very high flow if at all. Weibel's model gives a maximum Reynolds number of about 3500 for a flow of 60 $L\cdot min^{-1}$, and Olson's model yields a Reynolds number of 8500 for maximum flows of 120 $L\cdot min^{-1}$. Therefore, even at maximal flow rates, the Reynolds number is below that expected to result in fully developed turbulence. Consequently, we need not concern ourselves further with the energy losses accruing from the entrance length for turbulence.

The consequence of the energy requirements of a changing flow profile has been dealt with in detail by Olson et al (7). They calculated the entrance lengths for parabolic flow for each generation of bronchial airways at three flow rates; 30, 60, and 120 $L\cdot min^{-1}$. This was done both for their own asymmetrical series model, derived to fit the empirical data of several other groups of workers in addition to their own, and for the symmetrical model of Weibel.

Figure 6 shows entrance length as a ratio of geometrical length against airway generation for three flow rates for the Olson model and for one flow rate (60 $L\cdot min^{-1}$) for the Weibel model. The broken horizontal line is at the level where entrance length/geometrical length is unity. The results for the Weibel model fit within those of the Olson model for most flow rates and agree reasonably well at 60 $L\cdot min^{-1}$ for the higher generations. When entrance length/geometrical length is greater than unity, parabolic laminar flow cannot develop in that airway.

The inset for Fig. 6 shows an expanded section of the graph for airway generations higher than 10. Parabolic flow does not develop before the tenth generation even during quiet breathing, an observation verified by Pedley et al. (13,14). Thus, much of the airway tree can be classified by entrance length, in which inertial forces are important. The pressure drop down a length of tube

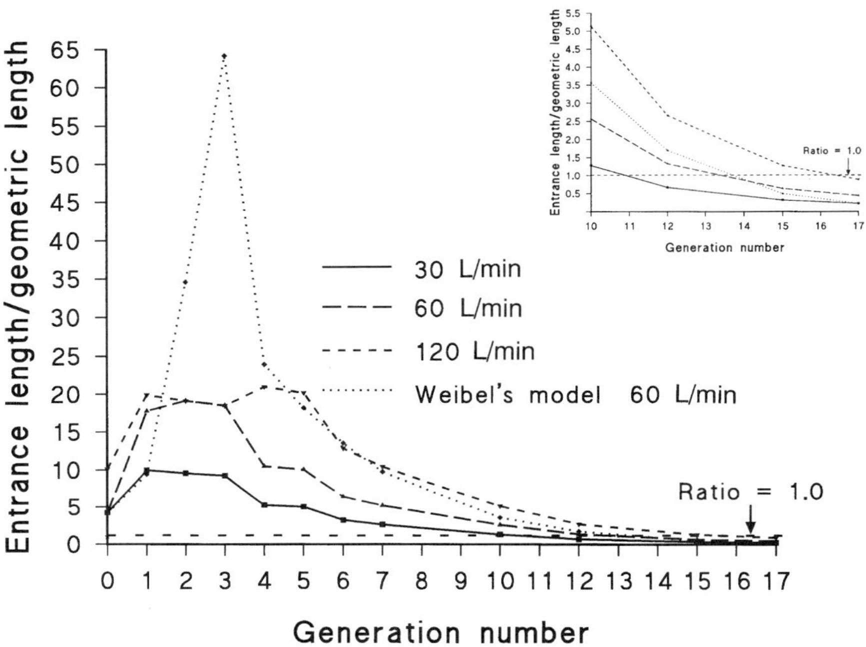

Figure 6 The ratios of entrance length to geometrical length as a function of airway generation. Inset: expanded portion for airway generations above 10. See text for details.

that is entirely entrance length is given by Olson et al. (7) as 1.63 times the pressure drop for Poiseuille flow in the same length of tube. They estimated that during quiet breathing in air at 1 atm absolute, as much as 75% of the pressure required to move air down the airway is used for changing the flow profiles.

Diving Application

The effect of gas density on entrance length is given in Fig. 7 for flow rates equivalent to quiet breathing. It is apparent that at a gas density 7 times that of 1 atm air, approximately equivalent to heliox at 45 atm absolute with 0.4 atm oxygen (the condition during saturation diving to 450 m), the whole of the lung is effectively entrance length. Parabolic velocity profiles do not develop and the energy requirements of inspiration even in quiet breathing is increased as a consequence.

Pedley et al. (14) derived an equation to account for the effect of entrance length on pressure drop down the lower airways.

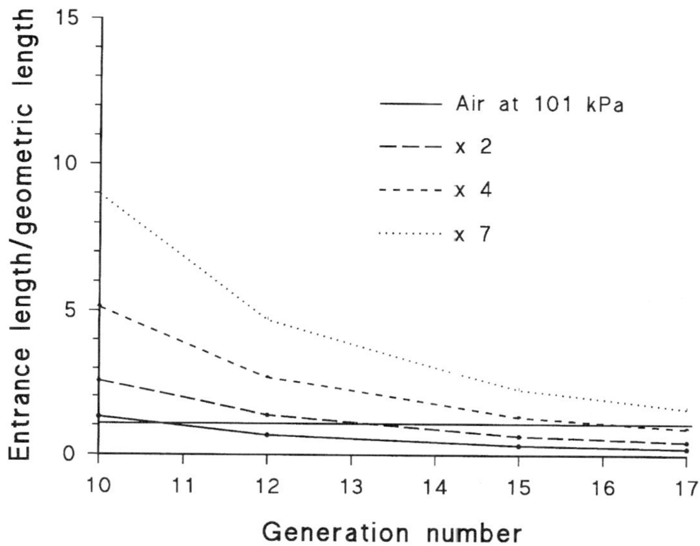

Figure 7 Effect of increased ambient pressure (in atm) on entrance length for generations greater than 10.

$$\Delta P = K(\mu\rho)^{1/2}\dot{V}^{3/2} \tag{4}$$

Equation (4) shows that because of entrance length effects, pressure drop down the lower airway should relate to the square root of both gas density and viscosity. Dividing Eq. (4) by $\dot{V}$, we see that flow resistance through entrance regions of the airways is proportional to the square root of flow, viscosity, and density.

$$R = K\cdot(\mu\rho\dot{V})^{1/2} \tag{5}$$

At elevated gas density, the majority of the lung is involved in entrance-length flow (Fig. 7), so Eq. (5) should be particularly applicable to deep diving. This applicability is discussed further in Chap. 12 in this volume. The models of Pedley et al. have been discussed in more detail in an earlier version of this series (15), with particular reference to the influence of flow patterns on gas mixing.

The notion that respiratory resistance varies as the square root of gas density has become a rule of thumb among diving scientists and practitioners, originating with a presentation by Jere Mead (16) at a diving symposium. However, Mead's 1955 paper notes that in subjects studied between the surface and

4 atm, airflow resistance increased approximately threefold. Because tissue resistance is generally included in resistance measurements and because tissue resistance is not dependent on gas density, the sensitivity of overall resistance to gas density should be less than airway-only resistance. "Taking tissue resistance into account, for a fourfold increase in density, the total pulmonary resistance should be approximately doubled."

We thus should not assume that Eq. (5) substantiates the rule of thumb about the dependence of resistance on the square root of gas density. Pedley's model does not explicitly deal with tissue resistance, as did Mead. Furthermore, as explained in Sec. IV.B of this chapter, there may be factors other than gas density that influence measured airway resistance at depth.

III. Dimensionless Analysis of Flow

Casts of mammalian airways show that the structure of respiratory airways is complex. Consequently, gas flow within them is also complex, containing a mixture of flow types, with bifurcations that present different profiles to each phase of ventilation and an orifice of variable size at the larynx.

In studies of fluid dynamics, complex problems are simplified by using dimensionless parameters. Reynolds number is one such dimensionless coefficient (Sec. II.A). Another is the Euler number, which is addressed in the following section; several other dimensionless numbers can be defined using dimensional homogeneity (17).

Plots of one dimensionless number against another give rise to a whole family of curves that apply for all flow regimes. An example of such a plot is a Moody diagram depicting the frictional resistance to flow as a function of Reynolds number and tube roughness. Such curves are useful because, once empirically determined values for any two dimensionless coefficients have been plotted for known conditions, the effect of changed conditions (such as an increase in fluid density) can be read from the plot.

From Table 1 it is evident that, on inspiration, most of the flow energy is dissipated in the upper airways. An important structure of the upper airway is the larynx, which, as we have pointed out, may act as an orifice at high enough flow rates, thereby accentuating energy dissipation. Some of the characteristics of inspiratory flow, described below, suggest that orifice flow may develop during inspiration of dense gases.

Figure 8 shows two types of orifices and the flow lines through them. The diameter of the pipe leading to the orifice is given as D, the diameter of the flow path through the orifice is d, and β is the angle which the orifice makes with the wall of the pipe. To pass through the constriction, the flow stream must narrow and the flow lines converge to a point called the vena contracta (c). The position of this, the narrowest point of the stream, is determined partly by the shape of the orifice. In some conditions the vena contracta is beyond the actual orifice simply because the momentum of the fluid resists changes in velocity. The cross-sectional area of the flow lines at c, A_c, divided by the cross-sectional area at d, A_d, is known as the coefficient of contraction, C_c.

In both orifice types shown in Fig. 8, eddy currents appear downstream of the orifice through a process called *flow separation*. Once formed, the eddy currents are stable and remain as long as the flow remains unchanged. Eddies cause a reduction in downstream pressure through energy dissipation; lateral pressure is reduced where the eddies are formed. In a changing flow, as during inspiration, eddies might be expected to develop as flow increases to a maximum and disperse as flow dies away. As shown below, the presence of eddies may have consequences for airway stability when the inhaled gas has a high density.

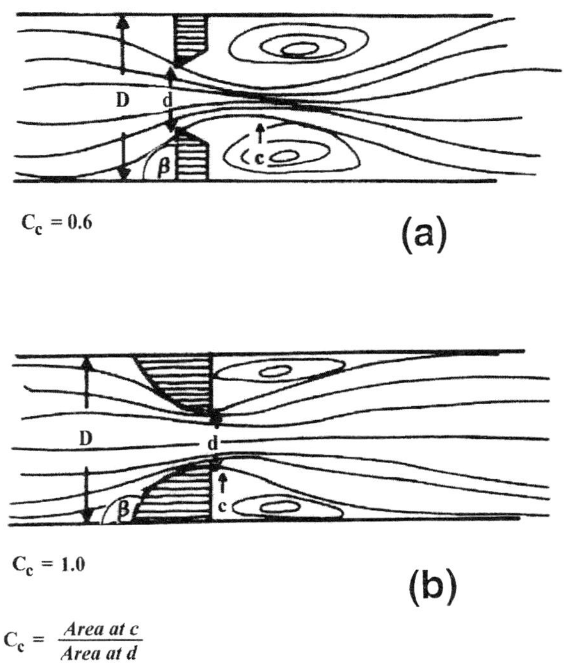

Figure 8 Orifices with (a) $\beta=90°$ and (b) β greater than 90°. When β is 90°, the coefficient of contraction is small and the region of eddy formation is large.

A. Coefficient of Discharge

The coefficient of discharge (C_d) is a dimensionless descriptor of orifice flow defined over the whole range of flow as:

$$C_d = \frac{\dot{V}}{A}\sqrt{\frac{\rho}{2\Delta P}} \tag{6}$$

where ρ is gas density, and ΔP, $\dot{V}$, and A are pressure drop, flow, and area of the orifice, respectively.

Figure 9 shows a graph of C_d against Reynolds number for all types of flow, including orifice flow, through a constriction of diameter d in a tube of diameter D. The relationships on this figure have been redrawn from Rouse (17) and are for four sizes of orifice for which β is 90° and for a venturi for which d/D is 0.5.

At a Reynolds number greater than about 10,000, C_d becomes constant at a value that depends on the orifice geometry and the coefficient of contraction (C_c) as given by Eq. 7.

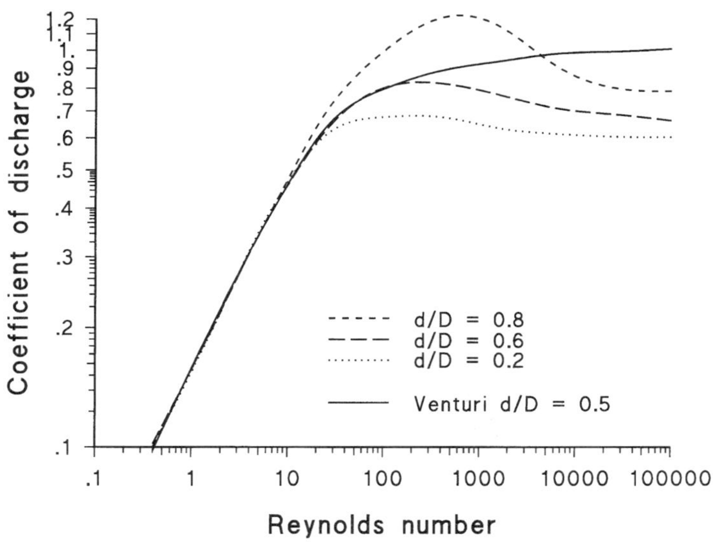

Figure 9 C_d versus Reynolds number for all types of flow through a constriction of diameter d in a tube of diameter D for four sizes of orifice for which β is 90° and for a venturi with $d/D = 0.5$.

$$C_d = \frac{C_c}{\sqrt{1 - C_c^2 \cdot (d/D)^4}} \tag{7}$$

The graph can be divided into regions of low, high, and intermediate Reynolds number.

When the Reynolds number is less than 10, the relationship is linear. Solving for pressure drop across the orifice for a low Reynolds number gives

$$\Delta P = K_3 \cdot \mu \cdot \frac{\dot{V}}{d^3} \tag{8}$$

Thus, at very low Reynolds numbers, inertial forces are unimportant; the pressure drop depends on viscosity and not on density. It should be noted that in constricted pipes, the change from viscosity dependence to density dependence occurs at much lower values of Reynolds number than for flow in unconstricted pipes (for example, 10 versus 2000).

At higher values of Reynolds number, C_d is a constant and the pressure drop across the orifice is given by

$$\Delta P = K_4 \cdot \rho \cdot \frac{\dot{V}^2}{d^4} \tag{9}$$

The pressure drop depends on density but not on viscosity.

Table 1 shows that the likely range of values for Reynolds number at the larynx lies within the intermediate region $10 < Re < 10{,}000$. Within this region, the pressure drop across the orifice changes from being dependent on d^3 to being dependent on d^4, from being dependent on viscosity to being dependent on density, and from being dependent on $\dot{V}^1$ to being dependent on $\dot{V}^2$.

IV. Airway Resistance

The above concepts were developed in studies of mechanical piping systems using instruments and methods not easily applied to human subjects. For human studies, instrumentation must be noninvasive and minimally obtrusive. The most convenient way to explore the linkage between the physical properties of a gas and respiratory function in humans is through a measurement of airway or respiratory resistance. Respiratory resistance represents the sum of airway and tissue flow resistance, whereas airway resistance is not affected by the viscous resistance of pulmonary tissue. In such measurements, the relationships among the three variables of ΔP, $\dot{V}$, and ρ pertain to the entire respiratory system or just the airways respectively.

The regions of the respiratory system that contribute the major portion of airway resistance are involved in nonlaminar flow even at 1 atm and are therefore affected by gas density. That fact is accentuated at depth. Pedley et al. (15) developed the following equation to describe density and flow dependence of transrespiratory pressures:

$$\Delta P = a \cdot (\rho^{1/2} \cdot \dot{V}^{3/2}) + b \cdot (\rho \cdot \dot{V}^2) \tag{10}$$

where the first term describes flow in lower airways [governed by entrance regions for laminar flow, Eq. (4)] and the second term represents a combined kinetic energy term and a term for flow in the upper airways, which is largely transitional or turbulent. This latter term comes from Darcy's formula (found in any fluid dynamics text) defining pressure drops in straight, constant-diameter pipes. The Darcy equation,

$$\Delta P = \frac{\rho f l v^2}{2D} \tag{11}$$

where f is a friction factor, l is pipe length, D is pipe diameter, and v is mean linear velocity applies to both laminar and turbulent flow. Figure 10 is a three-dimensional plot of Eq. (10), with the coefficients a and b set equal to 0.2 and 0.35, respectively.

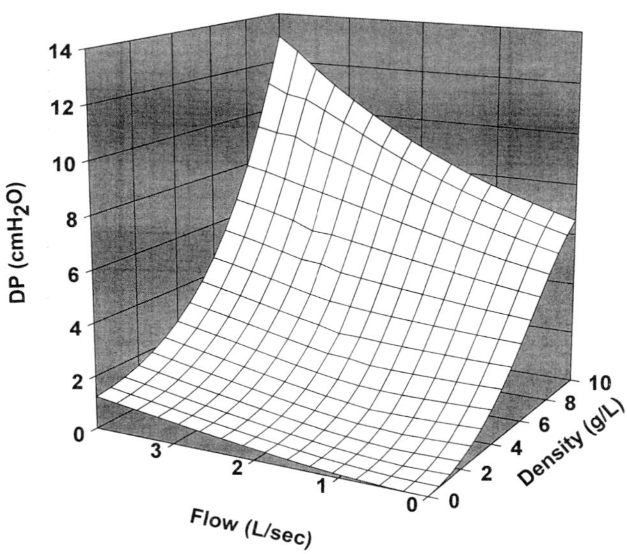

Figure 10 The dependence of pressure drop across the airways versus gas density and flow, with the coefficients in Eq. (12) being $a = 0.2$ and $b = 0.35$.

Airway resistance is obtained by dividing ΔP by $\dot{V}$, just as in Eq. (5). Consequently, expressing Eq. (10) as a resistance results in:

$$R = a \cdot (\rho\dot{V})^{1/2} + b \cdot (\rho\dot{V}) \tag{12}$$

Thus we expect resistance to range from (1) being proportional to the square root of density and flow to (2) being linearly dependent on density and flow. The actual curvilinearity of the relationships depends upon the relative values of the coefficients *a* and *b*.

A. Resistance Measurements

At 1 atm, there are at least five methods of measuring respiratory resistance, although one, a direct measurement of alveolar pressure (18), is not suitable for human studies. The four remaining techniques are the plethysmographic method of DuBois et al. (19); the subtraction method using esophageal pressure (20); the forced oscillation method (21), including variants based on swept sines and random noise (22); and the oldest method, the interrupter technique (23,24). The interrupter method is based on the equilibration of alveolar and mouth pressure during a brief occlusion of the airway. Although dated, the technique still finds application in modern studies because of the minimal amount of subject cooperation required (25–27).

B. Variability in Density Dependence

There have been few measurements of respiratory resistance at simulated depths of 300 msw or deeper. Clarke et al. (28) used the interrupter technique to measure resistance in resting divers at depths to 450 msw during heliox breathing. They found resistance rising approximately linearly with gas density, with values as high as 9 $cmH_2O \cdot L^{-1} \cdot s$. Surprisingly, the resistance in some divers increased twice as fast with density as in others on the dive team. Divers with the highest rates of increased resistance had significant smoking histories (Fig. 11).

In later work, a swept sines forced oscillation technique using the oscillator of Jackson and Vinegar (29) was used to measure respiratory resistance in divers at depths to 305 msw (30). As in the preceding study, the rate of resistance increase with gas density was twice as high in some divers as in others, rising as high as 7 $cmH_2O \cdot L^{-1} \cdot s$. Once again, the divers with higher resistance had considerable smoking histories.

It seems likely that if other methods of measuring resistance at depth had been used in the above studies, even greater changes in resistance might have been observed, since both the interrupter and forced oscillation techniques are less sensitive to differences in airway diameter than whole-body plethysmography and esophageal balloon catheters (31).

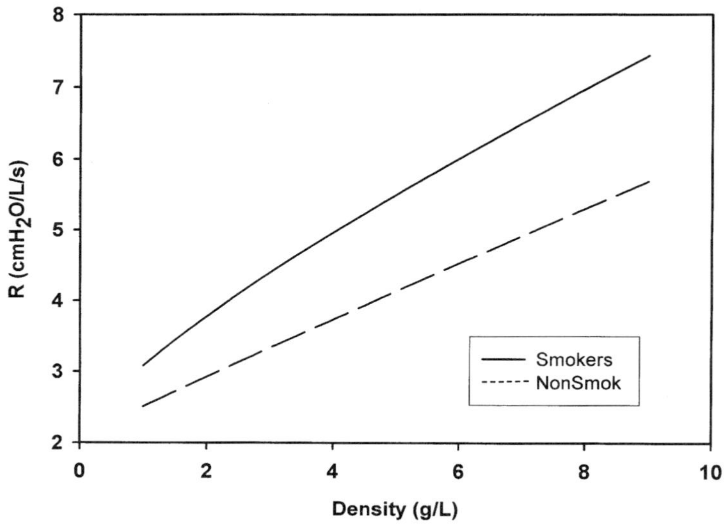

Figure 11 Regression of respiratory resistance against gas density for three smokers (solid line) and three nonsmokers (broken line) on a saturation dive to 450 msw.

Owing to the relatively small numbers of subjects (10 total) in the above hyperbaric studies, we lack the confidence of large numbers found in the usual studies of smokers. Unfortunately, substantiation may be a long while in coming, since deep research dives devoted to respiratory studies are relatively rare, and the presence of smokers in the population of research divers is becoming even rarer. Nevertheless, further discussion of those dive results illustrates interesting concepts in the respiratory mechanics of deep diving, as described below.

C. Mechanisms of Density Dependence

None of the techniques for measuring resistance are particularly sensitive to smoking histories at 1 atm in normal, asymptomatic smokers (32). Only small and variable differences in respiratory impedance between smokers and nonsmokers have been reported by Michaelson et al. (22), Kjeldgaard et al. (33), Hayes (34), and Peslin et al. (35). It appears, therefore, that the hyperbaric environment may somehow increase the sensitivity of resistance measurements or that undetectable differences in airway geometry at 1 atm absolute becomes accentuated at depth. As shown below, the latter possibility has support in the basic equations determining airway resistance.

Fluid Dynamics

As a reminder, the resistance to flow through a tube is determined by geometrical factors and mean gas velocity as well as gas density and viscosity. The following equation describes those relationships.

$$R = \frac{l \cdot \rho \cdot v^2}{2D \cdot \dot{V}} \cdot \mathrm{Re}^{-.25} \tag{13}$$

where l and D are tube length and diameter, respectively, in centimeters, ρ is gas density in grams per liter, v is mean gas velocity in centimeters per second, $\dot{V}$ is volumetric flow rate in liters per second, and Re is Reynolds number. In tube flow, velocity (v) is related to flow by the following equation.

$$v = \frac{\dot{V}}{\pi\left(\frac{D}{2}\right)^2}$$

Equation (13) describes the resistance of a tube containing fully developed turbulent flow. The equation is rewritten from Eq. (20) in Pedley et al. (15) and is valid for Reynolds numbers up to at least 100,000. The relation of Eq. (13) to the Darcy equation [Eq. (11)] becomes obvious when the Darcy equation is divided by flow to obtain resistance.

Both Eqs. (2) and (13) show that airway diameter has a pronounced effect on airway resistance when flow is either laminar or turbulent, respectively. When flow is density-dependent—i.e., turbulent as in Eq. (13) or controlled by entrance effects—an increase in gas density (ρ) amplifies the resistance increase for a given degree of airway narrowing. In other words, elevated gas density acts as a gain control, accentuating the effect of diameter changes.

If we substitute Eq. (1) for Reynolds number in Eq. (13), we can express the result in terms of its most fundamental variables.

$$R = 0.763 \cdot \left(\frac{l}{D^{4.75}}\right) \cdot \mu^{.25} \cdot \dot{V}^{.75} \cdot \rho^{.75} \tag{14}$$

Figure 12 is a plot of Eq. (14) for 2 $\mathrm{L \cdot sec^{-1}}$ flows of air through tubes 1.2 and 1.4 cm in diameter and 12 cm long. Air viscosity was assumed to be 188 μpoise. Density increased by an increase in ambient pressure, and viscosity changes with pressure were assumed to be negligible. Reynolds number for the larger tube began at 10,643 at a $\rho = 1.1\ \mathrm{g \cdot L^{-1}}$, and increased to 106,426 at a $\rho = 11.1\ \mathrm{g \cdot L^{-1}}$. For the smaller tube, Reynolds number began at 12,416 and rose to 124,163.

The key feature of Fig. 12 is the difference in inclination of the two curves; that is, the magnitude of the difference between the flow resistances of the two tubes was amplified by increases in gas density. Note the resemblance of Fig. 12 to Fig. 11.

Before accepting that airway narrowing could be responsible for the differing increases in resistance with increased gas density in deep-diving smokers, some thought must be given to the probable sites of narrowing in smokers. One possible site is the nose (36). However, in the interrupter and forced oscillation measurements of Clarke et al., the nose was clamped shut. We therefore focus our attention on intrathoracic airways.

When one speaks of the density dependence of resistance, it is usually in the context of studies of the small peripheral airways. When normal individuals breathe a low-density helium-oxygen gas mixture at 1 atm, airway resistance drops and peak flow rates and flow rates at mid–lung volume both increase. Not surprisingly, at high gas densities, the opposite is true; flow rates drop (37). This effect of density is attributed to the fact that the major sites of flow resistance are in the large airways, where flow is turbulent. The only form of flow that is not density-dependent is fully developed laminar flow—a pattern that may occur in small airways, where gas velocities are small owing to the combined volume of the many airways, and airway diameters are 2 mm or less,

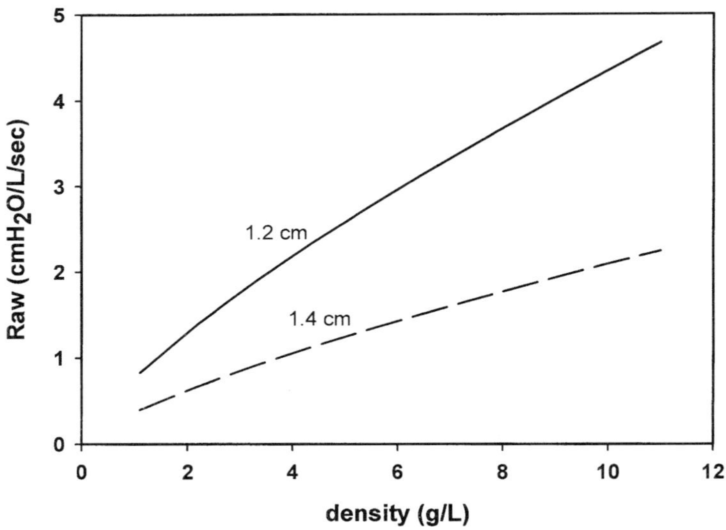

Figure 12 Plot of Eq. (14) for 2 L·sec^{-1} flows of air through tubes 12 cm long having diameters of 1.2 (solid line) and 1.4 cm (broken line).

making turbulence unlikely. Wood and Bryan (37) observed that ventilation with the dense gas sulfur hexafluoride raised lower pulmonary resistance in airways larger than 4 mm, but not in more peripheral airways. Presumably, flow in the lung periphery is fully laminar and therefore not density-dependent.

In asymptomatic smokers, it is the small peripheral airways that are usually affected by smoking. By use of a wedged bronchoscopic technique, peripheral airway resistance has been shown to vary widely among smokers, ranging from normal values to those found in asthmatics (38). For that reason, the percentage of gas flow that is laminar, and therefore density-independent, generally increases in smokers above that in nonsmokers. As a consequence, when a smoker inhales helium-oxygen gas mixtures, expiratory flow is increased as much as it is in normals (39–41). From this observation, we would anticipate that when gas density is increased, the resulting depression of flows and the increase in airway resistance would both be moderated in smokers, not accentuated, as the diving data suggest.

Equations of Motion

If we temporarily leave the subject of fluid dynamics and examine the equations of motion for the respiratory system, we do find phenomena similar to those observed in deep diving. As explained in Chapter 12, electrical analogs such as those of Fig. 13 and computer software for analyzing the time and frequency characteristics of electrical models are commonly used to describe the pressures and flows in oscillating mechanical systems.

Figure 13 is an analog of two serially aligned lung compartments, representing central and peripheral airways connected to a forced oscillation generator (e.g., a loudspeaker) at what would normally be the airway opening. Both the

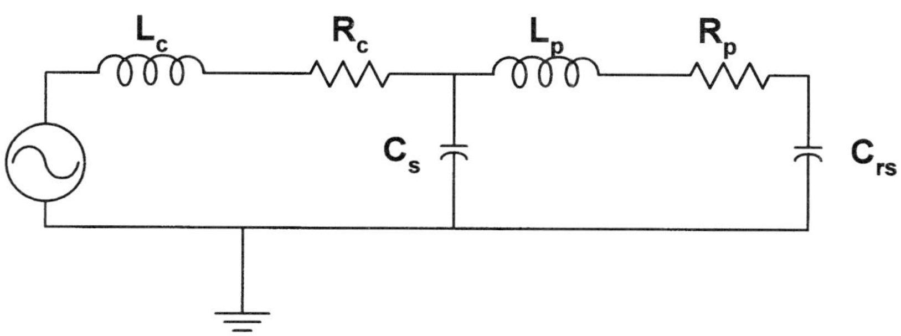

Figure 13 A two-compartment analog of serial inhomogeneity in a smoker. L, R, and C are inductances, resistances, and compliances, respectively. The subscripts c, p, and rs stand for central, peripheral, and respiratory system, respectively.

model and the nomenclature are taken from Mishima et al. (42), as were initial values for the various model components. In electrical terms, L is inductance, which is analogous to mechanical inertance (usually described by I), R is resistance, and C is compliance. (In keeping with electrical convention, we will use L in circuit diagrams such as Fig. 13. Also in keeping with convention, we use I when using the term *inertance* in a mechanical context.) The small letter c stands for central regions within the lungs, and p identifies peripheral components. Cs is a shunting compliance derived from airway wall tissue compliance. The only addition to the model of Mishima et al. was Crs, or respiratory system compliance. It was assumed to be equal to 0.1 $L \cdot cmH_2O^{-1}$, in accordance with Mead and Milic-Emili (43).

The inertance (I) of a fluid in a cylindrical tube such as the trachea is defined as:

$$I = \frac{\rho \cdot l}{A}$$

where ρ is gas density, l is the length of the tube, and A is the cross-sectional area of the tube (44). Inertance is a function of gas acceleration, which is unchanged with depth as long as $\dot{V}$ remains constant, and gas density, which is directly proportional to ambient pressure when the gas mixture remains constant. To simulate diving, we multiplied the normal 1 atm value of Lc by ambient pressure for simulated dives to 2.5, 4, 6, 8, 10, and 12 atm absolute. Both Rp and Lp were assumed to be unchanged by pressure. The normal value of Rc was multiplied by the square root of ambient pressure at each depth in accordance with long-standing estimates of gas density effects on respiratory resistance (16,37). Consequently, at 12 atm absolute, Lc rose to 0.18 $cmH_2O \cdot L^{-1} \cdot s^2$ ($12 \cdot 0.015$ $cmH_2O \cdot L^{-1} \cdot s^2$) and Rc increased to 4.78 $cmH_2O \cdot L^{-1} \cdot s$ ($12^{0.5} \cdot$ 1.38 $cmH_2O \cdot L^{-1} \cdot s$). Rp did not increase with ρ.

Input impedance (Z) was the ratio of voltage (the analog of pressure) on the oscillator side of Lc and the current (analog of flow) through Lc. Since the resulting impedance was complex valued, its real (Zr) and imaginary (Zi) components were determined. Resistance was then taken as the real component of input impedance at the resonant frequency (f_0) of the circuit; i.e., the frequency where Zi was zero. The resulting resistances are plotted as a function of ambient pressure up to 12 atm absolute in Fig. 14. Just as in the experimental dives, where forced oscillation measurements were made (30), the simulation for smokers (solid line) showed elevated resistances at pressures of 2 atm absolute and greater.

The preceding analysis teaches us that in interpreting measurements made of the respiratory system at depth, more than one approach may be required. An initial fluid dynamic analysis suggested that elevated resistances in smokers might be explained by the physics of turbulent flow through pipes. However,

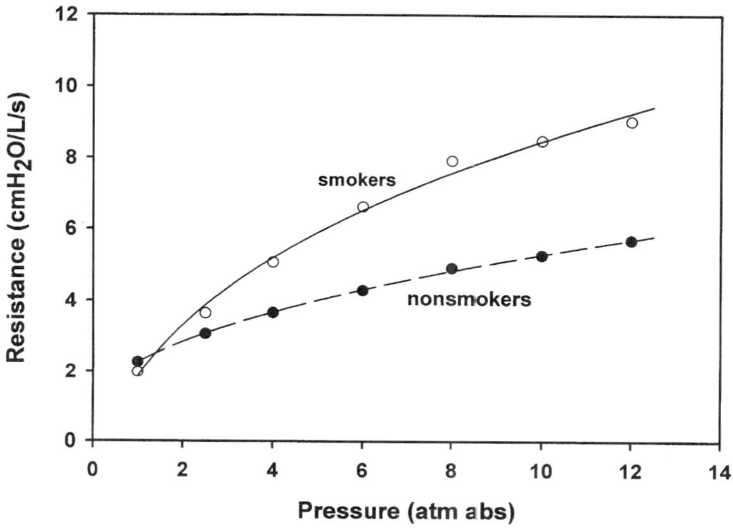

Figure 14 Predicted resistances based on the analogs of Fig. 13 as a function of ambient pressure for modeled smokers (Rp=5, solid line) and nonsmokers (Rp=1, broken line).

on closer inspection of the sites of airway narrowing in smokers, the fluid dynamic approach failed. Only by using simple electromechanical analogs of serial inhomogeneity were we able to gain insight into deep-dive measurements of respiratory resistance. In particular, respiratory analogs describe the consequences of oscillating flows in inertially loaded systems with more detail than comparably simple fluid dynamic models.

D. Computational Fluid Dynamics

The difficulty of explaining the apparent density dependence of resistance in deep-diving smokers by the usual arguments of fluid dynamics illustrates our ignorance of the dynamics of airway flow in small airways, especially as affected by the subclinical pathological changes induced by smoking.

The paucity of information regarding flow in small airways is not restricted to hyperbaria. Because of their size and location within the chest, small airways are amenable neither to direct measurements in situ nor to mechanical modeling (45). However, small airway flow can be simulated. A flow simulation involves obtaining numerical solutions to the three-dimensional, time-dependent Navier-

Stokes equations, which are nonlinear, second-order partial differential equations. These equations, coupled with those for mass and energy conservation, plus an appropriate equation of state, are assumed to be the complete equations of motion for fluids that obey the continuum condition. These solutions are the root of computational fluid dynamics (CFD), the dominant numerical field for continuum physics used to deal with the dynamics of large numbers of (on the order of 10^{23}) molecules.

In CFD, the mechanical and flow region to be analyzed is divided into a large number of cells or control volumes. The Navier-Stokes partial differential equations are rewritten as algebraic equations that relate simple physical parameters such as the velocity, temperature, and pressure of each cell to that of its neighbors. The resulting set of algebraic equations can then be solved iteratively to yield a description of flow throughout the region being analyzed.

CFD has been used in a variety of biomedical fields concerned with fluid flow; toxicology (46,47), anesthesiology (48), and neurology (49). The motivations for CFD simulations of flow in small respiratory airways are to describe flow at the locus for pathology in diseases affecting the small airways (50) and to learn how the details of airway geometry influence the distribution and deposition of aerosolized medications (51). Figure 15 shows graphical results from a three-dimensional lung airflow model depicting flow velocity at a single cross section in a single small-airway bifurcation. Velocity (in dimensionless units) ranges from zero (black in the right half of the figure) to maximum (white). The complex flow profiles are the result of airway curvature, which produces strong secondary flows (vortices, eddies, swirling). Such visualizations as Figs. 2, 3, and 15 support the current belief that flows within the larger airways of the lungs are exceedingly complex, and perhaps even chaotic, because of the constantly changing airway curvature and numerous bifurcations.

Because Reynolds numbers are less than 1000, flow in small airways is quasi-steady and laminar, but with velocity profiles that are highly skewed and inflected relative to similar flow in a section of straight tubing. In other words, the flow is complex but essentially laminar. We have no reason to believe that the fine detail of small-airway laminar flow has any effect on the density independence of small-airway flow.

The airway structures that produce such complex flow patterns may have evolved to ensure efficient gas mixing and distribution within the 50 m^2 of alveolar surface area contained within the adult human's 5- to 6-L thoracic volume (45,52). However, we do not know whether an anatomical design that may be optimized for gas mixing and flow distribution at 1 atm absolute remains equally effective at depth. CFD may provide a means for answering that question.

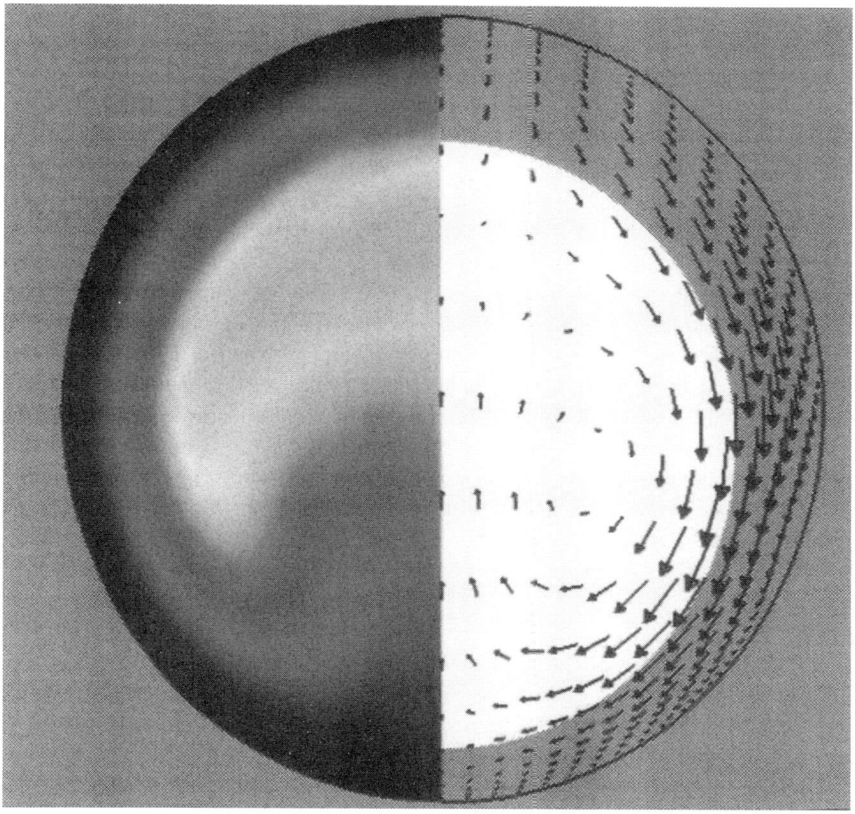

Figure 15 Velocity profiles and cross-flow vectors from a CFD simulation of laminar flow through a model bifurcation during quasi-steady flow typical of respiration. The flow is for a Reynolds number of 500. (*Courtesy of NSF Engineering Research Center, Mississippi State University.*)

CFD is a tool that might eventually help to explain how normal anatomical variation, increases in gas density, gas compressibility, and airway-wall compliance can translate into changes in the density dependence of airway resistance. Our initial hypothesis that the difference in respiratory resistance from one diver to another, for a given gas density, was due to variation in airway diameter is a gross and unlikely oversimplification. It is not satisfying that a more refined explanation based on gas inertance effects on serial inhomogeneity has not yet been mirrored by a fluid dynamic explanation involving inertial forces. We hope that CFD may provide the missing link between Newton's macroscopic equations of motion applied to diving and the Navier-Stokes equations for fluid flow.

The downside of CFD is that for large, time-dependent problems, such as a simulation of the beating heart or a breathing cycle in a complete bronchial tree, supercomputers with parallel processors and gigabyte memories are required. However, a great deal can be learned from computational simulation of flow through smaller subsystems, such as a cascade of lung bifurcations subjected to quasi-steady flow, as occurs around peak inspiration and expiration. Such simulations can be conducted on more modest machines, such as one of the Silicon Graphics Power Challenge series of compute servers.

The investment in time and dollars for supercomputer-based CFD simulations is typically rewarded with visually stunning three-dimensional images, as in Figs. 2, 3, and 15. This investment has heretofore been reserved for aerospace applications, where accurate calculations of drag can result in safer shuttle reentries or reduced fuel costs for supersonic fighters or subsonic commercial transports. The benefits from the application of CFD to medicine and diving are less certain but just as exciting.

E. Dive Phase–Related Airway Hysteresis

In a purely physical model of diving, the major variables are gas density, flow, and gas compressibility. Due to the small number of highly predictable variables, it is safe to assume that the mechanical aspects of the flow of compressed gases through human airways will eventually be fully described by CFD techniques. However, as stated in the introduction to this chapter, biological variability adds confounding factors to any purely physical interpretation of respiratory flow in divers. One notable example is the fact that airways are labile rather than static.

In analyzing the effects of breathing cold gas during exercise at hyperbaric pressures equivalent to a dive to 305 msw, Clarke et al. (53) noted that prior to the cold exposure, airway resistance was lower following a short stay at depth than it was during the compression phase of the dive. Similar changes in resistance were observed on an earlier dive to 457 msw (28). Increases in respiratory flow rates after the cessation of compression have been reported by Hamilton et al. (54), Dougherty and Schaefer (55), and Schaefer et al. (56).

Taylor and Clarke (57) explored these observations further during a saturation dive to 305 msw (31.3 atm absolute). They concurred with Clarke et al. (53) that divers' airways may compensate for breathing high-density gas by chronic bronchodilatation once a stable depth is reached. Alternatively, the steady increase in pressure during the compression phase of a dive may lead to an elevated resistance due to a subtle action of high pressure on bronchial smooth muscle (58). Conceivably, bronchoconstriction could subside after a short stay at depth, just as do symptoms of the high-pressure nervous syndrome (HPNS—a complex syndrome characterized by a generalized excitation of the central nervous system caused by the application of very high ambient pressures (59). Other potential HPNS-related changes in the control of respiratory flow at depth are described in Sec. VI.C of this chapter.

F. Subjective Effect of High Impedance

The simplest way to experience the effect of increased breathing resistance at normal room conditions is by forced nasal breathing. Normally, the resistance of 1 to 3.5 $cmH_2O \cdot L^{-1} \cdot s$ generated by the nares and nasopharynx of healthy adults (60,61) is unnoticeable at rest. However, when the nose becomes the only route for airflow, nasal impedance is enough to limit exercise capability severely (62). An instinctive switch from nasal to mouth breathing begins when respiratory flow rises toward the midrange of exercise ventilation (63) and upper airway resistance (61) exceeds 3.5 $cmH_2O \cdot L^{-1} \cdot s$

When they are breathing gas in a highly compressed atmosphere (30 atm absolute or so), divers become obligatory mouth breathers. This can prove unsettling to divers during a prolonged stay under pressure (so-called saturation dives may last a month or more), when they discover for the first time that air and food must simultaneously share the confines of the oral cavity. Even hungry divers prize oxygen more than food, so they tend to waste little time chewing. A way for nondivers to experience the deep saturation divers' dilemma without too much overstatement is to eat a full-course meal with nostrils clamped shut. The experience can be anxiety-provoking and risky.

The effects of increased gas density on ventilation can be investigated at 1 atm by having subjects inhale oxygenated mixtures of sulfur hexafluoride (SF_6), an inert gas with a density of about 5.5 $g \cdot L^{-1}$ BTPS. There are two drawbacks to this type of study: (1) it does not reproduce the reduced gas compressibility of hyperbaric exposures and (2) SF_6 is mildly anesthetic, with approximately one fourth the anesthetic potency of nitrous oxide (64). Interestingly, its psychophysical effects contrast sharply with those of nitrous oxide, or "laughing gas." In the parlance of divers, under room conditions, "SF_6 gives you a buzz. But it's not a happy buzz."

G. Work of Breathing

Mechanical work (W) is the product of force multiplied by displacement, or, for fluid systems, the change in system pressure (ΔP) multiplied by the change in system volume (ΔV). Expressed as an integral over an entire breath,

$$W = \oint P dV$$

with units of kgf·m or joules (J).

The work involved in breathing is normally a small fraction of the total energy expended by exercising humans. However, as a by-product of the effect of gas density on flow resistance, high ambient pressures increase the work of breathing (65,66). Buhlmann (67) reported that the work of breathing was doubled over that measured during eupnea at sea level, breathing air, when humans were compressed to 31 atm absolute (3.1 MPa) on helium. Underwater breathing apparatuses (Fig. 16) add their own work of breathing to that generated within the diver's airways.

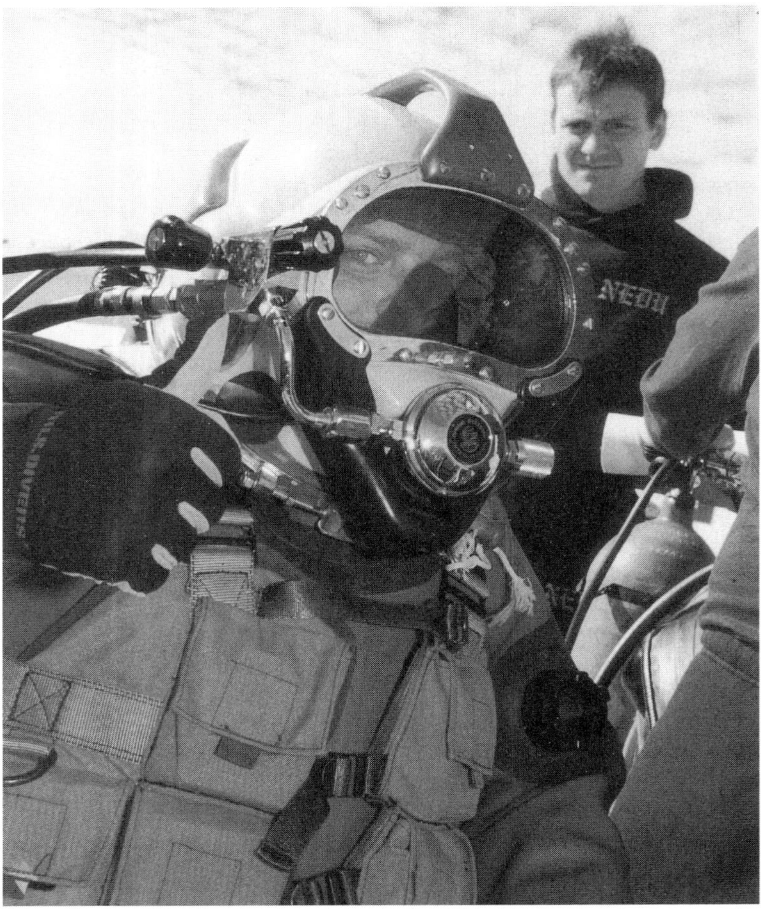

Figure 16 While his diving supervisor watches, a U.S. Navy deep sea diver gives a thumbs up during a communication check on his MK 21 diving helmet. The knurled knob on the left side of his regulator is a "dial-a-breath." When optimally adjusted, this knob minimizes the diver's work of breathing.

Ever since the pioneering work of Otis, Fenn and Rahn (68), who measured the external work of breathing, the concept of mechanical work and its time derivative, power, have frequently been used in respiratory and diving-related publications (69–71). Numerous modern publications such as that of Shikora et al. (72) describe the usefulness of work as an index of a patient's readiness for weaning from ventilatory support.

Unfortunately, the application of the phrase *work of breathing* to both clinical medicine and diving has not always been appropriate or dimensionally correct. As originally described, the work of breathing was measured by planimetry of a pressure-volume diagram obtained during a breath. The resulting area had units of joules, proper units for work. However, the modern literature contains work with units of both joules and joules per liter ($J \cdot L^{-1}$). To distinguish between these definitions, some papers refer to joules as the "work per breath" (73) while others use "work of breathing" to mean volume normalized work ($J \cdot L^{-1}$). Interestingly, $J \cdot L^{-1}$ is dimensionally equivalent to pressure. When the work of breathing is measured over a breath, the "work" in $J \cdot L^{-1}$ is actually the mean pressure due to flow resistance averaged over the entire volume history of the breath. This subject is explored further in Chapter 12, Sec. VI.C.

In spite of these dimensional ambiguities, the physical equivalence between work and energy has led to the pedagogic tenet that the energy expended by action of the respiratory muscles can be a significant fraction of the total energy expenditure during exercise.

The so-called oxygen cost of breathing, the metabolic representation of ventilatory energy expenditure, has been used in various estimates of respiratory efficiency (74). It is clearly elevated during hyperpnea (75) and inspiratory loaded breathing (76) but by itself does not limit exercise (77). As recently and succinctly summarized by Mead (78), it is "clear that respiratory limits are indeed encountered during maximal exercise. But these limitations are mechanical, and energy implications are secondary."

One of the most widely recognized mechanical limitations to ventilation is discussed in the following section.

V. Maximal Expiratory Flows

According to Mead (78), the earliest known description of expiratory flow limitation was written in 1892, when Willem Einthoven reported the clapping together of dog tracheas during attempts at coughing (79). According to Mead, pressures generated outside of the trachea by muscular contraction exceeded the internal pressures keeping the trachea open, allowing the tracheal walls to momentarily slap shut. This phenomenon defied quantitative explanation until Hyatt et al. (80) described flow maxima that varied directly with lung volume. From

Hyatt's work emerged the now familiar tool of maximal expiratory flow-volume (MEFV) curves, used clinically to define obstructive and restrictive patterns of pulmonary disease.

The 1960s saw the development of the concept of dynamic airway compression based upon the ''equal pressure point'' theory of Mead et al. (18) and the Starling resistor model of Pride et al. (81). Because of its apparent simplicity, we will devote attention to the more recent concept of tube wave-speed limitation (82). The wave-speed theory of flow limitation serves to explain and, in the authors' words, ''unify'' the previous observations. The cause of equal pressure or ''choke points'' such as those defined by Mead in the 1960s is now relatively well understood. As we see below, the wave-speed concept also explains the dependence of maximal flow on gas density, our primary concern in this chapter.

The premise of the wave-speed concept is that the velocity of fluid flowing in a tube cannot exceed the velocity of an elastic wave traveling along the tube walls. The velocity of that wave propagation is inversely dependent on the wall compliance; a floppy tube has a slow wave speed, meaning that a pressure pulse in the fluid must move more slowly through the tube than if the tube had rigid walls.

Wave speed (c) is defined as:

$$c = \sqrt{\frac{Y}{\rho}} \tag{15}$$

where Y is Young's elastic modulus of the tube at the cross section in question and ρ is gas density. Thus as gas density increases, c should decrease. Consequently, we would expect expiratory flows to be increasingly limited as gas density increases. Waves of pressure and flow propagating in this manner through the great blood vessels are called Moens-Korteweg waves, and c is the Moens-Korteweg wave speed (83).

Dawson and Elliott (82) expressed maximum expiratory flow as:

$$\dot{V}_{\max} = \sqrt{\frac{A^3}{\rho}E_{\mathrm{aww}}} \tag{16}$$

where E_{aww} is specific airway wall elastance (the inverse of airway wall compliance) at the ''choke point'' and A is airway cross-sectional area of the flow-limiting airway segment.

Figure 17 shows our predictions of the flow-volume relations for maximum expiratory flow-volume (MEFV) curves conducted at ambient pressures of 1, 2, and 8 atm absolute. The effort-dependent start of flow is not shown, since it is not part of the model. In the top panel of the figure, A was assumed

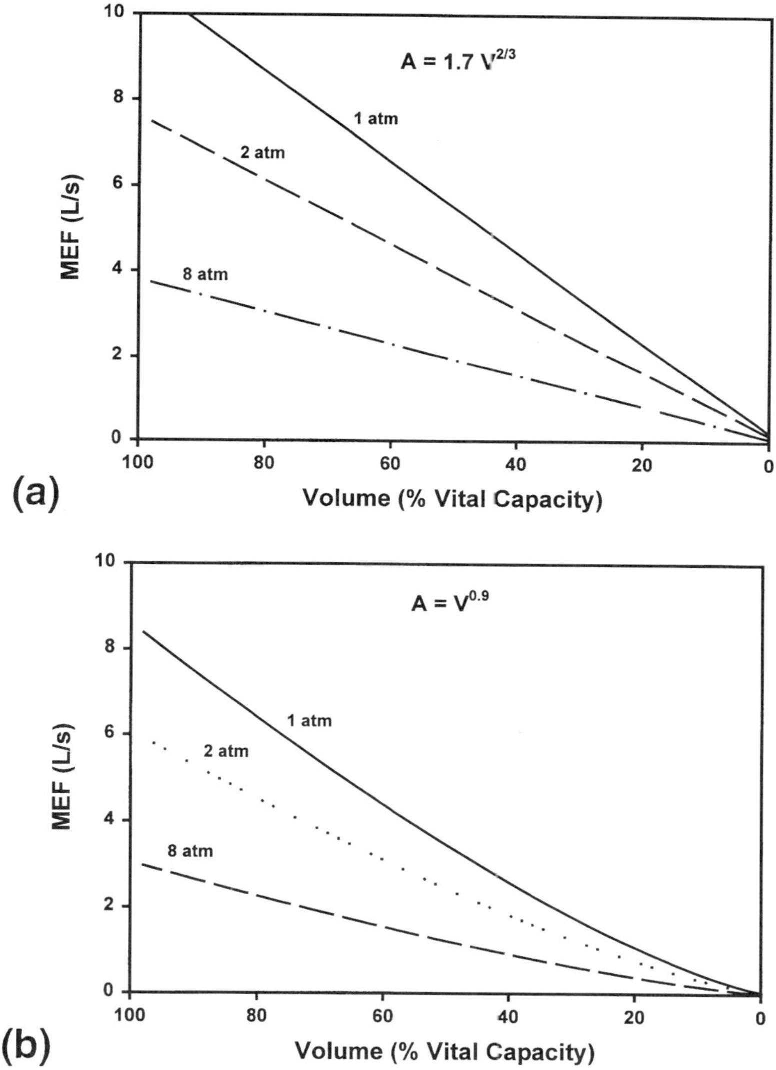

Figure 17 Predictions of the flow-volume relations for maximum expiratory flow-volume (MEFV) curves based on the wave-speed equation [Eq. (15)]. Predictions for ambient pressures of 1, 2, and 8 atm absolute. (a) A was assumed to vary with lung volume (V) to the ⅔ power. (b) A was assumed to vary with lung volume (V) to the 0.9 power.

to vary with lung volume (V) to the ⅔ power, as described by Hughes et al. (84) and Hahn et al. (85). When substituted into Eq. (16), the result is a linear $\dot{V}-V$ relation, with volume expressed as percent of the vital capacity. Increasing gas density causes a reduction in slope of that relation, thereby depressing maximum flow for any given lung volume.

In the lower frame of Fig. 17, the power of A's dependence on V is increased from ⅔ to 0.9, resulting in a curvilinear $\dot{V}-V$ relation, with a concavity typical of that seen in many clinical MEFV curves. Assuming that the majority of the lung volume comprises small peripheral airways, the $A-V$ relation demonstrated in the lower frame represents narrower than normal peripheral airways, with accentuation of that narrowing by reduction in lung volume. [The shape of the MEFV curves, and the inability to reliably attribute specific shapes to clinical history, is discussed in Hyatt et al.'s chapter on flow-volume relations (86) in Vol. 12 of this series].

Figure 18 is our plot of the maximum expiratory flow as seen in Fig. 17, at a lung volume of 3 L (60% of the vital capacity) versus gas density. It demonstrates the dependence of maximum flow on the square root of gas density. Figures 17 and 18 bear a striking resemblance to Fig. 19, parts (a) and (b), respectively, which show the overall patterns observed by Miller et al. (87,88) during chamber dives on air to a depth equivalence of 225 fsw ($\rho=8.9\ g\cdot L^{-1}$ at 37°C). This similarity leads us to the conclusion that the essential features of

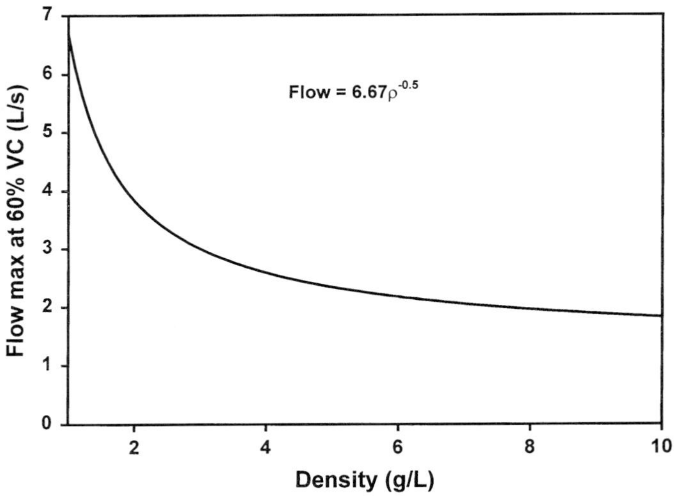

Figure 18 Plot of the maximum expiratory flow in Fig. 17 at a lung volume of 3 L (60% of the vital capacity) as a function of gas density, as described by Eq. (13).

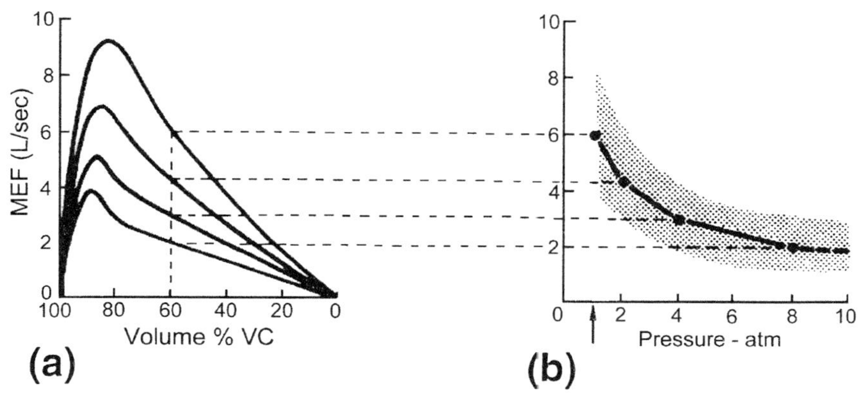

Figure 19 Maximum expiratory flow-volume curves performed at 1, 2, 4, and 8 atm. (From Ref. 87.)

expiratory flow limitation at depth can be explained by the concept of maximum wave speed in elastic walled airways.

A more complete model of maximal expiratory flow, yielding similar results for gas changes in density as our elementary analysis above, can be found in Lambert et al. (89). Both Lambert's paper and Hyatt's chapter on forced expiration in the *Handbook of Physiology* (90) should be consulted for a discussion of the limitations of even the most elaborate models.

VI. Inspiratory Flow Limitation

The first suggestion that inspiratory flow could be limited at 1 atm absolute in young, healthy subjects (91) was controversial; the evidence for dynamic airway compression on inspiration was not compelling. However, the author did propose, correctly we believe, that if inspiratory flow limitation were to occur in elastic-walled airways, it would be more likely to occur at depth than at the surface. The first real evidence of inspiratory flow limitation during dense gas breathing was revealed by Flook (92); potential mechanisms involving dynamic airway compression were presented in more detail by Flook and Fraser (93) and by Miller (94).

Inspiratory flow limitation cannot arise within the intrathoracic airway: during inspiration, pleural pressure is always subatmospheric and acts to hold the airways open; interdependence within the lungs transmits the effect of pleural pressure to all parts of the lungs. On the other hand, extrathoracic airways are surrounded by environmental pressure modified by muscular forces within the neck. The generation of subenvironmental pressure during inspiration causes a pressure drop across the extrathoracic airway. The magnitude of this pressure drop depends not only on flow but also on gas density. At some point in the airway, the gradient across the airway wall may be large enough to cause the airway to narrow. The chances of airway narrowing are enhanced by high flows and high gas density. In addition, if the flow rates are high enough for flow separation to occur at the larynx (Sec. III, Fig. 8), there will be a local severe decrease in pressure, which may cause the laryngeal aperture to narrow, perhaps even to close.

Olsen et al. (95) reported a reduction in the lumen of human trachea at transmural pressures as low as 10 kPa. Flook and Fraser (96) have shown that airflow through the excised human trachea is limited at transmural pressures as low as 3 kPa, with both the laryngeal orifice and deformation of the tracheal lumen contributing to the effect. To study the pressure drop down the airway for a range of flows, Olson et al. (97) used a cast of the upper airways prepared from a young male cadaver. They showed that, at inspiratory flows greater than about 1 $L \cdot sec^{-1}$, airway pressure reaches a minimum at the vocal cords, where eddy currents might be expected. Griscom and Wohl (98) observed narrowing of the extrathoracic trachea in adults during inspiratory maneuvers that generated intrathoracic pressures as low as 20 cmH_2O.

Gibson et al. (99) demonstrated inspiratory flow limitation in patients with tracheal obstruction. However, to our knowledge, only in diving can inspiratory flow limitation be demonstrated in young, healthy subjects.

A. Studies in Divers

To study inspiratory flow characteristics in divers, Flook and Fraser recorded flows, volumes, and pressures in divers breathing dense gases at 1 atm absolute, divers at depths to 56 m breathing air, and divers taking part in heliox saturation dives to 300 and 450 m. Data for a series of breaths ranging from slow to maximal inhalations were captured and stored using a computer-simulated oscilloscope (100). Some of the results are presented in Flook and Fraser (101) and Flook (102). A summary is presented here.

From pressure recordings, it was possible to separate the data for a fixed geometry-section such as a mouthpiece from the data for the variable-geometry section, the airway. Figure 20 shows pressure-flow curves for six divers breathing air at sea level (gas density 1.19 $g \cdot L^{-1}$), 18 m (density 3.3 $g \cdot L^{-1}$), and 56 m (density 7.85 $g \cdot L^{-1}$). For each depth, the characteristics of the fixed geometry of the mouthpiece assembly (circles) is shown together with those of the respiratory airway from mouth to alveoli (triangles). Flow is plotted as a percentage of each subject's average sea-level maximum flow. At depth, flow through the fixed-geometry section increases as pressure across that section in-

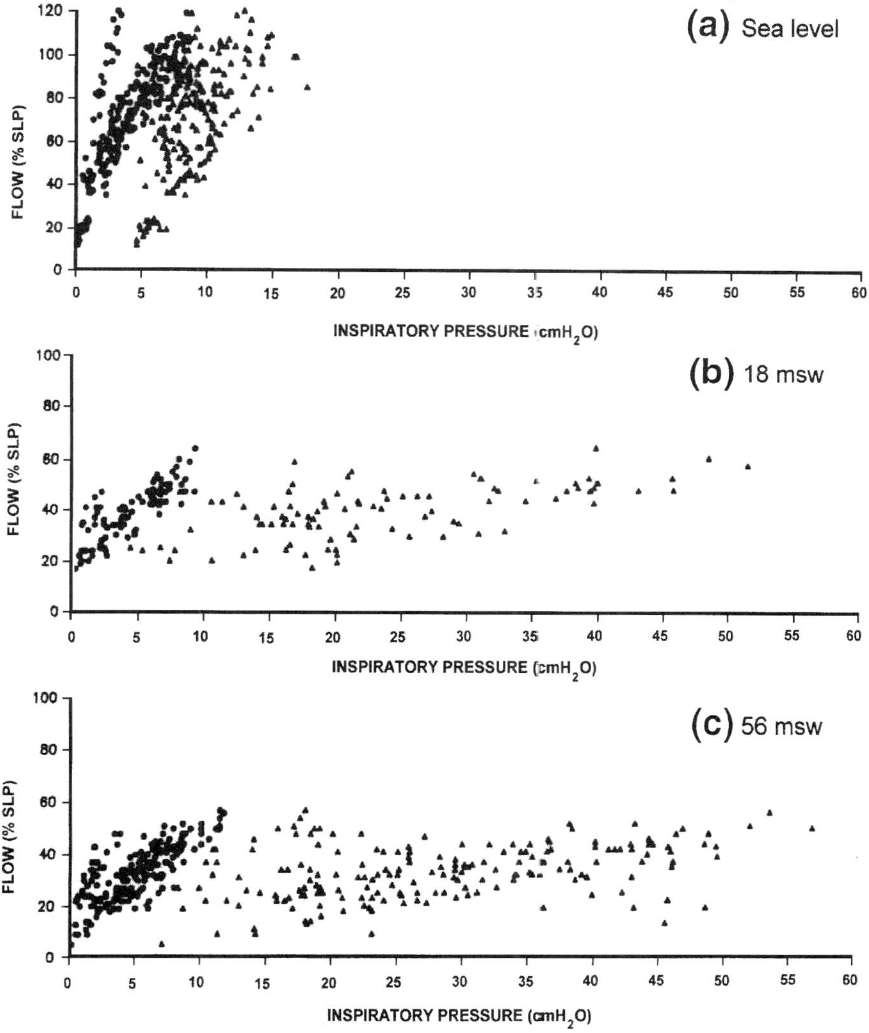

Figure 20 Pressure-flow curves for six divers breathing air at (a) sea level, (b) 18 msw, and (c) 56 msw. Circles: mouthpiece assembly. Triangles: respiratory airway from mouth to alveoli. Flow is plotted as a percentage of each subject's average sea-level maximum.

creases in keeping with inspiratory effect. However, flow through the airway eventually reaches a plateau and does not increase further with increasing effort.

Individual differences between subjects are apparent in Fig. 21, which shows respiratory resistance plotted against esophageal pressure for two of the divers. Diver 2 had a continuing increase in airway resistance as effort increased; his flow-pressure plot revealed flow limitation. Diver 6 showed no such increase in resistance and had no evidence of flow limitation.

The above data were plotted on a diagram of the coefficient of discharge (C_d) versus Reynolds number in Fig. 22. In the calculation of C_d, the diameter of the mouthpiece was 1.8 cm, area 2.5 cm^2; the diameter of the uncompressed pulmonary airway was taken as 1.7 cm, area 2.27 cm^2. The dependence of C_d on Reynolds number for the fixed geometry of the mouthpiece is expected for these high Reynolds numbers; the coefficient of discharge was constant. The C_d-Re relationship for the airway was not constant, and this has been taken to indicate variable geometry within the airway.

Flook and Fraser (96) also carried out studies using excised human tracheas. When a vacuum pump was used to create flow in the normal inspiratory direction, flow limitation was observed. Measurements were then repeated following the insertion of a cuff to hold the larynx open. Figure 23 shows the relationship between flow and driving pressure for 10 excised human tracheas both before (crosses) and after (circles) the laryngeal opening was fixed by insertion of the cuff. The cuff prevented flow limitation in all except one trachea. To accommodate the different flow rates resulting from different sizes of trachea, flow on Fig. 23 is shown as a percentage of flow when pressure drop down the trachea was very low, 0.1 kPa. It is assumed that no flow limitation occurs at that low transmural pressure.

The data showed that when free to change shape passively, the larynx contributed the major part of the flow limitation, with the trachea contributing a lesser part. In vivo, the larynx is under neural control, acting to increase the opening during inspiration, so the relative contribution to flow limitation of larynx and trachea may be different from those demonstrated in vitro.

The conclusions from this part of the chapter are that inspiratory flow limitation can occur in the extrathoracic airway. Both extrathoracic trachea and the larynx contribute, but the relative contributions are difficult to define.

In the work described above, the change in density was effected by a change in ambient pressure. When gas density was changed by a change in gas composition, always at 1 atm absolute, the results did not show such clear evidence of flow limitation. This seems to indicate that ambient pressure per se can have an effect over and above its effect on density. Why this should be is not known. However, analysis of the data on esophageal pressure showed that the respiratory muscles developed a maximum pressure, which was close to being a constant proportion of environmental pressures. Greater esophageal pres-

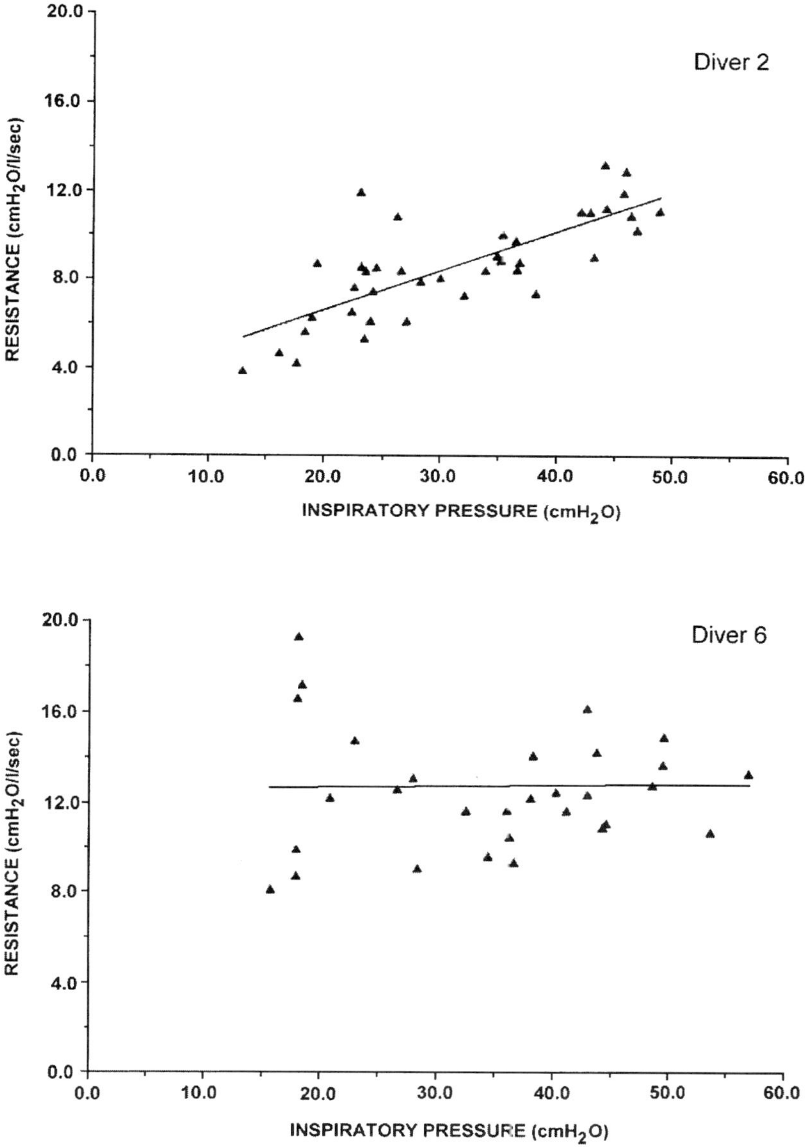

Figure 21 Respiratory resistance (triangles) as a function of esophageal pressure for two of the divers shown in Fig. 20. A best fit line is shown for each diver.

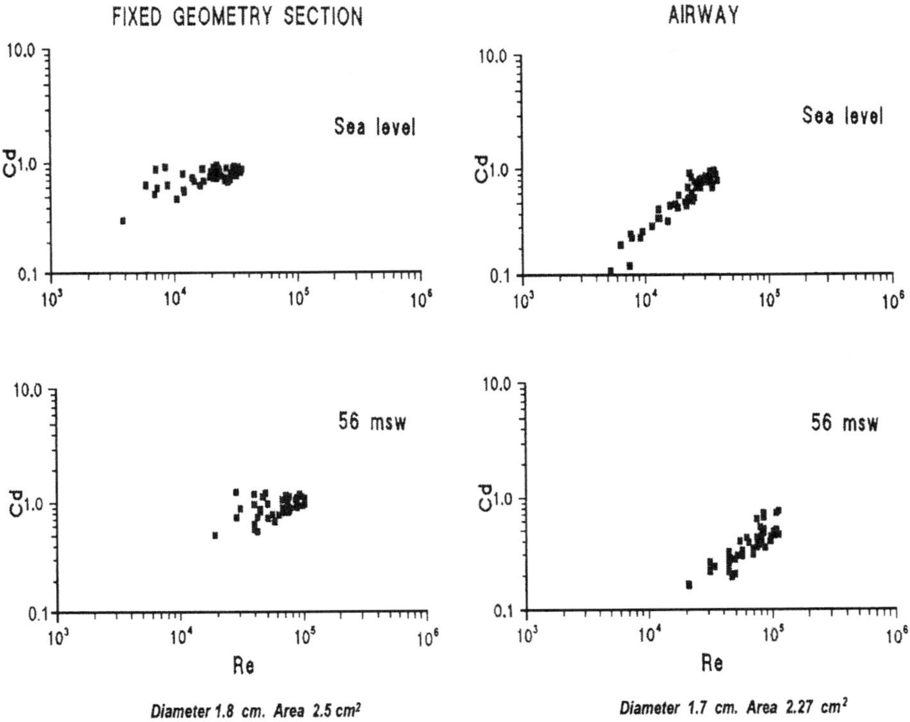

Figure 22 The data of Fig. 21 plotted on a diagram of the coefficient of discharge (C_d) versus Reynolds number. In the calculation of C_d, the diameter of the mouthpiece was 1.8 cm, area 2.5 cm^2, and the diameter of the uncompressed pulmonary airway was taken as 1.7 cm, area 2.27 cm^2.

sures, and therefore greater transmural pressures, were developed at higher environmental pressures (100).

B. Transient Airway Closure

The inspiratory flow-volume curves described above showed evidence of transient airway closure on some breaths at some depths for all subjects. Figure 24 shows the curves for two divers taking part in a deep heliox dive to 300 msw. The figure shows maximum inspiratory flow-volume curves recorded at sea level breathing air (density 1.15 $g \cdot L^{-1}$) and at 120, 270, and 300 msw breathing heliox (density 2.4, 4.8, and 5.3 $g \cdot L^{-1}$, respectively). The sharp notches evident

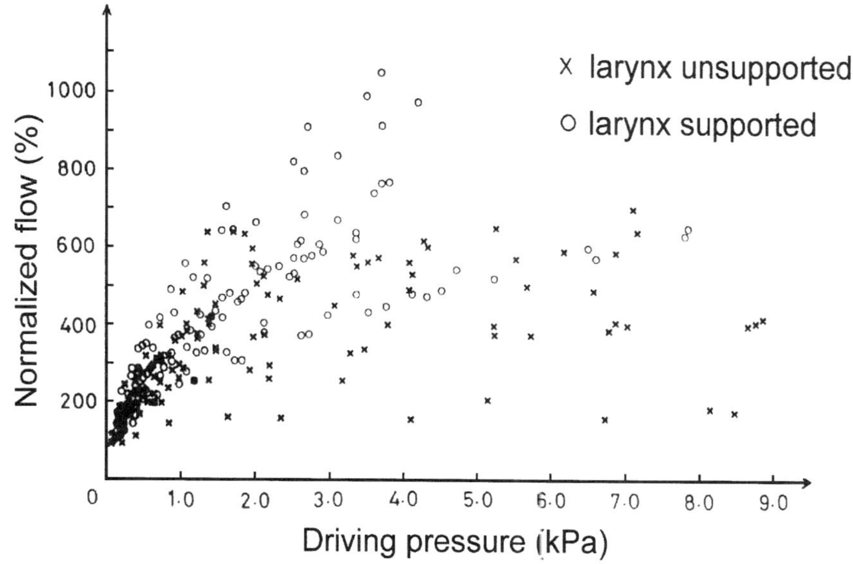

Figure 23 Maximal flow through excised human tracheae, with (○) and without (x) laryngeal support. Flow is expressed as a percentage of flow when pressure drop down the trachea was very low, 0.1 kPa.

on the curves taken at depth represent a sudden reduction in flow. In the diver in the upper figure, the effect always happened at the same lung volume for different depths. In the diver in the lower figure, the effect is seen at different lung volumes. Once again the effect of a change in density only (when density was changed by gas composition, not by pressure) was not so great, suggesting that pressure per se also played a role.

Figure 25 shows flow and esophageal minus mouth pressure (A) and flow with mouth pressure (B) for one of the lines in Fig. 24. The beginning and end of the notch, where flow drops, has been marked by dashed vertical lines. During the interruption in flow, mouth pressure returns to atmospheric pressure, indicating cessation of flow. This is more marked than the flow reduction, because once the airway has closed, the expansion of gas is registered as continuing flow for a time. For this reason the interruptions do not always show flow dropping to zero, because the airway reopens very quickly. During the interruption, esophageal pressure continues to become more negative as the inspiratory effort continues. Usually subjects are not aware of the interruption to flow. Interruptions

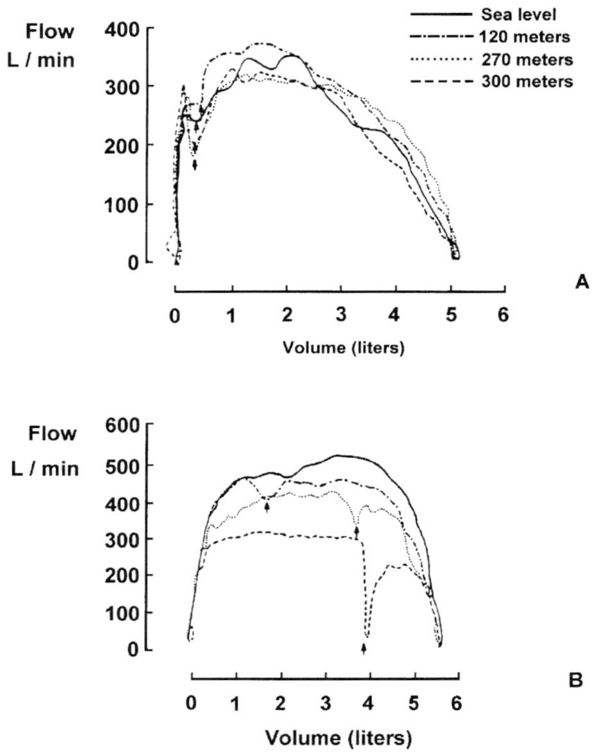

Figure 24 Maximum inspiratory flow-volume curves for two divers (A and B) in a deep heliox dive to 300 msw. The figure shows flow-volume curves recorded at sea-level breathing air (density 1.15 $g \cdot L^{-1}$) and at 120, 270, and 300 msw breathing heliox (density 2.4, 4.8, and 5.3 $g \cdot L^{-1}$, respectively). Arrows point to transient flow reductions.

are very brief, because once flow has stopped, the conditions that gave rise to the interruption have been removed.

At the moment of interruption, Reynolds number was calculated to exceed 10,000 for all breaths in all divers, suggesting that orifice flow was the dominant-flow type. The relationship between flow and gas density at the start of interruption was found to be

$$\text{Flow} = 0.95 \cdot \rho^{-0.42}$$

The relationship between density and peak flow at depth was found to be

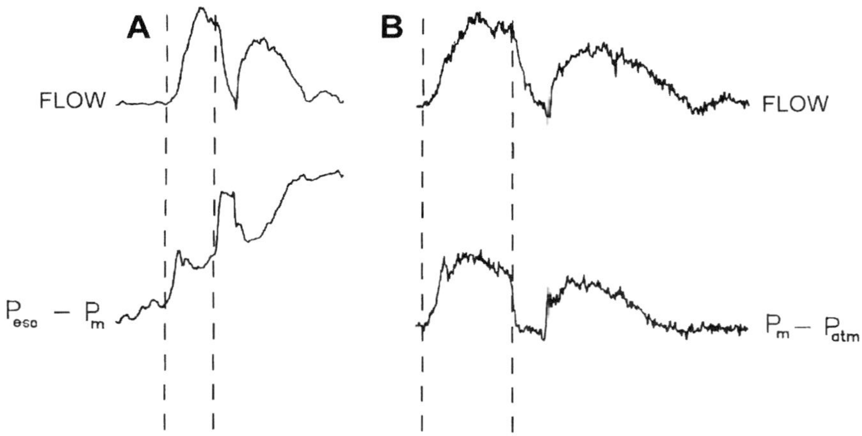

Figure 25 Time-based tracings of (A) flow and esophageal minus mouth pressure and (B) flow with mouth pressure for one of the curves in Fig. 24. The beginning and end of the notch, signifying a sudden flow reduction, have been marked by dashed vertical lines.

$$\text{Peak flow} = 0.99 \cdot \rho^{-0.47}$$

The similarity between these two equations might suggest that the dominant flow pattern at the moment of interruption is the same as that at peak flow. Theoretical considerations of orifice flow predict flow proportional to the square root of gas density. Thus, these results indicate that a high flow rate, the flow in the airway might be dominated by orifice flow.

During inspiration, the neural input to the vocal cords acts to increase the laryngeal aperture. If the vocal cords are indeed being closed briefly, it suggests that the mechanical forces are large enough to overcome neural control. As described earlier, a characteristic of orifice flow is flow separation—the development of eddies downstream of the orifice, with a very localized area of low pressure—as seen by Olson et al. (97). Flow separation is more likely in streamlined flow than in turbulent flow and is therefore more likely to occur in heliox than in air or nitrox.

C. The Effect of HPNS on Inspiratory Flow

The inspiratory flow curve shows regular oscillations when divers are suffering from the high-pressure nervous syndrome (HPNS) (96,100). The oscillations are readily distinguished from the flow interruptions discussed above by their regularity, by the fact that flow never drops close to zero, and by the fact that they become less marked as the diver acclimatizes to bottom depth during a prolonged saturation dive and then disappear once decompression starts. Neurological symptoms of HPNS follow a similar time course. Figure 26 shows flow traces for one diver on arrival at 450 msw, during the subsequent stay at that depth, and after decompression at 80 msw.

It was easily demonstrated that these oscillations did not result from hand tremor, a common manifestation of HPNS, by supporting the respiratory mouthpiece in a clamp, so that the only contact with the diver while recording was his mouth on the stiff mouthpiece. Further evidence that the oscillations arise within the respiratory system is the prolongation of inspiration when the oscillations are most marked. The mean inspiratory flow rate was reduced by the oscillations.

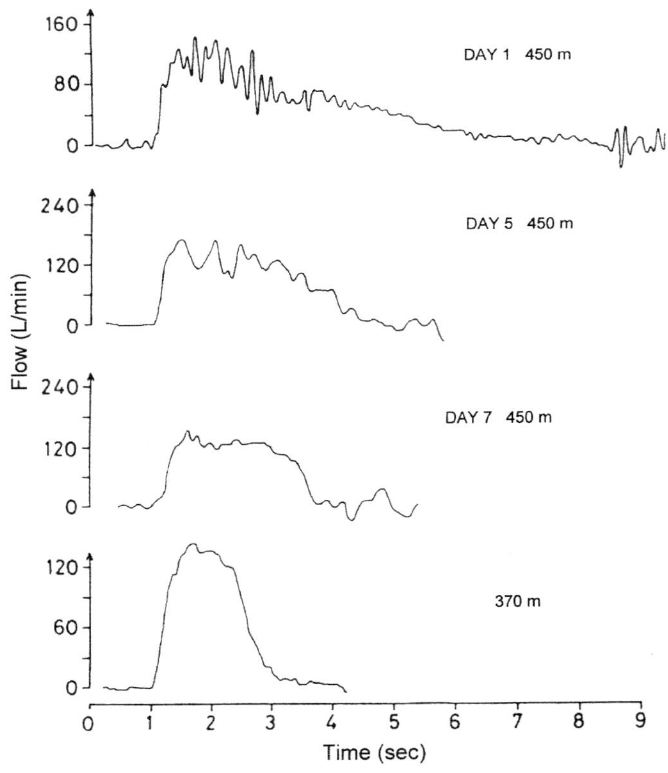

Figure 26 Flow traces for one diver on arrival at 450 msw, during the subsequent stay at that depth, and after decompression at 80 msw.

The mean frequency of flow oscillations was 7.1 Hz, fitting neatly in the center of the 5 to 10-Hz range for HPNS limb tremor given by Spencer et al. (103). The frequency tended to decrease with increased lung volume, suggesting that the oscillations may have been affected by the mass of the contained gas in a similar way that an increased mass reduces Parkinsonian limb tremor (104).

Tarasiuk and Grossman (105) reported what they called ''tremor-associated activity'' (TAA) in the cervical ventral roots of newborn rats, describing one of the triggering factors to be respiratory activity. At pressure, normal respiratory effort was often followed by a burst of electrical activity. Because the spinal roots enervate most of the respiratory muscles, Tarasiuk and Grossman believe that TAA may play a role in respiratory difficulties reported by divers at high pressures. Consequently, a potential explanation for the effect of HPNS on inspiratory flow is that HPNS may interfere with the neural input to the upper airway muscles or the neural input to the vocal cords. This interference would affect the muscular support of the airway and the laryngeal opening.

VII. Gas Compressibility

A. Background

Gas compressibility (C_g) is one of the six elements identified in the DuBois (106) electrical analogy of the respiratory system (Fig. 27). In humans, application of this model to respiratory transfer impedance (Ztr) data has been proposed as a means to estimate airway and tissue properties noninvasively. This approach requires forced oscillation measurements to be taken between frequencies of 2 and at least 64 Hz. Impedance measurements at frequencies of 250 Hz or more

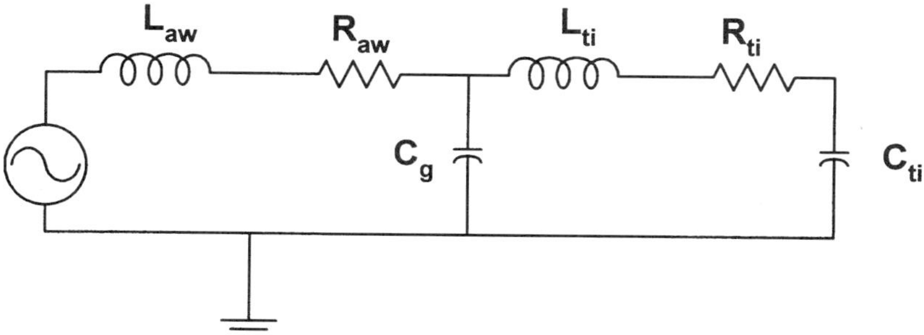

Figure 27 Electrical analogy of a diver's respiratory system divided into airway (aw), tissue (ti), and gas (g) components. *L*, *R*, and *C* represent inductance (inertance), resistance, and compliance.

are being successfully used to make clinically relevant inferences about human pulmonary disease (107) and the serial distribution of airway diameters (108). These measurements typically require prior knowledge of alveolar gas compressibility (*Cg*) (109).

Compressibility of alveolar gas varies directly with lung volume and inversely with ambient pressure. Assuming isothermal conditions and ignoring nonideal gas effects, Boyle's law yields:

$$P1 \cdot V1 = (P1 + \Delta P) \cdot (V1 - \Delta V) \tag{17}$$

Solving for ΔV and dividing by ΔP, we obtain:

$$\frac{\Delta V}{\Delta P} = \frac{V1}{(P1 - \Delta P)} \tag{18}$$

which is the definition of gas compliance. As long as ΔP is small compared with ambient pressure, gas compliance is essentially equal to lung volume ($V1$) divided by atmospheric pressure ($P1$) in atmospheres. For a lung volume of 3 L at 1 atm absolute, C=0.003 L·cmH$_2$O^{-1} or 0.03 L·kPa^{-1}. The expected change in gas compliance as a function of ambient pressure is shown for 3- and 7-L volumes in Fig. 28. As ambient pressure increases, compressibility declines dramatically, with the majority of the decrease occurring within the first 4 atm (30.6 msw).

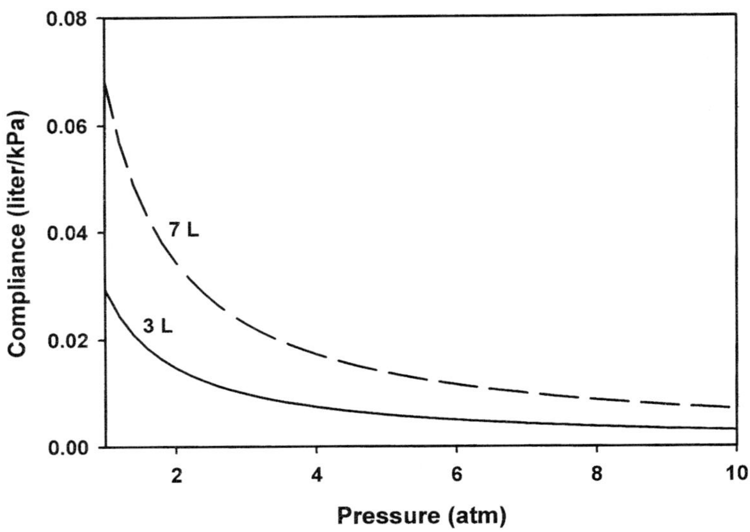

Figure 28 Gas compressibility versus depth based on Eq. (18).

In diving, gas inertance increases as gas compliance decreases. To estimate the combined effect of these changes on impedance measurements, we evaluated input impedance for the DuBois model shown in Fig. 27 using initial parameter estimates for air breathing from Lutchen et al. (110). The estimate for airway inertance increased directly with ambient pressure, and alveolar gas compressibility was assumed to decrease proportionately, as in Fig. 28. Values for tissue components were assumed unchanged by ambient pressure. The result is shown in Fig. 29: both the frequency and amplitude of the peak in the real component of impedance (antiresonance peak), top panel, increases with atmospheric pressure. Two high-frequency resonances, defined by zero crossings of the imaginary impedance axis (bottom panel), similarly shift to higher frequencies.

Inertance is directly dependent upon gas density, and therefore upon ambient pressure. Parameter estimates based on a three-parameter (respiratory system resistance, inertance, and compliance) model fits to input impedance data gathered in four divers at depths to 305 msw (30) showed inertance increasing an average of 0.0017 $cmH_2O \cdot L^{-1} \cdot s^2$ for each $g \cdot L^{-1}$ increase in gas density (unpublished observations), comparable to the density dependence of inertance assumed in Fig. 29.

Lutchen et al. (110) pointed out that the value of C_g required to fit their input impedance data at 1 atm (~0.001 $L \cdot kPa^{-1}$) was too small to represent the compliance of alveolar gas. In substituting a more realistic alveolar compliance of 0.03 $L \cdot kPa^{-1}$ in the model of Fig. 26, the antiresonance peaks in Fig. 29 disappear. Lutchen et al. considered the antiresonance peaks of Fig. 29 to be due to acoustical impedance.

It is not unexpected that at high frequencies, pulmonary impedance should be controlled by acoustical phenomena. However, that fact poses difficulties in predicting changes in pulmonary resonant phenomena as a function of diving depth. The characteristic frequencies of vibration for closed cylindrical tubes are determined by the tube length and the speed of sound in the vibrating medium, as in the following equation (111):

$$f_n = \frac{2n - 1}{4} \cdot \frac{c}{l} \tag{19}$$

where n is the nth harmonic, c is sound speed, and l is the length of the closed cylinder.

The free-field sound speed in gas is:

$$c = \sqrt{\frac{\gamma \cdot P}{\rho}} \tag{20}$$

where γ is the ratio of specific heats, P is ambient pressure, and ρ is gas density. For an ambient pressure of 1 atm (1.013×10^5 Pa) and a gas density for air at

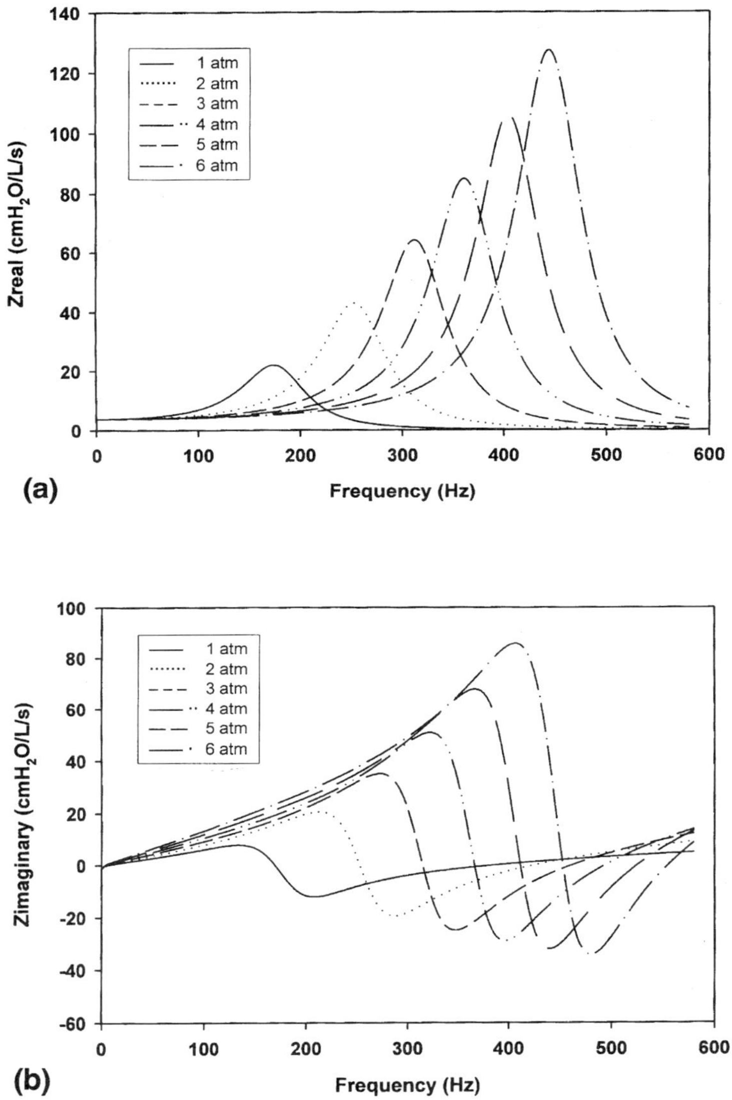

Figure 29 Impedance spectra versus depth for ambient pressures of 1 to 6 atm. Both (a) the real component of impedance and (b) the imaginary component are shown, based on the model shown in Fig. 27.

0°C of 1.293 g·L^{-1}, c is 331 m·s^{-1}. For a dive with an unchanging gas mixture such as air, both P and ρ increase in concert as depth increases, such that c remains unchanged. Therefore, we might expect no change in f_n as depth increases.

On the other hand, the speed of sound through the pulmonary parenchyma can be described as a weighted mixture of sound speed in gas and in tissue (112). Oddly, the result is a speed ranging between 25 and 75 msw, far lower than either the free-field velocity or the sound speed in soft tissue (1500 m/sec). From first principles, Rice (112) derived the following to describe the speed of sound propagating across lung lobes:

$$c = \left[\left(\frac{1-h}{\gamma P} + \frac{h}{Bt}\right) \cdot ((1-h)\rho_g + h\rho_t)\right]^{-\frac{1}{2}} \tag{21}$$

where h is tissue fraction, and Bt is tissue stiffness. When c is plotted against atmospheric pressure (Fig. 30), the result is a monotonic increase in the speed of sound through the lungs. This relation matched Rice's experimental data gathered at ambient pressures ranging from 0.11 to 7 atm.

Coincidentally, Eq. (21) once again reveals a square-root dependency; sound speed increases as approximately the square root of the increase in at-

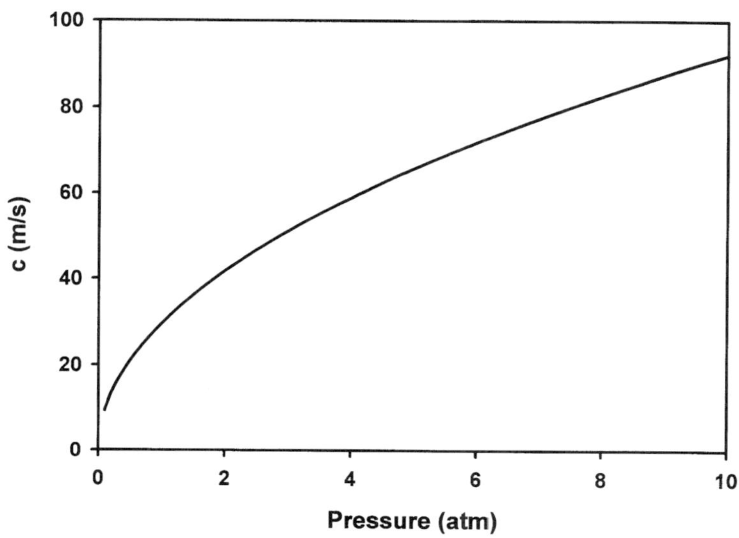

Figure 30 The speed of sound propagating across lung lobes as a function of ambient pressure. From Eq. (21).

mospheric pressure. Curiously, the increase in gas density with increasing pressure has little influence on the speed of translobar sound. The controlling density is that of lung tissue, which does not change with pressure.

To our knowledge, there are few if any measurements of resonant frequencies in lungs at increased pressure. However, if the standard model of vibrating gas columns in rigid tubes [Eq. (19)] is at all applicable to Rice's observations, we would expect resonant frequencies to increase with pressure, as seen in Fig. 29, because of the increase in the speed of sound through the lung parenchyma.

In light of all of the above, there are three plausible effects of hyperbaric pressure on pulmonary resonant frequencies. Simultaneous increases in ambient pressure and gas density may cause an increase in resonant frequency, no change, or even a decrease in the frequency of vibration. We will have to leave the final judgment in the hands of experimenters who conduct their research under hyperbaric conditions.

B. Cough and Speech

The above discussions concern the effect of gas compressibility on probes of pulmonary anatomy, specifically the forced oscillation technique for obtaining pulmonary impedance data. Gas compressibility becomes significant physiologically in the production and transmission of sound waves in speech and may be significant in cough (112,113), especially at altitude (114).

The influence of both the density and compressibility of gas on speech in highly compressed helium atmospheres remains one of the most vexing problems attending deep saturation diving, because of severe speech distortion by hyperbaric helium environments (115). Depth-related speech distortion is only partially mitigated by electronic means through so-called speech unscramblers (116–118).

VIII. Diffusion Resistance

Just as increasing gas density increases flow resistance, it also increases diffusion resistance. It is generally assumed that diffusion coefficients of gases decrease inversely with increase in hyperbaric pressure, as predicted from the Chapman-Enskog equation (119). That is, the product of molecular diffusivity (D) and ambient pressure (P) is constant. There are exceptions, such as that of the binary mixture of methane in argon over the pressure range from 1 to 100 atm absolute (120). However, at least within the range of 7 to 90 atm absolute, the diffusion of oxygen in helium and nitrogen does follow predictions (121). Binary diffusion coefficients at 37°C for a breathable helium-oxygen mixture decrease from 0.782 $cm^2 \cdot s^{-1}$ at 1 atm to 0.0091 $cm^2 \cdot s^{-1}$ at 90 atm, with the product of $D \cdot P$

being roughly 0.82. Binary diffusion coefficients at 37°C for a nitrogen-oxygen mixture decrease from 0.231 $cm^2 \cdot s^{-1}$ at 1 atm to 0.0004 $cm^2 \cdot s^{-1}$ at 90 atm, with $D \cdot P$ being approximately 0.25. The potential role of reduced diffusivity at depth has been explored by Van Liew et al. (122).

In spite of the increase in diffusion resistance in dense, hyperbaric atmospheres, there has been little evidence of gas-exchange perturbations in animals or humans (123,124). As summarized by Pedley et al. (15), dense gas seems to accentuate gas mixing in distal airways, with convection delivering oxygen close enough to the alveolar membranes to offset the increase in diffusion resistance. Exactly how gas density might accentuate convection in the distal airways and alveolar sacs is not clear but may well involve inertial effects on distal penetration of the relatively high-velocity gas in the central core during laminar flow reversal (Fig. 4) or hysteresis of alveolar wall motion, resulting in inertially influenced secondary flows within alveoli (125). Unlike the universally accepted maleficence of flow resistance, increases in diffusion resistance seem to exert little influence on gas exchange.

IX. Respiratory Muscle Fatigue

Taken to the extreme, the breathing of high-density gases can stress the respiratory system to the point of respiratory collapse. Animals exposed to atmospheric pressures as high as 270 atm frequently manifest symptoms of respiratory distress all too familiar to practitioners dealing with severe pulmonary disease. Hallmark signs of such ultrahyperbaric exposures in animals are mouth breathing and gasping (126), presternal depression (127), and pursed-lips breathing (128).

Presumably, subjects reduce respiratory flows and pressures in the face of elevated impedance to minimize the risk of respiratory muscle fatigue. Signs of fatigue can develop in normal human subjects after only 1 min of maximal isocapnic ventilation (on the order of 195 $L \cdot min^{-1}$) with no external respiratory impedance, seemingly through a fatigue-induced decrease in diaphragmatic contractility (129). That respiratory muscles can fatigue during prolonged exercise has been shown by a number of researchers (130–133). Power spectral shifts in diaphragmatic and intercostal electromyograms (EMGs) of human divers observed over 12 days at 46 atm absolute in HeO_2 ($\rho = 8.7$ $g \cdot L^{-1}$) and $N_2/He/O_2$ ($\rho = 11.1$ $g \cdot L^{-1}$) resemble the EMG changes observed in animals at 101 atm absolute and may indicate signs of respiratory muscle fatigue (134).

A. Narcotic Influences

It is clear that gas density is not the only factor influencing the tolerance of the respiratory system to hyperbaria. Various types of narcosis attenuate the debilitating effects of density. Mice who succumb at pressures of 15 MPa (149 atm absolute) in a helium-oxygen atmosphere have survived at 20 MPa showing no signs of respiratory difficulty when nitrous oxide was added to the breathing mixture (135). Similar effects have been experienced when mildly narcotic mixtures of nitrogen were added to the gas mixture. Cats would die at simulated depths of 1000 msw, 101 atm absolute breathing helium-oxygen (density = 18 $g \cdot L^{-1}$) but other cats did relatively well when breathing a trimixture containing nitrogen, in spite of the higher gas density (29 $g \cdot L^{-1}$) of the trimix (136). Hyperpnea is minimal or nonexistent when significant nitrogen partial pressures exist, perhaps sparing the respiratory muscles from the fatiguing respiratory pressures generated during hyperpnea.

Nitrogen may extend survival at great depth and may also minimize dyspnea during exercise at more moderate depths. Salzano et al. (137) had divers perform incremental exercise at simulated depths of 47 to 66 atm absolute (4.75 to 6.67 MPa) breathing either heliox or a mixture of helium, oxygen, and nitogen. Gas density ranged from 1.1 to 17.1 $g \cdot L^{-1}$. Work-limiting dyspnea was infrequent but occurred more often when nitrogen was absent from the gas mix than when it was present, even though gas mixes containing nitrogen had much greater gas densities than did the heliox mixtures.

Clarke (138) performed a post hoc probabilistic analysis of 12 years of diving results from the Navy Experimental Diving Unit, comparing gas density and gas mixture with dive outcome. It was observed that for equivalent gas densities, working dives in a partial nitrogen atmosphere resulted in approximately 50% fewer dive terminations due to respiratory events, such as dyspnea or hypercapnia, than did dives in heliox atmospheres. Fothergill et al. (139) recently reported on the ability of both nitrous oxide at 1 atm (Fig. 31) and nitrogen atmospheres at depth (140) to blunt the sensory effects of exercise in the presence of respiratory resistances.

B. Endogenous Opiates in Ventilatory Control

Beta endorphin is a naturally occurring neuropeptide serving as a neurotransmitter in the central nervous system. It is apparently released during stress and heavy exercise (141–143) and is found in increased concentrations in the cisternal cerebrospinal fluid of unanesthetized goats breathing through inspiratory resistors (144).

The action of beta endorphin is frequently deduced by study of the action of its best-known antagonist, naloxone. Beta endorphin seems to depress carbon dioxide responsiveness in rats, an inference based on the stimulatory effect of naloxone applied directly to the rat medulla (145). It leads to reductions in ventilatory drive during fatiguing inspiratory resistive loading (146), triggered in some instances by respiratory muscle acidosis (147). Just as other opiates dull the dyspnea of chronic obstructive pulmonary disease (COPD) (148–150),

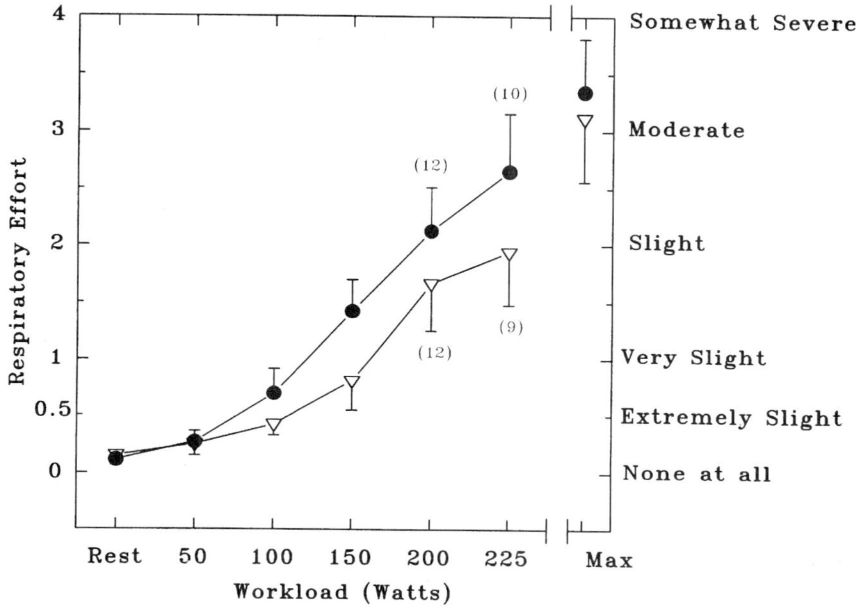

Figure 31 The sensation of respiratory effort at 1 atm absolute increases with workload but is reduced across all work rates when nitrous oxide is inhaled. Circles: air breathing. Triangles: 23% nitrous oxide. (From Ref. 139.)

beta endorphin dulls the perception of dyspnea during acute respiratory distress in normal adults (151) and asthmatics (152). It has been known since 1981 that, in some COPD patients, naloxone restores the ability to compensate for a flow-resistive load (153).

In the sense of being flow-limited, a normal diver mimics a COPD patient when breathing a dense gas. His ventilation is reduced below normal levels, and carbon dioxide is retained. However, to the present authors' knowledge, the role of endogenous opiates has yet to be explored during diving.

The works cited in the present section raise the intriguing possibility that the reductions in ventilation observed during diving, and the tolerance of high arterial carbon dioxide during respiratory loading, may be modified through the chemical mediation of endogenous opioids released as a result of respiratory stress. One may hypothesize that the administration of an opiate receptor antagonist to a diver should increase expired minute ventilation ($\dot{V}_E$), decrease partial pressure of carbon dioxide in alveolar blood (P_ACO_2), and possibly increase dyspnea. (In diving, dyspnea can have a protective effect, causing a highly motivated diver to reduce provocative workloads before he loses consciousness from hypoventilation and excessive retention of carbon dioxide.) Although highly speculative, it is conceivable that the sometimes remarkable differences between so-called carbon dioxide retainers and nonretainers (154) may ultimately be due to differing sensitivities to, or differing production rates of, endogenous opiates like beta endorphin.

X. Ventilation-Perfusion Inequalities

In 1967 Chouteau and Cousteau observed signs of hypoxia in goats exposed to pressures of up to 56 atm absolute, signs that were remedied by increasing oxygen partial pressure in the goats' breathing mixture (155). These observations were eventually shown to be an artifact due to an effect of inert gas on paramagnetic oxygen analyzers (156), which led to an overestimation of the oxygen partial pressure in the goats' chamber. However, before the discovery of this artifact, early attempts to explain the goat hypoxia episodes were based on the previously revealed concept of stratified inhomogeneity (157) in dense gas atmospheres. Stratification was defined as incomplete mixing between fresh and stale gas in the peripheral airways and alveoli.

To search for evidence of stratified inhomogeneity, Herb Saltzman of Duke University initiated careful studies of gas exchange in resting human subjects at pressures up to 8.6 atm absolute and gas densities to 7.7 g/L (BTPD). (This is one of the few studies where arterial blood samples have been drawn at depth). Saltzman et al. (123) reported no signs of impaired oxygen transfer or inhomogeneity, although they cautioned that inhomogeneity could not be ruled out by their measurements. They suspected that dense gas may have improved gas exchange relative to 1 atm by alteration of ventilation/perfusion ratios. Wood and Bryan (37) had already suggested that dense gas may encourage a uniform distribution of ventilation. Saltzman et al. (123) also made the curious observation that increases in partial pressure of carbon dioxide in arterial blood ($PaCO_2$) correlated better with increases in ambient pressure than with gas density.

Spurred by his experimental findings at Duke, Saltzman later spent a 1-year sabbatical in the laboratory of John West and Peter Wagner at the University of California–San Diego Medical School (158), where he began modeling the effect on gas exchange of alveolar ventilation/perfusion ($\dot{V}A/\dot{Q}$) abnormalities at high ambient pressure. This interest in the study of hyperbaric influences on arterial partial pressure of oxygen (P_{O_2}) and partial pressure of carbon dioxide (P_{CO_2}) eventually led to the highly successful multiple inert gas elimination technique (MIGET) (159).

Below, we explore more recent indications that diving should, at least in some circumstances, lead to alterations of ventilation/perfusion matching within the lungs.

A. Exercise-Induced Hypoxemia

It is now accepted that strenuous exercise can lead to mismatching of $\dot{V}_A/\dot{Q}$ in normal human subjects. In a large percentage of elite endurance athletes, mismatching results in hypoxemia (160–164). Although $\dot{V}_A/\dot{Q}$ mismatching is the primary contributor to increases in the alveolar-arterial oxygen difference (AaD_{O_2}), diffusion limitation also plays a role (165).

One potential source of diffusion limitation, and perhaps of $\dot{V}_A/\dot{Q}$ mismatching as well, is pulmonary edema. After exhausting exercise, highly trained athletes accumulate interstitial fluid in their lungs (166). Indeed, perivascular edema, and perhaps parenchymal interstitial edema, have been found in animals following heavy exercise (167).

B. Head-Out Immersion

Disturbances to gas exchange occur during head-out immersion, where hydrostatic forces cause a halving of functional residual capacity (FRC) due to elevation of the diaphragm (168) and redistribution of blood into the intrathoracic vascular bed (169,170). Closing volume (CV) is also increased (171,172). These changes would be expected to result in low $\dot{V}_A/\dot{Q}$ regions and shunt, with arterial desaturation. Indeed, Cohen et al. (173) and Prefaut et al. (172) have seen reductions in Pa_{O_2} during head-out immersion and have inferred alterations in $\dot{V}_A/\dot{Q}$ distributions, the usual cause of such hypoxemia. However, in the work of Derion et al. (174), using the multiple inert gas elimination technique (MIGET) for measuring continuous $\dot{V}_A/\dot{Q}$ ratios, increases in shunt were minimal and both Pa_{O_2} and $\dot{V}_A/\dot{Q}$ distributions were virtually unchanged. Since the above study was done at 1 atm, we do not know if $\dot{V}_A/\dot{Q}$ ratios remain similarly stable under hyperbaric conditions.

C. Hyperbaria

Based on methods predating the MIGET, in 1973 Miller and Winsborough (175) reported that although alterations in $\dot{V}_A/\dot{Q}$ occurred in healthy young men during heavy exertion at depth, the cause was relative hypoventilation as opposed to just an increase in gas density. However, as gas is compressed, density is not the only parameter that increases. Inertance, a reflection of the volumetric mass of the gas and the acceleration to which it is subjected during breathing, also increases in direct proportion to atmospheric pressure as long as gas mixtures remain unchanged. Clarke et al. (176) performed modeling studies suggesting that dense gas by itself may not exacerbate preexisting uneven ventilation, but that increases in gas inertance could accentuate, improve, or have no effect on ventilation evenness and perhaps on ventilation-perfusion inequalities, depending on respiratory frequency and the resonant frequency (f_0) of the diver's respiratory system.

Exercising divers are routinely hypercapneic. It is not unusual to see end-tidal carbon dioxide of 50 to 60 mmHg in divers doing moderate work at depth (154). Hypoventilation is undoubtedly a primary contributor to hypercapnea, but altered $\dot{V}_A/\dot{Q}$ matching and gas phase diffusion may also contribute. Using the MIGET, Morgan et al. (177) found that during exercise in the dry at 40 msw, hypercapnia was accompanied by both hypoventilation and increased $\dot{V}_A/\dot{Q}$ mismatch. There was also evidence of impaired intraalveolar carbon dioxide diffusion.

Clarke and Fothergill (178) reported on visual symptoms occurring in exercising divers under well-controlled hyperbaric conditions (simulated depths from 30 to 305 msw) that appeared to be due to a reduced oxygen supply to the brain. These symptoms included concentric visual field contraction (tunnel vision), graying, vertigo, and scintillating scotomata. Headache and severe dyspnea were often associated with the visual symptoms. Although a reduction in cerebral blood flow could not be ruled out, a more likely candidate was arterial hypoxemia. However, this suggestion is rather tenuous because the divers were extremely fit and were exercising in the oxygen-enriched atmosphere of a hyperbaric chamber during saturation dives. The oxygen partial pressure within the chambers was tightly controlled at 0.45 atm absolute—certainly not a value that would lead to a suspicion of hypoxemia.

This was not the first time hypoxia had been suspected during a deep saturation dive. Salzano et al. (137) also suspected hypoxia during their hyperoxic *Atlantis III* dive, a deep saturation dive to 66 atm absolute, equivalent to 650 msw. Noting marked elevations in lactic acidosis at depth, the authors speculated that there may have been an increase in anaerobic metabolism during the dive, in spite of an elevated Pa_{O_2}. During and after the highest workload of that dive, each subject reported unpleasant sensations similar to "those of general hypoxia: dizziness, inability to coordinate muscle movements of the legs, and an inner feeling of shakiness." These symptoms were not noted in previous, shallower dives in the *Atlantis* series. However, the earlier dives also exposed the divers to lower work rates and lower nitrogen partial pressures, so it is difficult to say whether the absence of symptoms in the earlier dives were due to the lower pressure (47 atm), the lower nitrogen, or to the lower work rates.

If cardiac output in fit divers is elevated to exercise demands and ventilation is reduced due to a learned response to resistive loaded breathing and a low chemosensitivity to carbon dioxide (154,179) (see Chap. 8 of this volume), then there can be two simultaneous outcomes. One is carbon dioxide retention resulting from hypoventilation, and the other is $\dot{V}_A/\dot{Q}$ mismatching due to a gross imbalance in cardiac output and ventilation. The former could lead to headache and dyspnea, while the latter could lead, in the extreme, to visual signs of hypoxemia. In other words, the events described by Morgan et al. (177) may also have been at work during the contemporaneous studies of Clarke and Fothergill (78) and perhaps in the earlier work of Salzano et al. (137).

D. Diving

Diving, of course, includes all of the above provocations; hyperbaric exposure, heavy exercise, and head-out immersion. (Head-out immersion has a hydrostatic equivalent in full immersion: breathing through a scuba regulator while fully immersed in a vertical position; Chap. 14). It would thus be surprising if $\dot{V}A/\dot{Q}$ mismatching, Pa_{O_2} reductions, and perhaps even edema did not occur under some conditions during diving. Fortunately, if gas-exchange perturbations occur, they are either of little consequence or relatively rare.

The first cases of clinical pulmonary edema in scuba divers were not reported until the 1980s (180,181). There have also been some reports of pulmonary edema in swimming (182), especially after heavy fluid loading (183). Hampson and Dunford (184) reported on six cases encountered over a 7-year period of likely or confirmed noncardiogenic pulmonary edema following scuba diving. Combining their data with those of Pons (182) and Wilmhurst (180,181), a total of 20 cases of pulmonary edema in scuba divers were available, with over half accompanied by cough and dyspnea; in some cases the dyspnea was severe. In a number of cases, pulmonary edema was confirmed radiographically, with resolution of signs within as little as 12 hr. All of the divers were healthy prior to the dive, and the incident dives were otherwise uneventful except for often being associated with cold water. Some divers reported multiple incidents, even in relatively warm water.

The causes of pulmonary edema in swimming and diving are not certain at this point. However, water immersion, heavy exercise, and fluid loading may all be contributing factors. Whether or not the startling but uncommon events described by Clarke and Fothergill (178) can be attributed to arterial hypoxemia secondary to subclinical edema or to other causes of presumed $\dot{V}A/\dot{Q}$ mismatching will have to be answered by further study.

XI. Conclusion

In the introduction, we marveled that in spite of an absence of hereditary disposition or environmental prods, men who dive have succeeded in tolerating increases in pressure over sixty times greater than that experienced by other living persons. This chapter demonstrates that during the breathing of respirable gas mixtures at depth, at least four physical factors are changed from their surface values. Gas compressibility is decreased and ambient pressure, gas inertance, and density are all increased. Gas-density effects receive the most attention in the literature and in this chapter, but it would be a mistake to ignore the influence of the other changes upon the human cardiorespiratory system. Gas inertance can theoretically redistribute gas flow within the airways (176), and gas compressibility influences the transmission of sound through the lungs and vocal tract.

The work of Flook, Fraser, and others demonstrate the existence of several factors that compromise inspiratory flow over and above the direct effects of gas density. These effects include limitation of inspiratory flow due to dynamic airway compression in the upper airway; transient interruption of flow due to closure of the upper airway, most probably at the vocal cords; and prolongation of inspiration with associated reduced average flow due to the presumed effects of HPNS. These effects are strong evidence for the case that ventilation of the lungs is limited during the inspiratory phase in diving. During air breathing by normal subjects at 1 atm absolute, ventilatory limitation occurs only during expiration.

Interestingly, Claude Lenfant, Executive Editor of the *Lung Biology in Health and Disease* series, was the first to exploit hyperbaria as a means for studying gas exchange and ventilation/perfusion ratios (185). Over 34 years later, hyperbaria is not so much a tool for studying these ratios as it is an object of study in its own right. As we have seen, gas exchange in general is unperturbed by considerable increases in atmospheric pressure and gas density. However, there is evidence suggesting that our understanding of gas exchange at depth, especially during strenuous exercise, remains incomplete. In addition to the references given in Sec. X.A, the interested reader should refer to Wagner and Gale (186) for an early review of ventilation/perfusion inequalities during exercise.

We have virtually ignored the potential influence of high ambient pressures per se. Throughout this chapter, pressure has occasionally been proposed as a cause for phenomena that are not reproduced in experiments conducted with dense gases at 1 atm absolute (123) (Sec. VI.A and B). Nevertheless, evidence of the effect of pressure within the human diving range on cellular and physiological systems is relatively scarce. HPNS represents the one major pathology unique to diving that is clearly identified with the rate of pressure application [reviewed by Bennett and Rostain (59)]. Lately, however, there have been suggestions that pressure might exert a direct effect on the mammalian respiratory center (105) or on the cell membranes of red blood cells (RBCs) leading to increases in RBC aggregation (187). The latter authors (187) report significant changes during human dives as remarkably shallow as 20 msw.

Clearly, if it is convincingly demonstrated that hydrostatic pressure can alter both excitable and nonexcitable cells at depths within the normal human diving range, we must carefully reconsider what we believe about the effects of diving on the human respiratory system. It would then seem all the more remarkable that our penetration of the ocean depths is as successful as it is.

Acknowledgments

We would like to thank the following for their review of and contributions to this chapter: Boyd Gatlin, Ph.D, Aerospace Engineering, Mississippi State University; Jeff Hammersley, M.D., Pulmonary Medicine, School of Medicine, Ohio State University; Marc Jaeger, M.D., School of Medicine, University of Florida; Andrew Jackson, Ph.D., Boston University; Hugh VanLiew, Ph.D, Navy Experimental Diving Unit, formerly State University of New York at Buffalo.

References

1. Vose RS, Schmoyer RL, Steurer PM, Peterson TC, Heim R, Karl TR, Eischeid J. The Global Historical Climatology Network: long-term monthly temperature, precipitation, sea level pressure, and station pressure data. ORNL/CDIAC-53, NDP-041. Oak Ridge National Laboratory, Oak Ridge, TN: Carbon Dioxide Information Analysis Center, 1992.
2. West JB. Highest inhabitants in the world. Nature 1986; 324:517.
3. West JB. Prediction of barometric pressures at high altitudes with the use of model atmospheres. J Appl Physiol 1996; 81:1850–1854.
4. Stänescu DC, Pattijn J, Clément J, van de Woestijne KP. Glottis opening and airway resistance. J Appl Physiol 1972; 32:460–466.
5. England SJ, Bartlett D Jr, Daubenspeck JA. Influence of human vocal cord movements on airflow and resistance in eupnea. J Appl Physiol 1982; 52:773–779.
6. Moin P, Kim J. Tackling turbulence with supercomputers. Sci Am 1997; 276:62–68.
7. Olson DE, Dart GA, Filley GF. Pressure drop and fluid flow regime of air inspired into the human lung. J Appl Physiol 1970; 28:482–494.
8. Weibel ER. Morphometry of the Human Lung. Berlin: Springer, 1963.
9. Otis AB, Bembower WC. Effect of gas density on resistance to respiratory flow in man. J Appl Physiol 1949; 2:300–306.
10. Maio DA, Farhi LE. Effect of gas density on mechanics of breathing. J Appl Physiol 1967; 23:687–693.
11. Pao RHF. Fluid Mechanics. New York: Wiley, 1967.
12. Olson DE. Essentials of Engineering Fluid Mechanics. Scranton, PA: International Textbooks, 1961.
13. Pedley TJ, Schroter RC, Sudlow MF. Energy losses and pressure drop in models of human airways. Resp Physiol 1970; 9:371–386.
14. Pedley TJ, Schroter RC, Sudlow MF. The prediction of pressure drop and variation of resistance within the human bronchial airways. Resp. Physiol 1970; 9:387–405.
15. Pedley, TJ, Schroter RC, Sudlow MF. Gas flow and mixing in the airways. In: West JB, ed. Bioengineering Aspects of the Lung. New York: Marcel Dekker, 1977: 163–265.
16. Mead J. Resistance to breathing at increased ambient pressures. In: Goff LG, ed. Proceedings of the Symposium on Underwater Physiology. Washington, DC: National Academy of Sciences, National Research Council, 1955:112–120.
17. Rouse H. Elementary Mechanics of Fluids. New York: Wiley, 1946.
18. Macklem PT, Mead J. Resistance of central and peripheral airways measured by a retrograde catheter. J Appl Physiol 1967; 22:395–401.

19. DuBois AB, Botelho SY, Comroe JH. A new method for measuring airway resistance in man using a body plethysmograph: values in normal subjects and in patients with respiratory disease. J Clin Invest 1956; 35:327–335.
20. Mead J, Whittenberger JL. Physical properties of human lungs measured during spontaneous respiration. J Appl Physiol 1953; 5:779–796.
21. DuBois AB, Brody AW, Lewis DH, Burgess BF. Oscillation mechanics of lungs and chest in man. J Appl Physiol 1956; 8:587–594.
22. Michaelson ED, Grassman ED, Peters WR. Pulmonary mechanics by spectral analysis of forced random noise. J Clin Invest 1975; 56:1210–1230.
23. Von Neergaard K, Wirz K. Die Messung der Strömungwiderstände in den Atemwegen des Menschen in besondere bei Asthma und Emphysema. Z Klin Med 1927; 105:51–82.
24. Vuilleumier P. Über ein Methode zur Messung des intraaalveolären Druckes und der Strömungswiderstände in Atemwegen des Menschen. Z Klin Med 1944; 143: 698–717.
25. Chowienczyk PJ, Lawson CP, Lane S, Johnson R, Wilson N, Silverman M, Cochrane GM. A flow interruption device for measurement of airway resistance. Eur Respir J 1991; 4:623–628.
26. Carter ER, Stecenko AA, Pollack BH, Jaeger MJ. Evaluation of the interrupter technique for the use of assessing airway obstruction in children. Pediatr Pulmonol 1994; 17:211–217.
27. Phagoo SB, Wilson NM, Silverman M. Evaluation of the interrupter technique for measuring change in airway resistance in 5-year old asthmatic children. Pediatr Pulmonol 1995; 20:387–395.
28. Clarke JR, Jaeger MJ, Zumrick JL, O'Bryan R, Spaur WH. Respiratory resistance from 1 to 46 ATA measured with the interrupter technique. J Appl Physiol 1982; 52:549–555.
29. Jackson AC, Vinegar A. A technique for measuring frequency response of pressure, volume, and flow transducers. J Appl Physiol 1977; 43:523–536.
30. Clarke JR, Flynn ET. The simultaneous measurement of resistance, elastance, and inertance at depths to 305m (abstr). Undersea Biomed Res 1990; 17(suppl):82.
31. Phagoo SB, Watson RA, Silverman M, Pride NB. Comparison of four methods of assessing airflow resistance before and after airway narrowing in normal subjects. J Appl Physiol 1995; 79:518–525.
32. Lándsér FJ, Clément J, Van de Woestijne KP. Normal values of total respiratory resistance and reactance determined by forced oscillations. Influence of smoking. Chest 1982; 81:586–591.
33. Kjeldgaard JM, Hyde RW, Speers DM, Reichert WW. Frequency dependence of total respiratory resistance in early airway disease. Am Rev Respir Dis 1976; 144: 501–508.
34. Hayes DA, Pimmel JM, Fullton, JM, Bromberg PA. Detection of respiratory mechanical dysfunction by forced random noise impedance parameters. Am Rev Respir Dis 1979; 120:1095–1100.
35. Peslin R, Hannhart B, Pino J. Impédance mécanique thoraco-pulmonaire chez des sujets fumeurs et non fumeurs. Bull Eur Physiopathol Respir 1981; 17:93–105.

36. Dessi P, Sambuc R, Moulin G, Ledoray V, Cannoni M. Effect of heavy smoking on nasal resistance. Acta Otolaryngol 1994; 114:305–310.
37. Wood LDH, Bryan AC. Effect of increased ambient pressure on flow-volume curve of the lung. J Appl Physiol 1969; 27:4–8.
38. Wagner EM, Bleecker ER, Permutt S, Liu MC. Peripheral airways resistance in smokers. Am Rev Respir Dis 1992; 146:92–95.
39. Dosman J, Bode F, Urbanetti J, Martin R, Macklem PT. The use of a helium-oxygen mixture during maximum expiratory flow to demonstrate obstruction in small airways in smokers. J Clin Invest 1975; 55:1090–1099.
40. Hutcheon M, Griffin P, Levison H, Zamel N. Volume of isoflow: a new test in detection of mild abnormalities of lung mechanics. Am Rev Respir Dis 1974; 110: 458–465.
41. Malo JL, LeBlanc P. Functional abnormalities in young asymptomatic smokers with special reference to flow volume curves breathing various gases. Am Rev Respir Dis 1975; 111:623–629.
42. Mishima M, Kawakami K, Higashiya K, Fukunaga T, Ooka T, Kuno K. Frequency characteristics of airway and tissue impedances in respiratory diseases. J Appl Physiol 1991; 71:259–270.
43. Mead J, Milic-Emili J. Theory and methodology in respiratory mechanics with glossary of symbols. In: Fenn WO, Rahn H, eds. Handbook of Physiology: I. Respiration. Washington, DC: American Physiological Society, 1964:363–376.
44. Peslin R, Fredberg JJ. Oscillation Mechanics in the Respiratory System. In: Handbook of Physiology: III The Respiratory System 1984:145–177.
45. Hammersley JR, Olson DE. Physical models of the smaller pulmonary airways. J Appl Physiol 1992; 76:2402–2414.
46. Kimbell JS, Gross EA, Joyner DR, Godo MN, Morgan KT. Application of computational fluid dynamics to regional dosimetry of inhaled chemicals in the upper respiratory tract of the rat. Toxicol Appl Pharmacol 1993; 253–263.
47. Godo MN, Morgan KT, Richardson RB, Kimbell JS. Reconstruction of complex passageways for simulations of transport phenomena: development of a graphical user interface for biological applications. Comput Methods Prog Biomed 1995; 97–112.
48. Myers MR. A numerical investigation into factors affecting anesthetic distribution during spinal anesthesia. J Biomech 1996; 139–149.
49. Gonzalez CF, Cho YI, Ortega HV, Moret J. Intracranial aneurysms: flow analysis of their origin and progression. AJNR 1992; 181–188.
50. Gatlin B, Cuicchi C, Hammersley J, Olson D, Reddy R, Burnside G. Computation of converging and diverging flow through an asymmetric tubular bifurcation. ASME Fluids Engineering Division Summer Meeting, June 22–26, 1997.
51. Gatlin B, Cuicchi C, Hammersley J, Olson D, Reddy R, Burnside G. Particle paths and wall deposition patterns in laminar flow through a bifurcation. ASME Fluid Engineering Division Summer Meeting, June 22–26, 1997.
52. Boyden EA. Segmental Anatomy of the Lungs. New York: McGraw-Hill, 1955.
53. Clarke JR, Bradley ME, Flynn ET. Pulmonary function during cold gas breathing at depths to 305 m. In: Bove AA, Bachrach AJ, Greenbaum LJ, eds. Underwater

and Hyperaric Physiology: IX. Proceedings of the Ninth International Symposium on Underwater and Hyperbaric Physiology. Bethesda, MD: Undersea Medical Society, 1987:359–371.
54. Hamilton RW Jr, MacInnis JB, Noble AD, Schreiner HR. Saturation diving to 650 feet. Technical Memorandum B-411. Tonawanda, NY: Ocean Systems Inc, 1966: 87–123.
55. Dougherty JH Jr, Schaefer KE. Pulmonary functions during saturation-excursion dives breathing air. Aerospace Med 1968; 39:289–292.
56. Schaefer KE, Carey CR, Dougherty JH Jr. Pulmonary function and respiratory gas exchange during saturation-excursion diving to pressures equivalent to 1000 feet of seawater. In: Lambertsen CJ, ed. Underwater Physiology: IV. Proceedings of the Fourth Symposium on Underwater Physiology. New York: Academic Press, 1971: 357–370.
57. Taylor NAS, Clarke JR, Pulmonary function hysteresis during compression to and decompression from 31.3 ATA. Aca Physiol Scand 1993; 148:371–378.
58. McWhirter J. The effect of helium pressure on guinea-pig isolated tracheal smooth muscle (abstr). J Physiol London 1979; 295:28P–29P.
59. Bennett PB, Rostain JC. The High Pressure Nervous Syndrome. In Bennett, PB, Elliott EH, eds. The Physiology and Medicine of Diving, 4th ed. London: Saunders, 1993:194–237.
60. Speizer FE, Frank NR. A technique for measuring nasal and pulmonary flow resistance simultaneously. J Appl Physiol 1964; 19:176–178.
61. Warren DW, Mayo R, Zajac DJ, Rochet AH. Dyspnea following experimentally induced increased nasal airway resistance. Cleft Palate Craniofac J 1996; 33:231–235.
62. Morton AR, King K, Papalia S, Goodman C, Turley KR, Wilmore JH. Comparison of maximal oxygen content with oral vs nasal breathing. Aust J Sci Med Sport 1995; 27:51–55.
63. Niinimaa V, Cole P, Mintz S, Shephard RJ. Oronasal distribution of respiratory airflow. Respir Physiol 1981; 43:69–75.
64. Östlund A, Linnarsson D, Lind F, Sporrong A. Relative narcotic potency and mode of action of sulfur hexafluoride and nitrogen in humans. J Appl Physiol 1994; 76: 439–444.
65. Jammes Y, Burnet H, Cosson P, Lucciano M. Bronchomotor response to cold air or helium-oxygen at normal and high ambient pressures. Undersea Biomed Res 1988; 15:179–192.
66. Vorosmarti J, Bradley ME, Anthonisen NR. The effects of increased gas density on pulmonary mechanics. Undersea Biomed Res 1975; 2:1–10.
67. Bühlmann AA. Respiratory resistance with hyperbaric gas mixtures. In: Lambertsen CJ, Greenbaum LJ Jr, eds. Proceedings of the Second Symposium on Underwater Physiology. Washington, DC: National Academy of Sciences, National Research Council Publication, 1963:98–107.
68. Otis AB, Fenn WO, Rahn H. The mechanics of breathing in man. J Appl Physiol 1950; 2:592–607.
69. Cooper EA. Suggested methods of testing and standards of resistance for respiratory protective devices. J Appl Physiol 1960; 15:1053–1061.

70. Morrison JB, Taylor NA. Measurement of static and dynamic pulmonary work during pressure breathing. Undersea Biomed Res 1990; 17:453–467.
71. Taylor NA, Morrison JB. Pulmonary flow-resistive work during hydrostatic loading. Acta Physiol Scand 1991; 142:307–312.
72. Shikora SA, Bistrian BR, Borlase BC, Blackburn GL, Stone MD, Benotti PN. Work of breathing: reliable predictor of weaning and extubation. Crit Care Med 1990; 18:157–162.
73. Wheatley JR, West S, Cala SJ, Engel LA. The effect of hyperinflation on respiratory muscle work in acute induced asthma. Eur Respir J 1990; 3:625–632.
74. Milic-Emili J, Petit JM. Mechanical efficiency of breathing. J Appl Physiol 1960; 15:359–362.
75. Aaron EA, Johnson BD, Seow CK, Dempsey JA. Oxygen cost of exercise hyperpnea: measurement. J Appl Physiol 1992; 72:1810–1817.
76. Cala SJ, Wilcox P, Edyvean J, Rynn M, Engel LA. Oxygen cost of inspiratory loading: resistive vs elastic. J Appl Physiol 1991; 70:1983–1990.
77. Aaron EA, Johnson BD, Seow CK, Dempsey JA. Oxygen cost of exercise hyperpnea: implications for performance. J Appl Physiol 1992; 72:1818–1825.
78. Mead J. Mechanics of lung and chest wall. In: West JB, ed. Respiratory Physiology, People and Ideas. New York: Oxford University Press, 1996:173–207.
79. Einthoven W. Über die Wirkung der Bronchialmuskeln, nach eine neuen Methode untersucht, und über Asthma nervosum. Pfluegers Arch Gesamte Physiol Menschen Tiere 1892; 51:367–445.
80. Hyatt RE, Schilder DP, Fry DL. Relationship between maximum expiratory flow and degree of lung inflation. J Appl Physiol 1958; 13:331–336.
81. Pride NB, Permutt S, Riley RL, Bromberger-Barnea B. Determinants of maximal expiratory flow from the lungs. J Appl Physiol 1967; 23:646–662.
82. Dawson SV, Elliot EA. Wave-speed limitation on expiratory flow—a unifying concept. J Appl Physiol 1977; 43:498–515.
83. MacDonald D. Blood Flow in Arteries. Baltimore MD: Williams & Wilkins, 1974.
84. Hughes JMB, Hoppin FG Jr, Mead J. Effect of lung inflation on bronchial length and diameter in excised lungs. J Appl Physiol 1972; 32:25–33.
85. Hahn HL, Graf PD, Nadel JA. Effect of vagal tone on airway diameters and on lung volume in anesthetized dogs. J Appl Physiol 1976; 41:581–589.
86. Hyatt RE, Rodarte JR, Mead J, Wilson TA. Changes In Lung Mechanics, Flow-Volume Relations. In: Macklem PT, Permutt S, eds. The Lung In the Transition Between Health and Disease. New York: Marcel Dekker, 1979:73–112.
87. Miller JN, Wangensteen OD, Lanphier EH. Ventilatory limitations on exertion at depth, In: Lambertsen CJ, ed. Underwater Physiology, Proceedings of the Fourth Symposium On Underwater Physiology, New York: Academic Press, 1971:317–323.
88. Miller JN, Lanphier EH, Wangensteen OD. Respiratory limitations to work in diving and their significance to the design of underwater breathing apparatus. Med Sport 1971; 24:231–237.
89. Lambert RK, Wilson TA, Hyatt RE, Rodarte JR. A computational model for expiratory flow. J Appl Physiol 1982; 52:44–56.
90. Hyatt RE. Forced expiration. In: Fishman AP, Macklem PT, Mead J, eds. Handbook

of Physiology, Sec 3. The Respiratory System, Vol III. Mechanics of Breathing, Part 1. 1986:295–314.
91. Vail EG. Respiratory mechanics—airway collapse. Aerospace Med 1971; 42:975–979.
92. Flook V. Physics and physiology in the hyperbaric environment. Clin Phys Physiol Meas 1987; 8:197–230.
93. Flook V, Fraser IM. Inspiratory flow limitation in divers. Undersea Biomed Res 1989; 16:305–311.
94. Miller JN. Physiological limits to breathing dense gas. In: Lundgren CEG, Warkander DE, eds. Physiological and Human Engineering Aspects of Underwater Breathing Apparatus. Bethesda, MD: Undersea and Hyperbaric Medical Society, 1989:5–18.
95. Olsen CR, Stevens AE, Pride NB, Staub NC. Structural basis for decreased compressibility of constricted trachea and bronchi. J Appl Physiol 1967; 23:35–39.
96. Flook V, Fraser IM. Pressure-flow characteristics of human trachea in vitro (abstr). Undersea Biomed Res 1990; 17(suppl):80.
97. Olson DE, Iliff LD, Sudlow MF. Some aspects of flow in the central airways. Bull Physio-Pathol Respir 1972; 8:391–408.
98. Griscom NT, Wohl MEB. Trachael size and shape: effects of change in intraluminal pressure. Radiology 1983; 149:27–30.
99. Gibson GJ, Pride NB, Empey DW. The role of inspiratory dynamic compression in upper airway obstruction. Am Rev Respir Dis 1973; 108:1352–1360.
100. Fraser IM. Some characteristics of human inspiratory flow of particular relevance to breathing at raised environmental pressure. PhD Thesis, University of Aberdeen, Scotland, 1992.
101. Flook V, Fraser IM. Resistance to breathing—diver's lungs the main problem? In Flook V, Brubakk AO, eds. Lung Physiology and Divers' Breathing Apparatus. Aberdeen, Scotland: BPCC-AUP Aberdeen Ltd, 1992:45–67 (available from Best Publishing).
102. Flook V. Characteristics of inspiratory flow. In Jones JG, Hanning CD, eds. The Upper Airways. Baillière's Clinical Anaesthesiology, vol. 9. London: Baillière Tindall, 1995:251–265.
103. Spencer JW, Findling A, Bachrach AJ, Gelfand R, Lambertsen CJ, Karreman G. Tremor and somatosensory studies during chamber He-O_2 compressions to 13.1, 25.2. 37.3 and 49.4 ATA. J Appl Physiol 1979; 47:804–812.
104. Stuart DGE, Eldred E, Wild WO. Comparisons between the physiological shivering and parkinsonian tremors. J Appl Physiol 1966; 21:1918–1924.
105. Tarasiuk A, Grossman Y. Pressure-induced tremor-associated activity in ventral roots in isolated spinal cord of newborn rats. Undesea Biomed Res 1990; 17:287–296.
106. DuBois AB, Brody AW, Lewis DH, Burgess BF. Oscillation mechanics of lungs and chest in man. J Appl Physiol 1956; 8:587–594.
107. Chalker RB, Celli BR, Habib RH, Jackson AC. Respiratory input impedance from 4 to 256 Hz in normals and chronic airflow obstruction: comparisons and correlations with spirometry. Am Rev Respir Dis 1992; 146:570–576.
108. Jackson AC, Habib RH, Suki B, Wood SA, Mitzner W. Serial distribution of

airway diameters from input impedance and computed tomography. Ann Biomed Eng 1995; 23:740–749.
109. Lutchen KR, Everett JR, Jackson AC. Impact of frequency range and input impedance on airway-tissue separation implied from transfer impedance. J Appl Physiol 1993; 74:1089–1099.
110. Lutchen KR, Giurdanella CA, Jackson AC. Inability to separate airway from tissue properties by use of human respiratory input impedance. J Appl Physiol 1990; 68: 2403–2412.
111. Kinsler LE, Frey AR. Fundamentals of Acoustics. 3d ed. New York: Wiley, 1982.
112. Rice DA. Sound speed in pulmonary parenchyma. J Appl Physiol 1983; 54:304–308.
113. Leith DE, Butler JP, Sneddon SL, Brain JD. Cough. In: Fishman AP, ed. Handbook of Physiology: The Respiratory System. Bethesda, MD: American Physiological Society, 1986:315–335.
114. Jaeger MJ. Coughing and forced expiration at reduced barometric pressure (abstr). Fed Proc 1972; 31:322.
115. Jack MA, Duncan G. The helium speech effect and electronic techniques for enhancing intelligibility in a helium-oxygen environment. Radio Electron Eng 1982; 52:211–233.
116. Giordano TA, Rothman HB, Hollien H. Helium speech unscramblers—a critical review of the state of the art. IEEE Trans Audio Electroaccoust 1973; AU-21: 436–444.
117. Boll SF. Suppression of acoustic noise in speech using spectral subtraction. IEEE Trans Acoust Speech Signal Proc 1979; ASSP-27:113–120.
118. Mendel LL, Hamill BW, Crepeau LJ, Fallon E. Speech intelligibility assessment in a helium environment. J. Acoust Soc Am 1995; 97:628–636.
119. Van Liew HD, Paganelli CV, Sponholtz DK. Estimation of gas-phase diffusivities in hyperbaric environments. Undersea Biomed Res 1982; 9:175–181.
120. Reid RC, Prausnitz JM, Sherwood TK. The Properties of Gases and Liquids, 3d ed. New York: McGraw-Hill, 1977.
121. Paganelli CV. Gas-phase diffusion of O_2 in helium and nitrogen under pressure. In: Bove AA, Bachrach AJ, Greenbaum LJ, eds. Underwater Physiology IX. Proceedings of the Ninth Symposium on Underwater and Hyperbaric Physiology. Bethesda, MD: Undersea Medical Society Inc, 1987:439–446.
122. Van Liew HD, Thalmann ED, Sponholtz DK. Hindrance to diffusive gas mixing in the lung in hyperbaric environments. J Appl Physiol 1981; 51:243–247.
123. Saltzman HA, Salzano JV, Blenkarn GD, Kylstra JA. Effects of pressure on ventilation and gas exchange in man. J Appl Physiol 1971; 30:443–449.
124. Martin RR, Zutter M, Anthonisen NR. Pulmonary gas exchange in dogs breathing SF_6 at 4 atm. J Appl Physiol 1972; 33:86–92.
125. Cinkotai FF. Fluid flow in a model alveolar sac. J Appl Physiol 1974; 37:249–251.
126. Halsey JM, Kent DW, Egger EI. Pressure studies with mice up to 270 ATA. In: Lambertsen DM, ed. Underwater Physiology: V. Proceedings of the Fifth Symposium on Underwater Physiology. Bethesda, MD: Federation of American Societies for Experimental Biology, 1976:245–249.

127. Parc J, Michaud A, Le Chuiton J, Michel A, Barthelemy L, Balouet G. Very deep diving experiments on miniature pigs. In: CJ Lambertsen, ed. Underwater Physiology: V. Proceedings of the Fifth Symposium on Underwater Physiology. Bethesda, MD: Federation of American Societies for Experimental Biology, 1976: 251–262.
128. Imbert G. Apports de l'experimentation animale en physiologie hyperbare et en plongée profunde. Bull Inst Océano (Monoco) 1982; 3(spécial):73–107.
129. Hamnegard CH, Wragg S, Kyroussis D, Mills HG, Polkey M, Moran J, Road J, Bake B, Green M, Moxham J. Diaphragmatic fatigue following maximal ventilation in man. Eur Respir J 1996; 9:241–247.
130. Leith DE, Bradley M. Ventilatory muscle strength and endurance training. J Appl Physiol 1976; 41:508–516.
131. Bye PTP, Farkas GA, Roussos C. Respiratory factors limiting exercise. Ann Rev Physiol 1983; 45:439–451.
132. Grassino A, Macklem PT. Respiratory muscle fatigue and ventilatory failure. Ann Rev Med 1984; 35:625–647.
133. Belman MJ, Gesser GA. Ventilatory muscle training in the elderly. J Appl Physiol 1988; 64:899–905.
134. Lenoir P, Jammes Y, Giry P, Rostain JC, Burnet H, Tomei C, Roussos C. Electromyographic study of respiratory muscles during human diving at 46 ATA. Undersea Biomed Res 1990; 17:121–137.
135. Halsey MJ, Kent DW, Egger EI. Pressure studies with mice up to 270 ATA. In: Lambertsen CJ, ed. Underwater Physiology: V. Proceedings of the Fifth Symposium on Underwater Physiology. Bethesda, MD: Federation of American Societies for Experimental Biology, 1976:245–249.
136. Burnet H, Lenoir P, Jammes Y. Changes in respiratory muscle activity in conscious cats during experimental dives at 101 ATA. J Appl Physiol 1992; 73:465–472.
137. Salzano JV, Camporesi EM, Stolp BW, Moon RE. Physiological responses to exercise at 47 and 66 ATA. J Appl Physiol 1984; 57:1055–1068.
138. Clarke JR. Diver tolerance to respiratory loading during wet and dry dives from 0 to 450 m. In: Flook V, Brubakk AO, eds. Lung Physiology and Diver's Breathing Apparatus. Aberdeen, Scotland: BPCC-AUP, Aberdeen Ltd, 1992:33–44.
139. Fothergill DM, Carlson NA. Effects of N_2O narcosis on breathing and effort sensations during exercise and inspiratory resistive loading. J Appl Physiol 1996; 81: 1562–1571.
140. Fothergill DM, Carlson NA. The role of gas density, high pressure, and inert gas narcosis on exercise tolerance and psychophysical perceptions of exertion (abstr). Undersea Biomed Res 1995; 17(suppl):70.
141. Surbey GD, Andrew GM, Cervenko FW, Hamilton PP. Effects of naloxone on exercise performance. J Appl Physiol 1984; 57:674–679.
142. Goldfarb AH, Hatfield BD, Armstrong D, Potts J. Plasma beta-endorphin concentration: response to intensity and duration of exercise. Med Sci Sports Exerc 1990; 22:241–244.

143. Hoffmann P, Jonsdottir IH, Thorén P. Activation of different opioid systems by muscle activity and exercise. News Physiol Sci 1996; 11:223–228.
144. Scardella AT, Parisi RA, Phair DK, Santiago TV, Edelman NH. The role of endogenous opiods in the ventilatory response to acute flow-resistive loads. Am Rev Respir Dis 1986; 133:26–31.
145. Trouth CO, Bada FJ, Barnard DG, Pan Y, Holloway JA, Millis RM, Bernard DG. Naloxone application to the ventral medulla enhances the respiratory response to increased inspired carbon dioxide. Life Sci 1991; 49:193–200.
146. Petrozzino JJ, Scardella AT, Li JK-J, Krawciw N, Edelman NH, Santiago TV. Effect of naloxone on spectral shifts of the diaphragm EMG during inspiratory loading. J Appl Physiol 1990; 68:1376–1385.
147. Petrozzino JJ, Scardella AT, Edelman NH, Santiago TV. Respiratory muscle acidosis stimulates endogenous opioids during inspiratory loading. Am Rev Respir Dis 1993; 147:607–615.
148. Woodcock AA, Gross MA, Gellert A, Shah S, Johnson M, Geddes DM. Effects of dihydrocodeine, alcohol, and caffeine on breathlessness and exercise tolerance in patients with chronic obstructive lung disease and normal blood gases. N Engl J Med 1981; 305:1611–1616.
149. Sackner MA. Effects of hydrocodone bitartrate on breathing pattern of patients with chronic obstructive pulmonary disease and restrictive lung disease. Mt Sinai J Med 1984; 51:222–226.
150. Light RW, Muro JR, Sato RI, Stansbury DW, Fischer CE, Brown SE. Effects of oral morphine on breathlessness and exercise tolerance in patients with chronic obstructive pulmonary disease. Am Rev Respir Dis 1989; 139:126–133.
151. Akiyama Y, Nishimura M, Kobayashi S, Yoshioka A, Yamamoto M, Miyamoto K, Kawakami Y. Effects of naloxone on the sensation of dyspnea during acute respiratory stress in normal adults. J Appl Physiol 1993; 74:590–595.
152. Bellofiore S, Di Maria GU, Privitera S, Sapienza S, Milic-Emili J, Mistretta A. Endogenous opiods modulate the increase in ventilatory output and dyspnea during severe acute bronchoconstriction. Am Rev Respir Dis 1990; 142:812–816.
153. Santiago TV, Remolina C, Scoles V III, Edelman NH. Endorphins and the control of breathing: ability of naloxone to restore-flow-resistive load compensation in chronic obstructive pulmonary disease. N Engl J Med 1981; 304:1190–1195.
154. Lanphier EH, Camporesi EM. Respiration and exercise. In: Bennett PB, Elliott DH, eds. The Physiology and Medicine of Diving, 4th ed. London: Saunders, 1993:77–120.
155. Chouteau J. Respiratory gas exchange in animals during exposure to extreme ambient pressures. In: Lambertson CJ, ed. Underwater Physiology: IV. Proceedings of the Fourth Symposium on Underwater Physiology. New York: Academic Press, 1971:385–397.
156. Rokitka MA, Rahn H. Physical performance of mouse colonies as a measure of inert gas narcosis, oxygen toxicity, and the Chouteau effect. In: Schilling CW, Beckett MW, eds. Underwater Physiology: VI. Proceedings of the Sixth Symposium on Underwater Physiology. Bethesda, MD: Federation of American Societies of Experimental Biology, 1978:241–250.

157. Cumming G, Crank J, Horsfield K, Parker I. Gaseous diffusion in the airways of the human lung. Resp Physiol 1966; 1:58–74.
158. West JB. Pulmonary blood flow and gas exchange. In: West JB, ed. Respiratory Physiology: People and Ideas. New York: Oxford University Press, 1996:165.
159. Wagner PD, Saltzman HA, West JB. Measurement of continuous distributions of ventilation-perfusion ratios: theory. J Appl Physiol 1974; 36:533–537.
160. Powers SK, Williams J. Exercise-induced hypoxaemia in highly trained athletes. Sports Med 4:46–53, 1987.
161. Powers SK, Dodd S, Lawler J, Landry G, Kirtley M, McKnight T, Grinton S. Incidence of exercise-induced hypoxemia in elite endurance athletes at sea level. Eur J Appl Physiol 1988; 58:298–302.
162. Wagner PD. Ventilation-perfusion matching during exercise. Chest 1992; 101: 192S–198S.
163. Schaffartzik W, Poole DC, Derion T, Tsukimoto K, Hogan MC, Arcos JP, Bebout DE, Wagner PD. $\dot{V}_A/\dot{Q}$ distribution during heavy exercise and recovery in humans: implications for pulmonary edema. J Appl Physiol 1992; 72:1657–1667.
164. Lama IL, Wolski LA, Coutts KD, McKenzie DC. The relationship between test protocol and the development of exercise-induced hypoxemia (EIH) in highly trained athletes. Eur J Appl Physiol 1996; 74:330–335.
165. Hopkins SR, McKenzie DC, Schoene RB, Glenny RW, Robertson HT. Pulmonary gas exchange during exercise in athletes: ventilation-perfusion mismatch and diffusion limitation. J Appl Physiol 1994; 77:912–917.
166. Caillaud D, Serrecousine O, Anselme F, Capdevilla X, Prefaut C. Computerized tomography and pulmonary diffusing capacity in highly trained athletes after performing a triathlon. J Appl Physiol 1995; 79:1226–1232.
167. Schaffartzik W, Arcos J, Tsukimoto K, Mathieucostello O, Wagner PD. Pulmonary interstitial edema in the pig after heavy exercise. J Appl Physiol 1992; 75: 2535–2540.
168. Agostoni E, Gurtner G, Torri G, Rahn H. Respiratory mechanics during submersion and negative-pressure breathing. J Appl Physiol 1966; 21:251–258.
169. Arborelius M Jr, Balldin UI, Lilja B, Lundgren CEG. Regional lung function in man during immersion with the head above water. Aerospace Med 1972; 43:701–707.
170. Lundgren CEG, Farhi LE. Pulmonary circulation in diving and hyperbaric environment. In: Weir EK, Reeves JT, eds. Pulmonary Vascular Physiology and Pathophysiology. New York: Marcel Dekker, 1989:199–240.
171. Bondi KR, Young JM, Bennett RM, Bradley ME. Closing volumes in man immersed to the neck in water. J Appl Physiol 1976; 40:736–740.
172. Prefaut C, Ramonatxo M, Boyer R, Chardon G. Human gas exchange during water immersion. Respir Physiol 1978; 34:307–318.
173. Cohen R, Bell WH, Saltzman HA, Klystra JA. Alveolar-arterial oxygen pressure difference in man immersed up to the neck in water. J Appl Physiol 1971; 30: 720–723.
174. Derion T, Guy HK, Tsukimoto K, Schaffartzik W, Prediletto R, Poole DC, Knight DR, Wagner PD. Ventilation-perfusion relationships in the lung during head-out immersion. J Appl Physiol 1992; 72:64–72.

175. Miller JN, Winsborough M. The effect of increased gas density upon $\dot{V}_A/\dot{Q}$ and gas exchange during expiratory flow-limited exercise. Forsvarsmedicin 1973; 9: 321–331.
176. Clarke JR, Fisher MA, Jaeger MJ. Inertance as a factor in uneven ventilation in diving. In: Bachrach AJ, Matzen MM, eds. Underwater Physiology: VII. Proceedings of the Seventh Symposium on Underwater Physiology. Bethesda, MD: Undersea Medical Society Inc, 1981:225–233.
177. Morgan BE, Breinbauer B, Stolp BW, Simonds D, Dear G de L, Castellano JM, Moon RE. Mechanisms of hypercapnia during exercise at 40 msw (abstr). Undersea Hyperbaric Med 1996; 23(suppl):76–77.
178. Clarke JR, Fothergill DM. Apparent cerebral hypoxia during exercise in hyperoxic atmospheres (abstr). Undersea Hyperbaric Med 1996; 23(suppl):22.
179. Kerem D, Daskalovic YI, Arieli R, Shupak A. CO_2 retention during hyperbaric exercise while breathing 40/60 nitrox. Undersea Hyperbaric Med 1995; 22:339–346.
180. Wilmshurst PT, Nuri M, Crowther A, Betts JC, Webb-Peploe MM. Recurrent pulmonary edema in SCUBA divers—prodrome of hypertension: a new syndrome. In: Bachrach AJ, Matzen MM, eds. Underwater Physiology: VIII. Proceedings of the Eighth Symposium on Underwater Physiology, Bethesda MD: Undersea Medical Society, 1984:327–342.
181. Wilmshurst PT, Nuri M, Crowther A, Betts JC, Webb-Peploe MM. Cold-induced pulmonary oedema in scuba divers and swimmers and subsequent development of hypertension. Lancet 1989; 1:62–65.
182. Pons M, Blickenstorf D, Oechslin E, Hold G, Greminger P, Franzeck UK, Russi EW. Pulmonary oedema in healthy persons during scuba-diving and swimming. Eur Respir J 1995; 8:762–767.
183. Weiler-Ravell D, Shupak A, Goldenberg I, Halpern et al. Pulmonary oedema and haemoptysis induced by strenuous swimming. Br Med J 1995; 311–362.
184. Hampson NB, Dunford RG. Pulmonary edema of scuba divers. Undersea Hyperbaric Med 1997; 24:29–33.
185. Lenfant C. Measurement of factors impairing gas exchange in man with hyperbaric pressure. J Appl Physiol 1964; 19:189–194.
186. Wagner PD, Gale GE. Ventilation-perfusion relationships. In: Whipp BJ, Wasserman K, eds. Exercise, Pulmonary Physiology and Pathophysiology. New York: Marcel Dekker, 1991:121–142.
187. Taylor WF, Marcinik EJ, Chen S, Yedgar S. Red blood cell aggregation and maximum skin blood flow during saturation diving (abstr). FASEB J 1995; 9: A643.

2

Pulmonary Fitness for Diving

TOM S. NEUMAN

University of California, San Diego, Medical Center
San Diego, California

I. Introduction

As there is in most human behaviors, there is some risk associated with diving activities. No sport or occupation is completely safe. The question that therefore must be raised is whether an activity is "safe enough" for the benefits derived from that activity. In trying to assess the risk of diving in relation to the pulmonary system, two major concerns must be addressed in considering pulmonary fitness to dive.

The first is simple aerobic capacity. Diving is a sport or occupation that has a wide range of possible ventilatory requirements. Scuba diving in warm, clear Caribbean waters with a gentle current propelling the diver along requires little if any exertion. On the other hand, the exertion required to swim against a strong current with full scuba gear and with a significant surge, in cold water, while towing a disabled buddy could easily exceed the functional abilities of even the most "fit" individual. Obviously a significant ventilatory limitation could prevent one from performing at the level necessary for reasonably safe diving activities. Furthermore, the unique stresses of the underwater environment can also serve to decrease ventilatory function secondary to effects of the water environment itself and the physiological derangements produced by the underwater breathing apparatus. Thus, the combined issues of variable functional requirements and the physiological effects of immersion, increased gas density, and the effects of equipment all demand a minimum degree of pulmonary fitness to dive.

The second major concern that must be addressed in assessing pulmonary fitness to dive is the consideration whether specific lung diseases might predispose the diver to injuries unique or nearly unique to the diving environment. Specifically, will airway disease, or, for that matter, structural lung disease of any sort predispose the diver to pulmonary barotrauma and subsequent systemic air embolism? An associated consideration would be whether lung disease or the medications used to treat such disease could interfere with the pulmonary vasculature sufficiently to allow bubbles (i.e., venous gas emboli) to more easily cross the pulmonary capillary filter and produce unexpected neurological decompression sickness or decompression sickness precipitated by arterialization of what otherwise would be asymptomatic venous gas emboli.

II. Ventilatory Capacity (Exercise Requirements of Normal Aquatic Activities)

Oxygen consumption is the most useful measure of assessing the requirements of exertion as well as providing a yardstick for assessing the functional cardiorespiratory requirements of any activity. Various studies have looked at oxygen consumption of underwater swimming activities, and they provide a range to estimate what may be the ventilatory requirements for such activities (1–4). Taking the mean of these studies, to swim at 0.6, 1.0, and 1.2 knots requires $\dot{V}_{O_2}$'s of 1.0, 1.7, and 2.4 L/min, respectively. Thus, as can been seen, swimming at what is approximately 1.4 mi/hr requires a fairly high oxygen consumption. At an oxygen consumption in this range, a respiratory quotient of 1 can reasonably be assumed; therefore a $\dot{V}_{O_2}$ of 2.4 L/min can be assumed to represent a $\dot{V}CO_2$ of the same or nearly the same 2.4 L/min. By definition, the fractional content of carbon dioxide (CO_2) in alveolar gas (FA_{CO_2}) is equal to the volume of CO_2 in the alveolar gas divided by the total volume of alveolar gas, or

$$FA_{CO_2} = VACO_2/VA \tag{1}$$

Correcting for the different units in which these values are usually reported, assuming standard barometric pressure, and assuming alveolar P_{CO_2} is essentially the same arterial P_{CO_2}, the following equation can be derived:

$$Pa_{CO_2} = 863\ [V_{CO_2}(\text{L/min at STPD})/VA(\text{L/min at BTPS})] \tag{2}$$

Solving the equation for a Pa_{CO_2} of 30 to 40 mmHg reveals that an alveolar ventilation of 50 to 70 L/min is necessary if one is to be able to sustain a $\dot{V}_{O_2}$

of 2.4 L/min. Alveolar ventilation, however, is only a portion of total minute ventilation ($\dot{V}_E$), with the remaining portion being dead-space ventilation ($\dot{V}_D$). Thus:

$$\dot{V}_E = \dot{V}_A + \dot{V}_D \tag{3}$$

As the ratio of dead-space ventilation to tidal volume varies inversely with the total ventilation and since the $\dot{V}_D$ itself changes with alterations in $\dot{V}_E$, it is impossible to predict the total $\dot{V}_E$ required for a given $\dot{V}O_2$; however, assuming a $\dot{V}_D$ of 10%, $\dot{V}_E$ requirements at STPD are approximately 55 to 80 L/min for levels of exertion that might reasonably be required of a scuba diver in adverse conditions. An alternative method of estimating the $\dot{V}_E$ necessary for a given level of exercise can be made from the work of Harries (5) in his studies of world-class athletes. He observed the following relationship:

$$\dot{V}_{O_2MAX} = \dot{V}E_{MAX} * 0.026 + 0.44 \tag{4}$$

where $r = .94$. Solving for a $\dot{V}_{O_2}$ of 2.4 L yields essentially the same estimate as that made previously.

There are, however, effects of immersion, increased gas density, and the added work of breathing due to diving equipment that now must be considered in addition to the simple ventilatory requirements of a given level of exercise. Various studies (6–10) have looked at changes in maximum voluntary ventilation (MVV) or maximum breathing capacity (MBC) with increasing depth. Although there is considerable variability in the data for more extreme depths, at approximately 100 FSW (dry), it appears these values are reduced by about one-half compared with surface values. Immersion further decreases MVV by approximately 15% (11). If at depth, as has been reported for conditions at 1 atm, individuals can sustain a $\dot{V}_E$ of only about 70% of MVV (12–15), it should be apparent that in order to sustain a moderate $\dot{V}_{O_2}$ at 100 FSW, for all intents and purposes normal pulmonary function is necessary, even without considering the added work of breathing due to the immersion and the underwater breathing apparatus.

Although not strictly in the category of what would generally be described as pulmonary function, there are additional problems associated with obtaining adequate gas exchange in very deep diving. The best-studied phenomenon, which is probably secondary to intrapulmonary diffusion limitation, has been termed "Chouteau hypoxia" and was described in a series of experiments with goats in deep chamber dives (16,17). Gas mixtures were initially nearly normoxic. At increasing depths, animals developed problems that were ameliorated by relatively minor increments in the $P_{I_{O_2}}$. The problems would then develop again as atmospheric pressure was raised, and it would again be ameliorated by increasing the PI_{O_2} until, at pressures greater than 100 bar, several animals died from what appeared to be pulmonary O_2 toxicity. Whether these observations are due to the direct effects of increases in gas density due to changes in the diffusion coefficient of oxygen mixed in a diluent gas or to technical problems with the experiment remains to be determined; however, it does appear as if alveolar gas exchange may be limited by problems with intrapulmonary diffusion at great depth. Whether humans can ever descend to depths where these issues represent practical problems is as yet unknown.

In summary then, it appears that normal or nearly normal ventilatory capacity is necessary for levels of activity that can reasonably be expected to occur during some diving activities. Clearly, in extremely protected environments and benign circumstances, less function would be required; however, that functional level would have to be dictated by those specific circumstances.

Unfortunately, determining "normal" pulmonary function is not simple. However, for practical purposes, it can be defined as no more than two standard deviations from the mean values of a healthy reference group (18) (Table 1). Individuals with low normal values or with values below the definition of normal can be referred for further exercise testing to make sure that they have the necessary ventilatory and gas-exchange capacity to undertake the level of exercise that may be anticipated, taking into account the effects of immersion, depth, and the breathing apparatus.

The second major concern facing the diver with regard to pulmonary fitness to dive is the potential risk for pulmonary barotrauma that underlying lung disease may present. Whereas the risk of not being fit enough if caught in a strong current is readily apparent, it may be difficult to appreciate whether there is increased risk of air embolism because of an abnormal distribution of ventilation or altered airway function.

Table 1 Lower Limits of Normal of Various Pulmonary Function Tests

Test	Lower limit of normal
Vital capacity	< 75% of predicted
Functional residual capacity	< 70% or above 130% predicted
Residual volume	< 65% or above 135% predicted
Total lung capacity	< 80% or above 120% predicted
Forced expiratory volume (1 sec)	< 80% predicted
FEV_1 /FVC	< 85% predicted
FEF_{25-75}	< 65% predicted

III. Asthma

Asthma is the most common pulmonary disorder that must be evaluated in a diver or diving candidate. Yet, defining asthma can be difficult due to the various asthma "syndromes." For practical purposes, asthma may be defined as a disorder or disorders "characterized by increased responsiveness of the airways (i.e., hyper-reactivity) to various stimuli and by resultant smooth muscle contraction and obstruction" (19).

One of the more common asthma syndromes is "atopic" asthma. This is most frequently characterized by onset in childhood and by its association with multiple other allergies (e.g., allergic rhinitis or dermatitis). Attacks tend to be precipitated by sensitizing agents. Children who develop this asthma syndrome early in life do not necessarily have persistent asthma into their adult years. In one study, only 15% of 10-year-old children whose asthma began before the age of 2 had persistent wheezing (20). On the other hand, if the precipitating cause of attacks was infection, it was found that only 50% of children were considered to be free from asthma when reexamined 20 years later (21). Adults do not seem to do as well as children. There is a much lower percentage of individuals who become free of disease with time (22–24), and the proportion of severe to mild cases seems to rise steeply with age (25); but whether this represents the additional impact of cigarette smoking, urban environments, and occupational exposures is unclear. Frequently exacerbations cannot be ascribed to a specific precipitating agent or event. This syndrome has been called *intrinsic asthma*; however, the syndromes are often not clearly different (26,27). Another frequently seen syndrome is exercise-induced asthma, the cause of which remains unclear. However, some evidence now suggests that the underlying etiology is cold stimulus to the tracheobronchial tree in susceptible individuals (28,29).

Other less common syndromes are the aspirin-sensitivity triad (nasal polyps, urticaria, and asthma following aspirin ingestion), occupational asthma, and cough asthma.

Thus, asthma is not a single disease but rather an increased degree of airway responsiveness (i.e., obstruction) to a heterogeneous group of stimuli associated with a highly variable degree of smooth muscle contraction, mucus production, and the presence of inflammatory mediators. As already mentioned, the factors that precipitate attacks vary tremendously, but—equally important—the actual location of obstruction also appears to vary with different patients depending upon what one believes to be measured by various pulmonary function tests.

Most importantly, there is considerable difference in the reversibility of the airway obstruction seen in asthmatic patients. Some asthmatics demonstrate completely normal pulmonary function tests (PFTs) between attacks (30). Others, although asymptomatic, show evidence of airway obstruction even after vigorous therapy. Under such circumstances, the distinction between chronic obstructive pulmonary disease (COPD) and reactive airway disease (RAD)—i.e., asthma—becomes blurred.

As a result of these differences, recommendations concerning diving must take into consideration the individual patient's specific asthma syndrome, history, and response to treatment.

The major concern of many practitioners advising asthmatics about diving is that such an individual might be dangerously susceptible to pulmonary barotrauma and cerebral air embolism during even a normal ascent. Liebow et al. (31) suggested that under certain conditions partial pulmonary obstruction in large airways could lead to arterial gas embolism (AGE). Similarly, Schaefer and colleagues (32) demonstrated that overpressurization of the lung could lead to AGE, and Colebatch et al. (33) demonstrated decreased compliance to be associated with AGE. All of these factors can occur in asthmatics. Additionally, some asthmatics have significant noncommunicating air spaces, as demonstrated by differences in measured lung volumes compared by helium dilution techniques and whole-body plethysmography (34). Moreover, the acute asthmatic is usually hyperinflated. It also has been demonstrated that not only overpressurization but also overinflation is required to produce AGE (32). Finally, a more sophisticated study on asthmatics by Wagner and co-workers (35) revealed that even in supposedly asymptomatic individuals, marked abnormalities of ventilation/perfusion ratios could exist. This experiment demonstrated that as many as half of the lung units were behind completely closed airways, which had low $\dot{V}_A/\dot{Q}$ ratios (due to collateral ventilation).

Epidemiological data are hard to interpret as, according to experts, asthma is considered, in general, to be a contraindication to diving. Nonetheless, in Australia and New Zealand (36), asthma was found to be present in 9% of the scuba fatalities. A study from the Divers' Alert Network (DAN) (37) revealed that as many as 12% of AGE victims have asthma. In an additional study by authors from DAN (38), a fourfold increase in relative risk for dysbarism was noted in asthmatic divers. Finally, an examination of other data suggests that perhaps as many as 50% of air embolisms are not associated with panic, out-of-air, or breath-holding ascents (39). In other words, apparently half of the incidents of arterial gas embolism appear to occur in divers without an obvious precipitating behavioral cause. This would imply that undetected underlying lung disease may play a role in these accidents. Thus, there is a solid rationale and perhaps some epidemiological data to suggest that it would be unsafe for the asthmatic to dive, and this explains the reluctance on the part of many physicians to suggest that asthmatics can dive with an acceptable level of risk.

On the other hand, closer analysis of the above data and additional studies can yield different interpretations. In the years the University of Rhode Island collected diving fatality statistics, only one of 2132 deaths occurred in an individual with asthma; furthermore, no other information concerning the death was available, nor was it clear what role asthma may have played in that individual's death (40–49). Examining the Australian and New Zealand data more closely, Douglas Walker (50), referring to alleged overrepresentation of asthmatics (51) in diving fatalities, states: "This appears to be untrue in relation to Australia and New Zealand'' (50). Reexamining all the combined DAN data reveals that there is little evidence for excess risk (52). Indeed the 95% confidence interval of the odds ratio (relative risk) for all asthmatics is 0.80 to 2.99 (not significant); for current asthmatics, it is 0.65 to 5.33 (53) (n.s.) (Table 2). Similarly, analysis of pulmonary function in approximately forty cases of air embolism at the Marine Science Center on Catalina Island over a 5-year period revealed only one asthmatic (54), and analysis of 18 consecutive fatalities in Los Angeles County between 1985 and 1990 did not reveal any asthmatic victims (55). Investigators reviewing the records of the Institute of Naval Medicine in England did not find asthmatics in the 140 cases of AGE they investigated from 1965 to 1985 (56). Importantly, in the studies done in the United States (57–59), asthmatics appear to be represented in the diving population in much the same numbers as seen in the nondiving population.

Perhaps because differences in the interpretation of these studies are possible, the international community does not uniformly agree that asthmatics should be restricted from diving. In the past, the British SubAqua Club allowed members with extrinsic asthma to dive, although they prohibited those with exercise-induced asthma to dive. It was felt that those needing bronchodilators regularly or those on steroids should not dive. They recommended that asthmatics not dive within 48 hr of wheezing; however, in a study of asthmatic

Table 2 Risk of Asthma and Diving

Diving injury	Relative risk	Confidence interval (95%)	*p* value
All asthmatics			
Age	1.58	0.80–2.99	n.s.
Type II DCS	0.74	0.43–1.24	n.s.
Current asthmatics			
Age	1.98	0.65–5.33	n.s.
Type II DCS	1.16	0.51–2.59	n.s.

divers conducted via questionnaire from a diving magazine, nine individuals wheezed daily, dove within 1 hr of wheezing, and logged more than 1200 dives without incident (60). In the same study, 104 asthmatic divers reported more than 12,000 dives without an AGE. More recent recommendations (61), are similar with specific suggestions made concerning medications, exercise testing, and the use of peak airflow meters for self-monitoring.

Review of papers historically quoted to support the recommendations that asthmatics not dive reveals interesting inconsistencies. In the report by Liebow et al. (31), it is hypothesized a broncholith in a large airway was the cause of a fatal air embolism in an escape trainee; yet this does not account for the findings of bilateral barotrauma noted on autopsy. In the previously mentioned report by Wagner et al. (33), which is often used to justify the exclusion of all asthmatics from diving because even asymptomatic asthmatics have marked abnormalities of $\dot{V}_A/\dot{Q}$ distribution (62), the seven "asymptomatic" patients had profoundly abnormal airflows and/or volumes. Finally, at two recent symposia, it was the consensus opinion of the participants (predominantly physicians and researchers interested in diving medicine) that asthma did not appear to measurably increase the risk of diving-related pulmonary barotrauma (63,64) and that the limiting factor for asthmatics is adequate exercise capacity. What then are reasonable conclusions in light of these disparate data? First, there are insufficient data to uniformly restrict diving for asthmatic individuals. Second, there appears to be a group of asthmatic divers who dive at an acceptable level of safety. Third, there still may be a slightly increased risk of pulmonary barotrauma in asthmatic divers. In light of the above, it seems reasonable to make the following recommendations (pending the availability of additional data):

1. Individuals with asthma who have normal pulmonary function testing (normal flow rates) defined as within two standard deviations of established norms can be considered candidates to dive.
2. Individuals with exercise- or cold-induced asthma in general should not dive unless airway reactivity can be completely controlled by appropriate medications. Additionally, an appropriate exercise or cold challenge (at a level of exertion well above that expected during scuba diving) should be performed without evidence of airway reactivity.
3. Following an episode of asthma, an individual should not dive until it has been determined (usually by the use of a peak airflow meter) that airway function has returned to normal.

In summary, it must be realized that asthmatic individuals are a heterogeneous group. The stimuli that produce bronchospasm differ from individual to individual, and the degree of airway obstruction varies tremendously even in the same person. Thus, helping an asthmatic patient decide whether or not to dive must be individualized, taking into account not only the severity of the patient's disease but also his or her level of understanding and willingness to accept the risk. It does appear, however, that individuals with normal airway function (whether or not on medication) appear to be at low risk for idiopathic pulmonary barotrauma and subsequent air embolism.

IV. Chronic Obstructive Pulmonary Disease, Chronic Bronchitis, and Emphysema

The issues of diving with chronic obstructive pulmonary disease (COPD) are quite similar to the issues in diving with asthma. Similar theoretical arguments exist for the individual with COPD in relation to increased risk for AGE except that the person with COPD always has abnormal airway function. Thus, the individual who dives with COPD has an increased theoretical risk at all times rather than only at the time of an "attack."

Practically, however, by the time individuals with chronic lung diseases become significantly symptomatic, they are generally incapable of developing an exercise level appropriate for diving activities; consequently, it is quite unusual to see a diver with clinically significant COPD. Furthermore, COPD is usually a disease that takes decades of exposure to tobacco smoke to develop; therefore it most often affects older individuals, again making divers or diving candidates with COPD relatively rare in the practice of diving medicine. Thus, by the time COPD is clinically evident, such major physiological abnormalities have developed that these individuals probably ought to be advised, on the basis of their exercise capacity, not to dive. Therefore, the issue of advising an individual with COPD is really the issue of advising an asymptomatic individual with abnormal PFTs. An additional factor to be considered is that some patients with COPD have a component of reactive airway disease as well; therefore their degree of pulmonary obstruction can vary with external stimuli, and their airway obstruction is also treated with bronchodilating drugs. If asthmatics with abnormal airway function are to be advised not to dive on the basis of exercise tolerance, then individuals with clear-cut pulmonary function evidence of COPD should also be advised not to dive. As noted previously, this is generally defined as PFTs more than two standard deviations from the norm. Keeping in mind the limitations of available normative data and that by the above criteria 5% of normal persons will test "abnormally," individuals with low-normal values but with a clinical history suggestive of chronic lung disease should undergo more extensive testing. It is important, however, to note that observations in submarine escape trainees (SET) reveal that PFTs lack any useful predictive value for barotrauma and, specifically, PFTs with minor evidence of obstructive physiology are not a risk factor (65,66). Thus, using PFTs as criteria for diving to reduce the risk of pulmonary barotrauma may not be justified.

V. Pneumothorax

The definition of a pneumothorax is a collection of air within the pleural space. There are a variety of ways in which this condition can be classified; however, to advise a diving candidate who has had a pneumothorax, it is probably best to consider whether the pneumothorax was spontaneous, iatrogenic, or traumatic. Spontaneous pneumothorax occurs in a patient without any obvious antecedent trauma and without any previous surgical (invasive) intervention. In a population of young, otherwise healthy individuals without any readily apparent underlying lung disease, pneumothoraces are usually caused by congenital subapical blebs that rupture into the pleural space. Such individuals are usually tall, thin, male cigarette smokers between 20 and 30 years of age (67). Overdistention of distal air spaces by partial bronchial obstruction acting as a one-way valve is another purported mechanism for the development of a pneumothorax. As this process continues, air spaces are disrupted and air then dissects along the bronchovascular sheaths to the mediastinum. Finally, air can either enter soft tissues of the neck (causing subcutaneous emphysema) or rupture into the pleural space, resulting in a pneumothorax (68). This mechanism is thought to be the basis for the development of subcutaneous emphysema in some patients during asthma attacks. Additionally, spontaneous pneumothoraces can also occur in the presence of more severe underlying parenchymal lung disease. It appears that any diffuse interstitial lung disease predisposes to pneumothoraces (e.g., eosinophilic granuloma, sarcoidosis, pneumoconiosis, interstitial pneumonitis, etc.). Additionally, spontaneous pneumothraces are also common in patients with COPD (especially bullous emphysema) (69).

Once a person has developed a spontaneous pneumothorax, recurrences are likely. In one study (70) of individuals without apparent underlying lung disease who developed a pneumothorax, 40% developed a second. The range of time between the first and second episodes was from 4 to 35 months with a mean of approximately 1.5 years. Of those who developed a second pneumothorax, approximately one-third developed a third. Evidence that spontaneous pneumothoraces are a recurrent process is also found in another study (71) of individuals without apparent underlying lung disease treated with tube thoracostomies. Approximately 50% had an ipsilateral recurrence. The average time span to recurrence in that group was 2.3 years, and approximately two-thirds of those who developed a second pneumothorax developed a third.

A traumatic pneumothorax can be seen after either blunt or penetrating trauma. Blunt trauma can cause rib fractures that lacerate the lung surface; however, there are other mechanisms that can produce pneumothorax in conjunction with blunt trauma. Penetrating trauma can cause pneumothorax from direct lung injury or from a leak from the chest wall.

Iatrogenic pneumothoraces may be caused by any invasive thoracic procedures, such as subclavian line placement, thoracocentesis, transthoracic needle aspiration of the lung, and, of course, thoracotomy. Iatrogenic pneumothorax can also be seen secondary to positive-pressure ventilation.

Almost any pneumothorax may be converted to a tension pneumothorax. This occurs when the defect in the pleura or the chest wall acts as a one-way valve, allowing air to be continually or repeatedly introduced into the pleural cavity. Progressive collapse of the involved lung can occur and the mediastinum may be shifted to the uninvolved side, compressing the contralateral lung and compromising venous return to the heart. A tension pneumothorax can rapidly cause death (72).

The above analysis provides only a theoretical basis to advise divers who have had a previous spontaneous pneumothorax not to dive. If a pneumothorax were to occur under water at nearly any depth, changes in barometric pressure while rising to the surface could cause a simple pneumothorax to develop into a tension pneumothorax, which could result in death. It is also clear that recurrences can and do arise after several years; thus, even though a pneumothorax has not occurred for 2 to 3 years, there is no assurance that it will not recur at some time in the future. Finally and perhaps equally important, the presence of apical subpleural blebs (the cause of most spontaneous pneumothoraces) suggests that there may be poorly ventilated areas of the lung that trap air and pose a risk for AGE. For these reasons, a history of spontaneous pneumothorax with or without underlying lung disease is generally considered a contraindication to diving (62,73–76). There are, however, authorities who find the above arguments overly restrictive (77) and who feel that after a suitable period of time, individuals who have had a previous spontaneous pneumothorax may resume diving. Inasmuch it has been difficult to obtain dependable statistics in a condition where approximately 5% of the population is affected (asthma), it is highly unlikely that meaningful data on a condition as uncommon as a spontaneous pneumothorax will soon be available.

It would seem that resolved traumatic pneumothoraces due to isolated injury to the chest wall should not pose a risk to a diver; however, a traumatic pneumothorax may also be associated with an underlying lung injury. Should the injury be severe enough to lead to radiographic changes, it may well have been severe enough to have caused areas of air trapping to develop. Consequently, some authorities believe such individuals are best advised not to dive. However, further diagnostic testing might be able to define those at greatest risk (78).

An iatrogenic pneumothorax can be secondary to either a pulmonary or nonpulmonary procedure. A pneumothorax due to nonpulmonary procedures—such as a subclavian line placement or cardiac or mediastinal surgery during which the pleura was opened—should not be a contraindication to diving. If the pneumothorax was secondary to a pulmonary procedure, it is probably not the pneumothorax per se but rather the underlying lung disease or the effect of the surgery on the lung that is the issue. Stapling devices are generally used for suture lines in the pulmonary parenchyma; thus surgeons may not need to follow anatomical planes with precision. Lung architecture may be distorted and lead to the areas of air trapping. As a result of this reasoning, individuals who have had previous pulmonary surgery are generally advised not to dive. From a practical point of view, any lung disease, procedure, or event that results in air trapping is generally considered a contraindication to diving (62,73–76).

The above arguments for increased risk are almost entirely theoretical. There does not appear to be, anywhere in U.S. diving fatality statistics, a single well-reported case that has been attributed to a tension pneumothorax or an arterial gas embolism ascribed to a previous spontaneous pneumothorax or previous thoracic surgery (40–49). Whether this is because of limited excess risk or because such individuals do not dive remains to be determined. Thus, these contraindications to diving have to be evaluated in consideration of the diver's maturity, level of understanding, responsibility, and willingness to accept potentially increased risk.

VI. Decompression Sickness

The final issue that must be taken into account in advising an individual to dive, insofar as pulmonary fitness is concerned, is whether a lung disease or the treatment of such disease may predispose the diver to decompression sickness (DCS). A superficial analysis of the relation between lung pathology and DCS might lead one to question whether any relation ought to exist. Decompression sickness is generally thought to be due to processes associated with the development of a gas phase in a variety of body tissues and due to secondary effects of the gas phase, be they anatomical, rheological, or biochemical. It is now clear, however, that the lung plays a role in DCS and that the transpulmonary passage of venous gas emboli (vge) occurs more frequently than had previously been considered (see Chap. 9). Arterialization of gas, whether it is due to vge or pulmonary barotrauma, has been suggested to promote the development of DCS in a variety of anatomical ways and a variety of pathophysiologic ways as well. Thus, processes that affect the ability of the lung to act as a bubble filter or that might predispose to clinically silent but biochemically or rheologically important AGE (secondary to PBT) can be a factor in the development of DCS. Thus, any alteration in the vasculature of the lung that permits the transfer of vge to the systemic circulation might cause an increased susceptibility to DCS, or any alteration in the parenchyma or airways that allowed AGE to occur more easily might cause an increased susceptibility to DCS. The only pulmonary abnormality for which any data exist is once again asthma. Asthma might predispose to DCS by either of the above-mentioned mechanisms that allow for the arterialization of gas. As noted in the preceding section, it appears that asthma does not measurably increase the risk of overt AGE. Nonetheless, if asthma were to increase the incidence of subclinical AGE, it might be manifest as an increase in the incidence of DCS. Similarly, asthmatics who use $beta_2$ agonists might have a higher incidence of DCS due to the passage of what otherwise might have been asymptomatic vge through a "porous" pulmonary vascular bed produced by the pulmonary vasodilatory effect of $beta_2$ agonists.

Unfortunately, there are very few data available that help to test either or both of the above hypotheses. Table 3 is a compilation of the statistics available from 1988–1991 about all forms of dysbarism seen in asthmatic divers (52). These data were derived from annual DAN accident reports. As the data are presented, a "worst case" has been assumed (i.e., the "current" and "past history" groups do not overlap) and, as can be seen, the data do not indicate asthma to be an independent risk factor for codes 1 to 5, which probably represent the bulk of the cases of DCS. In another analysis, Mebane (79) looked at the incidence of dysbarism (AGE and DCS) in a group of DAN members compared to an unselected control population. In the DAN group, the calculated risk was 1:5100. This was significantly different from the risk for an unselected English group, but there was no difference in the incidence in dysbarism compared with other unselected groups (80). Thus, it appears from the bulk of the studies available, that in spite of an appealing physiological rationale, there is either no difference in the incidence in DCS in asthmatic divers or the risk of DCS is only marginally increased.

In summary, then, it appears that common pulmonary disorders are a major factor in diving only insofar as their effect upon exercise tolerance is concerned. Theoretical concerns about the risk of gas embolism and DCS appear not to be supported by the currently available data.

Table 3 Nonfatal Diving Accidents, 1988–1991

		Victims with history of asthma	
	All cases	Current number (%)	Past number (%)
Code 1 (Prob Type I DCS)	192	4 (2.1)	7 (3.6)
Code 2–5 (Prob Type II DCS)	1214	18 (1.5)	45 (3.7)
Code 6 (Prob AGE)	148	2 (1.4)	7 (4.7)

References

1. Lanphier EH. Oxygen Consumption in Underwater Swimming. Washington DC: U.S. Navy Experimental Diving Unit, formal report. 1954:14–54.
2. Donald KW, Davidson WM. Oxygen uptake of booted and "fin swimming'' divers. J Appl Physiol 1954; 7:31–37.
3. Goff LG, Frassetto R, Specht H. Measurements of respiratory responses and work efficiency of underwater swimmers utilizing improved instrumentation. J Appl Physiol 1956; 9:219–221.
4. Goff LG, Brubach HF, Specht H. Measurements of respiratory responses and work efficiency of underwater swimmers utilizing improved instrumentation. J Appl Physiol 1957; 10:197–202.
5. Harries M. Ventilatory requirements presented at Are Asthmatics Fit to Dive Symposium. Elliott DH, ed. UHMS West Palm Beach, FL, June 1995.
6. Jato DA, Farhi LE. Effect of gas density on mechanics of breathing. J Appl Physiol 1967; 23:687–693.
7. Wood LDH. Ventilatory dynamics under hyperbaric states. In: Lambertsen CJ, Greenbaum LJ Jr, eds. Proceedings of the 2nd Symposium on Underwater Physiology (publ 1181). Washington, DC: National Academy of Sciences—National Research Council, 1990:108–123.
8. Seusing J, Drube HC. Die Bedeutung der Hyperkapnie fur das Auftreten des Tiefenrausches. Klin Wochenschr 1960; 38:1088–1090.
9. Morrison JB, Butt WS. Effect of underwater breathing apparatus and absolute air pressure on divers' ventilatory capacity. Aerospace Med 1972; 42:881–888.
10. Fagraeus L, Linnarsson D. Maximal voluntary and exercise ventilation at high ambient air pressures. Forsvarmedicin 1973; 9:275–278.
11. Stolp BW. Maximum Voluntary and Exercise Ventilations in the Open Ocean to Pressures of 5.0 ATA. Master's thesis, University of Southern California, Los Angeles, CA, 1979.
12. Zocche GP, Frittis HW Jr, Cournand A. Fraction of maximum breathing capacity available for prolonged hyperventilation. J Appl Physiol 1960; 15:1073–1074.
13. Tenny SM, Reese RE. The ability to sustain great breathing efforts. Respir Physiol 1968; 5:187–201.
14. Shephard RJ. The maximum sustained voluntary ventilation in exercise. Clin Sci 1967; 32:167–176.
15. Freedman S. Sustained maximum voluntary ventilation. Respir Physiol 1970; 8: 230–244.
16. Chouteau J. Experimentation animale de plongee profonde en melanges synthetiques realisee au CEMA, au GERS, et au CERTSM. In: Fractus X, ed. Third International Conference on Hyperbaric and Underwater Physiology. Paris: Doin, 1972:8–12.
17. Chouteau J, Impert G, Leppechon JC. Physiologie comparee de divers mammiferes aux hautes presions en atmosphere oxygene-helium. Maroc Med 1972; 52R:448–449.
18. Clausen J. Pulmonary function testing. In: Bardow RA, Moser KM eds. Manual of

Clinical Problems in Pulmonary Medicine, 3d ed. Boston: Little, Brown, 1991:11–20.

19. Report of the Working Group on Definition of Asthma. In: Porter R, Birch J eds. Identification of Asthma. CIBA Foundation Study Group No. 38, January 13–14, 1971. Edinburgh: Churchill-Livingstone, 1971.
20. William H, McNickol KN. Prevalence, natural history and relationship of wheezy bronchitis and asthma in children: An epidemiologic study. Br Med J 1969;4:321.
21. Rackeman FN, Edwards MC. Asthma in children: A follow-up study of 688 patients after an interval of 20 years. N Engl J Med 1952; 246:815.
22. Derrick EH. The significance of the age of onset of asthma. Med J Aust 1971; 1: 1317.
23. Ogilvie AG. Asthma: A study in prognosis of 1000 patients. Thorax 1962; 17:183.
24. Smith. Survey of rural children with asthma and hay fever. J Allergy Clin Immunol 1971; 47:28.
25. Pearson RSB. Natural history of asthma. Acta Allergol 1958; 12:277.
26. Bernstein IL, Siegal SC, Brandon ML, et al. A controlled study of cromolyn sodium sponsored by the Drug Committee of the American Academy of allergy. J Allergy Clin Immunol 1972; 50:235.
27. Lindblad JR, Farr RS. The incidence of positive intradermal reactions and the demonstration of skin sensitizing antibody to extracts of ragweed and dust in humans without history of rhinitis or asthma. J Allergy Clin Immunol 1961; 32:392.
28. Deal EC, McFadden ER, Ingram RH, Strauss RH. Heat loss vaporization of water and exercise-induced asthma. Am Rev Respir Dis 1978; 117:328.
29. Zebellos RJ, Shturman-Ellstein R, McNally JF, et al. The role of hyperventilation in exercise-induced bronchoconstriction. Am Rev Respir Dis 1978; 118:277.
30. Bates D, Macklem P, Christie R eds. Spasmodic asthma. In: Respiratory Function in Disease, 2d ed. Philadelphia: Saunders, 1971.
31. Liebow AA, Stark JE, Vogel J, Schaeffer KE. Intrapulmonary air-trapping in submarine escape training casualties. U.S. Armed Forces Med J 1959; 10:265.
32. Schaefer KE, McNulty WP, Carey C, Liebow AA. Mechanisms in development of interstitial emphysema and air embolism on decompression from depth. J Appl Physiol 1958; 13:15.
33. Colebatch HJH, Smith MM, Ng CKY. Increased elastic recoil as a determinant of pulmonary barotrauma in divers. Respir Physiol 1976; 26:55.
34. Farr RS, Spector SL. Management of the difficult asthmatic. In: Stein M, ed. New Directions in Asthma. Park Ridge, IL: American College of Chest Physicians, 1975.
35. Wagner PD, Dantzker DR, Iacovoni VE, et al. Ventilation-perfusion inequality in asymptomatic asthma. Am Rev Respir Dis 1978; 118:511.
36. Edmonds C. Asthma and diving. SPUMS J 1991; 21:70–74.
37. 1987 Report on Diving Accidents. Divers' Alert Network. Durham, NC: Duke University Medical Center, 1990.
38. Wells JH, Moon RE. What is the risk of pulmonary barotrauma due to asthma in SCUBA divers (abstr)? J Allergy Clin Immunol 1993; 91:172.
39. Dick AP, Massey EW. Neurologic presentation of decompression sickness and air embolism in sport divers. Neurology 1985; 35:667.
40. Schench HV, McAniff JJ. United States Underwater Fatality Statistics, 1972. U.S.

Department of Commerce, NOAA. U.S. Government Printing Office Report No. URI-73-8, December 1973.
41. Schench HV, McAniff JJ. United States Underwater Fatality Statistics, 1973. U.S. Department of Commerce, NOAA. U.S. Government Printing Office Report No. URI-SSR-75-9, May 1975.
42. Schench HV, McAniff JJ. United States Underwater Fatality Statistics, 1974. U.S. Department of Commerce, NOAA. U.S. Government Printing Office Report No. URI-75-10, April 1976.
43. Schench HV, McAniff JJ. United States Underwater Fatality Statistics, 1972. U.S. Department of Commerce, NOAA. U.S. Government Printing Office Report No. URI-77-11, March 1977.
44. Schench HV, McAniff JJ. United States Underwater Fatality Statistics, 1972. U.S. Department of Commerce, NOAA. U.S. Government Printing Office Report No. URI-78-12, December 1978.
45. McAniff JJ. United States Underwater Fatality Statistics, 1970–78. National Underwater Accident Data Center, University of Rhode Island. Report No. URI-SSR-80-13, September 1980.
46. McAniff JJ. United States Underwater Fatality Statistics, 1970–79. National Underwater Accident Data Center, University of Rhode Island. Report No. URI-SSR-80-14, August 1981.
47. McAniff JJ. United States Underwater Fatality Statistics, 1970–79 (including a preliminary assessment of 1981 fatalities). National Underwater Accident Data Center, University of Rhode Island. Report No. URI-SSR-82-15, December 1982.
48. McAniff JJ. United States Underwater Fatality Statistics, 1970–81 (including a preliminary assessment of 1982 fatalities). National Underwater Accident Data Center, University of Rhode Island. Report No. URI-SSR-83-16.
49. McAniff JJ. United States Underwater Fatality Statistics, 1970–82 (including a preliminary assessment of 1983 fatalities). National Underwater Accident Data Center, University of Rhode Island. Report No. URI-SSR-84-17.
50. Walker D. Asthma and Diving. SPUMS J 1994; 24:88–90.
51. Gorman D. Fitness for Diving, a review of critical issues. SPUMS J 1994; 24:2–4.
52. Neuman TS, Bove AA, O'Connor R MD, et al. Asthma and diving. Ann Allergy 1994; 73:344–350.
53. Corson KS, Dovenbarger JA, Moon RE, et al. Risk assessment for asthma for decompression illness. Undersea Biomed Res 1991; 18(suppl);16–17.
54. Sipsey J. Correlation of dive injury/accident/illness due to medical/physical problems, or is there a lack of problems due to present absolute/relative contraindications for diving. UMS Workshop on Physical Standards for Diving. Bethesda, MD, May 15–16, 1986.
55. Shanker H, Spector H. Relationship between asthma and scuba diving mortality (abstr). J Allergy Clin Immunol 1991; 87:313.
56. Shanker H, Spector SL. Exercise induced asthma and scuba diving. Insights Allergy 1992; 7:2–8.
57. Neuman TS, Powers AT, Osborne DE. The prevelance of asthma, diabetes

and epilepsy in a population of divers. Undersea Biomed Res 1988; 15(suppl): 62–63.
58. Corson KS, Moon RE, Nealen ML, et al: A survey of diving asthmatics. Undersea Biomed Res 1988; 1992(19) (suppl):18–19.
59. Bove AA, Neuman TS, Kelsen S, et al. Observations on asthmas in the recreational diving population. Undersea Biomed Res 1992; 19(suppl):18.
60. Farrell PJS, Glanvill P. Diving practices of scuba divers with asthma. Br Med J 1990; 300:166.
61. Farrell PJS. Asthma and diving in England. In: Elliott DH, ed. Are Asthmatics Fit to Dive Symposium. UMHS, Palm Beach, FL, June 1995.
62. Linaweaver PG. In: Schilling CW, Carlston CB, Mathias RA, eds. The Physician's Guide to Diving Medicine. San Pedro, CA: Best Publishing, 1984:499–500.
63. Elliott DH, ed. Medical Assessment of Fitness to Dive, Proceedings of an International Conference. London: Biomedical Seminars, 1995:334.
64. Elliott EH, ed. Are Asthmatics Fit to Dive Symposium. UHMS, Palm Beach, FL, June 1995.
65. Benton PJ. Vitalography as a predictor for pulmonary barotrauma. In: Elliott D, ed. Medical Assessment of Fitness to Dive. Flagstaff, AZ: Best Publishing, 1995:118–122.
66. Brooks GJ, Pethybridge RJ, Pearson RR. Lung function reference values for FEV_1, FVC, FEV_1/FVC ratio and FEF_{75-85} derived from the results of screening 3788 Royal Naval Submariners and submarine candidates by spirometry. In Proc XIV EUBS Annual Meeting, Aberdeen, Scotland, 1994.
67. Editorial. Br Med J 1976; 2:1407–1408.
68. Clausen JL. Pneumothorax. In: Bordow RA, Moser KM, eds. Manual of Clinical Problems in Pulmonary Medicine, 3d ed. Boston: Little, Brown, 1991:62–67.
69. Stradling P, Poole G. Conservative management of spontaneous pneumothorax. Thorax 1966; 21:145–149.
70. Seremetis MG. The management of spontaneous pneumothorax. Chest 1970; 57: 65–68.
71. Gobbel WG, Rhea WG, Nelson IA, Daniel RA. Spontaneous pneumothorax. J Thorac Cardiovasc Surg 1963; 46:331–345.
72. Noble D. Some particulars of treatment in a case of pneumothorax. Br Med J 1973; 2:425–426.
73. Becker GD, Parell GJ. Medical examination of the sport scuba diver. Otolaryngol Head Neck Surg 1983; 91:246.
74. Neblett LM. Otolaryngology and sport scuba diving: Update and guidelines. Ann Otol Rhinol Laryngol 1985; 94(suppl 115):2.
75. Edmonds C, Lowry C, Pennefeather eds. Medical standards. In: Diving and Subaquatic Medicine, 2d ed. Mossman, Australia: Diving Medical Center, 1981:448–474.
76. Kindwall EP. Medical examination of the diver. In: Strauss R, ed. Diving Medicine. New York: Grune & Stratton, 1976:341–347.
77. Watt SJ. Current criteria of pulmonary fitness to dive. In: Elliott EH, ed. Medical Assessment of Fitness to Dive. Flagstaff, AZ: Best Publishing, 1995:114–118.

78. O'Hara V. Pulmonary considerations. Second UMS Workshop on Physical Standards for Diving. Bethesda, MD, May 15–16, 1986.
79. Mebane YG. Recreational diving medical standards: DAN in the United States. In: Elliott EH, ed. Medical Assessment of Fitness to Dive. Flagstaff, AZ: Best Publishing 1995:14–118.
80. Marroni A. Recreational diving medical standards: DAN in the United States. In: Elliott EH, ed. Medical Assessment of Fitness to Dive. Flagstaff, AZ: Best Publishing, 1995:40–43.

3

Immersion Effects

CLAES E. G. LUNDGREN

State University of New York at Buffalo
Buffalo, New York

I. Introduction

In common usage, the terms *immersion* and *submersion* are synonymous (1). However, in texts on respiratory physiology, *immersion* appears to be the preferred term when water surrounding the body exerts a pressure on it that is different from the gas pressure prevailing in the lungs. This is the situation considered in this chapter on immersion effects on lung function, although secondary effects, such as the thermal stress caused by cold water, are also discussed.

Depending on the intensity of the immersion stress—which may be modest, as in head-out immersion, or intense, as when somebody who is well below the surface attempts to breathe through a long tube—the effects range from mild modifications of respiratory mechanics to life-threatening injuries. This presentation first addresses the physics of immersion and then the basic effects of immersion on respiratory mechanics, respiratory control, and pulmonary circulation, and it is noted that there is interaction between these influences. Finally, in Sec. V, ''Function and Dysfunction,'' these effects are considered in the perspective of applied physiology.

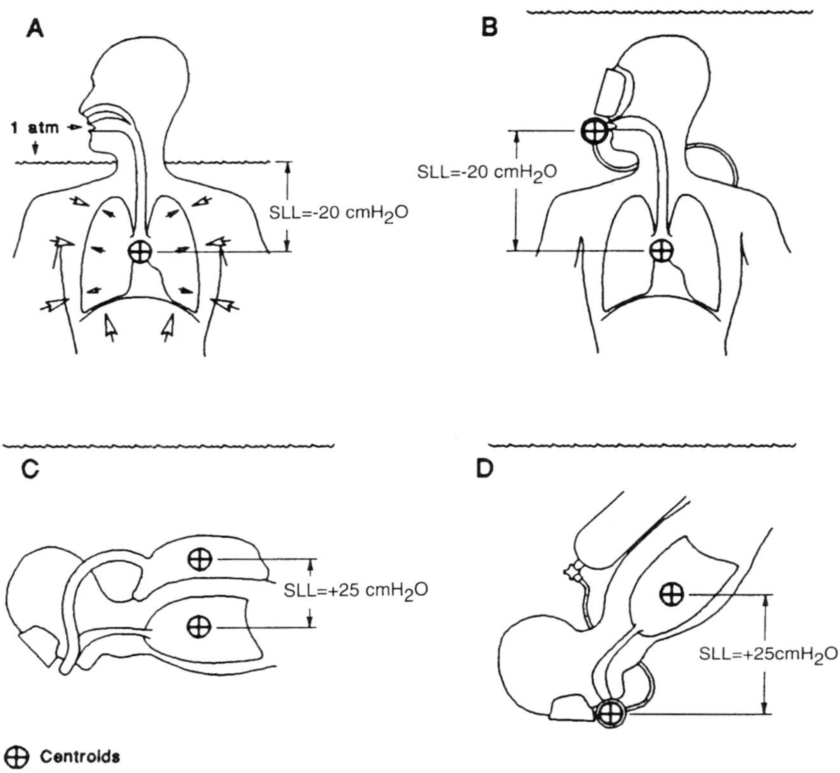

Figure 1 (A) Upright head-out immersion: negative static lung loading (SLL) amounts to -20 cmH_2O (-2kPa) caused by difference between gas pressure in the lungs (equal to pressure at water surface: 1.0 atm, 101 kPa) and pressure at chest centroid (1.02 atm, 103 kPa). Sizes of arrows illustrate relative magnitude of gas pressures and hydrostatic pressures. Note symbol for pressure centroid. (B) Upright posture under water with use of mouth-positioned scuba regulator; negative SLL caused by pressure (depth) difference between pressure centroids of scuba valve membrane in regulator (which sets lung-gas pressure) and diver's chest. (C) Prone posture under water using diving gear with rebreathing bag; negative SLL set by pressure (depth) difference between pressure centroids of rebreathing bag (which sets lung gas pressure) and diver's chest. (D) Head-down posture under water; positive static lung loading set by pressure (depth) difference between pressure centroids of scuba valve membrane in regulator and diver's chest. (From Ref. 84.)

II. The Physics of Immersion

Important immersion effects are caused by differences in pressure exerted by the water column acting on the outside of the body and the gas pressure acting in the lungs. Depending on body posture and type of breathing gear (if any), the water pressure on the chest may either be higher than the gas pressure in the lungs or vice versa. As an introduction to these concepts, Fig. 1A illustrates the commonplace situation of an upright person in head-out immersion, the pressures exerted on the chest and in lungs being shown schematically. The gas pressure in the lungs is less than the water pressure on the chest. This situation, also known as negative static lung loading (SLL), forces the subject to perform negative-pressure breathing.

The situation just described has a parallel in that of the upright, fully submersed diver wearing a scuba regulator at the mouth level (Fig. 1B) or a prone diver with a rebreathing bag on the back (Fig. 1C). By contrast, other postures or types of breathing gear may cause positive SLL—i.e., the diver performs positive-pressure breathing (Fig. 1D). Both negative and positive SLL may have undesirable effects.

The static mechanical properties of the respiratory system cause it to assume certain dimensions when the airways are open and the respiratory muscles are relaxed. These dimensions are then defined by the balance between forces in the lungs, which are recoiling inward, and in the chest wall, which is recoiling outward. The volume assumed by the system at these dimensions is known as the functional residual capacity (FRC). It stands to reason that any differences between the pressures on the chest and in the alveoli, induced by immersion, would change the normal balance, with negative SLL reducing the FRC and positive SLL increasing it. Before going into the quantitative aspects of this, it will be helpful to introduce the concept of the chest pressure centroid as used in studying respiratory mechanics during immersion. The pressure centroid is the location on the chest at which the infinite number of different hydrostatic forces acting on the chest can be represented by one force. The pressure centroid is typically determined experimentally. One method is to have the subject submersed and breathing from a scuba regulator through flexible hoses. (The membrane on the regulator is acted upon by the water pressure so as to deliver breathing gas at exactly the water pressure to which the membrane is exposed.) The regulator is moved stepwise in the vertical plane until a location is found at which the subject exhibits the same thoracic relaxation volume, or rather the same expiratory reserve volume, as in air. This location may be marked on the subject's chest for subsequent reference during experimentation. When this is performed in the upright posture, the centroid is typically found about 14 cm below the sternal notch (2,3); in the horizontal position, it is 7 cm dorsal of a horizontal plane through the sternal notch. (3,4) The exact position relative to these anatomical landmarks is likely to be influenced by body size. One important aspect is that, in order not to bias the measurements, the subject should be wearing some kind of strapped-on breathing mask, since the muscle activity required to bite on to a mouthpiece may prevent full relaxation of the respiratory muscles and jeopardize identification of the relaxation volume (3,4).

III. The Lung and Chest

The first comprehensive study of respiratory mechanics during immersion was made by Agostoni et al (5), from whose work Fig. 2A, B, and C and Fig. 3A and B were borrowed. The ensuing comments to these figures are based on the analysis made by the same authors. The values of pressure (which are mean values from measurements in two subjects) are quoted here to give an idea of the magnitude of the pressures developed in the interplay between the respiratory system and the hydrostatic forces. The pressure changes typically generated within the healthy respiratory system during breathing rarely exceed ±30 $cmH_2.O$ (3 kPa). By comparison, the pressures differences that can be imposed on the system by hydrostatic forces during immersion can be very large in

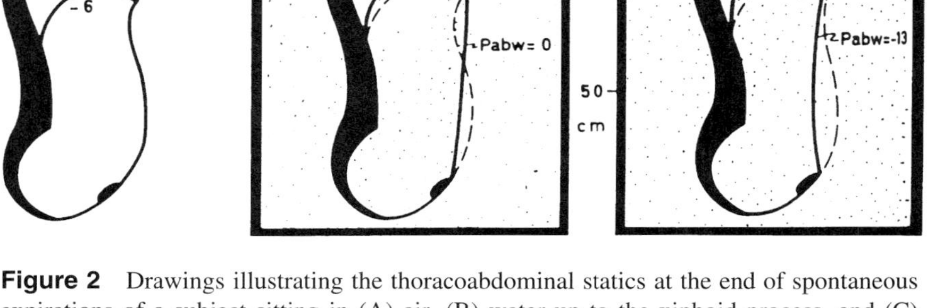

Figure 2 Drawings illustrating the thoracoabdominal statics at the end of spontaneous expirations of a subject sitting in (A) air, (B) water up to the xiphoid process, and (C) water up to the neck. The broken lines in (B) and (C) indicate the profile of condition (A) for comparison. The values of pressure in cmH_2O are the mean values recorded in two subjects. P_{rc}, P_{di}, and P_{abw} indicate, respectively, the average pressure across the rib cage, the diaphragm, and the abdominal wall; further details in text. (From Ref. 5.)

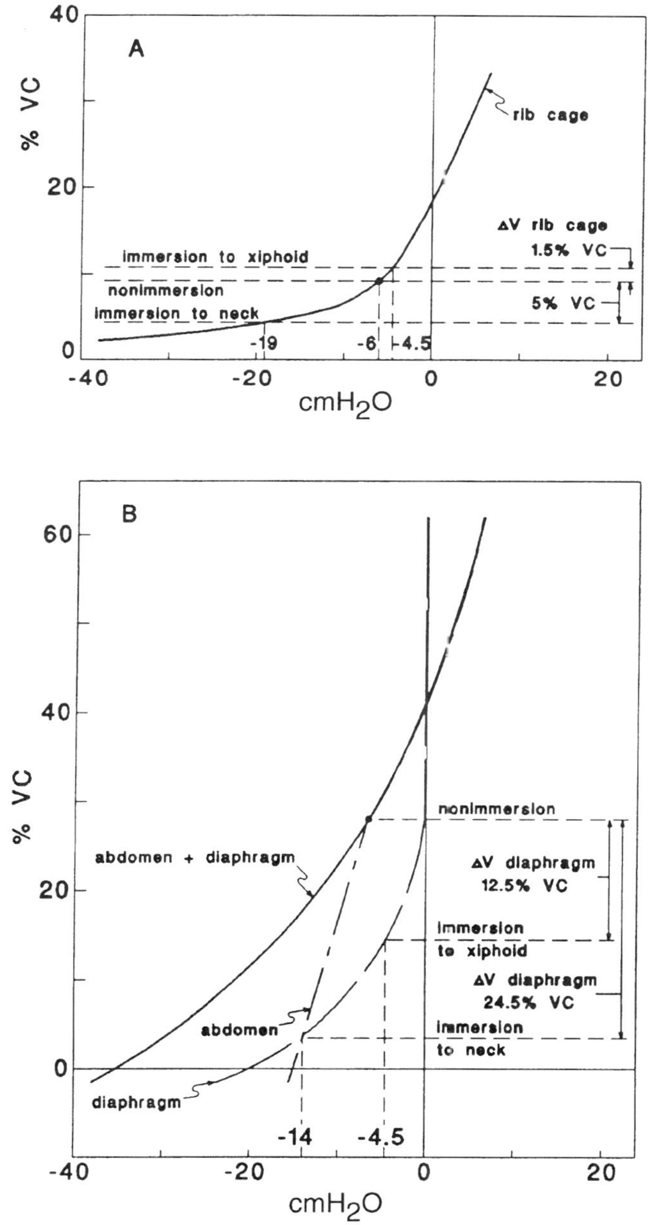

Figure 3 Volume-pressure curves of (A) relaxed rib cage and (B) abdomen-diaphragm of same two subjects as in Fig 2; further details in text. (Modified from Ref. 5.)

certain accident scenarios, as described further on in this chapter. The situation at the end of a relaxed expiration—i.e., at FRC, in nonimmersion is shown in Fig. 2A. The weight of the abdominal content pulls down on the diaphragm so as to stretch the lung, which sets the pleural pressure at −6 cmH_2O (−0.6 kPa). The diaphragm is relaxed and the transdiaphragmatic pressure is zero. On immersion to the xiphoid process, the weight of the abdominal viscera is fully balanced by the water column—i.e., subdiaphragmatic pressure is zero and the diaphragm is somewhat elevated, resulting in pleural and transdiaphragmatic pressures of −4.5 cmH_2O (−0.45 kPa). Thus, the end-expiratory pressure across the rib cage changes from −6 to −4.5 cmH_2O (−0.6 to −0.45 kPa) (Fig. 2A and B), and the rib cage expands somewhat. This expansion corresponds to a volume increase equivalent to 1.5% of VC (Fig. 3A). At the same time, the transdiaphragmatic pressure changes from 0 to −4.5 cmH_2O (−0.45 kPa) (Fig. 2A and B), and this causes the diaphragm to move up, resulting in a volume reduction of 12.5% of VC (Fig. 3B). Thus, when the upright subject is immersed to the xiphoid, the net volume change caused by the two elements, the chest wall and diaphragm, that delineate the chest cavity amounted to a decrease by 11%. The same kind of analysis applies to the case of immersion to the neck. As abdominal content is put under increased pressure, the abdominal wall is pushed in and the diaphragm is displaced in a craniad direction. The transdiaphragmatic pressure changes from 0 to −14 cmH_2O (−1.4 kPa) (Fig. 2A and C). This causes a decrease in chest (lung) volume equivalent to 24.5% of VC (Fig. 3B). Simultaneously, the transmural pressure of the rib cage changes from −6 to −19 cmH_2O (−0.6 to −1.9 kPa). This results in a volume reduction corresponding to 5% of VC (Fig. 3A). The sum of these volume reductions, 29.5% of VC, are in good agreement with the reductions in ERV to about 70% of nonimmersed control values directly recorded in these subjects as well as in numerous other studies.

Tension in the abdominal wall during head-out immersion serves to limit the reduction of chest volume. As pointed out by Agostoni et al. (5), in the upright person, the dome of the diaphragm is about 25 cm below the water surface, while the transdiaphragmatic pressure (Pdi) is only −14 cmH_2O (−1.4 kPa) (Fig. 2C). This is possible because the abdominal wall, pushed in by the water column and recoiling outward, generates tension that balances an additional pressure difference (P_{abw}) of −13 cmH_2O (−1.3 kPa). During head-out immersion, relaxed expiration stretches the diaphragm to a position that, in the nonimmersed state, would be achieved only by a maximal expiration. Yet, as discussed by Agostoni et al. (5), the stretching of the diaphragm apparently does not induce any increase in its neurogenic tonus.

Considering the effects of immersion on static lung volumes, one should expect the external hydrostatic load to limit the expansion of the chest (and lungs) during maximal inspiratory effort. The limit in nonimmersion is set by the opposing forces of the outward-directed pull of the inspiratory muscles (tending to generate negative pressure in the chest) and the recoil directed inward (generating positive pressure) of the chest wall and the lung. It stands to reason that if additional positive pressure is exerted by the water acting on the chest, the expansion of the respiratory system will be somewhat limited. This has been given as the major reason for the frequently reported reduction of about 6% in vital capacity (VC) during head-out immersion (Table 1). However, the VC is determined by the volume span achieved with maximal inspiratory and expiratory efforts. During nonimmersion, the residual volume (RV) is determined by the balance between the (at this volume level) outward-directed elastic recoil (negative pressure) of the chest wall and the inward-directed (positive) pressure generated by lung recoil and expiratory muscle effort. The additional positive pressure exerted by water surrounding the chest should cause some further reduction in lung volume (RV) at maximal expiratory effort, thus tending to increase the volume span between maximal inspiration and expiration—i.e., the VC. It is noteworthy that these effects of immersion on chest and lung mechanics seem to balance each other, so that, if they alone were to determine VC, it would not be changed by immersion (6). This notion is supported by the observation that when erect subjects were placed in a water container with a rubber sleeve separating the torso from the legs and only the torso (and arms) were immersed while leaving the legs dry, the VC was the same as during nonimmersion (6,7). Thus, the dominating and possibly only factor reducing VC during whole-body, head-out immersion is the redistribution of blood from the periphery into the chest. This is in contrast to the teachings of earlier studies, which employed graphical treatment of the pressure-volume curves of the respiratory system to arrive at the mechanical and circulatory contributions, respectively, to the VC reduction during immersion. Thus two-thirds of a 9% reduction in VC during immersion was ascribed to mechanical limitation of chest expansion and one-third to blood shift (5).

Additional support for the notion that blood redistribution is the main factor causing the VC reduction during immersion is derived from the observation that this reduction can be almost completely eliminated if arterial stasis is applied to the subject's arms and legs before immersion, as shown in Fig. 4. Similarly, Bondi et al. (8) found that arterial tourniquets applied to the extremities modified the immersion VC from being 9.9% less than (nonimmersed) control values to only 1.9%. Thus, in these experiments, the immersion effect on VC can be ascribed to be more than 80% (1–1.9/9.9) due to blood redistribution. It should be recognized that applying tourniquets to arms and legs would still allow blood from a large soft-tissue mass, in particular the gluteal region, to affect VC during immersion. Oddly, attempts at circulatory isolation of the extremities were less successful in the hands of Hamilton and Mayo (9) who recorded VC reductions due to immersion of 7.6% with cuffs off and 4.7% with

Table 1 Changes in VC, ERV, and RV During Head-Out Water Immersion Reported in the Literature

		Δ VC		Δ ERV		Δ RV	
Study	Ref.	%	No. of subj.	%	No. of subj.	%	No. of subj.
Agostoni et al.	5	−9[b]	2	−69[a]	8	−16[c]	4
Baer et al.	32	9	8	—	—	—	—
Balldin et al.	54	−8[a]	2	—	—	—	—
Beckman et al.	85	−3[b]	7	−64[b]	7	—	—
Bondi et al.	8	−10[a]	10	−71[a]	10	−9[a,c]	10
Brozek et al.	86	—	—	—	—	n.s.[c,g]	9
Burki	10	−10[b]	8	—	—	n.s.[c]	6
Carey et al.	87	n.s.	8	−48[b]	8	n.s.[c]	8
Craig and Ware	88	−4[b]	21	—	—	n.s.[c]	21
Craig and Dvorak	89	−9[b]	11	—	—	—	—
Dahlbäck	7	−4[a]	6	−66[a]	6	n.s.[d]	6
Dahlbäck and Lundgren	37	−8[a]	20	−73[a]	20	—	—
Dahlbäck et al.	6	−6[a]	5	−75[a]	5	n.s.[d]	5
Flynn et al.	90	−3[b]	5	−53[b]	5	−7[b,c]	5
Girandola et al.	91	−9[b]	20	−61[b]	20	+7[b,d]	20
Guyett et al.	46	−5[b]	7	—	—	n.s[c]	7
Hamilton and Mayo	9	−8[a]	20	—	—	—	—
Hong et al.	13	n.s.	7	−70[b]	7	—	—
Hong et al.	12	−8	4	−71[b]	4	—	—
Jarrett	92	−4[a]	5	−75[a]	5	−10[a,c]	5
Jarrett	4	—	—	—	—	−8[a,c]	3
Kurss et al.	11	0–9[f]	3–9	—	—	—	—
Löllgen and von Nieding	93	−15[a]	5	—	—	—	—
Prefaut et al.	29	n.s.	5	—	—	n.s.[c]	5
Prefaut and Chardon	94	−8[a]	14	−59[a]	14	—	—
Robertson et al.	36	−4[a]	9	−69[a]	9	−13[a,c,e]	9
Robertson et al.	95	−6[a]	9	−67	9	n.s.[e]	9

[a] Mean of individual changes in percent calculated from original values.
[b] Difference in percent of the absolute mean values.
[c] RV measured by dilution technique.
[d] RV measured by dilution technique with extra deep breaths.
[e] RV measured with body plethysmograph.
[f] Depending on water temperature.
n.s. = nonsignificant, $p>0.05$.
Source: Modified from Ref. 23.

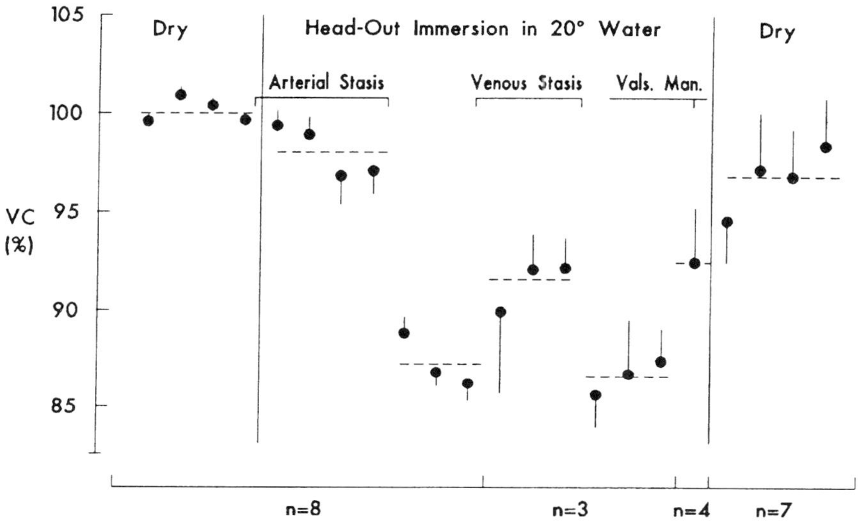

Figure 4 Vital capacity (VC) during head-out immersion (seated) in water at 20°C. Data given in percent of nonimmersed (dry) control values. Effects of periods of arterial and venous occlusions by tourniquets on arms and legs and of the Valsalva maneuver are shown. Values are means ±SE from three to eight experiments (see abscissa) in three or four subjects. Dashed lines indicate mean values for measurements obtained during related time span. (From Ref. 11.)

cuffs on. Application of venous (as opposed to arterial) stasis after immersion allows some of the blood that has been pooled in the chest to be redistributed to vascular beds peripheral to the occlusion cuffs Removal of blood from the chest in this manner, albeit incomplete, caused initial VC reductions of 10.2 (10) and 12.7% (11) to be lessened to 7 and 8.4% (Fig. 4), respectively.

Another way to demonstrate, at least qualitatively, the role of blood shifts for VC changes during immersion is to record VC before and immediately after performing the Valsalva maneuver, which will reverse some of the blood shift into the chest. Thus, in one study (11), the VC during head-out immersion at 86.5% of nonimmersed VC increased to 92.5% post-Valsalva (Fig. 4)—i.e., 40% of the VC reduction appears to have been due to intrathoracic blood pooling that could be eliminated by the Valsalva maneuver, while another study employing the same technique ascribed about 60% of the VC reduction to be due to blood redistribution (12). However, it seems questionable whether this technique would be able to completely eliminate the hydrostatically caused blood shift at the moment of VC measurement. As already mentioned, other measuring techniques indicate that nearly all of the VC reduction during immersion is due to the blood shift.

It appears that the immersion effects on VC are very dependent on the water temperature (11). Thus measurements during head-out immersion in thermoneutral water (35°C) yielded VC values at 94.6% ± 0.2% SE of dry control values ($p < 0.005$); in water at a cool 20°C, the VC was 91.1% ± 0.5% ($p < 0.005$); while in warm water (40°C), the VC values were 98.0% ; pm 0.2% of control and not significantly different from the preimmersion values (Fig. 5). These profound effects of temperature, mediated via blood shifts, suggest that the wide variation in immersion-induced VC changes reported in the literature (Table 1) is to a large extent due to differences, between studies, in thermal balance, and hence in vasomotor tone as influenced by water temperatures and duration of the immersion. In the following discussion, the water temperature employed in the various immersion studies quoted was thermoneutral unless otherwise stated.

As for immersion in the nonerect posture, it stands to reason that the VC showed no decrement in subjects who were submersed in the horizontal position (breathing through a tube) with the sternum immediately below the surface. With

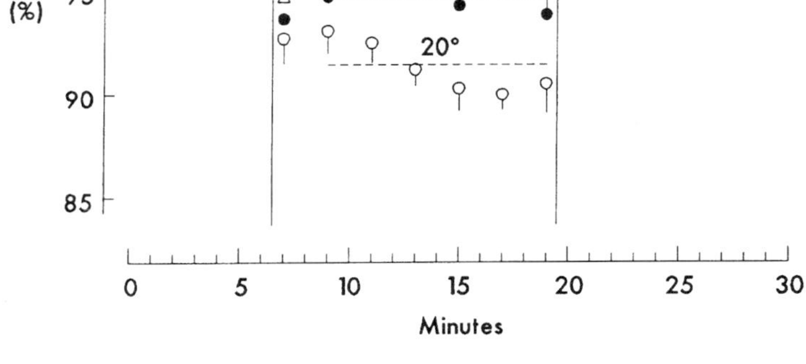

Figure 5 Vital capacity (VC) in subjects sitting immersed, head out, in water at temperatures of 20°, 35°, and 40°C, respectively. Data given in percent of nonimmersed (dry) control values. Mean values ±SE are given for nine subjects. Dashed lines indicate mean values for measurements obtained during related time span. (From Ref. 11.)

increasing depth, the VC was gradually more reduced, reaching 68% of nonimmersed control values at a depth of 40 cm to the sternum (13).

It is universally agreed that head-out immersion in the upright posture reduces the expiratory reserve volume (ERV), and the reductions cited range from 48 to 75% (Table 1). This reduction can be attributed to the hydrostatic pressure causing the earlier mentioned craniad displacement of the diaphragm to a position close to full expiration (see Ref. 12). A discrepancy between ERV during normal breathing in the resting state and the volume (V_R) above RV reached at sustained respiratory muscle relaxation with open glottis has been reported by Taylor and Morrison (14). While ERV and V_R were the same in nonimmersion, head-out immersion in their upright subjects caused reductions in ERV by 58% and in V_R by 87%. The lesser reduction of FRC was interpreted as the result of maintained inspiratory muscle tone. It was reasoned that this would serve the purpose of reducing respiratory work, since tidal breathing would occur at a more favorable (higher compliance) section of the pressure-volume curve of the respiratory system and the larger lung volume would be conducive to less flow-resistive work (14). Adjustments in SLL from −30 to +30 cmH_2O (−3 to +3 kPa) caused very similar changes in ERV both during exercise and at rest in three prone subjects (Fig. 6). Thus, relative to neutral

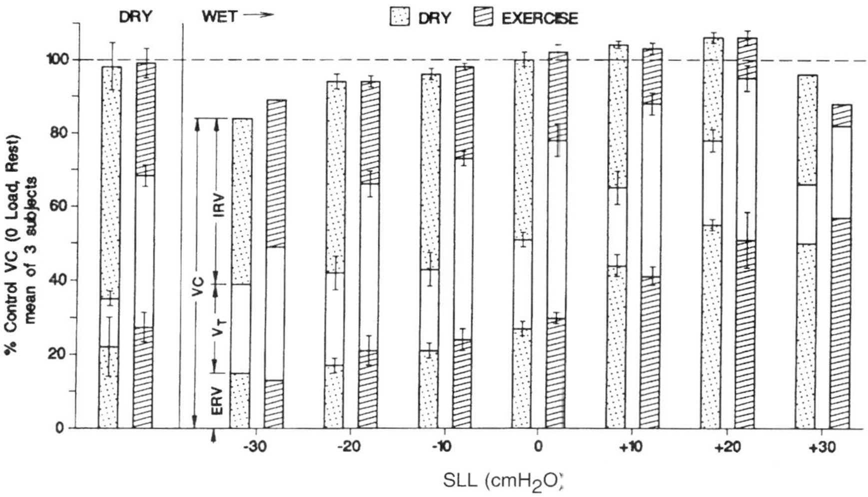

Figure 6 Influence of static lung loading (SLL) on spirogram. Values (mean ±SD) are presented as percent of control vital capacity (0 SLL, rest). Ergometer exercise was at 191 W in nonimmersed (dry) experiments and 141 W in submersed (wet) experiments. Difference in ergometer settings was roughly eliminated by hydrodynamic work in wet experiments. (Modified from Ref. 15.)

SLL, the ERV was more reduced as the the SLL became more negative and gradually rose as the SLL became more positive, both during rest and exercise (15).

With regard to immersion effects on the residual volume (RV), it was argued above that the hydrostatic load could be expected to help the erect subject to achieve a deeper maximal expiration, thus reducing the RV. However, most studies have found RV to be relatively unaffected by immersion (Table 1). This could be due to changes in the mechanical properties of the lungs brought about by engorgement of the pulmonary vasculature. This engorgement may cause stiffening of the lungs (see Sec. III. C, "The Parenchyma") as well as enhanced air trapping, as discussed in more detail in Sec. V, "Function and Dysfunction."

The effects of positive static lung loads, such as those encountered when a scuba diver with the breathing regulator at the mouth level assumes a more or less vertical, head-down position (see Fig. 1D), has been studied less intensively than the more common situation of erect head-out immersion. However, as might be expected, increased intraluminal airway pressure tends to increase lung volumes. Thus, vital capacity was normalized when erect subjects, immersed to the mouth level, were provided breathing air at lung (chest) centroid pressure, and so were the relaxation volume and the functional residual capacity (they became identical) (14). Further increases in mouth pressure to centroid pressure plus 0.98 kPa ($\approx$10 $cmH_2.O$) led to additional increases in VC and ERV (See Fig. 6).

A. Respiratory Muscles and Respiratory Control

The reduction in FRC during immersion results when the ERV becomes smaller. This change can be expected to influence the operating length and therefore the tension development of the respiratory muscles as noted by Reid et al. (16). The same authors recorded diaphragmatic and intercostal electromyographic (EMG) activity during immersion to the hip level (control), to the xiphoid, and to the shoulder level in seated subjects. Immersion to the xiphoid pushed the abdomen in and expanded the rib cage at end expiration. This increased the diaphragm's operating length, giving it a contractile advantage, and shortened the inspiratory intercostals so as to give them a contractile disadvantage. Peak EMG activity in both muscle types was reduced, and both tidal volume and respiratory frequency were unchanged. With immersion to the shoulders, both types of inspiratory muscles were placed at a contractile advantage. This resulted in further reduction in inspiratory EMG activity, and breathing frequency and tidal volumes were still unchanged. This global response preserved the ventilation pattern, as also evidenced by essentially unchanged alveolar carbon dioxide pressures. An unchanged respiratory minute volume and end-tidal carbon dioxide pressure were also observed by Chang and Lundgren (17) under very similar conditions of head-out immersion. Furthermore, an unaltered carbon dioxide sensitivity was demonstrated in the same study. The preservation of the ventilatory performance at the nonimmersed level during immersion was interpreted as possibly being the result of a mechanoreceptive reflex originating in afferent information from the lungs or diaphragm and serving to adjust all inspiratory muscle activity (16). The observations just mentioned were obtained in resting, spontaneously breathing subjects. In a different study, the same kind of compensation was also present in subjects voluntarily taking somewhat larger and faster than eupneic breaths (18). However, during maximal exertion and head-out immersion, a 6% reduction in ventilation was observed in the subjects of Dressendorfer et al. (19), although maximal oxygen uptake was not different than that in nonimmersed control runs. A reduction in maximal voluntary ventilation by 12% was also noted and, like the lowering of the maximal exercise ventilation, it was ascribed to increased airway resistance, as discussed further on. A marked change in breathing pattern, with potentially serious consequences for safety (see Sec. V, ''Function and Dysfunction''), may be induced in resting individuals who are suddenly immersed in cold water.

Carbon dioxide retention is a potential threat to the diver's performance and safety (see also Chap. 6). The ability of divers to recognize acute CO_2 exposure during immersion and by what mechanism they would detect it were studied by Fothergill et al. (20). The subjects were immersed to the neck and exercised at 75 W while being exposed to a 10-min linear increase from 0 to 6% in inhaled CO_2 followed by 5 min of breathing 6% CO_2. Two water temperatures were used—namely, 18°C and 34°C. The subjects, who had undergone a preparatory familiarization exposure to hypercarbia, used a rating scale to quantify symptoms. Hypercarbia was recognized at lower end-tidal P_{CO2} levels in the cold water than in the warmer water. Moreover, even though the minute ventilation, tidal volumes, and end-tidal P_{CO2} levels were similar in the two water temperatures, the level of hypercarbia was rated higher in the cold water than in the warmer water. Most subjects used nonrespiratory symptoms to rank their level of hypercarbia. Symptoms such as dizziness and visual distortions were more common in the cold immersions. The authors proposed that cold exposure, which may cause arousal and increase attentiveness, may have contributed to the earlier recognition and the higher ratings of hypercarbia during the immersions in cold water than that in the warmer water.

B. Airways

Ventilation, maximal voluntary ventilation, and maximal oxygen uptake were studied by Dressendorfer et al. (19) in subjects exercising on a cycle ergometer while immersed head out with the chest in a nearly horizontal position immediately below the surface. These subjects had a normal maximal oxygen uptake while the lung ventilation was reduced by 11% and the maximal voluntary ventilation by 12% as compared with nonimmersed control runs. The authors ascribed the reduced ventilation to increased airway resistance. To support this interpretation, they quote work by Hong et al. (12), who noted a 25% increase, and Agostoni et al. (5), who reported a 58% increase in airway resistance, in both cases ascribable to the narrowing of the airways that comes with the reduction in FRC during head-out immersion. Similarly, it can be calculated from data published by Löllgen et al. (21) that flow resistance during eupnea increased about 57% during head-out immersion. Increases in pulmonary resistance during erect head-out immersion in the subjects of Morrison and Taylor (22) was from 0.18 (nonimmersion) to 0.44 $kPa{\cdot}L^{-1}$ (at 0.5 $L{\cdot}sec^{-1}$)—i.e., a 144% increase. The increases in resistance during head-out immersion reported by Dahlbäck (23) amounted to 31% for functional resistance and 56% for end-tidal resistance. These increases were not significantly different from what he recorded during thorax immersion, namely, 22 and 73%, respectively. Hence, he concluded that the increase in flow resistance was strictly due to the hydrostatic compression of the lungs, which would narrow airways larger than 2 mm in diameter, where 90% of the flow resistance is created (24). However, when flow is tested under a wider range of the pulmonary volume envelope, a more nuanced picture emerges. Expiratory flows obtained by maximal effort in flow-volume recordings performed by Prefaut et al. (25) showed increased flows (relative to nonimmersion) in the upper volume range and decreased flows at low lung volumes in subjects undergoing head-out immersion. The increased flow was suggested to be due to the water pressure, which added to the expiratory effort under the condition of effort-dependent flow that is present at large lung volumes. This is so because, at large lung volumes, pulmonary recoil is strong, which directly and indirectly (via lowered pleural pressure) makes the airways well distended. The reduced maximal-effort flow at low lung volumes during immersion was ascribed to a reduction in lung recoil (which is caused by vascular engorgement as explained in Sec. III.C, "The Parenchyma" below). It is well known that an increased lung compliance is particularly critical at low lung volumes, where effort-independent flow develops. Moreover, the extrathoracic airways should be subjected to some compression from the water column acting on the neck. How large this compression is has apparently not been measured, but it is noteworthy that, as shown by Mead and Whittenberger (26), the flow resistance of an isolated human trachea increases substantially when exposed to external pressures. From their measurements, it can be deduced that an external overpressure of, for instance, 10 mmHg ($\approx$ 14 cmH_2O or 1.4 kPa) would increase flow resistance by 130% at a flow of 1 L/sec.

C. The Parenchyma

The negative static lung loading inherent in head-out immersion and the hydrostatic balancing out of the blood column below heart level cause pulmonary vascular engorgement, as noted earlier. An increase in pulmonary vascular (capillary and/or venous) pressures has been given as an explanation for immersion-induced reductions in pulmonary compliance of respectively 50 (27) and 30% (6). An erectile effect of increased intravascular pressure on excised lungs was first described by von Basch in 1887 (28). This was, as mentioned earlier, the proposed mechanism behind a reduction in recoil (increased compliance) at low lung volumes and an increase in recoil (reduced compliance) at large lung volumes in response to head-out immersion in erect subjects (29). Thus, the picture with regard to the pulmonary elastic behavior during immersion is unclear. This is especially so since esophageal pressure was measured by balloon technique in the studies just mentioned and this technique may not yield valid data regarding pleural pressure in the presence of central vascular congestion (30). Direct measurements of pulmonary pressure/volume relationships in open-chested dogs during substantial experimental increases in left atrial pressure showed only small decreases in compliance, which were confined to the upper lung-volume range (31).

Dynamic compliance obtained during eupneic breathing at FRC fell 36% as an immediate effect of head-out immersion in experiments performed by Baer et al. (32). This is in close agreement with similar studies reporting reductions of 37 (23) and 34% (33), respectively. In two of the studies mentioned above, additional drops in dynamic compliance by 13.2 (32) and 21% (33), respectively, were noted as immersion was continued for 25 to 30 min. Moreover, in the same time span, FRC declined by 7.6% in the study of Baer et al. (32), who proposed as one explanation for these changes an increase in fluid, either intravascularly or interstitially, in the lung. It is interesting to consider this notion in the context of cases of pulmonary edema observed in swimmers and divers, as is discussed further on in this chapter.

D. Distribution of Ventilation

The distribution of ventilation during head-out immersion in the sitting posture (compared with nonimmersion) has been studied with different techniques. Employing ^{133}Xe-radiospirometry and comparing one relatively large apical region with a large basal region, Arborelius et al. (34) found a decreased ventilation in dependent parts of the lung and an increase in the apical regions, indicating a somewhat more uneven ventilation distribution during immersion. Under similar experimental conditions, a generally more uneven ventilation was also found with a multiple-breath nitrogen elimination method by Lichtneckert and Lundgren (35).

Support for the notion of reduced ventilation in some lung areas during immersion is also lent by other types of measurements. Thus, closing volume increases (8), as does the amount of air trapped behind closed airways. The trapped gas volume has been measured at 0.2 L (36) and 0.03 to 0.290 L (37). Some of this air trapping is due to tidal breathing at a reduced FRC, leading to less distended and thus more easily collapsible airways (see Ref. 24). About 75% of the air trapping can be ascribed to pulmonary vascular congestion (7), which causes airway closure at larger lung volumes (38, 39). Vascular congestion appears to induce closure primarily in airways with diameters below 2 mm (24, 40). By contrast, the patency of larger airways is reduced primarily by the hydrostatic compression of the chest and the lungs during immersion. Another factor that may contribute to the narrowing of the airways in dependent parts of the lung is the increased weight of the blood-engorged lung, which is likely to raise pleural pressure around those dependent parts.

IV. The Central Circulation

Head-out immersion in thermoneutral water causes a redistribution of blood from the periphery into the chest of about 0.7 L (41). Partly, this may be an effect of the water pressure increasing cardiac afterload by acting on all tissues outside the chest, so as to make the tissue pressure, including vascular pressures, higher than intrathoracic pressure and partly it is due to the fact that the external water column balances the hydrostatic pressure of the blood column between the heart and the feet. The feet are, from the circulatory point of view, lifted up to the level of the air-water interface. The space taken up by the centralized volume of blood is, as mentioned above, largely responsible for the reduction of about 6% in VC in water at thermoneutral temperature. The larger reduction in VC in cold water and the smaller reduction in warm water are, as noted above, caused by intrathoracic pooling of larger and smaller blood volumes, respectively (11). This effect of temperature, which is independent of hydrostatic forces, is apparently the result of changes in vasomotor tone.

A. Distribution of the Intrathoracic Blood Pool

Since the blood that is redistributed due to immersion must be accommodated by the blood-containing structures of the chest, the question arises as to the compliance of these structures. From the measurements of intrathoracic blood deposition and changes in right atrial pressure recorded by Arborelius et al. (41) in subjects immersed to the neck in thermoneutral water, vascular compliance values of between 0.42 and 0.78 ml·mmHg^{-1}·kg body weight were calculated by Lundgren and Farhi (42). These numbers are relatively close to values of 0.9 and 1.2 ml·mmHg^{-1}·kg body weight arrived at by Echt et al. (43) when they were manipulating the intrathoracic blood pool in their subjects by expanding and reducing the circulating blood volume and by norepinephrine administration, respectively.

Radiographic measurements indicate that during immersion, the (diastolic) size of the heart increases by between about 180 (44) and 250 ml (45). Consequently, this would account for between about 25 and 35% of the redistributed volume. The remaining 450 to 500 ml are accommodated by the vasculature in the chest and lungs. Pulmonary capillary volume was observed to increase 70% corresponding to 51 ml, by Löllgen et al. (21) and 47% by Guyatt et al. (46). These changes would account for only about 10% of the 500 ml just mentioned. However, a quantitatively more important role for the pulmonary capillaries is suggested by measurements by Farhi and Linnarsson (47) of the so-called equivalent lung tissue volume, which can be calculated to correspond to a capillary volume increase of 200 ml due to head-out immersion as compared with the suspended semierect posture during nonimmersion (42).

B. Pulmonary Blood Flow

The increased diastolic filling of the heart during head-out immersion (sitting) in water at 36°C has been shown to cause transmural pressure increases in the right atrium and pulmonary artery of about 13 mmHg (1.7 kPa) (41). The increased preload in the same resting subjects resulted in a stroke volume enlargement of 35% (relative to sitting nonimmersed), and this induced increases in cardiac output of 32%. Likewise, an increase in cardiac output of 30% was found under very similar conditions by Löllgen et al. (21) and of between 20 and 40% by Begin et al. (48). An increase of 62% was recorded by Farhi and Linnarsson (47) in subjects whose cardiac outputs during immersion were similar to those of the studies just cited but considerably lower during nonimmersion. The authors attributed this low nonimmersed cardiac output to the fact that their subjects were suspended in a harness in a relaxed half-standing posture in which blood pooling in dependent parts of the body was more pronounced than during sitting.

The effects of head-out immersion on the distribution of the blood flow to the lung in the upright posture has been studied with ^{133}Xe-radiospirometry (25,34) and with injected tagged albumin particles and scintigraphy (45). Observations, common to these studies were increases in blood flow to the apical regions and decreases in the basal regions of the lungs, probably because of several contributing factors. Increased pulmonary blood flow and the enhanced filling of apical vessels, which would result from the increase by 12 mmHg in mean pulmonary arterial pressure recorded by Arborelius et al. (41), would favor apical perfusion. The latter authors also pointed to the earlier-mentioned reduced ventilation or frank air trapping and consequent hypoxia in dependent lung regions, which is common in head-out immersion. The hypoxia thus elicited would induce local vasoconstriction and shifting of blood flow toward the better ventilated apical regions of the lungs. This is consistent with the observation that when the subjects breathed oxygen instead of air, the perfusion distribution was not changed by immersion (41). Other factors tending to increase vascular resistance and reduce perfusion in dependent lung regions include an increase in pleural pressure due to (1) lowered compliance, (2) reduced lung distension, (3) closing of airways with a resulting increase in alveolar pressure, and (4) increased weight of the lungs due to vascular engorgement. The functional implications of immersion-induced changes in ventilation/perfusion distribution are discussed further on in this chapter.

V. Function and Dysfunction

When evaluating the effects of immersion, consideration must be given to both respiratory comfort and function. Indeed, the optima for these two criteria do not necessarily coincide in all individuals. So, for instance, have studies of divers' response to respiratory impediment shown that some individuals will react to negative static lung loading by exhibiting hypoventilation and dangerous CO_2 accumulation without experiencing any discomfort, while others breathe more vigorously and maintain nearly normal CO_2 levels but do so at the expense of suffering dyspnea (49).

A. Respiratory Comfort

A number of studies have addressed the question: What breathing gas pressure is preferred by the immersed subject? Primarily the erect posture has been studied, but also the horizontal. One important difference between studies is that in some, the subjects have been breathing through a mouthpiece exposing the extrathoracic airways, the cheeks, and the lips to transmural pressure differences, while others have used face masks, thus counterbalancing the pressure in the nasopharynx and oral cavity. One study compared mouthpiece breathing with mask breathing (50). Yet another study used a hood-like arrangement that allowed pressure on the face as well as the neck region to be equal to mouth pressure (51). The significance of these different diver-equipment interfaces is that, having to bite on to a mouthpiece in order not to lose it when mouth pressure is high, may modify respiratory muscle tone, at least at rest, while this is not the case with the mask approach (4). Another difference between studies is that in some only resting conditions were investigated, while in others hyperpnea was induced by exercise or CO_2 loading. Typically, a range of breathing gas pressures (measured at the mouth) were tried in these studies and the subjects indicated what pressure they preferred. The results are summarized in Table 2.

Table 2 Preferred P_{mouth} (cmH_2O)

Study	Interface	Posture	Eupnea	Hyperpnea	Exercise	Remarks
Paton & Sand (52)	MP	V, HU Hz	−19 to −24 0–0	−24 tc −29	−14	
Thompson & McCally (82)	MP, FM	V, HU	−14 to−22			Sliding SLL @ 1 atm
Thalmann et al. (15)	FM	Hz, Pr	+10		+10	SLL −30, −20, −10, 0, +10, +20 cmH_2O @ 15 & 190 fsw
Norfleet et al. (50)	MP, FM	V, HU	0		0	SLL 0, −20 cmH_2O @ 15 & 190 fsw
Hickey et al. (2)		V, HU	0 to +10		0 to +10	SLL −20, −10, 0, +10 cmH_2O @ 15 & 190 fsw
Taylor & Morrison (51)	Helmet	V, HU	0		0	SLL −24 and 0 cmH_2O @ 1.02 & 6.05 atm
Derion et al. (83)	MP	V, HU			−24, +4	SLL −24, +4 cmH_2O
		Hz, Pr			−3, +17	SLL −3, +17 cmH_2O; Ex. to exhaustion @ 1 atm
Lundgren & Warkander (81)	Pr		+10		+10	SLL −10, 0, +10 cmH_2O @ 1 atm & 190 fsw

Key: MP, mouthpiece; FM, face mask; V, vertical posture; U, head up; Hz, horizontal; Pr, prone; SLL, static lung loading; Ex, exercise.

Preferred breathing gas pressure is given relative to the chest (or lung) pressure centroid, which is taken to be located 14 cm below the sternal notch (2,3) and 7 cm behind (upright posture) a vertical line through the sternal notch (3,4). For studies that give another reference point such as the external auditory meatus (52), the data were recalculated for the table.

The tendency for airway closure and air trapping during head-out immersion (i.e., negative SLL), mentioned earlier, may have a secondary undesirable effect during oxygen breathing. Thus, subjects breathing oxygen for 1 or 2 hr in a thermoneutral bath exhibited reductions in vital capacity by 42 (53) and 22.4% (54), respectively. The explanation offered for these results was that absorption atelectases were formed, a notion gaining support in both studies from the fact that the subjects suffered cough attacks and that they complained of chest tightness. However, the actual lung volume lost by collapse of alveoli is uncertain. The possibility of reflex inhibition or pain limiting the deep inspiration in a VC measurement must be entertained. Nonetheless, repeated deep inhalation led to normalization of the VC in these studies. The difference in results between the two studies, as proposed by Dahlbäck and Balldin (53), also supports the atelectasis theory. The subjects in the study showing the largest reduction in vital capacity (despite a briefer oxygen exposure) were older (32 to 41 years) than in the other series (20 to 37 years), and the tendency for airway closure increases with age, especially in immersion (55). Moreover, the immersion depth in the study on the older subjects was deeper by 5 to 6 cm (53). The importance of the immersion effect was further underscored in this study since, when the subjects were provided with oxygen to breathe at a positive pressure of 1.5 kPa (15 cmH_2O), the reduction in VC was only one-fifth of what it had been when they were breathing oxygen without positive pressure. In addition, the subjects were free of discomfort.

A practically interesting corollary to the study mentioned above was made in divers swimming for 30 min in the prone posture and using two types of closed-circuit oxygen breathing gear, one with the rebreathing bag on the diver's back and one with the bag on the front of the chest (56). Not only was the rating of perceived exertion less favorable with the back-mounted bag but marked reductions (0.8 to 1.9 L) in vital capacity were also recorded with this gear, which exposed the divers to an SLL of about -20 cmH_2O (-2 kPa). With the chest-mounted bag exerting an SLL of $+10$ to $+20$ cmH_2O ($+1$ to $+2$ kPa), reductions in vital capacity were largely prevented, as were discomfort and coughing.

Rapid immersion in cold water has been found to increase minute ventilation during the first 0.5 to 1.0 min by between 360 and 520% (57,58). These observations were obtained in water temperatures from 0° (58) to 13.5°C (57), with no clear temperature correlation. The increases are caused by elevation in both respiratory rate and tidal volume (Fig. 7) (58). The extremely strong respiratory drive may pose the danger of drowning if an individual falls into cold water and does not surface rapidly enough. Indeed, the maximal voluntary breath-holding time after sudden submersion in 0°C water may be reduced by as much as 75% as compared with nonsubmersion (59). However, if the subject's head is above the surface, a few minutes of continued immersion will allow the ventilation to decrease, although it remains elevated at a level com-

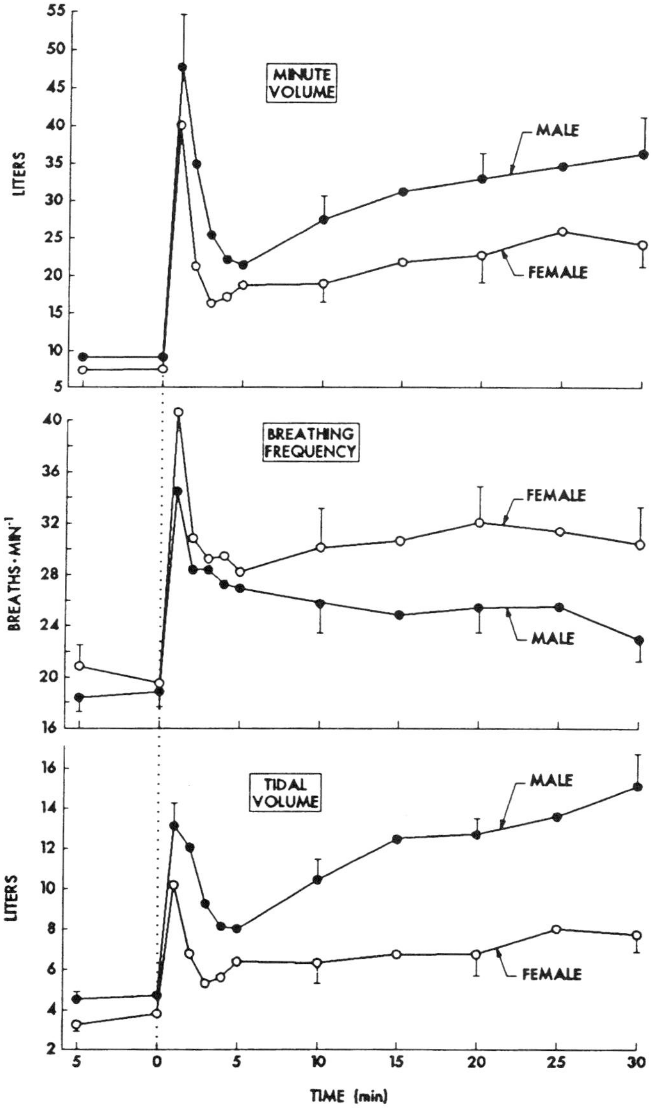

Figure 7 Ventilatory changes of 21 lightly clothed, nonexercising humans in response to rapid immersion (at zero time) in 0°C water. Representative standard errors are indicated. (From Ref. 58.)

mensurate with the cold-induced increase in metabolism (58). The initial increase is a hyperventilation with mean end-tidal carbon dioxide pressures of about 27 mmHg (3.6 kPa) in water at 10°C (60) and about 32.5 mmHg (4.3 kPa) in water at 15°C (61). These drops in end-tidal carbon dioxide levels can be prevented by vigorous exercise during immersion (60,61). Due to extremely rapid onset of the cold-induced hyperventilation and the fact that it can be prevented by heating the skin in a sauna before immersion, the mechanism has been described as a reflex initiated by stimulation of the skin's cold receptors (60,61). Observations by Keatinge and Nadel (62) in decerebrate cats suggest that the ventilatory response is mediated at the midbrain level. Furthermore, since the same authors observed the hyperventilation in human subjects exposed to very cold showers, it may be concluded that immersion per se is not a requirement for the response. The relatively rapid moderation of the hyperventilation during continued immersion in cold water can probably best be ascribed to receptor adaptation. However, an element of habituation was also noted by Keatinge and Evans (61) in subjects who were exposed to head-out immersion in water at 15°C eight times in the course of 14 days. The fall in end-tidal P_{CO_2} observed in the first immersions was eliminated or replaced by a slight rise in the eighth immersion.

B. Engorgement of the Central Circulation

An extreme form of immersion-induced negative SLL will result from attempts to descend below the surface while breathing through a long breathing tube with the open, upper end sticking out of the water. Since the maximal (static) inspiratory pressure that a healthy adult can generate is about 150 cmH_2O (15 kPa) (63), this sets an absolute depth limit beyond which it would be impossible to inspire. Indeed, as vividly described by Stigler (64), his attempts in 1911 at breathing through a tube at 2.5 m of depth were not only unsuccessful but brought on ''delirium cordis'' and severe cardiac dilatation. It is satisfying to note that, later the same year, Stigler was still part of the Viennese medical community, explaining, at a scientific meeting, the mechanism by which immersion influences central circulation (65). He lucidly described how blood is forced from extrathoracic organs into the chest and that each beat of the left ventricle has to overcome the pressure added on the extrathoracic vessels by the external water column. In Stigler's experiment on himself, this extra load of 2.5 m of water was equivalent to about 180 mmHg (24 kPa). The notion that the pressure of the external water column is added to the normal arterial pressure was confirmed by Lanari et al. (66), who performed direct arterial pressure measurements in subjects breathing through a tube at a submersion depth of 1 m. The blood redistribution also increases preload, mere head-out immersion (compared to nonimmersion) having been reported to boost right atrial and pulmonary arterial transmural pressure gradients by 13 mmHg (1.7 kPa) (41). It was Stigler's contention, apparently backed by some animal experimentation, that the immersion effect at 2 m of depth would be fatal within 1 min in humans (65). It follows that the snorkel—i.e., the breathing tube favored by skin divers—is not suitable for enhancing the diving depth. Its function is to allow a prone swimmer to breathe in a comfortable (face-down) head position while the chest is close to the surface.

C. Pulmonary Edema

The first report on pulmonary edema as a result of immersion was published in 1981 by Wilmshurst et al. (67), who briefly discussed hemodynamic studies and cold-pressor tests performed in three divers who had developed this condition on several occasions while diving. Measurements were also performed in divers who had never had pulmonary edema. Based on the results, it was proposed that persons denoted as ''labile'' hypertensives with an exaggerated constrictor response to cold would be particularly likely to develop pulmonary edema in response to the increases in preload and afterload and the expansion of the central blood volume that occurs with diving (67). After a study, published in 1984 (68), of four divers who had developed pulmonary edema, Wilmshurst et al. (69) went on to experiment on 11 persons who had had (up to seven) episodes of pulmonary edema when scuba diving or swimming at the surface. They were compared with divers who had not suffered pulmonary edema. Exposure to cold and/or raised partial pressure of oxygen caused pathological vasoconstriction in all individuals in the pulmonary edema group, nine of them also displaying signs of cardiac decompensation, in one case with severe pulmonary edema. Reactions in the control group were physiologically unremarkable, and there were no untoward reactions. The divers in the edema group were followed up for an average of 8 years, at which time seven had become hypertensive. It was the authors' contention that there was a clear relationship between the occurrence of pulmonary edema during immersion and exposure to cold and that an abnormal reactivity to cold exposure was a prerequisite for developing pulmonary edema while immersed (69).

The results of the studies by Wilmshurst et al., referred to above, were not entirely repeatable in a later investigation by Pons et al. (70). From an inquiry among 1250 scuba divers in Switzerland, they identified four persons with documented episodes and one with a history suggestive of pulmonary edema on several occasions when scuba diving or swimming. They measured forearm vascular resistance, levels of vasoactive hormones, and left ventricular function at room temperature and during cold exposure and found no difference between subjects with histories of pulmonary edema and healthy controls. Moreover, while all the subjects of Wilmshurst et al. (69) experienced their episodes of pulmonary edema in waters with temperatures below 12°C, some of the subjects of Pons et al. (70) had their symptoms when immersed in water at 20.6°C. One problem in determining how crucial a role cold water temperature plays is that the diver may have been using a suit that more or less effectively protected him or her against the cooling effect of the water. When conditions are otherwise conducive to pulmonary edema, cold exposure may not be a prerequisite. Overhydration may have played an important role in initiating pulmonary edema and hemoptysis in 8 persons in a group of 30 young men who, as part of a military fitness program, performed a strenuous swimming time trial in the sea (71). The swimmers wore only bathing suits and fins and the water temperature was 23°C. Symptoms developed within the first 45 min of the swim. The fact that all the swimmers had drunk about 5 L of water (to counteract anticipated dehydration) during the 2 hr preceding the swim is, as pointed out by the authors, probably a factor in these cases. However, two of the subjects who had symptoms later experienced repeated episodes of pulmonary edema during less strenuous swimming and without fluid overload. The other six swimmers did not have any recurrences when continuing their swim training, but they avoided fluid overloading.

In another case related by Hampson and Dunford (72), a 60-year-old woman on medication for essential hypertension developed pulmonary edema on 2 consecutive days while diving in the warm waters (27°C) off Cozumel (Mexico). However, after shifting her diving activities to the waters of Australia and using a wet suit, she had no further problems in seven subsequent dives. Cold may not have been an important factor in some of the other cases described by Hampson and Dunford (72), since, while their episodes of pulmonary edema developed in the cool waters of Puget Sound, the divers were probably well protected by insulating dry suits.

Despite uncertainties about what the exact combination of circumstances is that, during immersion, will produce an incident of pulmonary edema, several contributing mechanisms are mentioned by the authors who discuss the etiology of this phenomenon. Thus, immersion per se is thought to be important because, in the head-up position, it causes increased preload and afterload and pulmonary vascular engorgement (67–69,72). These changes are likely to be further strengthened during cold-water immersion both because of increased peripheral resistance and increased intrathoracic blood pooling (67–69) Some authors feel that increased capillary permeability is not a likely explanation for the development of this form of edema (70,72). An argument given for this notion is that, typically, the symptoms resolve rapidly once the diver is out of the water (72). However, the fact that several case histories include production of hemoptysis—specifically, expectoration of bloody froth—speaks for increased capillary permeability (68,70,72). In this context, it is interesting that an analysis of West et al. (73) suggests that even a physiological act such as heavy (terrestrial) exercise may bring the pulmonary capillaries close to stress failure and cause protein leakage and frank hemorrhage. An individual disposition for hydrostatic pulmonary edema is also a likely factor, since, as pointed out by Hampson and Dunford (72), a diver or swimmer would often have a history of several episodes. Yet diving under similar conditions, both earlier and later, the diver may have been spared. Advanced age is one possibly predisposing factor according to the same authors, who, quoting from the literature (69,70,72), cite the age of divers with histories of pulmonary edema during immersion to have been, on the average, 42.7 ± 2.7 years (SE) while a large group of divers with other types of diving injuries averaged 35.5 ± 0.4 years.

The frequency of scuba divers who have experienced immersion-dependent pulmonary edema seems to be quite low—e.g., 4 to 5 of 1250 individuals in the study by Pons et al. (70). However, in a recent study, Shupak et al. (74) diagnosed what was termed *swimming-induced pulmonary congestion* in 21 (60%) of 35 young men undergoing a fitness training program and strenuous swim tests. This diagnosis was based on a total of 29 events of self-reported shortness of breath and coughing. These cases exhibited significantly lower oxygen saturation—i.e., 96 to 91% versus 99%—than that among unaffected swimmers. Dynamic spirometry (FVC and FEV_1) also showed significant decreases after swimming in the individuals with breathing difficulties. Remarkably, the individuals who were to be afflicted later on also had some subnormal spirometry values (FVC, FEV_1 $FEF_{25-75}\%$ and MEF_{25}) during screening for the program. Thus, they started out with lower spirometry values and suffered further deterioration in those values during swimming, in contrast to the swimmers who did not report breathing problems. The apparently lower frequency of immersion-induced breathing problems in scuba divers than in surface swimmers can possibly be explained by differences in exercise intensity, cold exposure, and static lung loading. Recreational scuba divers usually do not exert themselves severely while submersed, and they tend to dress so as to stay warm, which may not have been possible for the swimmers in the military swim training programs. Moreover, in the normal swimming position and when exploring the bottom at a dive site, the diver is typically in a prone position and a mouth-held scuba regulator tends to deliver gas at a less negative static lung load than is experienced by the swimmer at the surface. An exception would be if the scuba diver spends an extended period of time in the upright posture. For instance, hanging onto a line during decompression stops in the water, he or she may be exposed to a large negative static lung load (see Fig. 1B). Likewise, if the diver swims at the surface, the weight of the air tanks on his or her back is likely to force the diver to assume a relatively upright posture, in which case the immersion effect may be quite pronounced, especially if the diver also uses a snorkel, which invites lying deeper in the water (so as to reduce the weight of the air tanks).

As for other pulmonary injuries that may be considered for the purpose of differential diagnostics, decompression-or barotrauma-trauma–related mechanisms are out of the question in the case of the surface swimmers and also in that of many of the divers, since the symptoms would often start before ascent.

D. Gas Exchange

The effect of immersion-induced blood redistribution into the chest was explained above, and it was noted that this may result in increases in cardiac output of 30% or more in the resting individual. Such a hyperkinetic circulation will have interesting effects on the exchange of inert gases. The gases of particular interest in the context of diving are nitrogen and helium. Since these gases are relatively poorly soluble in blood, the rate at which they are taken up or eliminated is primarily determined by the blood flow through the lungs (cardiac output) and not by lung ventilation (75). This notion is illustrated by experiments in which the tissue nitrogen elimination (via the lungs) was recorded in oxygen-breathing subjects sitting nonimmersed or immersed in water to the neck under thermoneutral conditions (76). Compared with nonimmersion, the nitrogen yield during immersion was higher by about 40% at the end of the first 30 min and by 29% after 2 hr of oxygen breathing (76). Under similar conditions, elimination of ^{133}Xe from a deposit in the anterior tibial muscle was increased by as much as 130% (77).

Warm-water immersion can further enhance nitrogen elimination (76), and this technique has been used to obtain a protective effect against experimental decompression sickness in humans. Of 10 nonimmersed subjects breathing oxygen for 25 min before a standard decompression to altitude, 9 developed decompression sickness while only 2 of the same subjects developed symptoms when the decompression was preceded by oxygen breathing during 25 min of head-out immersion in water at 37°C (78). From a practical point of view, it is important to realize that the immersion effect may also enhance the uptake of gas while a diver is exposed to high pressures of inert gas. A technical solution (79) to the problem of preventing or controlling immersion effects that may be transmitted to a diver's chest cavity is shown in Fig. 8.

The effects on oxygen uptake, which may be caused by changes in ventilation perfusion distribution due to immersion, have been particularly well analyzed in studies by Prefaut et al. (25,55). They identified three types of respiratory pattern in different subjects (Fig. 9) and found that, if an individual's expiratory reserve volume (ERV) during head-out immersion was larger than his or her closing volume (CV), the difference in alveoloarterial oxygen pressure [$P(A\text{-}a)O_2$] would diminish compared to nonimmersed conditions (Fig. 10). This was due to the dominating effect in these individuals of an improved diffusing capacity (55). This improvement is brought about by an expansion of the pul-

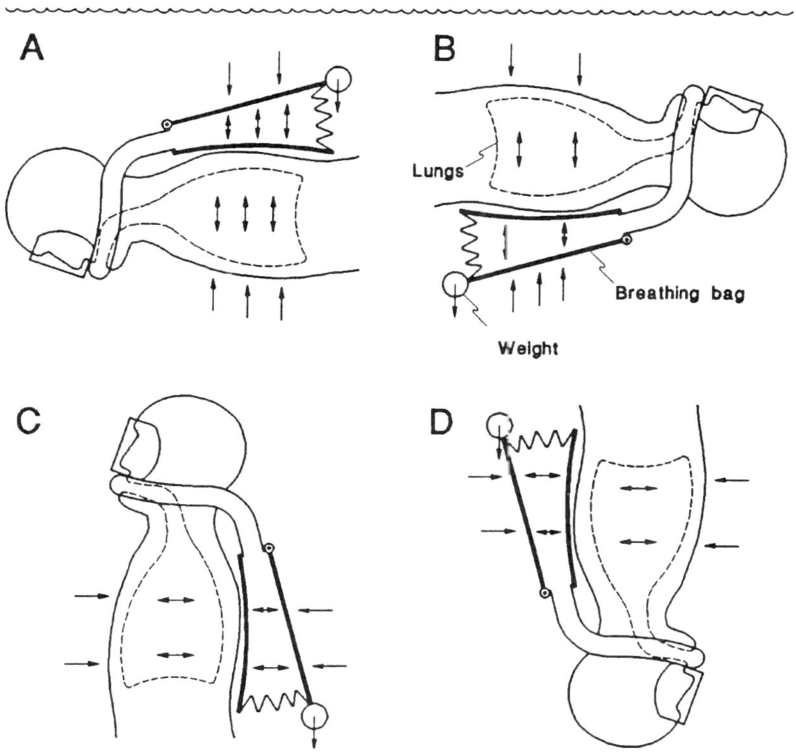

Figure 8 Schematic illustrating a technical solution (79) for counteracting the immersion effect induced by depth differences between a diver's chest and a rebreathing bag (bellows). The number of arrows symbolizes the hydrostatic pressure or gas pressure. (A) Prone posture: potential negative SLL (cf. Fig. 1C) is counteracted by weight on hinged side of bellows, which increases gas pressure in bellows and lungs to balance high water pressure on chest. (B) Supine posture: weight pulling on hinged side of bellows reduces gas pressure in bellows and lungs to match low water pressure on chest. (C, D) Vertical postures: weight on hinged side of bellows is essentially right above or below hinge and exerts very little positive or negative pressure on bellows, which is subject to the same water pressure as the chest.

monary vascular bed that is caused by the intrathoracic blood pooling during head-out immersion. Additionally, as mentioned above, increased pulmonary arterial pressure and blood flow (41) enhance perfusion of apical regions, resulting in a more even ventilation-perfusion distribution. In individuals whose ERV was less than the CV, the $P(A\text{-}a)O_2$ difference increased during immersion

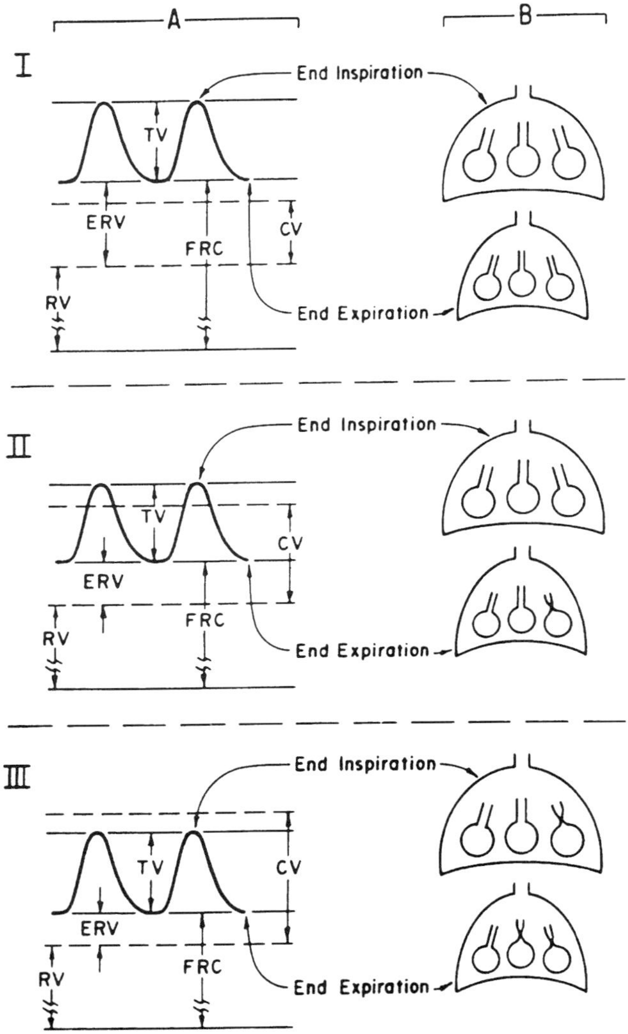

Figure 9 Illustration of three types (I, II, and III) of respiratory pattern during immersion, as described by Prefaut et al. (55). The relationship between breathing range (ERV + TV) and closing volume (CV) and effects on patency of airways during breathing cycle are shown. The A panels represent hypothetical spirograms and show relative positions of end inspiration and expiration [i.e., tidal volume (TV)], upper limit of functional residual capacity (FRC), expiratory reserve volume (ERV), residual volume, (RV), and closing volume (CV). The B panels represent lungs and lung units with open or closed airways at end inspiration or end expiration. Panels IA and B refer to a young,

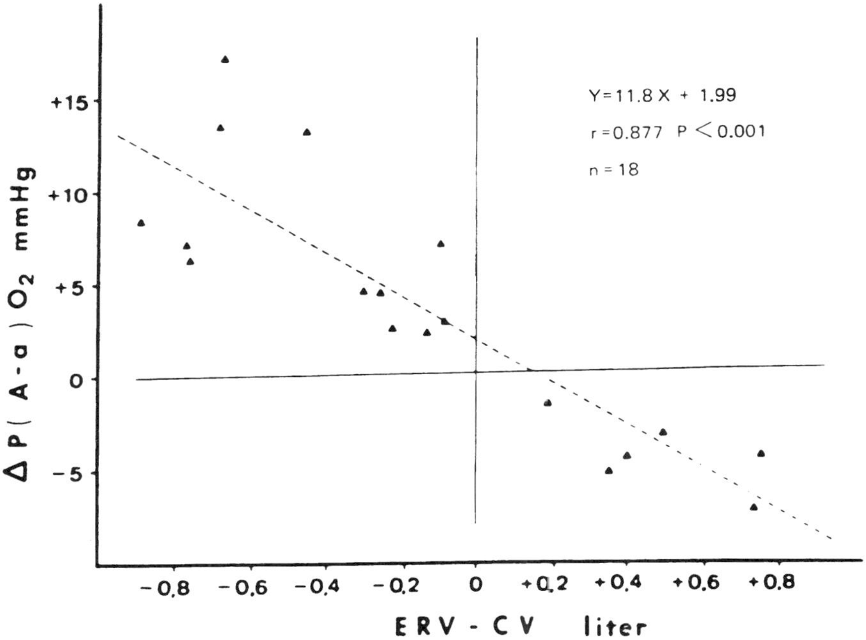

Figure 10 Relationship between $P(A\text{-}a)O_2$ in water minus $P(A\text{-}a)O_2$ in air and expiratory reserve volume (ERV) minus closing volume (CV) in water. (From Ref. 55.)

as air trapping exerted its effects throughout the respiratory cycles (Fig. 10). In addition, the diffusing capacity of such individuals was reduced during immersion, apparently due to temporary loss of exchange area in closed-off lung regions. The distinguishing features between persons whose breaths were taken above CV and those whose breaths dipped into the CV was that the former were young and/or of light build while the latter were older and/or overweight,

---

healthy, nonimmersed person whose entire breathing cycle is outside the CV envelope; panels IIA and B represent a situation of immersion that reduces ERV and increases CV so that breathing occurs partially within the CV envelope: some airways close toward the end of expiration. Panels IIIA and B show a situation in, for instance, an older and/or overweight person in whom immersion causes substantial enlargement of the CV, so that breathing occurs wholly within the CV envelope and the airways of some lung units remain closed even at end inspiration. (From Ref. 96; Shiraki K and Yousef M K, eds., Man in Stressful Environments—Diving, Hyper and Hypobaric Physiology, 1987, Courtesy of Charles C. Thomas, publisher, Springfield, Illinois.)

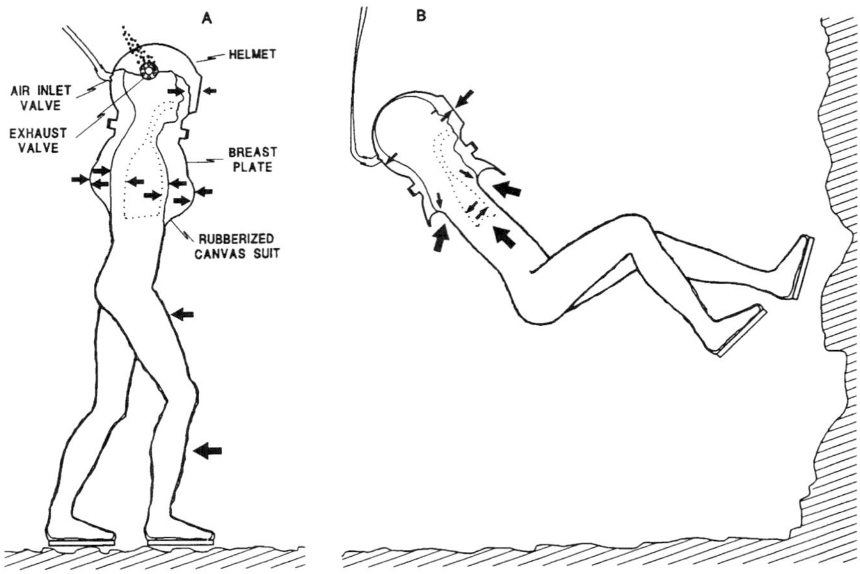

Figure 11 (A) Cross section of diver in heavy suit showing that gas pressure in the helmet and the lungs is determined by the water pressure acting on the air volume in the suit surrounding the chest. Relative magnitudes of air and water pressures are illustrated by size of arrows. (Modified from Ref. 84.) (B) Schematic of chest-squeeze incident in diver suffering a fall without adequate air supply from the surface to equilibrate air pressure in the suit with rapidly increasing water pressure.

both these characteristics being conducive to airway closure, as pointed out by Prefaut et al. (55). These subject-dependent reactions to immersion were offered as an explanation for increases in $P(A\text{-}a)O_2$ differences observed in earlier studies (21,80). Furthermore, the study by Prefaut et al. (55) showed that when the subjects voluntarily modified their respiration, so as to maintain the ERV above CV, or when they breathed under positive end-expiratory pressure, the blood gas problems were effectively counteracted. This observation lends objective support to the notion that the design of breathing gear and its usage should preferably be such that the diver is minimally exposed to negative SLL.

Carbon dioxide exchange appears not to be very sensitive to moderate changes in SLL, although they may still be subjectively significant. Thus, five subjects exposed to submersed exercise in the prone posture at a (simulated) depth of 190 ft had an average (significant) increase in Pa_{CO_2} of about 3 mmHg when the SLL was changed from +10 to −10 cmH_2O. This carbon dioxide retention was apparently caused by an average reduction of 9.6% in ventilation, from 50 L•min^{-1} to 46 L•min^{1} (81).

E. Chest Squeeze

In order to breathe freely, a diver must be supplied with breathing gas at a pressure essentially equal to that of the water at his or her chest pressure centroid. This can be achieved, for instance, by using the scuba breathing regulator described above, drawing air from portable gas tanks or by pumping breathing gas down from the surface to the diver. The latter method is used in conventional "hard-hat" diving. In this case, the gas pressure in the helmet, from which the diver is breathing, is regulated to equal the water pressure on the chest. This is done by the diver who manually adjusts an exhaust valve on the helmet so as to keep the suit somewhat inflated around the chest. The pressure of the air in the suit and in the helmet is thus determined by the water pressure on the chest (Fig. 11A). This type of "heavy" diving gear is the classical outfit of the working diver, but it does put the diver at the risk of suffering the mother of all immersion accidents. If the diver experiences a fall to a substantially greater depth under water and the airflow to the suit (and helmet) is not high enough to make up for the compression (due to rapidly increasing water depth) of the air in the helmet-suit assembly, his or her chest may be subjected to enormous, crushing pressure differentials (Fig. 11B). Since the helmet is rigid, the water pressure will tend to force the diver's torso and body fluids into the helmet. An uncompensated depth increase of say 10 m (equivalent to 33 fsw or 101 kPa) will exert a total force across a 500-cm^2 neck opening in the helmet of 4.9 kN or 1100 lb$_f$. Another mechanism that may cause this type of injury occurs if the air hose is severed high above the diver and the check valve in the helmet's air inlet does not seal adequately. The hose then acts as a long snorkel and the air pressure in the helmet and hence in the lungs falls to equal the water pressure at the upper end of the hose, again generating a potentially very large body-to-helmet pressure difference. The effects are known as whole-body or chest squeeze.

VI. Concluding Remarks

Astute clinical observation must have inspired the old head nurse who made it a house rule never to allow a patient with an ailing heart to take a full tub bath. Cases of acute cardiac failure and pulmonary edema resulting from the immersion effect were probably vivid in her memory. Yet, considering the fact that our species probably has practiced swimming throughout its existence, it is remarkable that we seem to be lacking even anecdotal accounts of as dramatic an occurrence as the immersion-induced pulmonary edema, capable of causing se-

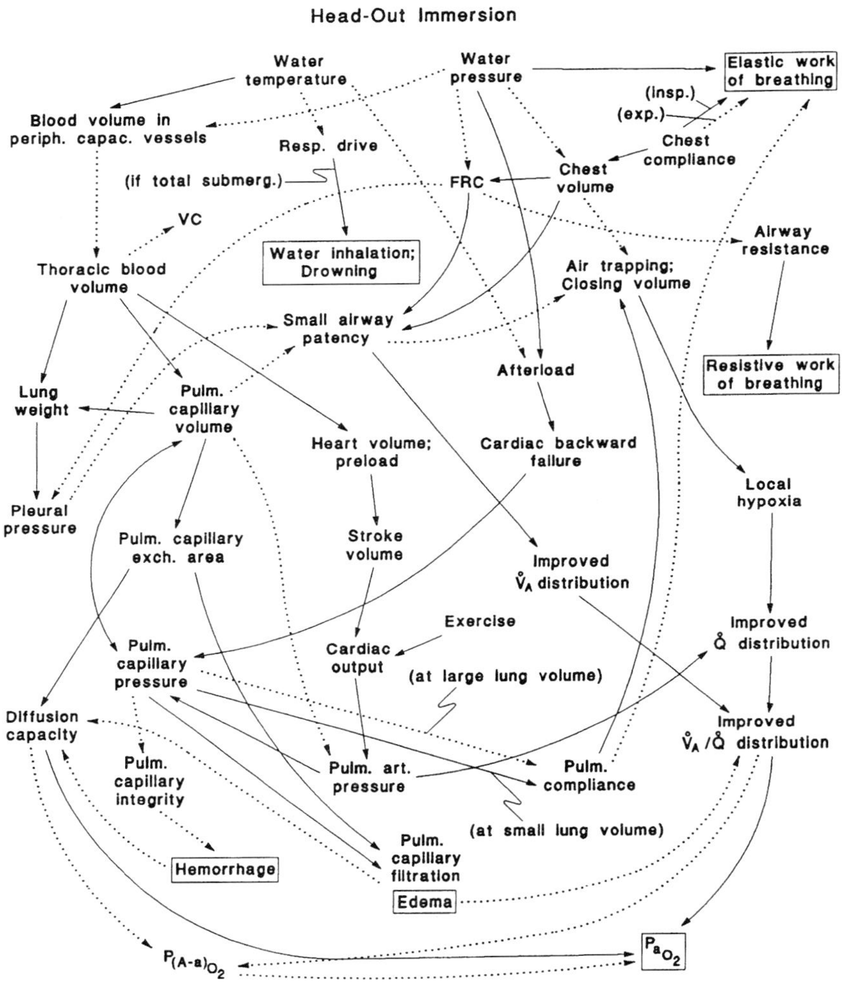

Figure 12 This diagram shows the interaction between circulatory and respiratory effects of immersion. Some aspects of the circulatory and respiratory sequences of events are not discussed in the text, since they are treated in standard physiology texts. Solid arrows indicate positive influences (e.g., increased water temperature causing increased blood volume to be pooled in peripheral capacitance vessels); dotted arrows indicate negative influences (e.g., increased water pressure causing decreased chest volume). A framed item is one in which changes are of potential applied significance.

vere hypoxia (e.g., Ref. 72) and even loss of consciousness (69). It is equally surprising that despite the fact that the history of balneology goes back at least to the nineteenth century, the first scientific report on this phenomenon is only 18 years old (67).

As for the physiological mechanisms behind this phenomenon and other effects of immersion, they can, as the foregoing text attempts to show, largely be traced to studies over the last 45 years of adjustments in pulmonary circulation and respiratory mechanics and the interaction between the two. The diagram in Fig. 12 is intended to give an overview of the salient features of these mechanisms as invoked by upright head-out immersion.

References

1. Roget's International Thesaurus, 4th ed. Revised by R L Chapman. New York: Thomas Y Crowell Co, 1977.
2. Hickey D D, Norfleet W T, Påsche A J, Lundgren C E G. Respiratory function in the upright, working diver at 6.8 ATA (190 fsw). Undersea Biomed Res 1987; 14(3):241–262.
3. Taylor N A S, Morrison J B. Lung centroid pressure in immersed man. Undersea Biomed Res 1989; 16(1):3–19.
4. Jarrett A S. Effect of immersion on intrapulmonary pressure. J Appl Physiol 1965; 20:1261–1266.
5. Agostoni E, Gurtner G, Torri G, Rahn H. Respiratory mechanics during submersion and negative pressure breathing. J Appl Physiol 1966; 21 (1):251–258.
6. Dahlbäck G O, Jönsson E, Linér M H. Influence of hydrostatic compression of the chest and intrathoracic blood pooling on static lung mechanics during head out immersion. Undersea Biomed Res 1978; 5(1):71–85.
7. Dahlbäck G O. Influence of intrathoracic blood pooling on pulmonary air trapping during immersion. Undersea Biomed Res 1975; 2(2):133–140.
8. Bondi K R, Young J M, Bennett R M, Bradley M E. Closing volumes in man immersed to the neck in water. J Appl Physiol 1976; 40:736–740.
9. Hamilton W F, Mayo J P. Changes in the vital capacity when the body is immersed in water. Am J Physiol 1944; 141:51–53.
10. Burki N K. Effects of immersion in water and changes in intrathoracic blood volume on lung function in man. Clin Sci Mol Med 1976; 51:303–311.
11. Kurss D I, Lundgren C E G, Påsche A J. Effect of water temperature on vital capacity in head-out immersion. In: Bachrach A J, Matzen M M, eds. Underwater Physiology VII. Bethesda, MD: Undersea Medical Society Inc., 1981:297–301.
12. Hong S K, Cerretelli P, Cruz J C, Rahn H. Mechanics of respiration during submersion in water. J Appl Physiol 1969; 27(4):535–538.
13. Hong S K, Ting E Y, Rahn H. Lung volumes at different depths of submersion. J Appl Physiol 1960; 15(4):550–553.
14. Taylor N A S, Morrison J B. Lung volume changes in response to altered breathing

gas pressure during upright immersion. Eur J Appl Physiol Occup Physiol 1991; 62(2):122–129.

15. Thalmann E D, Sponholtz D K, Lundgren C E G. Effects of immersion and static lung loading on submerged exercise at depth. Undersea Biomed Res 1979; 6(3): 259–290.
16. Reid M B, Banzett R B, Feldman H A, Mead J. Reflex compensation of spontaneous breathing when immersion changes diaphragm length. J Appl Physiol 1985; 58(4):1136–1142.
17. Chang L P, Lundgren C E G. Maximal breath-holding time and immediate tissue CO_2 storage capacity during head-out immersion in humans. Eur J Appl Physiol 1996; 73:210–218.
18. Banzett R B, Lansing R W, Reid M B. Reflex compensation of voluntary inspiration when immersion changes diaphragm length. J Appl Physiol 1985; 59(2):611–618.
19. Dressendorfer R H, Morlock J F, Bakker D J, Hong S K. Effects of head-out water immersion on cardiorespiratory responses to maximal cycling exercise. Undersea Biomed Res 1976; 3(3):177–187.
20. Fothergill D M, Taylor W F, Hyde D E. Physiological and perceptual responses to hypercarbia during warm and cold water immersion. Undersea Hyperbar Med 1998; 25(1): 1–12.
21. Löllgen H, Nieding G von, Horres R. Respiratory and hemodynamic adjustment during head out water immersion. Int J Sports Med 1980; 1:25–29
22. Morrison J B, Taylor N A S. Measurement of static and dynamic pulmonary work during pressure breathing. Undersea Biomed Res 1990; 17(5):453–467.
23. Dahlbäck G O. Lung mechanics during immersion in water with special reference to pulmonary air trapping. Thesis. Sweden: Institute of Physiology and Biophysics, University of Lund, 1978: 1–62.
24. Burger E J, Macklem P T. Airway closure: demonstration by breathing 100% O_2 at low lung volumes and N_2 washout. J Appl Physiol 1968; 25:139–148.
25. Prefaut C H, Dubois F, Roussos C H, Amaral-Marques R, Macklem P T, Ruff F. Influence of immersion to the neck in water on airway closure and distribution of perfusion in man. Respir Physiol 1979; 37:313–323.
26. Mead J, Whittenberger J L, Physical properties of human lungs measured during spontaneous respiration. J Appl Physiol 1953; 5:779–796.
27. Bondurant S, Hickam J B, Isley J K. Pulmonary and circulatory effects of acute pulmonary vascular engorgement in normal subjects. J Clin Invest 1957; 36:55–66.
28. Basch S von. Über eine Funktion des Capillardruckes in den Lungenalveolen. Wiener Med Blätter 1887; 15:465–467.
29. Prefaut C, Eulo L H, Anthonisen N R. Human lung mechanics during water immersion. J Appl Physiol 1976; 40:320–323.
30. Bondurant S, Mead J, Cook C D. A re-evaluation of effects of acute pulmonary vascular engorgement on pulmonary compliance in normal subjects. J Appl Physiol 1960; 15:875–877.
31. Borst H G, Berglund E, Whittenberger J L, Mead J, McGregor M, Collier C. The effect of pulmonary vascular pressures on the mechanical properties of the lungs of anesthetized dogs. J Clin Invest 1957; 36:1708–1714.
32. Baer R, Dahlbäck G O, Balldin U. Pulmonary mechanics and atelectasis during

immersion in oxygen breathing subjects. Undersea Biomed Res 1987; 14(3):229–240.

33. Sterk W. Respiratory mechanics of diver and diving apparatus. Thesis. The Netherlands: University of Utrecht, Physiological Laboratory, Drukkerij Elinkwijk 1973: 1–129.
34. Arborelius M Jr, Balldin U I, Lilja B, Lundgren C E G. Regional lung function in man during immersion with the head above water. Aerospace Med 1972; 43(7): 701–707.
35. Lichtneckert S J A, Lundgren, C E G. An index of alveolar ventilation. J Appl Physiol 1963; 18:639–645.
36. Robertson C H Jr, Engle C M, Bradley M E. Lung volumes in man immersed to the neck: dilution and plethysmographic techniques. J Appl Physiol: Respir Environ Exerc Physiol 1978; 44:679–682.
37. Dahlbäck G O, Lundgren C E G. Pulmonary air-trapping induced by water immersion. Aerospace Med 1972; 43(7): 768–774.
38. Hughes J M B, Rosenzweig D Y. Factors affecting trapped gas volume in perfused dog lungs. J Appl Physiol 1970; 29:332–339.
39. Zidulka A, Despas P J, Milic-Emili J, Anthonisen N R. Pulmonary function with acute loss of excess lung water by hemodialysis in patients with chronic uremia. Am J Med 1973; 55:134–141.
40. Hughes J M B, Rosenzweig D Y, Kivitz P B. Site of airway closure in excised dog lungs: histologic demonstration. J Appl Physiol 1970; 29:340–344.
41. Arborelius M Jr, Balldin U I, Lilja B, Lundgren C E G. Hemodynamic changes in man during immersion with the head above water Aerospace Med 1972; 43:592–598.
42. Lundgren C E G, Farhi L E. Pulmonary circulation in diving and hyperbaric environment. In: Weir E K, Reeves J T, eds. Pulmonary Vascular Physiology and Pathophysiology. New York: Marcel Dekker, 1989: 199–240.
43. Echt M, Düweling J, Gauer O H, Lange L. Effective compliance of the total vascular bed and the intrathoracic compartment derived from changes in central venous pressure induced by volume changes in man. Circ Res 1974; 34:61–68.
44. Lange L, Lange S, Echt M, Gauer O H. Heart volume in relation to body posture and immersion in a thermo-neutral bath: a roentgenometric study. Pflügers Arch 1974; 352:219–226.
45. Risch W D, Koubenec H J, Beckmann U, Lange S, Gauer O H. The effect of graded immersion on heart volume, central venous pressure, pulmonary blood distribution and heart rate in man. Pflügers Arch 1978; 374:115–118.
46. Guyatt A R, Newman F, Cinkotai F F, Palmer J I, Thompson M L. Pulmonary diffusing capacity in man during immersion in water. J Appl Physiol 1965; 20(5): 878–881.
47. Farhi L E, Linnarsson D. Cardiopulmonary readjustments during graded immersion in water at 35°C. Respir Physiol 1977; 30:35–50.
48. Begin R, Epstein M, Sackner M A, Levinson R, Dougherty R, Duncan D. Effect of water immersion to the neck on pulmonary circulation and tissue volume in man. J Appl Physiol 1976; 40:293–299.
49. Warkander D E, Norfleet W T, Nagasawa G K, Lundgren C E G. Physiologically

and subjectively acceptable breathing resistance in divers breathing gear. Undersea Biomed Res 1992; 19:427–445.
50. Norfleet W T, Hickey D D, Lundgren C E G. A comparison of respiratory function in divers breathing with a mouthpiece or a full face mask. Undersea Biomed Res 1987; 14(6):503–526.
51. Taylor N A S, Morrison J B. Effects of breathing-gas pressure on pulmonary function and work capacity during immersion. Undersea Biomed Res 1990; 17(5):413–428.
52. Paton W D M, Sand A. The optimum intrapulmonary pressure in underwater respiration. J Physiol 1947; 106:119–138.
53. Dahlbäck G O, Balldin U I. Positive-pressure oxygen breathing and pulmonary atelectasis during immersion. Undersea Biomed Res 1983; 10(1):39–44.
54. Balldin U I, Dahlbäck G O, Lundgren C E G. Changes in vital capacity produced by oxygen breathing during immersion with the head above water. Aerospace Med 1971; 42 (4):384–387.
55. Prefaut C H, Ramonatxo M, Boyer R, Chardon G. Human gas exchange during water immersion. Respir Physiol 1978; 34:307–318.
56. Dahlbäck G O, Balldin U I. Pulmonary atelectasis formation during diving with closed-circuit oxygen breathing apparatus. Undersea Biomed Res 1985; 12(2):129–137.
57. Malkinson T J, Martin S, Simper P. Cooper K E. Expired air volumes of males and females during cold water immersion. Can J Physiol Pharmacol 1981; 59:843–846.
58. Hayward J S, Eckerson J D. Physiological responses and survival time prediction for humans in ice-water. Aviat Space Environ Med 1984; 55(3):206–212.
59. Hayward J S, Hay C, Matthews B R, Overweel C H, Radford D D. Temperature effect on the human dive response in relation to cold water near-drowning. J Appl Physiol: Environ Exercise Physiol 1984; 56:202–206.
60. Cooper K E, Martin S, Riben P. Respiratory and other responses in subjects immersed in cold water. J Appl Physiol 1976; 40(6):903–910.
61. Keatinge W R, Evans M. The respiratory and cardiovascular response to immersion in cold and warm water. Q J Exptl Physiol 1961; 46:83–94.
62. Keatinge W R, Nadel J A. Immediate respiratory response to sudden cooling of the skin. J Appl Physiol 1965; 20(1):65–69.
63. Ringqvist T. The ventilatory capacity in healthy subjects. Scand J Clin Lab Invest 1966; 18 (suppl 88):1–179.
64. Stigler R. Die Kraft unserer Inspirationsmuskulatur. Pflügers Arch 1911; 139:234–254.
65. Stigler R. Die physiologische Bedeutung von Differenzen zwischen extra-und intrathoracalem Drucke. Zentralbl Physiol 1911; 255(23):1095.
66. Lanari A, Lambertini A, Lanari Zubaiur F, Bromberger Barnea B. Las modificaciones de la presion intratorarica, arterial sistemica y venosa periferica durante la sumersion. Medicina (Buenos Aires) 1960; 20(5–6):159–163.
67. Wilmshurst P, Nuri M, Crowther A, Betts J, Webb-Peploe M M. Forearm vascular responses in subjects who develop recurrent pulmonary oedema when scuba diving: a new syndrome. Br Heart J 1981; 45:349.

68. Wilmshurst P T, Nuri M, Crowther A, Betts J C, Webb-Peploe M M. Recurrent pulmonary edema in scuba divers; prodrome of hypertension: a new syndrome. In: Bachrach A J, Matzen M M, eds. Underwater Physiology VIII. Bethesda, MD: Undersea Medical Society, 1984:327–339.
69. Wilmshurst P T, Nuri M, Crowther A, Webb-Peploe N M. Cold Induced pulmonary oedema in scuba divers and subsequent development of hypertension. Lancet 1989; 1:62–65.
70. Pons M, Blickenstorfer D, Oechslin E, Hold G, Greiminger P, Franzeck U K, Russi E W. Pulmonary oedema in healthy persons during scuba-diving and swimming. Eur Respir J 1995; 8:762–767.
71. Weiler-Ravell D, Shupak A, Goldenberg I, Halpern P, Shoshani O, Hirschhorn G, Margulis A. Pulmonary oedema and hemoptysis induced by strenuous swimming. Br Med J 1995; 311:661–662.
72. Hampson N B, Dunford R G. Pulmonary edema of scuba divers. Undersea Hyperbar Med 1997; 24(1):29–33.
73. West J B, Tsukimoto K, Mathieu-Costello O, Prediletto R. Stress failure in pulmonary capillaries. J Appl Physiol 1991; 70(4):1731–1742.
74. Shupak A, Weiler-Ravell D, Adir Y, Kerem D, Daskalovic Y, Ramon Y, Abramovich A. Pulmonary congestion induced by strenuous swimming: a field study (abstr). Undersea Hyperbar Med 1998; 25(suppl):27.
75. Farhi L E. Elimination of inert gas by the lung. Respir Physiol 1967; 3:1–11.
76. Balldin U I, Lundgren C E G. Effects of immersion with the head above water on tissue nitrogen elimination in man. Aerospace Med 1972; 43:1101–1108.
77. Balldin U I, Lundgren C E G, Lundvall J, Mellander S. Changes in the elimination of ^{133}xenon from the anterior tibial muscle in man induced by immersion in water and by shifts in body position. Aerospace Med 1971; 42:489–493.
78. Balldin U I. The preventive effect of denitrogenation during warm water immersion on decompression sickness in man. Försvarsmedicin (Sweden) 1973; 9:239–243.
79. Arborelius M M, Lundgren C. Improvement on breathing apparatus for underwater use. US Patent No. 2896 616.
80. Cohen R, Bell W H, Saltzman H A, Kylstra J A. Alveolar-arterial oxygen pressure difference in man immersed to the neck in water. J Appl Physiol 1971; 30:720–723.
81. Lundgren C E G, Warkander D E. Effects of combined breathing impediments on divers' respiratory performance. Final Report submitted to US Navy, Naval Medical Research and Development Command. Contract N000149310509, 1997.
82. Thompson L J, McCally M. Role of transpharyngeal pressure gradients in determining intrapulmonary pressure during immersion. Aerospace Medicine 1967; 38(9):931–935.
83. Derion T, Reddan W G, Lanphier E H. Static lung load and posture effects on pulmonary mechanics and comfort in underwater exercise. Undersea Biomed Res 1992; 19:85–96.
84. Lundgren C E G. Gas physiology in diving; breathing underwater: ventilatory needs. In: Fregly M J, Blatteis C M, eds. Handbook of Physiology, Section 4, En-

vironmental Physiology, Vol II. New York: For the American Physiological Society by Oxford University Press, 1996.
85. Beckman E L, Coburn K R, Chambers R M, DeForest R E, Augerson W S, Benson V G. Physiologic changes observed in human subjects during zero G simulation by immersion in water up to neck level. Aerospace Med 1961; 32:1030–1041.
86. Brozek J, Henschel A, Keys A. Effect of submersion in water on the volume of residual air in man. J Appl Physiol 1949; 2:240–246.
87. Cary C R, Schaefer K E, Alvis H J. Effect of skin diving on lung volumes. J Appl Physiol 1956; 8:519–523.
88. Craig A B Jr, Ware D E. Effects of immersion in water on vital capacity and residual volume of the lungs. J Appl Physiol 1967; 23(4):423–425.
89. Craig A B Jr, Dvorak M. Expiratory reserve volume and vital capacity of the lungs during immersion in water. J Appl Physiol 1975; 38(1):5–9.
90. Flynn E T Jr, Camporesi E M, Nunneley S A. Cardiopulmonary responses to pressure breathing during immersion in water. Pressure Vol II. Department of Physiology, State University of NY at Buffalo. 1975; 79–94.
91. Girandola R N, Wiswell R A, Mohler J G, Romero G T, Barnes W S. Effects of water immersion on lung volumes: implications for body composition analysis. J Appl Physiol: Respir Environ Exerc Physiol 1977; 43(3):276–279.
92. Jarrett A S. The effect of immersion on the lung volumes. Report No. FPRC/1221 1963; Flying Personnel Research Committee, RAF Institute of Aviation Medicine, Farnborough, Hants, England.
93. Löllgen H, von Nieding G. Heart synchronous oscillations in the alveolar plateau and closing volume. Scand J Respir Dis 1976; suppl 95:13–21.
94. Prefaut C H Jr, Chardon G. Modifications relatives des gas du sang du volume de fermeture au cours de l'immersion. Rev Med Sub Hyp 1977; 61:48–50.
95. Robertson P C, Anthonisen N R, Ross D. Effect of inspiratory flow rate on regional distribution of inspired gas. J Appl Physiol 1969; 26:438–443.
96. Lundgren C E G, Norfleet W T. Respiratory function in hyperbaric environments. In: Shiraki K, Yousef M K, eds. Man in Stressful Environments: Diving, Hyper- and Hypobaric Physiology. Springfield, IL: Charles C Thomas, 1987:21–40.

4

Temperature Effects

EDWARD T. FLYNN, JR.

University of Pennsylvania
Philadelphia, Pennsylvania

I. Introduction

One of the most important functions of the airways is to condition the inspired gas stream before it reaches the gas-exchanging surfaces. Conditioning includes raising (or lowering) the inspired gas temperature to body temperature, saturating the gas stream with water vapor, and removing particulates. Of nearly equal importance is the recovery of heat and moisture from the gas stream during exhalation to conserve body heat and prevent airway drying. In fact, these two processes are closely coupled and each has important influences on the other.

The possibility that conditioning of the inspired gas might pose practical problems for divers was first recognized in the late 1960s by Webb and Annis (1,2), Tauber and Rawlins (3,4), and Varene, L'Huillier, and Jacquemin (5,6). Until that time, divers had not experienced problems even though they operated routinely in very cold water and breathed gases close to water temperature. The basis of concern was the development of saturation diving. Saturation diving allowed the diver to break through the old depth barrier of 300 ft of seawater (fsw) to dive safely to depths of 1000 fsw and beyond.

Based on measurements of respiratory heat loss (RHL) by Webb and Annis (1) in divers immersed in cold water at 200 fsw (7 ata),* Tauber et al. (3) predicted that somewhere between 600 and 800 fsw (19 to 25 ata), inspired gas near 0°C would have the thermal capacity to remove essentially all of the metabolic heat produced by the diver. This would be true over the full range of exercise, since oxygen consumption and respiratory minute ventilation increase in constant proportion to each other. Any extra heat generated by additional exercise would be dissipated by the simultaneously increased respiratory minute volume. Experiments by Hoke et al. and Goodman et al. (7,8) quickly bore out the basic accuracy of Tauber's predictions. In addition, these experiments demonstrated that the airways themselves were affected by the cold gases and that divers were often forced to stop work because of airway narrowing and excessive airway secretions.

This chapter discusses the basic principles of respiratory heat and mass transfer under pressure, the studies that have been conducted in animals and humans to define the nature and extent of the problem of respiratory heat loss in divers, and the engineering techniques that have been developed to assist the diver in conditioning the inspired gas.

II. Respiratory Heat and Mass Transfer Under Pressure

The process of respiratory heat and mass transfer under hyperbaric conditions is identical to the process at normal barometric pressure; only the magnitude of the exchange is different. The basic process is the same whether the inhaled gas is cold and must be warmed or whether it is hot and must be cooled. Both hot- and cold-gas breathing conditions are encountered in diving, but the inhalation of hot gas is relatively unusual. Accordingly most of the discussion that follows focuses on the inhalation of cold gas.

A. General Principles

During inspiration, the inspired gas is warmed progressively to body temperature as it passes over the warm mucous membranes of the nose, mouth, pharynx, larynx, and tracheobronchial tree. During its transit, water vapor is also added progressively to the gas stream to ensure full saturation at body temperature. The process of heat- and water-vapor transfer during inspiration cools the mu-

*The atmosphere (atm) is the principal unit of pressure used in this chapter. 1 atm=33.08 fsw=10.13 msw=101.325 kPa=0.101325 MPa. ata=atmospheres absolute.

cosa, creating a longitudinal temperature gradient from the airway opening to the distal airways.

Upon expiration, the process of heat and mass transfer is reversed. The warm, saturated alveolar gas returns heat to the cooler mucosa as it flows toward the airway opening. As the gas temperature falls from alveolar temperature, water vapor becomes supersaturated and condenses, returning additional heat to the mucosa. The recovery of heat from the expired gas stream rewarms the mucosa cooled by the previous inspiration, but only partially. The heat recovered is only a fraction of the heat lost during the preceding inspiration. Expired gas thus exits the body at a temperature below alveolar temperature but still above the inspired gas temperature (9–11). At the expired gas temperature, the expired gas stream is also observed to be slightly unsaturated (12,13).

For resting individuals at normobaric pressures, McCutchen and Taylor (14) observed that expired gas temperatures remained below body temperature (37°C) even with inspired gas temperatures as high as 55°C (for partially saturated gas) or 75°C (for dry gas). These results may be explained by the fact that at normobaric pressures, approximately 90% of the respiratory heat transfer is due to evaporation and condensation of water vapor. The evaporation of water vapor into the dry inspired gas cools the mucosa despite the fact that the inspired gas temperature is well above body temperature. This result would not be observed under hyperbaric conditions (see below).

In a steady state, the net result of the mucosal inspiratory heat loss and the subsequent partial expiratory heat gain is the creation of a longitudinal temperature gradient within the airways (15). Mean airway temperature rises steadily from the low inspired value at the airway opening to core body temperature at a point in the distal airways. At each axial location along the temperature gradient, the mucosal and airstream temperatures fluctuate over a small range with each inspiration and expiration. The extent to which cold gas can penetrate into the distal airways before warming is complete is of fundamental concern in cold-induced asthma and in respiratory injury that might result from exposure to extremely harsh environments, including diving. Studies conducted at normobaric pressures demonstrate that the degree of airway penetration increases with increased respiratory minute ventilation, increased thermal capacity and dryness of the inspired gas, and decreased inspired gas temperature (15,16).

The primary difference between respiratory heat and mass transfer under normobaric and hyperbaric conditions resides in the magnitude of the effect, which is increased under hyperbaric conditions. The increased transfer of heat under pressure is due principally to the direct linear relationship between the thermal capacity of the respired gas and the ambient pressure. The high thermal conductivity of some diving gases also contributes to the process at the local airway level.

B. Thermal Properties of Diving Gases

The magnitude of heat and mass transfer in the airways is determined by three variables: (1) the respiratory flow rate, (2) the temperature and humidity of the inspired gas, and (3) the physical properties of the respired gas mixture. The first two variables are a function of the diver's workload, the type of breathing apparatus employed, and the water temperature. The third is a function of the diver's depth and the composition of his or her gas mixture.

Air is the most common gas used for diving. Because of the narcotic properties of the nitrogen component, however, air diving is usually limited to 6 to 7 ata. Deeper than 7 ata, mixtures of helium and oxygen are employed. Helium-oxygen is not only nonnarcotic but much less dense than air, making it easier to breathe. In very deep diving (>30 ata), part of the helium may be replaced by hydrogen to further lighten the gas and to counteract symptoms of the high-pressure nervous syndrome. The oxygen content of the diver's mixture also varies with the diver's depth. Deeper than 10 ata, the diver's mixture is usually changed from a fixed fraction of oxygen (generally 12 to 21% oxygen) to a constant partial pressure of oxygen (generally 0.3 to 1.3 ata oxygen). This is to avoid problems with central nervous system oxygen toxicity. With a constant oxygen partial pressure, the oxygen content of the mixture will decrease with depth. At 30 ata, for example, a mixture might contain as little as 1 to 2% oxygen. In very deep diving, the inert gas component of the gas mixture dominates the heat- and mass-transfer process because so little oxygen is present.

Five physical properties of the gas mixture are important in respiratory heat and mass transfer: its viscosity (μ), density (ρ), thermal conductivity (k), constant-pressure specific heat (C_P), and water vapor diffusivity (D_{H_2O}). Table 1 shows these physical properties at 1 ata for air and the pure gases used to create diving gas mixtures (17,18). Several things are worth noting in Table 1. The physical properties of oxygen and nitrogen (and consequently air) are approximately the same. Helium and hydrogen are both much less dense than nitrogen or oxygen but have substantially higher specific heats. The product of density and specific heat (ρC_P), a measure of the specific heat of the gas on a per-liter basis (J/L·°K), however, is essentially the same for all the gases with the exception of helium, which has a slightly lower ρC_P product. The capacity of helium to remove heat convectively from the respiratory tract, therefore, will be slightly less than the capacity of nitrogen, oxygen, or hydrogen at the same ambient pressure (see below). The thermal conductivities of helium and hydrogen are six to seven times greater than those of nitrogen and oxygen. Finally, the water-vapor diffusivity into helium and hydrogen is more than three times its diffusivity into nitrogen or oxygen.

Very few of the physical properties of diving gas mixtures have actually been measured under pressure. Values are usually calculated from the mole

Table 1 Physical Properties of Air and Pure Gases Used to Make Diving Gas Mixtures (1 ata, 27°C)

Quantity	Air	Nitrogen	Oxygen	Helium	Hydrogen
Molar mass (g/mol)	28.97	28.01	32.00	4.00	2.02
Density (ρ) (g/L)	1.102	1.066	1.218	0.152	0.077
Specific heat (C_P) (J/g·°K)	1.007	1.039	0.919	5.196	14.286
ρC_P (J/L·°K)	1.110	1.107	1.119	0.790	1.100
Viscosity (μ) (g/cm·sec$\times 10^{-5}$)	18.6	17.9	20.8	20.0	9.0
Thermal conductivity (k) (J/sec·cm·°K$\times 10^{-5}$)	26.2	26.0	26.3	156.7	186.9
D_{H_2O}(cm^2/sec)	0.274	0.249	0.281	0.894	0.895
Prandtl no. (Pr)	0.715	0.715	0.727	0.663	0.688
Schmidt no. (Sc)	0.616	0.674	0.608	1.472	1.306

Sources: Refs. 17 and 18.

fractions of the various pure gases in the mixture (ρ, C_P, D_{H_2O}) or from mixture formulas (k, μ) and then projected to depth using known or predicted pressure relationships. Occasionally values are extrapolated from nearby experimental data. Several summaries of calculation methods, including comparisons with experimental data, are available (18–22). Of the five gas properties cited in Table 1, all but the specific heat (C_P) vary significantly with temperature. Only density and water vapor diffusivity, however, vary significantly with ambient pressure. The viscosity, thermal conductivity, and specific heat of a mixture can, for our purposes, be considered independent of ambient pressure.

At the temperatures and pressures encountered by divers, the diving gases demonstrate nearly ideal behavior. The density of a given gas mixture, therefore, will increase in direct proportion to the ambient pressure. A helium-oxygen mixture breathed at 30 ata, for example, has a density approximately thirty times greater than at 1 ata. This is the single most important factor governing respiratory heat loss at depth. Since a greater mass of gas is inhaled with each breath, a greater amount of heat is required to warm it.

In contrast to gas density, the water-vapor diffusivity in a gas mixture decreases with pressure. An inverse relationship ($D_{H_2O} \approx 1/P_B$) is predicted by the Chapman-Enskog theory and by a variety of derivative formulations (17). In experiments, D_{H_2O} is observed to closely follow the inverse relationship at both altitude and moderate depth (23,24). At deep depth, however, the reduction in D_{H_2O} is not quite as severe as predicted by the $1/P_B$ relationship. Paganelli and Kurata (24) observed a break from the $1/P_B$ relationship beginning at 4 ata with nitrogen and at 20 ata with helium. At 10 ata of nitrogen, values of D_{H_2O}

were 13% higher than predicted for the depth by the inverse relationship. A similar deviation (13%) was observed at 50 ata with helium. It is important to point out, however, that D_{H_2O} is still very much reduced at depth despite these deviations from the inverse relationship. At 10 ata of nitrogen, D_{H_2O} is only 11.7% of its value at 1 ata; at 50 ata of helium, it is only 2.2% of its value at 1 ata.

Another property of water vapor also deserves mention. The Poynting relationship predicts that the vapor pressure of water will be increased at pressure. At 50 ata, the calculated increase is approximately 3% (20,24). The actual increase, however, appears to be highly dependent on the nature of the gas in contact with the water, both in terms of its solubility and its deviation from ideal behavior. At 7 ata, the water content of saturated air at 37.8°C is approximately 2% greater than at 1 ata; at 41 ata, it is 12% greater (25). The water content of helium, on the other hand, appears to remain constant over the range of 1 to 41 ata (25). Because air cannot be used much deeper than 7 ata, where the observed pressure effect is small, and because helium appears to be devoid of a pressure effect altogether, we will ignore any effects of pressure on water-vapor pressure in the subsequent discussions.

Table 2 puts these various pressure and gas mixture effects into perspective. The table shows the calculated thermal properties of a helium-oxygen gas mixture with a constant oxygen partial pressure of 0.5 ata at depths ranging from 1 to 61.6 ata (2000 fsw). This gas mixture is typical of those used in deep saturation diving. Values given are relative to those at 1 ata (22). With a constant oxygen partial pressure, the oxygen content of the mixture decreases steadily from 50% at 1 ata to only 0.8% at 61 ata. The density of the mixture increases by a factor of 14.1—a large increase but substantially less than the 61.6 ata increase in ambient pressure. This is because the oxygen in the mixture is steadily being replaced by helium, a much lighter gas. Similarly, the specific heat, viscosity, and thermal conductivity of the mixture, normally independent of ambient pressure, either increase (C_P,k) or decrease (μ) as the oxygen content falls and the gas mixture becomes more like pure helium. This change is most prominent in the first 300 fsw of descent. Water-vapor diffusivity decreases with

Table 2 Physical Properties of 0.5 ata Oxygen in Helium at Depth Relative to 1 ata

Depth (fsw)	P_B (ata)	$\%O_2$	ρ	C_P	ρC_P	μ	k	D_{H_2O}
0	1.0	50.0	1.00	1.00	1.00	1.00	1.00	1.000
100	4.0	12.4	1.67	2.10	3.51	0.95	2.21	0.345
300	10.0	5.0	3.02	2.82	8.52	0.85	2.81	0.146
1000	31.3	1.6	7.63	3.37	25.71	0.80	3.16	0.048
2000	61.6	0.8	14.06	3.54	49.77	0.79	3.29	0.024

ambient pressure, reaching 2.4% of the 1 ata value at 61 ata. This value is higher than expected from the 1/PB relationship and again reflects the fact that the gas is becoming more like pure helium, which has a higher value for D_{H_2O} than does oxygen. At 61.6 ata, the product of density and specific heat of the mixture is 50 times greater than at 1 ata.

C. Global Respiratory Heat Loss

Initial concerns in deep diving focused on the magnitude of the overall respiratory heat loss. Later, several studies examined the details of heat and mass transfer at the airway level. We will consider overall heat transfer first.

Respiratory heat loss results from both convective and evaporative heat transfer. Conduction and radiation heat play little or no role. The overall loss is equal to the difference in enthalpy between the expired and inspired gas. In equation form:

$$RHL = \dot{V}_E \rho_G C_{PG} (T_E - T_I) + \dot{V}_E \rho_G W_I C_{PV} (T_E - T_I) + \dot{V}_E \rho_G \lambda (W_E - W_I) \quad (1)$$

where: RHL = respiratory heat loss (J/min)*
$\dot{V}_E$ = respiratory minute ventilation (L/min, dry gas)
ρ_G = density of the dry gas (g/L)
C_{PG} = constant pressure specific heat of dry gas (J/g·°K)
C_{PV} = constant pressure specific heat of water vapor (J/g·°K)
T_E = expired gas temperature (°K)
T_I = inspired gas temperature (°K)
λ = latent heat of vaporization (J/g·°K)
W_E = water content of expired gas (g H_2O/g DRY GAS)
W_I = water content of inspired gas (g H_2O/g DRY GAS)

If the water vapor pressure is known, W can be calculated from:

$$W = (M_{H_2O}/M_{DRY\ GAS})(P_{H_2O}/P_B - P_{H_2O}) \quad (2)$$

where: M_{H_2O} = molar mass of water vapor (g/mole)
$M_{DRY\ GAS}$ = molar mass of the dry gas mixture (g/mole)
P_{H_2O} = water vapor pressure (torr)†
P_B = ambient barometric pressure (torr)

*1 W=60 J/min=0.0143 Kcal/min

†The water-vapor pressure of saturated gas may be calculated from the Antoine equation, where P_{H_2O} is the saturated vapor pressure (torr) and T is the temperature of the gas (°C):

$$P_{H_2O} = e^{\left(18.6686 - \frac{4030.183}{T + 235}\right)}$$

This relationship is accurate to within ± 0.05 torr over the 0 to 50°C range (26).

The first term in Eq. (1) is the amount of heat expended per minute to warm the dry component of the inspired gas from T_I to T_E. The second term is the amount of heat expended to warm the water vapor in the inspired gas from T_I to T_E. The third term is the latent heat associated with raising the water vapor content of the gas from W_I to W_E. The first two terms represent the convective component of respiratory heat transfer, while the third term represents the evaporative component. Both the convective and evaporative components increase with increased respiratory minute ventilation.

The convective component of respiratory heat loss is strongly driven by the product ρC_P and the magnitude of the inspired-expired temperature difference. The evaporative component is driven by the latent heat of vaporization of water and the magnitude of the inspired-expired gas–water content difference. To a first approximation, the latent heat of vaporization and the water content of the gas (see above) depend only on the temperature of the gas, not the ambient pressure. Evaporative losses, therefore, will remain relatively constant as pressure increases. On the other hand, convective losses will increase as the product ρC_P increases with depth. Accordingly, the evaporative heat loss, which accounts for approximately 90% of the respiratory heat loss at normobaric pressures, will constitute a progressively smaller fraction of the total heat loss as depth increases.

In most studies of hyperbaric respiratory heat loss, $\dot{V}_E$, T_E, and T_I have been measured, ρ and C_P calculated from the ambient pressure and mole fractions of the gas in the diver's breathing mixture, and W_E calculated assuming that the expired gas is fully saturated with water vapor at T_E. W_I is usually near zero, since diving gases must be kept very dry to avoid freeze-up of valves and regulators. In some instances, however, the gas is wet. Rebreathing systems are an example. In these instances, W_I is calculated assuming either full saturation of the gas with water vapor at T_I or less often from the product of the relative humidity of the inspired gas and its saturation water-vapor content. λ is known to vary with temperature. Most studies, however, assume a constant value of λ [as shown in Eq. (1)], rather than evaluating the inspired and expired gas separately with two values of λ. The latter is the more accurate technique.

Gas temperature at the airway opening is measured with fast-responding ($\tau \leq 0.1$ sec) thermistors or thermocouples. In most studies, T_I and T_E are measured separately with devices in both the inspired and expired gas streams, even though this arrangement puts the devices at a slight distance from the airway opening. When only one device is used to measure both T_I and T_E, water-vapor condensation on the device during expiration frequently degrades its time response, thereby limiting the usefulness of the measurement to short time periods (27,28). No hyperbaric studies to date have performed a volume-weighted integration of T_I and T_E over the respiratory cycle as suggested by Caldwell et al. (29), perhaps due to the experimental difficulty of implementing this technique properly (30). Reported values of T_I and T_E are simply the lowest and highest recorded values, respectively. For expiration, this is the temperature of the expiratory plateau. As with expired gas composition measurements, expired gas temperature rises rapidly from inspired levels during the initial stages of expiration to reach a plateau value that remains nearly constant for the remainder of the expiration (12,31–33).

Following the predictions of Tauber and Rawlins (3,4), Hoke et al. (7) were the first to systematically study the magnitude of the respiratory heat loss in divers breathing helium-oxygen mixtures deeper than 200 fsw (7 ata). Two divers were studied at six depths ranging from 0 to 1000 fsw (1 to 31 ata) in a warm (30°C), dry hyperbaric chamber. At each depth, the divers performed graded work on a bicycle ergometer while breathing either warm (27 to 32°C) or cold (0 to 7°C) gas delivered to the mouth from a heat exchanger. At each depth and gas temperature, RHL increased linearly with $\dot{V}_E$. The slope of the linear response was greater the deeper the diver's depth and the colder the breathing gas (Fig. 1).

Hoke et al. observed that a diver at the surface (1 ata) breathing 30°C gas at $\dot{V}_E$=40 L/min had a calculated RHL of 50 W (3000 J/min) and that 95% of this loss could be attributed to humidifying the inspired gas. With the same minute volume and gas temperature at depths of 800 and 1000 fsw (25 and 31 ata), calculated RHL increased to 150 to 200 W, a three- to fourfold increase over surface values.

With cold-gas breathing at $\dot{V}_E$=40 L/min at the surface, the RHL was about the same as with warm gas, 50 W. At 800 and 1000 fsw, however, RHL increased to 400 to 500 W, an 8 to 10-fold increase over surface values. The highest observed RHL, 778 W, a 16-fold increase, occurred during heavy work at 1000 fsw (31 ata) with a $\dot{V}_E$ of 64 L/min. With cold gas at 800 to 1000 fsw (25 to 31 ata), only 10% of the heat loss could be attributed to humidification of the inspired gas. Confirming the predictions of Tauber and Rawlins (3,4), 80 to 100% of the metabolic heat produced was lost to the environment through the lungs, resulting in a rapid fall in core body temperature.

Shortly after the study of Hoke et al., Goodman et al. (8) undertook a similar study, but with the divers immersed in water rather than being exposed in a dry environment. Three subjects wearing hot water–protective suits performed exercise on an ergometer while immersed in water of 35, 45, and 55 °F (1.7, 7.2, and 12.8°C) at depths of 450 to 1000 fsw (14.6 to 31.3 ata). Measured inspired gas temperatures were nearly equal to water temperature. The results were similar to those observed by Hoke et al. Calculated RHL showed a strong relationship to $\dot{V}_E$ and T_I. The highest observed heat loss was 394 W with a T_I of 3°C and $\dot{V}_E$=41 L/min at 850 fsw (26.8 ata).

A number of other hyperbaric studies have subsequently confirmed the accelerated loss of respiratory heat under pressure (34–45).

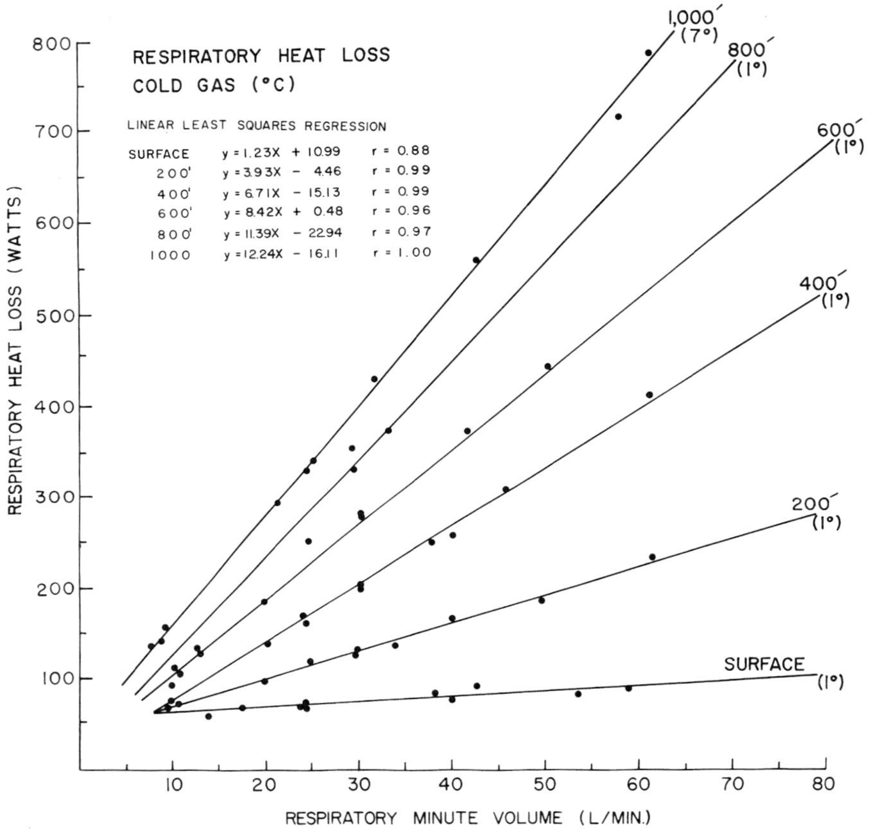

Figure 1 Respiratory heat loss as a function of respiratory minute ventilation during cold-gas inhalation at depth. Values of T_I are shown in parentheses. Respiratory heat loss increases as a function of both the respiratory minute ventilation and the depth. (From Ref. 7.)

There is general agreement, in both surface and hyperbaric respiratory heat-loss studies, that the relationship between expired temperature and inspired temperature is linear (46–50):

$$T_E = B + m\ T_I \tag{3}$$

where: B = the y intercept
m = the slope

This allows the convective term of Eq. (1) to be conveniently expressed only as a function of T_I:

$$\dot{V}_E \ \rho \ C_{PG} \ [B+(m-1) \ T_I] \tag{4}$$

Unfortunately, the various studies have not agreed on the values for the slope and intercept of this relationship. Results from key studies are shown in Table 3. The wide variability may be attributed to methodological errors, including sensor placement, slow sensor time constants, condensate on the expiratory sensor, and failure to volume-integrate the sensor output. Some differences may also be due to failure to take into account inspired humidity levels (47,48). It is also possible that the relationship between T_E and T_I is not truly linear but only appears to be so in the various studies because of the narrow range of environmental conditions studied. In this instance, different linear relationships could be found depending on which regions had been selected for study.

A very puzzling aspect of the relationship between T_E and T_I is the failure to observe any influence of $\dot{V}_E$ or ρC_P on it. Most studies show that the relationship is independent of either $\dot{V}_E$ or depth (6–8,27,48). This led Moore et al. (38) to describe the respiratory tract as a "simple temporal countercurrent heat exchanger.'' Only one study (50) has been able to demonstrate an effect of ρC_P. In that study, conducted with helium and then hydrogen as the diluent gas at a depth a 21 ata, T_E at a given T_I was significantly lower with the hydrogen mixture (see Table 3), reflecting its greater thermal capacity (6.29 versus 4.62 cal/L·°C).

The absence of good agreement on the relationship between T_E and T_I makes it difficult to describe the overall efficiency of the respiratory heat exchanger or to predict the relative risk of heat loss or gain in various environmental situations. The latter is of special interest in attempting to relate changes observed during very cold air breathing at normal pressure (1 ata) to the changes

Table 3 Normobaric and Hyperbaric Inspired/Expired Temperature Relationships

Study	P_B (ata)	Gas	$\dot{V}_E$ (L/min)	T_I (°C)	Relationship
Webb (46)	1	Air	Rest	−40–25	T_E=29.0+0.20 T_I
Houdas and Colin (47)	1	Air	Rest	5–50	T_E=24.6+0.32 T_I
Cain et al. (27)	1	Air	9–42	−20–20	T_E=31.9+0.11 T_I
Varene et al. (48)	1–30	Air/HeO_2	6–35	10–35	T_E=24.0+0.32 T_I[a]
Hoke et al. (7)	1–31	HeO_2	8–97	0–30	T_E=29.2+0.21 T_I
Goodman et al. (8)	14–31	HeO_2	5–44	2–13	T_E=24.4+0.32 T_I
Piantadosi (49)	20–56	HeO_2	Rest	12–33	T_E=25.4+0.28 T_I
Hayes et al. (43)	19–31	HeO_2	15–40	8–19	T_E=26.4+0.42 T_I
Burnet et al. (50)	21	HeO_2	Rest	10–30	T_E=28.2+0.23 T_I
	21	H_2O_2	Rest	10–30	T_E=27.5+0.19 T_I

[a]For RH ≤ 35%. For RH 35–65%, T_E = 26.0+0.25 T_I. For RH ≥ 65%, T_E = 27.0+0.20 T_I.

observed in divers at high ambient pressure. Varene's (51) graphical analysis is the best analytical tool available to date for both efficiency calculations and environmental comparisons. Nevertheless, it is critically dependent on the assumed relationship between T_E and T_I.

One measure of the efficiency of the respiratory heat exchanger is the ratio of the heat recovered during expiration to the heat lost during inspiration. A heat exchanger with 100% efficiency would warm gas to alveolar temperature during inspiration, then recover all of that heat during the subsequent expiration. In equation form:

$$\text{Efficiency} = \frac{\text{heat gain during expiration}}{\text{heat loss during inspiration}} \tag{5}$$

Substituting Eqs. (1) and (2) in Eq. (5), (1) ignoring the small amount of heat necessary to warm the water vapor in the inspired gas and (2) assuming that $P_B - P_{H_2O} = P_B$, the following expression can be derived:

$$\text{Efficiency} = \frac{C_P(T_A - T_E) + A/P_B(P_{A_{H_2O}} - P_{E_{H_2O}})}{C_P(T_A - T_I) + A/P_B(P_{A_{H_2O}} - P_{I_{H_2O}})} \tag{6}$$

where: T_A = alveolar temperature (°C)
$A = M_{H_2O}\lambda / M_{DRY\ GAS}$

When a linear relationship between T_E and T_I is selected that is invariant with $\dot{V}_E$ or P_B (as in Table 3), T_E and $P_{E_{H_2O}}$ are uniquely determined by T_I and are independent of the diver's depth. Figure 2 shows the calculated efficiency of the respiratory heat exchanger for two relationships, $T_E = 29.2 + 0.21\ T_I$ (7,46) and $T_E = 24 + 0.32\ T_I$ (48), for dry inspired air at 1 ata. With both formulations, the efficiency falls as the inspired gas becomes warmer. The assumed T_E/T_I relationship does make a substantial difference in calculated efficiency. The Varene relationship (48) yields higher efficiency values at a given T_I because the calculated T_E and $P_{E_{H_2O}}$ values are lower. Figure 3 illustrates what happens at depth. The efficiency of the heat exchanger with dry helium-oxygen at 31 ata is compared with dry air at 1 ata using the Hoke/Webb (7,46) T_E/T_I relationship. At 31 ata, the efficiency with helium-oxygen still decreases as the gas becomes warmer, but the slope of the relationship is very much reduced relative to the slope at 1 ata. As depth continues to increase further and the evaporative component becomes an even smaller fraction of the total heat exchange, the efficiency of exchange will approach the efficiency of the convective component, $T_A - T_E / T_A - T_I$, as a limit. This latter relationship (shown by the dotted line in Fig. 3) shows a very slight upward slope as inspired gas temperature increases.

The graphical analysis of Varene (51) may be used to compare the relative stress of different thermal environments. For illustration purposes, a simpler

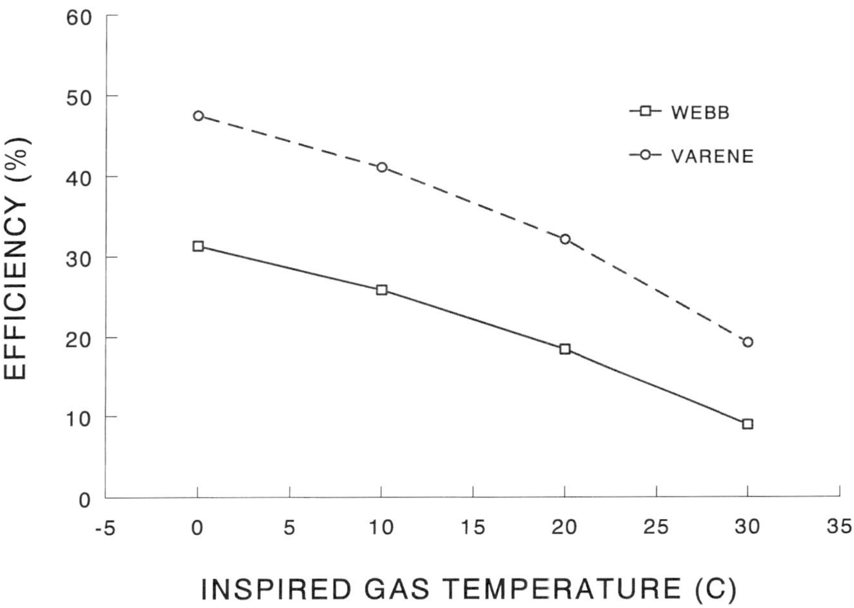

Figure 2 Efficiency of the respiratory heat exchanger with dry inspired air at 1 ata. Calculations were performed using Eq. (6) and the relationship $T_E = 29.0 + 0.20\ T_I$ from Webb (46) (solid line) or $T_E = 24 + 0.32\ T_I$ from Varene (48) (dotted line). The calculated efficiency decreases as the inspired temperature increases. The assumed T_E/T_I relation is an important determinant of the calculated efficiency.

approach can be adopted that does not rely on an assumed T_E/T_I relationship. This approach looks only at the cooling capacity (J/L_{BTPD}) of the gas—i.e., the amount of heat removed from the respiratory mucosa by the gas per liter as it flows from the airway opening to the alveoli. It can be considered a measure of the load placed on the heat exchanger by the environment. The heat exchanger will respond to this inspiratory load by recovering some of the heat during the subsequent expiration. The net heat loss can be determined by multiplying the cooling capacity by 1 minus the efficiency.

Figure 4 compares the cooling capacity (J/L_{BTPD}) of the inspired gas in three common environmental situations: dry air at 1 ata; dry air at 7 ata, the depth limit for air; and dry helium at 31 ata. The energy needed to saturate and warm 1 L of dry inspired gas to an alveolar temperature of 37°C is plotted as a function of the temperature at which it is inspired. For each environmental situation, the relationship between the cooling capacity and T_I is linear and has slope equal to $-\rho C_P$. All three curves converge at $T_I = 37°C$, where, for each

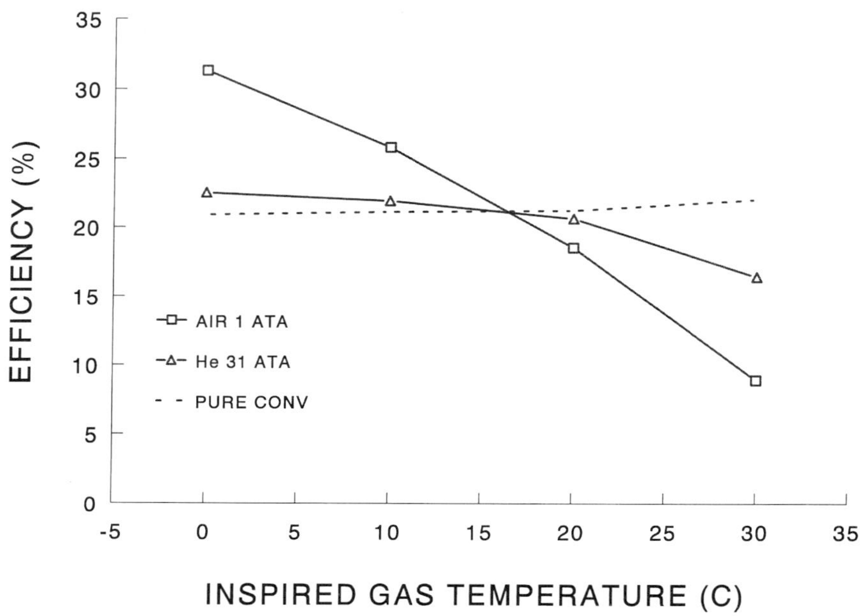

Figure 3 Efficiency of the respiratory heat exchanger with dry inspired gas at depth. Calculations were performed for air at 1 ata (open squares) and helium at 31 ata (open triangles) using Eq. (6) and the relation $T_E = 29.2 + 0.21\ T_I$ (7,46). The calculated efficiency decreases as the inspired temperature increases at both depths, but the response is considerably flatter at 31 ata, reflecting the reduced contribution of water vaporization. The dashed line shows the efficiency for convective heat transfer alone. For pure convection, the efficiency increases slightly with increasing inspired temperature. As the diver's depth increases, the efficiency curve approaches the pure convection curve as a limit.

gas, the only cooling (106 to 112 J/L) is related to the vaporization of water. Inspired temperatures greater than 37°C may still cool the respiratory mucosa. Cooling will continue until an inspired temperature is reached where the excess heat content of the gas equals the heat required for water vaporization. This temperature is well in excess of 100°C for air at 1 ata, but it is reduced to 50°C at 7 ata of air and to 41°C with helium at 31 ata. At $T_I = 0$°C, air at 7 ata imposes 2.7 times the inspiratory stress on the respiratory heat exchanger that air at 1 ata does; at 31 ata on helium, the stress is increased sevenfold. These numbers are lower than would be predicted from the ratios of ρC_P and reflect the contribution made by water vaporization to the overall heat-transfer process.

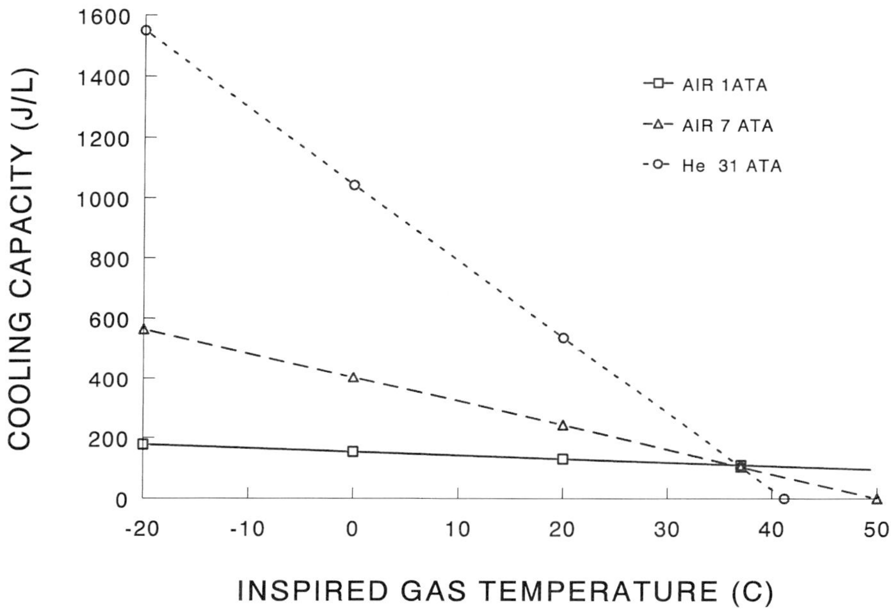

Figure 4 Cooling capacity of dry inspired gas as a function of inspired-gas temperature and depth. Curves are shown for air at 1 ata (open squares), air at 7 ata (open triangles), and helium at 31 ata (open circles). Cooling capacity is defined in the text. At each depth, the cooling capacity decreases linearly with increasing T_I. The slope of the relationship is $-\rho C_P$. All three curves interesect at $T_I=37°C$, where the only heat removal is related to the vaporization of water. At $T_I=0$, the cooling capacity of air at 7 ata is 2.7 times the capacity of air at 1 ata; at 31 ata on helium, the capacity is seven times the capacity on air at 1 ata. Heating of the airways by the inspired gas stream is predicted at $T_I=50°C$ on air at 7 ata and at $T_I=41°C$ on helium at 31 ata.

D. Local Airway Heat Exchange

Invasive measurement of the air and mucosal temperature in the upper airways of humans was first described by Seeley, Cole, and others in the early 1940s (52). The first invasive measurements of the lower airways were reported in 1946 (53). Since that time, numerous studies have been published of intra-airway temperatures in humans during hot- and cold-gas breathing at normobaric pressures, usually in the context of cold-induced asthma. These studies have shown that cold gas can penetrate the airways beyond the level of the subsegmental bronchi and that the magnitude of the temperature gradient observed in the airways is a function of the temperature, water content, and thermal capacity of the inspired gas as well as the respiratory minute ventilation (15,54,55).

In contrast, and despite the magnitude of the problem, there are no studies of heat and mass transfer at the airway level in humans under hyperbaric conditions. Only two studies in model systems and one study in dogs are available for examination (20,21,56–58).

When turbulent flow is well developed, heat transfer in long, smooth, straight pipes can be described by the relationship:

$$Nu = A\,(RePr)^{N} \tag{7}$$

where: Nu = Nusselt number = hcd/k (dimensionless)
A = a constant
Re = Reynolds number = $\rho vd/\mu$ (dimensionless)
Pr = Prandtl number = $C_P\mu/k$ (dimensionless)
N = an exponent
d = pipe diameter (cm)
v = gas velocity (cm/sec)
hc = convective heat-transfer coefficient ($J/cm^2 \cdot sec \cdot {}^\circ K$)
k = gas thermal conductivity ($J/sec \cdot cm \cdot {}^\circ K$)
μ = gas viscosity ($g/cm \cdot sec$)

Using the definition of the Nusselt number, Eq. (4) may be rearranged to solve directly for the convective heat transfer coefficient:

$$hc = k\,A\,(RePr)^{N}/d \tag{8}$$

Flow in most of the upper airway and major bronchi can be described as turbulent. However, with the short segment lengths, uneven branching, and curved paths characteristic of the tracheobronchial tree, flow can hardly be described as well developed. Nevertheless, Eq. (7) is believed to apply to the airways also, at least as a first approximation.

Linderoth and Nuckols (20,21,56) studied convective heat transfer in two bifurcating pipe models similar in configuration to the human tracheobronchial tree but larger in size. The models consisted of three segments with two bifurcations simulating the trachea, main stem bronchi, and lobar bronchi. Heat transfer was measured during the quasi–steady state flow of air or helium-oxygen at depths from 1 to 4 ata. Flow was either in the inspiratory or expiratory direction and was varied to produce Reynolds numbers varying from 200 to 34,000. Wall temperature was maintained at a constant value throughout the length of the model. Linderoth and Nuckols found that both inspiratory and expiratory heat transfer across the broad range of conditions could be described by the single relationship:

$$Nu = 0.0733\,(RePr)^{0.731} \tag{9}$$

Johnson (57) followed the work of Linderoth and Nuckols with a study in anesthetized, intubated dogs. Animals were exposed to air and helium-oxygen mixtures at depths ranging from 1 to 10 ata and to gas temperatures ranging from 2 to 27°C. Mucosal and airstream temperatures were measured in the trachea and in the main stem bronchi. Johnson again found that a single relationship could describe the data:

$$\text{Nu}=0.303\ (\text{RePr})^{0.786} \tag{10}$$

Heat transfer in the bifurcating pipe model of the lower airway was found to be three to four times greater than for smooth pipe, while the transfer rates in the dog were nearly ten times greater. The steadily increasing transfer moving from smooth pipe to the branching pipe model to the actual airway was attributed to the steadily increasing geometric complexity of the system.

Nuckols et al. (58) also studied convective heat transfer in a plastic cast of the human upper airway. The cast extended from the nasal and oral portals down to the bifurcation of the trachea. The heat transfer characteristics were measured for air, nitrogen, and helium at pressures ranging from 1 to 31 ata. The following relationships were observed:

$$\text{Nasal inhalation: Nu}=0.028\ (\text{RePr})^{0.854} \tag{11}$$

$$\text{Oral inhalation: Nu}=0.035\ (\text{RePr})^{0.804} \tag{12}$$

Again, both the oral and nasal passages showed enhanced heat transfer relative to smooth pipe. The nasal passage proved slightly more efficient in heat exchange than the oral passage. Nuckols et al. found that the ratio of oral to nasal conditioning capacity could be described as:

$$\eta_{\text{oral}}/\eta_{\text{nasal}}=1.04\ \text{Re}^{-0.05} \tag{13}$$

At low Reynolds numbers, characteristic of shallow diving, the oral passage had approximately 80% of the capacity of the nasal passage. At the high Reynolds numbers, characteristic of deep diving, this capacity ratio declined to approximately 60%. In humans at 1 ata, it has been observed that respiratory heat loss is greater during oral breathing than during nasal breathing but that the difference between the two is less than 10% (59).

Using the Linderoth-Nuckols equation for heat transfer in the lower tract [Eq. (9)], the convective heat-transfer coefficients in the trachea ($d=1.8$ cm) at $\dot{V}_E=40$ L/min can be calculated for the three representative environmental conditions discussed above: air at 1 ata, air at 7 ata and helium at 31 ata. The respective values for hc are 4.58×10^{-3}, 18.99×10^{-3}, and 71.20×10^{-3} J/sec·cm^2·°K. Relative to air at 1 ata, hc is increased 4.15-fold on air at 7 ata and 15.55-fold on helium at 31 ata. These increases, however, are less than the relative increases in the heat capacity of the gases (J/L·°K). The latter are increased 7- and 22-fold respectively under the same conditions. Greater penetration of cold gas into the airways, therefore, can be expected at depth (see below).

There have be no measurements of water vapor-transfer in the airways under hyperbaric conditions. Nuckols et al. (21,58), however, have reviewed a method where mass transfer can be inferred from measurements of heat transfer. This method relies on the Chilton-Colburn j-factor analogy, which assumes that similarities exist between heat and mass transfer under a wide range of gas-flow conditions.

According to the Chilton-Colburn analogy (60), the mass-transfer coefficient can be calculated from the convective heat-transfer coefficient as follows:

$$h_D = h_c (Pr/Sc)^{0.67} / \rho C_P \tag{14}$$

where: h_D = mass transfer coefficient (cm/sec)*
Sc = Schmidt number = $\mu/\rho D_{H_2O}$ (dimensionless)

This equation is frequently referred to as the Chilton-Colburn correction to the Lewis relation. Using the convective heat-transfer coefficients calculated above for the trachea at $\dot{V}_E$=40 L/min, the corresponding mass-transfer coefficients for air at 1 ata, air at 7 ata, and helium at 31 ata can be calculated as 4.57, 2.88, and 1.82 cm/sec, respectively. The h_D is reduced to 63% of the 1 ata value with air at 7 ata and to 40% with helium at 31 ata. The capacity of the respiratory heat exchanger to transfer water vapor to the gas stream, therefore, is progressively reduced at depth. Since the mass of water required to condition the gas is essentially constant and independent of depth for normal air and helium diving (see above), the inspired gas can be expected to penetrate deeper into the airways at depth before full conditioning is achieved.

For the evaluation of h_D, D_{H_2O} at 7 ata on air and 31 ata on helium was assumed to be 10% higher than the value predicted by the $1/P_B$ relationship (24). This increase over theory has the effect of reducing the Schmidt number, which otherwise would have remained constant with increasing depth. If the Schmidt number is held constant, the calculated values of h_D at 7 ata air and 31 ata helium are 2.84 and 1.71 cm/sec, respectively. This is a further 1% reduction in mass transfer for air at 7 ata and a further 7% reduction for helium at 31 ata, both calculations reflecting the lower assumed value for D_{H_2O}.

The extent to which cold gas can penetrate the airways in hyperbaric conditions remains undefined. Nuckols (21) used the convective and mass-transfer coefficients derived from his modeling efforts to predict the location of gas warming in the human respiratory system at 31 ata (Fig. 5). With inspired gas at 20°C and $\dot{V}_E$=20 L/min, conditioning was complete by the 12th bifur-

*This unit is the reduced form of the mass flux (g/sec) per unit area (cm^2) per unit of driving gradient (g/cm^3).

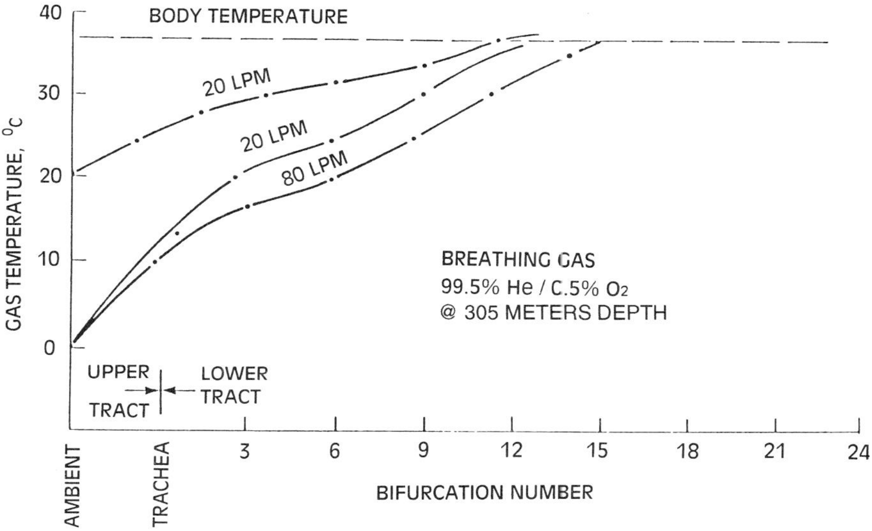

Figure 5 Gas conditioning in the human respiratory system during inhalation of cold helium-oxygen at 305 msw (31.1 ata). Cold helium-oxygen is predicted to penetrate deeply into the lung. Large increases in pulmonary ventilation or decreases in gas temperature increase the depth of penetration only slightly because of the low gas flows and high surface areas for exchange at this level of the airways. (From Ref. 21.)

cation. When the temperature was lowered to 0°C, only one additional airway generation was required to bring the gas to alveolar temperature. If $\dot{V}_E$ was increased to 80 L/min, however, conditioning was not complete until the 15th bifurcation. Nuckols assumed a constant airway wall temperature throughout. If a more sophisticated model incorporating an axial gradient of wall temperature had been used, the calculated penetration would have been further. More sophisticated models of heat mass transfer in the airways are available (61,62), but they have not been applied to the hyperbaric situation.

Unfortunately, there are no measurements of airway temperatures available in humans under hyperbaric conditions to confirm Nuckols' predictions. Jacquemin (6) measured esophageal temperature during cold-gas breathing at 5 ata. At esophageal depths of 17, 25, and 33 cm, temperatures remained considerably below 37°C and were inversely related to the respiratory minute ventilation. Similar esophageal effects were seen in a lost-bell survival study at 16 ata (63). Esophageal temperatures fell when respiratory gas heaters were removed and increased when they were put back on. McFadden (15) estimates that temperatures in the retrotracheal esophagus may be 8 to 9°C higher than the corresponding airway temperatures during the inhalation of cold gas at normobaric pressures. Presumably the difference would be at least as great under hyperbaric conditions.

Johnson (57) measured airway temperatures in anesthetized intubated dogs breathing air at 190 fsw (6.8 ata) and helium-oxygen at 300 fsw (10.1 ata). With inspired gas temperatures near 0°C, an axial gradient of both airway and wall temperature was observed. Temperatures in the distal left main stem bronchus were approximately 33°C on air at 1 ata and 23 to 25°C on both air at 6.8 ata and helium-oxygen at 10 ata. Measurements at more distal sites or deeper depths could not be made because of technical difficulties.

Johnson (57) made the interesting observation that airway wall temperatures did not immediately fall to new steady-state values upon institution of cold-gas breathing. The fall in airway temperature was exponential and had a fairly long time constant. Some 30 to 60 min was required to reach a new plateau. A similar finding was reported by McFadden and Pichurko (54) in humans at 1 ata. During either exercise or eucapnic hyperventilation in the cold, airway temperature declined steadily over the 4-min exposure period. Johnson (57) also reported the occurrence of a sudden exponential rise in airway temperature to a new steady-state plateau after 30 min of exposure to cold hyperbaric air, suggesting the possibility of airway vasodilation after some period of cold exposure. This effect was not seen with hyperbaric helium.

It should be pointed out that the predictions made by Nuckols (21) are in general agreement with the hypothesis put forward by Cole (52) and McFadden (15) that increasing demands on the respiratory heat exchanger are met not by increasing nasopharyngeal or bronchial blood flow but by pushing the site of final conditioning deeper into the lung. With each successive airway generation, the conditioning capacity increases because of the greater surface area, the slower gas flow, and the more immediate proximity of the gas stream to the airway wall. In the Nuckols model, only one airway generation was needed to deal with a 20°C decrease in inspired gas temperature at 31 ata.

There is considerable controversy in the literature as to whether the heat required to condition the inspired gas arises primarily from the nasopharyngeal and bronchial circulations or from the pulmonary circulation (54,64–66). The large heat fluxes associated with hyperbaric exposure suggest that the pulmonary circulation must be involved, at least at high heat loads (67). For example, Hoke et al. (7) observed a respiratory heat loss of 778 W at 1000 fsw in a diver breathing helium-oxygen at 5.5°C and working at an oxygen consumption rate of 2.6 L/min. The expired gas temperature was 31.2°C. The specific heat of blood is 4.08 J/ml·°C. Assuming that blood entered the exchanging area at 37°C and left at a temperature equal to the calculated mean airway temperature, 27.7°C [(37+18.3)/2], a flow of 1,226 ml/min would have been required to deliver the requisite heat. This flow is far greater than the nasopharyngeal and bronchial blood flows. Bronchial blood flow, for example, is estimated to be less than 1% of the resting cardiac output (68). Involvement of the pulmonary circulation is not surprising given the extent to which cold helium-oxygen is able to penetrate the lung (Fig. 5). Even at 1 ata, however, hyperventilation with air has been shown to be a viable technique for measuring pulmonary blood flow (69).

III. Pathophysiology of Cold-Gas Inhalation

A. Signs and Symptoms

Inhalation of cold gas at depth may produce a transient sensation of facial cold and dyspnea (41) followed by a more sustained sensation of intense cold (or pain) in the upper airways and a feeling of chest tightness or substernal discomfort. At low levels of heat loss, this discomfort is confined to the upper airways. At high levels of heat loss, the entire substernal area down to and including the epigastrium may be involved (42–44,67,70).

More important from the standpoint of diver safety is the increased flow of saliva that develops almost immediately upon initiating the cold-gas breathing episode and the excessive secretion of copious, thick respiratory tract mucus that follows shortly thereafter (7,8,43). These secretions can plug the diver's airway and breathing apparatus, cause acute respiratory difficulty, and stop an individual from working. The exact origin of the respiratory tract secretions is unknown, but it is likely that the nasal and oral pharynx as well as the trachea and bronchi are involved. Auscultation of the chest reveals coarse rhonchi that clear with coughing. Breathing warm gas will cause the reaction to subside, but up to 15 to 20 min of warm-gas breathing may be required (43). Therefore, simply returning power to a failed breath heater after the bronchorrhea is well established may not be sufficient to remove the diver from danger. There is marked individual variability in the susceptibility to this reaction, both in terms of its severity and the time of onset. Within a given individual, the reaction is reproducible on a subsequent exposure.

Hayes (43,71) noted that excessive mucus production was likely when the total respiratory heat loss exceeded 200 W. This is generally consistent with the observations of Piantadosi et al. (42), whose divers remained free of excessive production of mucus at respiratory heat losses up to 224 W at 1800 fsw (55.5 ata).

Other reactions include headache, visual disturbance, cough, and shivering. Shivering usually begins in the chest muscles, spreads to the abdomen then the back, and finally extends to the upper and lower limbs. Low back pain may result (41). In high-heat-loss situations, shivering may become uncontrollable and intense: shivering of the neck and jaw muscles may make it impossible for the diver to hold a mouthpiece.

B. Alterations in Pulmonary Mechanics

Hoke et al. (7) were the first to describe the pulmonary mechanical changes associated with cold-helium breathing at depths to 1000 fsw (31 ata). In the experiments described earlier, they measured FEV_1 after 5 and 55 min of exposure to 0 to 7°C gas while the divers remained breathing the cold helium. After 5 min of exposure, FEV_1 was unchanged from the corresponding warm-gas control value at depths to 200 fsw (7 ata). Deeper than 200 fsw, FEV_1 essentially fell linearly with increasing depth, to reach a low value of 60 to 70% of the warm control value at 800 fsw (25 ata), the severest thermal condition tested. Reductions in FEV_1 were also seen after 55 min of exposure, but the magnitude was substantially less than after 5 min of exposure despite an intervening 26-min period of exercise on cold gas at workloads of 30 to 120 W (Fig. 6).

Hoke et al. (7) also measured VC, FEV_1, MVV, and FIV_{25-75} before and immediately following each cold-gas breathing episode. These episodes were either 1 or 4 hr in duration and involved intermittent exercise. No change in any parameter was seen except for a 30% reduction in FIV_{25-75} in one subject at 850 and 1000 fsw (27 and 31 ata). The other subject showed no change in FIV_{25-75}.

Clarke et al. (72) examined pulmonary function immediately following 30 min of mild exercise ($\dot{V}_E$=30 L/min) in divers exposed to inspired helium-oxygen temperatures of 12, 22, and 32°C at 1000 fsw (31 ata). These temperatures corresponded to heat losses of 80, 159, and 229 W respectively, substantially less than the thermal loads imposed by Hoke et al. and more in line with maximal loads recommended for diving operations. Respiratory resistance was measured with an interrupter technique (73). Contrary to expectations, respiratory resistance decreased by 49 to 50% following exercise at the two lower temperatures. At 32°C, respiratory resistance was unchanged after exercise. Clarke et al. also looked at peak expiratory flow rate, FEV_1, FEV_1/FVC, and FEF_{25-75} following exercise. These measurements were made approximately 15 min after the subjects had resumed breathing warm gas. No change in any parameter from the pre-exposure control was noted. Clarke et al. concluded that for respiratory heat losses up to 230 W at 1000 fsw (31 ata), no compromise in pulmonary mechanical function was present.

Jammes et al. (44) measured total lung resistance (R_L) in three resting divers breathing warm (28.5 to 33°C) or cold (8°C) helium oxygen at pressures up to 25 ata. R_L was measured with the technique of Mead and Whittenberger (74). In contrast to the studies of Clarke et al. (72), they found a detectable increase in R_L at 2 to 3 ata, a 30 to 55% increase at 8 ata, and a 38 to 95% increase at 25 ata. A linear relationship was observed between the increase in R_L and the additional respiratory heat loss incurred when the diver switched

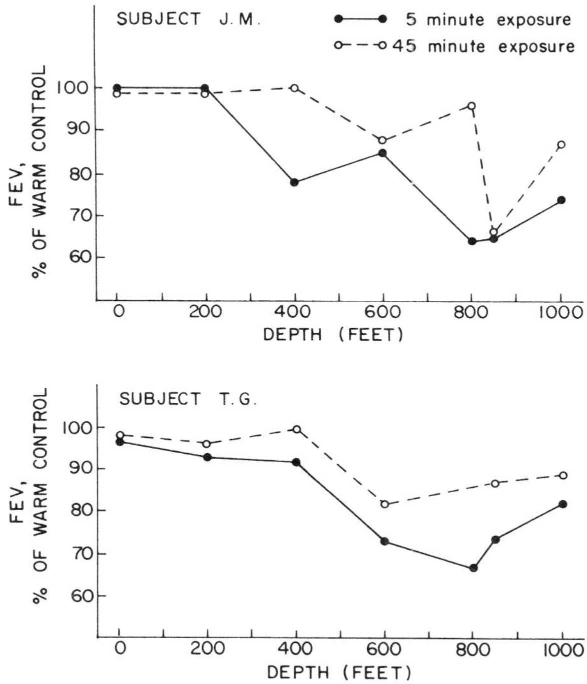

Figure 6 Change in FEV_1 after cold-gas inhalation at depth. Values shown are a percentage of the warm-gas control value determined at each depth. Inspired gas temperatures were 0°C from 0 to 850 fsw, then increased to 7°C at 1000 fsw. FEV_1 is decreased on cold gas deeper than 200 fsw. The decreases in FEV_1 are greater after 5 min on cold gas than after 45 min, despite the intervening period of heavy exercise and high respiratory heat loss (see text for details). (From Ref. 7.)

from warm to cold gas. At the deepest depth, the increase in RL could not be reversed by performing vital capacity maneuvers. At 8 ata and shallower, however, vital capacity maneuvers were frequently effective in reversing the increase in RL.

The most notable difference between the study of Clarke et al. (72) and Jammes et al. (44) is that Jammes' subjects remained at rest throughout the study while Clarke's subjects were studied after performing mild exercise. That exercise might exert some protective effect in this situation is suggested by the data of Hoke et al. (7) (Fig. 6). Following a period of sustained heavy exercise during which heat loss was high, Hoke et al. (7) observed that the reduction in FEV_1 was actually less than during the initial resting exposure to cold gas. This is consistent with the finding that exercise in normal subjects leads to bronchodilation (75).

Burnet et al. (45) extended the RL observations of Jammes et al. (44) to a total pressure of 46 ata, confirming previous findings in an additional four subjects. A significant increase in RL was observed in one or more subjects at inspired gas temperatures of 18 to 19°C at 46 ata, 17°C at 36 ata, 9 to 11°C at 21 ata, and 7.5°C at 12.5 ata. No change in RL was seen with 7°C gas at ambient pressures lower than 12.5 ata. A linear relationship was observed between the increase in RL and the degree of convective respiratory cooling. RL increased 20% when convective heat losses reached 1.4 kcal/min (98 W).

These hyperbaric observations may be compared to the pulmonary mechanical changes observed in normal men breathing cold air at 1 ata. At −30°C, Guleria (76) observed a doubling of inspiratory resistance and an 8% decrease in MBC in subjects at rest. No changes in FEV_1, MMEFR, dynamic compliance, or expiratory flow resistance were seen. At −18°C, Gilbert (55) was unable to detect any change in FEV_1 in exercising subjects with ventilations ranging between 36 and 56 L/min. At the same temperature, Deal (77) was also unable to detect any change in residual volume, FEV_1, or specific airway conductance 5 min after completion of exercise with minute ventilations in the vicinity of 100 L/min. At −9 and −10°C, Gilbert (78,79) was unable to detect any significant change in FEV_1 with eucapnic hyperventilation at 75 L/min. O'Cain (80), however, did see an 8% reduction in FEV_1 at −10°C when the rate of eucapnic hyperventilation was increased to 123 L/min. At −5°C, Decramer (81,82), using the forced-oscillation technique, observed a 20% increase in total lung resistance 1 min after completing 3 min of eucapnic hyperventilation at 60% of MBC. This effect lasted for approximately 4 min. No changes in slow vital capacity, FRC, FEV_1, peak expiratory flow rate, or plethysmographically determined airway resistance (Raw) were seen when these variables were measured 2 to 8 min posthyperventilation. To date, no one has attempted to correlate the normobaric and hyperbaric findings through the magnitude of the heat fluxes involved.

Divers usually breathe gases with an oxygen partial pressure above the normal value of 0.21 ata. At normobaric pressures, an elevation in the inspired oxygen partial pressure has been observed to blunt the bronchoconstrictive response to exercise in asthmatics (75,83). No effect is observed in normal subjects, however, and it is unlikely that the hyperoxic environment associated with diving offers any specific protection against cold-induced bronchoconstriction.

Recently, Thorsen et al. (84) have focused attention on the pulmonary mechanical changes associated with breathing dry gas. They reported a 4% reduction in FEV_1 and an 8.6% reduction in FEF_{25-75} following dives to 6 ata in which the divers breathed warm, dry air. Minimal changes were seen when these same dives were performed with warm, humid gas. Convective respiratory heat losses under these conditions were calculated to be minimal, but mucosal heat and water losses were increased in the dry-gas condition due to evaporative water loss.

The pathophysiological mechanisms underlying the pulmonary mechanical changes with cold-gas breathing are complex and only partially understood. A detailed discussion is beyond the scope of this chapter. Giesbrecht (85) provides an excellent recent review.

C. Alterations in Pulmonary Ventilation

At 1 ata, a voluntary change in respiratory pattern to one of low frequency and high tidal volume enhances the loss of respiratory heat (38,86). This is precisely the pattern adopted by divers when confronted by high gas density and respiratory flow resistance. Nevertheless, the breathing of cold gas itself appears to have no influence on the pattern of breathing. Systematic variations in respiratory frequency or tidal volume cannot be demonstrated with cold-gas breathing either at 1 ata (27,87) or at elevated pressure (7,44,50). Even with precise control of respiratory frequency with a metronome, Burnett et al. (50) were unable to discern any alteration in V_T or $\dot{V}_E$ with cold-gas breathing.

Studies of the ventilatory response to increased metabolic demand during cold-gas breathing at depth are extremely limited. Hoke et al. (7) were unable to discern any consistent effect of cold-gas breathing on the relationship between $\dot{V}_E$ and metabolic rate (measured as $\dot{V}_{CO_2}$) in exercising divers to depths of 31 ata (Fig. 7). These subjects were breathing cold helium while immersed in a warm-chamber environment. In resting subjects breathing cold gas while simultaneously exposed to a cold helium-oxygen environment at 21 ata, Piantadosi (41) observed a marked variation in the $\dot{V}_E/\dot{V}_{O_2}$ ratio, ranging from a low of 28 to a high of 44. Subjects with the lowest values of skin insulation had the highest ratios and therefore lost heat through both avenues at an accelerated rate. The $\dot{V}_E/\dot{V}_{O_2}$ patterns were similar to the hyperventilation sometimes seen during immersion in cold water and may not have been a specific effect of the inhaled gas but rather related to the cutaneous cold stress. In a subsequent study of resting divers at 43.4 and 55.5 ata breathing cold gas but immersed in a warm-chamber environment, Piantadosi et al. (42) observed a 16 to 22% decrease in the $\dot{V}_E/\dot{V}_{O_2}$ ratio when metabolic rate increased. It was unclear, however, whether this was a true decrease or an artifact of a nonzero intercept in the $\dot{V}_E/\dot{V}_{O_2}$ relationship.

Piantadosi (41,42) also observed that the respiratory heat loss associated with cold-gas breathing at depth was not well compensated. When subjects were immersed in a cold hyperbaric environment, metabolism increased to match skin losses but not respiratory losses. When the skin was kept warm and the only avenue of heat loss was through the respiratory system, core body temperature

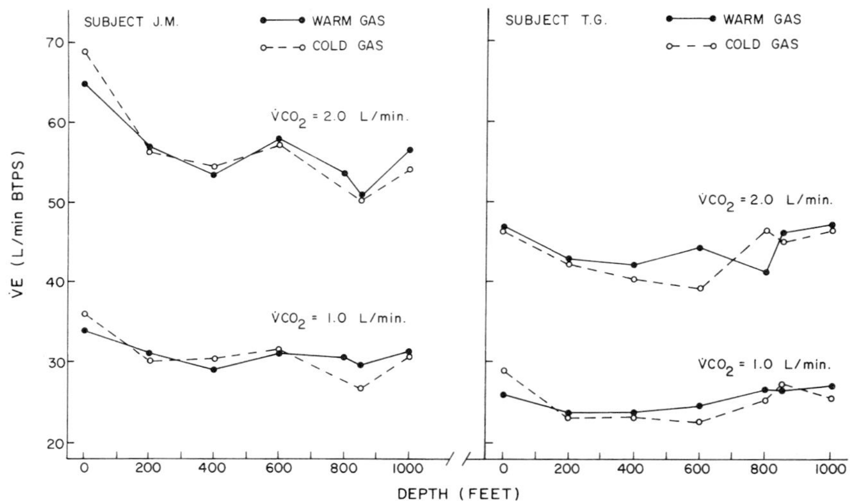

Figure 7 Pulmonary ventilation during warm- and cold-gas breathing as a function of depth. Pulmonary ventilation at 1 and 2 L/min CO_2 production is shown as a function of depth in two exercising subjects breathing either warm gas (closed circles) or cold gas (open circles). Cold-gas breathing does not appear to significantly alter the relationship between pulmonary ventilation and metabolism. (From Ref. 7.)

dropped without an increase in metabolic rate unless the rate of decrease in core temperature exceeded 0.7°C/hr. When metabolic rate did increase, the excess heat production was dissipated through the associated increase in pulmonary ventilation, allowing the core temperature to continue to drop. Similar results were reported by Timbal et al. (37).

There are no reported studies of pulmonary gas exchange during cold-gas breathing at hyperbaric pressures.

D. Pathological Changes

The rapid recovery of divers from the effects of cold-gas breathing once they are removed to a warm environment suggests that pathological changes, if present, are minimal. There have been no direct observations of the airways of humans following hyperbaric cold exposures. In tracheostomized dogs subjected to cold-gas breathing at depths of 190 and 300 fsw for prolonged periods and then autopsied, the upper trachea appeared dry and traumatized (57). It was uncertain whether this represented the effects of the cold-gas exposure or trauma related to the surgical procedure. Given the conditioning capacity of the upper airway and the fact that hyperbaric gases are almost always above freezing, the likelihood of significant injury to the larynx, tracheobronchial tree, or lung is low.

IV. Inspired Gas Temperature Limits

A. Historical Evolution

Following the initial cold-gas studies of Hoke et al. (7) and Goodman et al. (8), Braithwaite (88) developed a minimum inspired-gas temperature curve for use by the U.S. Navy. It was based primarily on Goodman's observation that divers in hot-water suits performing moderate work could breathe 2°C helium-oxygen at 21 ata for 90 min or more without major discomfort or task performance degradation. This temperature corresponded to an RHL of approximately 270 W at $\dot{V}_E$=40 L/min. Braithwaite refitted the T_E/T_I data obtained by Goodman to derive the relationship, $T_E = 24.4 + 0.32\ T_I$. He then used this relationship and the first term of Eq. (1) to calculate the inspired temperature at other depths that would produce the same heat loss per liter of ventilation as 2°C at 21 ata. The resultant curve is shown in Fig. 8. No account was taken of evaporative losses or the fact that losses would be substantially higher than 270 W during hard work.

The Braithwaite curve remained the standard for about 8 years. In the interim, accumulating operational and experimental experience suggested that the limits might be too low. In 1982, Hayes (43) reported a study demonstrating conclusively that the Braithwaite limits were inadequate to prevent the development of excessive respiratory secretions and dyspnea in working divers in hot-water suits. At 19 ata, Hayes observed excessive respiratory secretions after 15 to 20 min if T_I was allowed to go below 12°C (Braithwaite limit, −1°C). At 30 ata, secretions were observed in less than 5 min if T_I was set below 10°C. With T_I at or above the 13°C Braithwaite limit at 30 ata, secretions were still observed but could be managed by the divers if ventilation did not exceed 20 to 25 L/min.

Piantadosi (49) revisited the U.S. Navy limits in 1980 and again in 1982. He noted that a resting diver had a metabolic heat production of 56 W/m^2. In a hot-water suit, cutaneous heat loss was 50 W/m^2, leaving 6 W/m^2 to be lost through the respiratory system in thermal balance. He further observed that additional respiratory heat loss above 6 W/m^2 would not trigger the usual increase in metabolic rate that cutaneous loss did but rather resulted in a linear fall in rectal temperature proportional to the magnitude of the loss. He selected a core cooling rate of 0.25°C/hr to allow for a 4-hr exposure with no more than a 1°C temperature drop. This rate of cooling was equivalent to a heat-removal rate from body stores of 14 W/m^2, allowing a total respiratory heat loss of 20

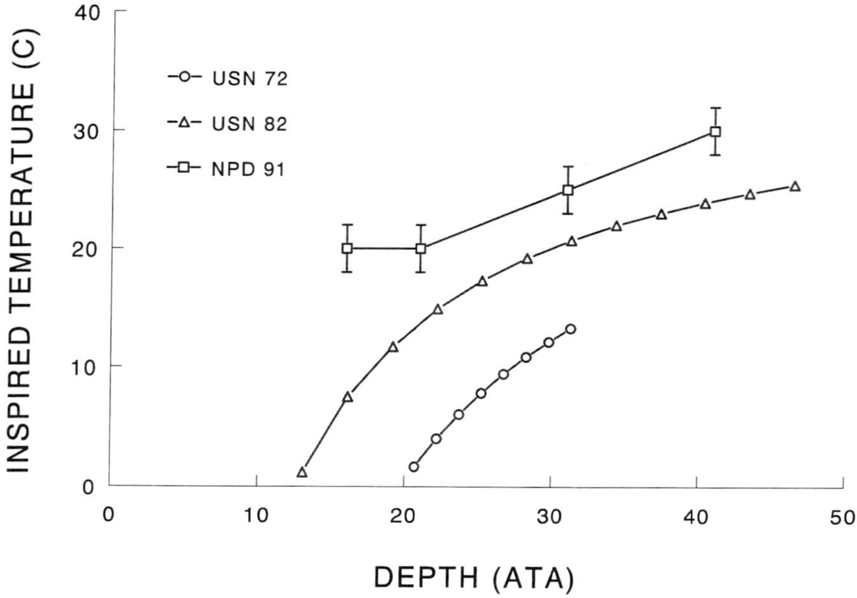

Figure 8 Inspired gas temperature limits as a function of depth. Curve labeled USN 72 is from Braithwaite (87). Curve labeled USN 82 is from Piantadosi (49) and gives the minimum values currently allowed by the U.S. Navy. The curve with error bars (NPD 91) is the Norwegian Petroleum Directorate 1991 Guideline (88).

W/m^2 (14+6). Inspired temperatures corresponding to this level of RHL were computed for the depths of interest using the first term of Eq. (1), a body surface area of 2 m^2, a $\dot{V}_E$=8 L/min BTPS, and T_E=25.4+0.28 T_I. Evaporative losses were not considered. Although computed for rest, these temperatures were considered applicable to work as well. With exercise, both respiratory heat loss and metabolic heat production will increase. Piantadosi calculated that unless the $\dot{V}_E/\dot{V}_{O_2}$ ratio exceeded 69 (an extremely high value), the diver would always gain body heat with exercise. This excess heat would be dissipated by slowing the flow of hot water to the suit. Piantadosi's analysis was based entirely on whole-body heat balance. No consideration was given to possible adverse effects on the lungs at ventilation rates higher than rest. The Piantadosi curve is shown in Fig. 8.

B. Current Standards

Minimum inspired gas temperature limits currently used by the U.S. Navy are shown in Fig. 8. These are essentially the limits developed by Piantadosi (49) and subsequently modified slightly in 1982. They are minimum limits and are designed to be exceeded whenever heating technology allows. The U.S. Navy limits are substantially lower than the limits currently given in the Norwegian Petroleum Directorate Guidelines (1991) (89) for North Sea operations. In that sector, gas heating is required deeper than 150 msw. The limits thereafter are given as follows:

150 msw (492 fsw)	20 ± 2°C
200 msw (656 fsw)	20 ± 2°C
300 msw (984 fsw)	25 ± 2°C
400 msw (1312 fsw)	30 ± 2°C

The Norwegian limits are more in line with current thinking about the needs for diver comfort and safety and also reflect improvements in gas heating technology.

No systematic work has been done to establish the upper limits for inspired gas temperature. The Norwegian Petroleum Directorate Guidelines (1991) state that the gas should never exceed 37°C. The x-intercept of Fig. 4 suggests that temperatures over 41°C at 31 ata might begin to prove stressful. The few warm-gas studies available for examination have used breath heaters either in the context of a "lost bell'' scenario to prevent hypothermia or in the context of rewarming hypothermic divers returning to the hyperbaric chamber environment. In lost-bell studies, divers at 16 ata tolerated gas at 34 to 39°C without difficulty in one study (90), while in two others some divers complained the gas was too hot even at 34.5°C (63,91,92). In the rewarming studies, two hypothermic divers were able to breathe humidified gas at 38 to 43°C at 26 ata continuously for 40 min without difficulty (43,70). In one wet study where 6 divers were immersed in 4 to 9°C water with hot-water suits and gas heaters at 51 ata, gas at less than 28°C was considered too cold, gas at 30 to 32°C to be comfortable, and gas at 33.5 to 34°C to be uncomfortably hot (93).

C. Gas Heating

To meet the inspired gas temperature limits outlined above, some form of gas heating is required for most deep diving operations.

In semiclosed and closed-circuit UBAs, some heat from the expired gas is retained in the circuit by the natural insulation of the hoses and breathing bag. Additional heat is provided by the exothermic reaction of the CO_2 scrubber. In these systems, the breathing-loop temperature will rise as a direct function of the diver's depth, and this alone may be sufficient in some circumstances to avoid excessive respiratory heat loss in some systems. Frequently, however, supplemental heat is provided by circulating hot water to the CO_2 canister or by simply flooding the entire rig with hot water (94). A metal sponge placed in the oronasal mask may trap some heat from the exhaled gas and return it to the subsequent inspiration. Semiclosed and closed-circuit systems have the additional advantage that the gas is humidified.

Historically, heating has proven more difficult in open-circuit demand systems. Not only must more heat be supplied than in closed systems but the heat exchanger must be placed in the gas supply line and may add breathing resistance. In addition, the gas is dry. For nearly all open-circuit systems, hot-water heating is currently used and engineering design has progressed to the point where this heating is very effective. Equipment may take the form of an in-line heat exchanger with the discharge water flowing through a rubber shroud over the intermediate pressure line and second-stage regulator. In some applications, simply the shroud itself has been found to provide a satisfactory result.

V. Summary

The specific heat (J/L·°K) of air at 1 ata is quite low. Accordingly, most of the respiratory heat exchange is related to the vaporization of water, and a very wide range of inspired gas temperatures (−40 to +75°C) can be tolerated without difficulty. At hyperbaric pressures, the reverse is observed. The specific heat of the gas mixture is elevated and the convective component of respiratory heat transfer dominates. Vaporization of water plays only a minor role. As the specific heat of the gas mixture increases with depth, the range of tolerable inspired gas temperature decreases. At deep depths, respiratory heat losses in an unprotected airway can approach the total metabolic heat production, resulting in the rapid development of hypothermia. Cold gases can also increase airway resistance and lead to a disturbing syndrome of airway pain, copious secretions, and dyspnea, which can become life-threatening for a diver in the water. Accordingly, most deep dives require some form of gas heating. Minimum inspired gas temperature limits have been established through a combination of study and practical experience. Upper bounds for inspired temperature are less well defined, although it is clear that temperatures only a few degrees above body temperature can be tolerated at the deepest depths.

References

1. Webb P, Annis WF. Respiratory heat loss with high density gas mixtures. Final Report on Contract NONR 4965(00). Washington, DC: Office of Naval Research, Department of the Navy, May 1966.
2. Webb P. Body heat loss in undersea gaseous environments. Aerospace Med 1970; 41:1282–1288.
3. Tauber JF, Rawlins JSP, Bondi KR. Theoretical thermal requirements for the Mark II diving system. Project M4306.02-6010B, Report No. 2. Bethesda, MD: Naval Medical Research Institute, Department of the Navy, August 1969.

4. Rawlins JSP, Tauber JF. Thermal balance at depth. In: Lambertsen CJ, ed. Underwater Physiology: Proceedings of the Fourth Symposium on Underwater Physiology. New York: Academic Press, 1971:435–442.
5. Varene P, L'Huillier J, Jacquemin C. Deperdition de chaleur par convection respiratoire: Application a l'environnment hyperbare. J Physiol (Paris) 1970; 62(suppl 2):326–327.
6. Jacquemin C, Varene P, L'Huillier J. Aspects respiratoires de l'environnment thermique hyperbare. J Physiol (Paris) 1971; 63:293–295.
7. Hoke B, Jackson DL, Alexander JM, Flynn ET. Respiratory heat loss and pulmonary function during cold-gas breathing at high pressures. In: Lambertsen CJ, ed. Underwater Physiology: V. Proceedings of the Fifth Symposium on Underwater Physiology. Bethesda MD: FASEB 1976:725–740.
8. Goodman MW, Colston JW, Smith NE, Rich EL. Hyperbaric respiratory heat loss study. Final Report on Contract N00014-71-C-0099. Washington DC: Office of Naval Research, Department of the Navy, October 1971.
9. Seeley LE. Study of changes in the temperature and water vapor content of respired air in the nasal cavity. Trans Am Soc Heat Vent Eng 1940; 46:259–290.
10. Burch G. Rate of water and heat loss from the respiratory tract of normal subjects in a subtropical climate. Arch Intern Med 1945; 76:315–327.
11. Webb P. Air temperatures in respiratory tracts of resting subjects in cold. J Appl Physiol 1951; 4:378–382.
12. Ferrus L, Guenard H, Vardon G, Varene P. Respiratory water loss. Respir Physiol 1980; 39:367–381.
13. Ferrus L, Commenges D, Gire J, Varene P. Respiratory water loss as a function of ventilatory or environmental factors. Respir Physiol 1984; 56:11–20.
14. McCutchan JW, Taylor CL. Respiratory heat exchange with varying temperature and humidity of inspired air. J Appl Physiol 1951; 4:121–136.
15. McFadden ER, Pichurko BM, Bowman HF, et al. Thermal mapping of the airways in humans. J Appl Physiol 1985; 58:564–570.
16. McFadden ER, Denison DM, Waller JR, et al. Direct recordings of the temperatures in the tracheobronchial tree in normal man. J Clin Invest 1982; 69:700–705.
17. Lide DR, ed. Handbook of Chemistry and Physics, 73d ed. Boca Raton, FL: CRC Press, 1992.
18. Reid RC, Prausnitz JM, Poling BE. The Properties of Gases and Liquids, 4th ed. New York: McGraw-Hill, 1987.
19. U.S. Navy Diving Gas Manual. NAVSHIPS 0994-003-7010, 2nd ed. Washington DC: Naval Sea Systems Command, Department of the Navy, 1971.
20. Linderoth LS. Heat and mass transfer in the human respiratory tract at hyperbaric pressures. Technical Report. Durham, NC: Duke University School of Engineering, May 1973.
21. Nuckols ML. Heat and water vapor transfer in the human respiratory system at hyperbaric conditions. Technical Report TR 364-81. Panama City, FL: Naval Coastal Systems Center, Department of the Navy, September 1981.
22. Homer LD, Kayar SR. Density, heat capacity, viscosity, and thermal conductivity of mixtures of CO_2, He, H_2, H_2O, N_2 and O_2. Technical Report 94-51. Bethesda, MD: Naval Medical Research Institute, Department of the Navy, July 1994.

23. Paganelli CV, Ar A, Rahn H, Wangensteen OD. Diffusion in the gas phase: The effects of ambient pressure and gas composition. Respir Physiol 1975; 25:247–258.
24. Paganelli CV, Kurata FK. Diffusion of water vapor in binary and ternary gas mixtures at increased pressures. Respir Physiol 1977; 30:15–26.
25. Deaton WM, Frost EM. Water content of compressed gases. Am Gas J, October 1941, p. 70. (Quoted in Ref. 20.)
26. Nishi Y, Gagge AP. Effective temperature scale useful for hypo- and hyperbaric environments. Aviat Space Environ Med 1977; 48:97–107.
27. Cain JB, Livingstone SD, Nolan RW, Keefe AA. Respiratory heat loss during work at various ambient temperatures. Respir Physiol 1990; 79:145–150.
28. Eschenbacher WL, Sheppard D. Respiratory heat loss is not the sole stimulus for bronchoconstriction induced by isocapnic hyperpnea with dry air. Am Rev Respir Dis 1985; 131:894–901.
29. Caldwell PRB, Gomez DM, Fritts HW. Respiratory heat exchange in normal subjects and in patients with pulmonary disease. J Appl Physiol 1969; 26:82–88.
30. Phelipeau D, Ferrus L, Varene P. Les echanges thermiques respiratoires chez l'homme en fonction de la temperature du gaz inspire. J Physiol (Paris) 78:163–169.
31. Hoppe P. Temperatures of expired air under varying climatic conditions. Int J Biometeorol 1981; 25(2):127–132.
32. Solway J, Richurko BM, Ingenito EP, et al. Breathing pattern affects airway wall temperature during cold hyperpnea in humans. Am Rev Respir Dis 1985; 132:853–857.
33. Guenard H, Timbal J, Varene P, Vieillefond H. La deperdition thermique par convection respiratoire en plongee profonde. Forsvarsmedicin 1973; 9:475–480.
34. L'Huillier, Jacquemin C, Varene P. La dissipation de chaleur par convection respiratoire en plongee. In: Fructus X, ed. Third International Conference on Hyperbaric and Underwater Physiology. Paris: Doin, 1972.
35. Varene P, Vieillefond H, Guenard H, L'Huillier J. Experience Sagittaire I: Le bilan thermique des plongeurs en atmosphere helium oxygene. Compte Rendu d'Etude No. 978, Laboratoire de Medecine Aerospatiale, Centre D'Essais en Vol, Bretigny sur Orge, France, October 1972.
36. Varene P, Timbal J, Vieillefond H, Guenard H, L'Huillier J. Energy balance of man in simulated dive from 1.5 to 31 ata. In: Lambertsen CJ, ed. Underwater Physiology: V. Proceedings of the Fifth Symposium on Underwater Physiology. Bethesda, MD: FASEB. 1976.
37. Timbal J, Vieillefond H, Guenard H, Varene P. Metabolism and heat losses of resting man in a hyperbaric helium atmosphere. J Appl Physiol 1974; 36:444–448.
38. Moore TO, Morlock JF. Quantification of heat loss from various routes in man dwelling in a wet/dry hyperbaric environment. Final report on Contract N00014-67-A-0387-0016. Washington, DC: Office of Naval Research, Department of the Navy, June 1976.
39. Moore TO, Morlock JF, Lally DA, Hong SK. Thermal cost of saturation diving: Respiratory and whole body heat loss at 16.1 ata. In: Lambertsen CJ, ed. Underwater Physiology: V. Proceedings of the Fifth Symposium on Underwater Physiology. Bethesda, MD: FASEB, 1976.

40. Varene P, Vieillefond H, Timbal J, et al. Energy balance of divers at work in helium-oxygen atmospheres. In: Shilling CW, Beckett MW, eds. Underwater Physiology: VI. Proceedings of the Sixth Symposium on Underwater Physiology. Bethesda, MD: FASEB, 1978.
41. Piantadosi CA, Thalmann ED. Thermal responses in humans exposed to cold hyperbaric helium-oxygen. J Appl Physiol Respir Environ Exerc Physiol 1980; 49: 1099–1106.
42. Piantadosi CA, Thalmann ED, Spaur WH. Metabolic response to respiratory heat loss-induced core cooling. J Appl Physiol Respir Environ Exerc Physiol 1981; 50: 829–834.
43. Hayes PA, Padbury EH, Florio JT, Fyfield TP. Respiratory heat transfer in cold water and during rewarming. J Biomech Eng 1982; 104:45–49.
44. Jammes Y, Burnet H, Cosson P, Lucciano M. Bronchomotor response to cold air or helium-oxygen at normal and high ambient pressures. Undersea Biomed Res 1988; 15:179–192.
45. Burnet H, Lucciano M, Jammes Y. Respiratory effects of cold-gas breathing in humans under hyperbaric environment. Respir Physiol 1990; 81:413–424.
46. Webb P. Heat loss from the respiratory tract in cold. Project No. 7-1951, Report No. 3. Ladd AFB, AK: Artic Aeromedical Laboratory, 1955.
47. Houdas Y, Colin J. Echanges thermiques et hydriques par les voies respiratoires de l'homme. Pathol Biol 1966; 14(3–4):229–238.
48. Varene P. Computation of respiratory heat exchanges. J Appl Physiol 1986; 61: 1586–1589.
49. Piantadosi CA. Respiratory heat loss limits in helium-oxygen saturation diving. Report No. 10-80. Panama City, FL: Navy Experimental Diving Unit, Department of the Navy, 1980.
50. Burnet H, Reynaud-Gaubert M, Lucciano M, Jammes Y. Relationship between inspired and expired gas temperatures in a hyperbaric environment. Respir Physiol 1992; 90:377–386.
51. Varene P, Kays C. A graphic analysis of respiratory heat exchange. J Appl Physiol 1987; 63:1374–1380.
52. Cole P. Modification of inspired air. In: Mathew OP, Sant'Ambrogio G, eds. Respiratory Function of the Upper Airway. New York: Marcel Dekker, 1988.
53. Pugitt CH, Riley RL. Determination of aqueous vapor tension inired air. Research Project X-475, Report No. 1. Pensacola, FL: Naval School of Aviation Medicine, Department of the Navy, 1946.
54. McFadden ER, Pichurko BM. Intra-airway thermal profiles during exercise and hyperventilation in normal man. J Clin Invest 1985; 76:1007–1010.
55. Gilbert IA, Fouke JM, McFadden ER. Heat and water flux in the intrathoracic airways and exercise-induced asthma. J Appl Physiol 1987; 63:1681–1691.
56. Linderoth LS, Kuonen EA, Nuckols ML, Johnson CE. Heat and mass transfer in the human respiratory tract at hyperbaric pressures. Final Report on Contract N00014-67-A-0251-00018. Washington, DC: Office of Naval Research, Department of the Navy, November 1975.
57. Johnson CE. Deep diving respiratory heat and mass transfer. Ph.D. dissertation. Durham NC: Duke University, 1976.

58. Nuckols ML, Zumrick JL, Johnson CE. Heat and water vapor transport in the human airways at hyperbaric conditions. J Biomech Eng 1983; 105:24–30.
59. Varene P, Ferrus L, Manier G, Gire J. Heat and water respiratory exchanges: Comparison between mouth and nose breathing in humans. Clin Physiol 1986; 6:405–414.
60. Chilton TH, Colburn AP. Mass transfer (absorption) coefficients: Prediction from data on heat transfer and fluid friction. Ind Eng Chem 1934; 26:1183–1187.
61. Hanna LM, Scherer PW. Regional control of local airway heat and water vapor losses. J Appl Physiol 1986; 61:624–632.
62. Ingenito EP, Solway J, McFadden ER, et al. Finite difference analysis of respiratory heat transfer. J Appl Physiol 1986; 61:2252–2259.
63. Tonjum S, Hamilton RW, Brubakk AO, et al. Project Polar Bear: Testing of diver thermal protection in a simulated "lost bell." Report 2-80. Bergen, Norway: Norwegian Underwater Institute, January 1980.
64. Baile EM, Dahlby RW, Wiggs BR, Pare PD. Role of tracheal and bronchial circulation in respiratory heat exchange. J Appl Physiol 1985; 58:217–222.
65. Solway J, Leff AR, Dreshaj I, et al. Circulatory heat sources for canine respiratory exchange. J Clin Invest 1986; 78:1015–1019.
66. McFadden ER. Heat and water exchange in human airways. Am Rev Respir Dis 1992; 146:S8–S10.
67. Hanson RdeG. Respiratory heat loss and other thermal problems of deep diving. J R Naval Med Serv 1975; 61:16–21.
68. Deffebach ME, Widdicombe J. The bronchial circulation. In: Chung KF, Barnes PJ, eds. Pharmacology of the Respiratory Tract. New York: Marcel Dekker, 1993.
69. Serikov VB, Rumm MS, Kambara K, et al. Application of respiratory heat exchange for the measurement of lung water. J Appl Physiol 1992; 72;944–953.
70. Garrard MP, Hayes PA, Carlyle RF, Stock MJ. Metabolic and thermal status of divers during simulated dives to 55 bars. In: Bachrach AJ, Matzen MM, eds. Underwater Physiology: VIII. Proceedings of the Eighth Symposium on Underwater Physiology. Bethesda, MD: Undersea Medical Society, 1984.
71. Hayes P. Cooling in divers following loss of hot water heating: Limits of endurance and the subsequent rewarming procedures. In: Kuehn, LA, ed. Thermal Constraints in Diving. The Twenty-Fourth Undersea Medical Society Workshop. Bethesda, MD: Undersea Medical Society, 1981.
72. Clarke JR, Bradley ME, Flynn ET. Pulmonary function during cold gas breathing at depths to 305 M. In: Bove AA, Bachrach AJ, Greenbaum LJ, eds. Underwater and Hyperbaric Physiology: IX. Proceedings of the Ninth International Symposium on Underwater and Hyperbaric Physiology. Bethesda, MD: Undersea and Hyperbaric Medical Society, 1987.
73. Clarke JR, Jaeger MJ, Zumrick JL, et al. Respiratory resistance from 1 to 46 ata measured with the interrupter technique. J Appl Physiol Respir Environ Exerc Physiol 1982; 52:549–555.
74. Mead J, Wittenberger JL. Physical properties of human lungs measured during spontaneous respiration. J Appl Physiol 1953; 5:779–796.
75. Schiffman PL, Ryan A, Whipp BJ, Hansen JE. Hyperoxic attenuation of exercise-induced bronchospasm in asthmatics. J Clin Invest 1979; 63:30–37.

76. Guleria JS, Talwar JR, Malhotra OP, Pande JN. Effect of breathing cold air on pulmonary mechanics in normal man. J Appl Physiol 1969; 27:320–322.
77. Deal EC, McFadden ER, Ingram RH, Jaeger JJ. Esophageal temperature during exercise in asthmatic and nonasthmatic subjects. J Appl Physiol Respir Environ Exerc Physiol 1979; 46:484–490.
78. Gilbert IA, Regnard J, Lenner KA, et al. Intrathoracic airstream temperatures during acute expansions of thoracic blood volume. Clin Sci 1991; 81:655–661.
79. Gilbert IA, Winslow CJ, Lenner KA, et al. Vascular volume expansion and thermally induced asthma. Eur Respir J 1993; 6:189–197.
80. O'Cain CF, Dowling NB, Slutsky AS, et al. Airway effects of respiratory heat loss in normal subjects. J Appl Physiol 1980; 49:875–880.
81. Decramer M, Demets M, Van de Woestijne KP. Effects of hyperventilation with cold air on respiratory impedence in normal subjects. Bull Eur Physiopathol Respir 1982; 18:105–106P.
82. Decramer M, Demets M. Van de Woestijne KP. Isocapnic hyperventilation with cold air in healthy non-smokers, smokers, and asthmatic subjects. Bull Eur Physiopathol Respir 1984; 20:237–243.
83. Resnick AD, Deal EC, Ingram RH, McFadden ER. A critical assessment of the mechanism by which hyperoxia attenuates exercise-induced asthma. J Clin Invest 1979; 64:541–549.
84. Thorsen E, Ronnestad I, Segadal K, Hope A. Respiratory effects of warm and dry air at increased ambient pressure. Undersea Biomed Res 1992; 19:73–83.
85. Giesbrecht GG. The respiratory system in a cold environment. Aviat Space Environ Med 1995; 66:890–902.
86. Burnet H, Bascou-Bussac M, Martin C, Jammes Y. Relationship between Cr and breathing pattern in mechanically ventilated patients. J Appl Physiol 1994; 77: 2703–2708.
87. Hartung GH, Myhre LG, Nunneley SA. Physiological effects of cold air inhalation during exercise. Aviat Space Environ Med 1980; 51:591–594.
88. Braithwaite WR. The calculation of minimum safe inspired gas temperature limits for deep diving. Report 12-72. Panama City, FL: Navy Experimental Diving Unit, Department of the Navy, 1972.
89. Guidelines for Evaluation of Breathing Apparatus for Use in Manned Underwater Operations in the Petroleum Activities. Stavanger, Norway: Norwegian Petroleum Directorate, 1991.
90. Magnusson J, Holmer I, Elnas S, Hamilton RW. Metabolic rate of divers in a simulated "lost bell'' survival test. In: Bachrach AJ, Matzen MM, eds. Underwater Physiology: VIII. Proceedings of the Eighth Symposium on Underwater Physiology. Bethesda MD: Undersea Medical Society, 1984.
91. Tonjum S, Pasche A, Onarheim J, et al. Cold exposure in heliox environment at 16 bars for 24 hours. In: Bachrach AJ, Matzen MM, eds. Underwater Physiology: VIII. Proceedings of the Eighth Symposium on Underwater Physiology. Bethesda, MD: Undersea Medical Society, 1984.
92. Brubakk AO, Tonjum S, Holand B, et al. Heat loss and tolerance time during cold exposure in heliox atmosphere at 16 ata. Undersea Biomed Res 1982; 9:81–90.

93. Pasche A, Tonjum S, Olsen CR, Holand B. Diver heating during simulated lockout dives at 500 msw. Eighth Annual Congress of the European Undersea Biomedical Society. Lubeck, Germany: Dragerwerk, 1982.
94. Bentz RL. A study of several approaches for supplying a diver with warm breathing gas. Report 105-72. Panama City, FL: Naval Coastal Systems Laboratory, Department of the Navy, 1972.

5

Oxygen Toxicity

JAMES C. PARKER and AUBREY E. TAYLOR

University of South Alabama
Mobile, Alabama

An increasing number of occupational and therapeutic conditions expose humans to high oxygen partial pressures. In addition, hyperbaric oxygen therapy has been used as a standard treatment for decompression sickness in divers for over thirty years (1). Saturation dives at pressures up to 45.4 atm (4.6 MPa) and durations of 4 weeks are now used in many commercial operations (2). These divers are exposed to high P_{O_2} during both work and lengthy decompression periods; they typically have circulating microbubbles in both veins and arteries during decompression (2). Subsequent recompression with oxygen rapidly reduces bubble size and restores perfusion to tissue vessels blocked by bubble microemboli.

Use of normobaric oxygen for the clinical treatment of respiratory failure and adult and infant respiratory distress syndromes (ARDS, IRDS) results in hyperoxic exposure in many critically ill patients. Medical applications of hyperbaric oxygen have increased steadily and have been used successfully to treat carbon monoxide poisoning (3), gas gangrene (4), diabetic gangrene (5), bacterial infections (4,6), skin grafts (1), burns (7), and soft tissue wounds (8), and air emboli produced either by rapid ascent of divers or by iatrogenic accidents during cardiopulmonary bypass or cardiac or pulmonary artery catheterization.

I. Cellular Mechanisms of Hyperoxic Damage

The evolution of oxidative metabolism in animals confers a tremendous advantage for the production of energy through the complete oxidative metabolism of glucose to produce the body's basic energy source, ATP. However, all living organisms exhibit variable signs of toxicity in the presence of excessive oxygen partial pressures. These effects range from anaerobic bacteria, which cease to grow when exposed to even minute amounts of oxygen, to the pathological pulmonary and neurological effects observed in higher animals' exposured to hyperoxia (9,10). Oxygen toxicity is generally considered to result from the formation of oxygen free radicals in excess of the quantity that can be detoxified by the available antioxidant enzyme systems in the tissues (11). Serious oxidative cell damage is normally prevented by (1) cellular mechanisms that minimize the production of reactive oxygen species; (2) compartmentation of free radicals in subcellular organelles; (3) conversion of free radicals to less reactive forms; and (4) rapid repair or replacement of injured cellular components (12).

A. Types of Oxygen Radicals

At ambient temperatures and pressures, oxygen reacts relatively slowly with organic compounds. However, the addition of sufficient energy can change the electron spin direction or pair the unpaired electrons in ground state oxygen to produce a highly reactive metabolite, singlet oxygen. Reactive oxygen metabolites are also formed by incomplete reduction of oxygen by one, two, and three electrons, are shown in Fig. 1. Free radicals are those intermediate reduction products of oxygen and organic molecules that have an unpaired electron (·).

Reactive intermediates of oxygen reduction include superoxide anions ($O_2\cdot^-$), hydrogen peroxide (H_2O_2), and hydroxyl radicals (OH·). Superoxide anion is a relatively weak oxidant that spontaneously dismutates into hydrogen peroxide with a half-time of 10^{-6} sec, but it also is capable of reducing ferric iron to its ferrous state. The dismutation reaction rate is increased ten thousand times by superoxide dismutase (13).

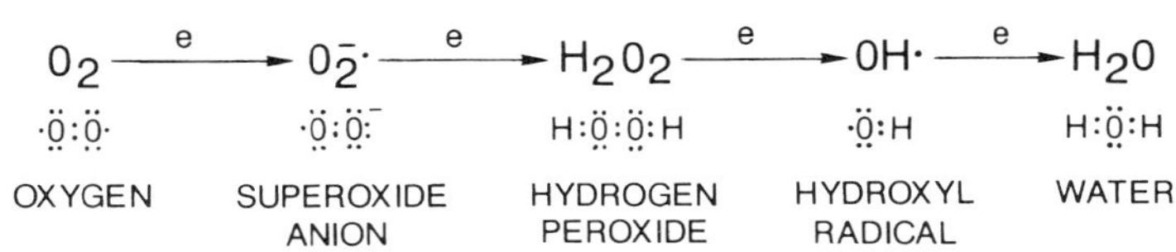

Figure 1 Reduction states of oxygen.

$$2O_2\cdot^- + 2H^+ \rightarrow H_2O_2 + O_2 \qquad (1)$$

H_2O_2 is the two-electron reduction intermediate of oxygen primarily formed from dismutation of superoxide. It reacts relatively slowly with organic compounds and passes through aqueous channels almost as easily as water. Thus, H_2O_2 can diffuse relatively large distances before reacting with tissue components (14). H_2O_2 produces cellular injury primarily through conversion to more reactive species such as the hydroxyl radical (OH·) in the presence of either Fe^{2+} or Cu^{2+} in the catalyzed Fenton reaction:

$$H_2O_2 + Fe^{2+} \rightarrow Fe^{3+} + OH\cdot + OH^- \qquad (2)$$

or in the Haber-Weiss reaction:

$$O_2\cdot^- + H_2O_2 \rightarrow O_2 + OH^- + OH\cdot \qquad (3)$$

OH· is extremely reactive, having a half-life of only one-billionth of a second. Since it reacts with the first available molecule it contacts, it does not diffuse far from its site of generation. OH· can also react with carbohydrates, proteins, and lipids to form peroxyl (ROO·) and alkyl (R·) radicals and undoubtedly causes most serious cellular damage.

A third potential source of OH· is the combination of superoxide with nitric oxide, another free radical, to form peroxynitrite anions.

$$O_2\cdot^- + NO\cdot \rightarrow ONOO^- \qquad (4)$$

$$ONOO^- + H^+ \rightarrow OH\cdot + NO_2\cdot \qquad (5)$$

NO· is produced in small amounts by endothelial cells by the action of NO synthase on L-arginine, but it can also be produced in large amounts by activated neutrophils and macrophages (9). Although NO· has a relatively long biological half-life of several seconds, it reacts with $O_2\cdot^-$ on a molar basis at three times the rate of the superoxide dismutase (SOD) catalyzed dismutation (15). The $ONOO^-$ produced has much the same reactivity as OH· and has considerable potential to initiate peroxidation reactions (16). However, the pro-oxidant effects of NO· depends upon the ratio of NO· to $O_2\cdot^-$ because NO· alone cannot initiate lipid peroxidation and quenches the chain reactions of lipid peroxidation by reacting with alkoyl and peroxyl radicals (15).

Hypohalous acids are also strong oxidants, generated when $O_2\cdot^-$ and H_2O_2 are produced by neutrophils, eosinophils, and macrophages through reactions with myeloperoxidase or eosinophil peroxidase (9). These hypohalous acids have 100 times the oxidizing potential of either $O_2\cdot^-$ or H_2O_2 and are major oxidants produced during an inflammatory response.

$$H_2O_2 + X^- + H^+ \rightarrow HOX + H_2O \qquad (6)$$

where X^- is Cl^-, Br^-, I^-, or SCN^-.

These hypohalous acids further react with amine groups to form chloramines, which have a lower oxidative potential but greater lipid solubility and membrane permeability.

$$RNH + HOCl \rightarrow RNHCl + H_2O \qquad (7)$$

B. Sources of Oxygen Radicals During Hyperoxia

At normal oxygen partial pressures, little $O_2\cdot^-$ is generated by most cells. But, the small fraction of incompletely reduced O_2 lost as $O_2\cdot^-$ can become a significant oxidant load at a high P_{O_2} (17). Cellular sources of reactive O_2 metabolites during hyperoxia include mitochondria, peroxisomes, microsomes, membrane and cytosolic oxidases, xanthine oxidase, arachidonic acid metabolism, and autooxidation of iron, hemoglobin, myoglobin, catecholamines and various coenzymes (9,14,18–20).

Mitochondrial Electron Transport Chain

Cytochrome oxidase reduces approximately 95% of the O_2 consumed to water by 4-electron reduction, but some 1 to 2% of the O_2 is converted to superoxide anions by electrons leaking from the mitochondrial electron transport chain (9,14). An efficient scavenging system usually maintains an $O_2\cdot^-$ concentration of only 8×10^{-12} M in mitochondria, so that only H_2O_2 leaks out of intact mitochondria (14). But H_2O_2 production by mitochondria increases linearly with O_2 tension from 0 to 60% and at an accelerated rate above this level (21). Although no $O_2\cdot^-$ production occurs at the cytochrome oxidase step, superoxide ''leak'' sites have been identified at the ubiquinone-cytochrome b and the NADH dehydrogenase regions in the electron transport chain (22) (Fig. 2). The relatively low ubiquinone content of the lung results in a lower tissue production of $O_2\cdot^-$ than in other tissues and undoubtedly enhances the lung's tolerance of hyperoxia (23).

Microsomes

The mixed-function oxidase system of electron transport and oxidase enzymes located in membranes of endoplasmic reticulum, nuclear membranes, and microsomes are also important sources of oxygen free radicals in tissues exposed to hyperoxia (14). Cytochromes P450 and b_5 are particularly high in Clara cells

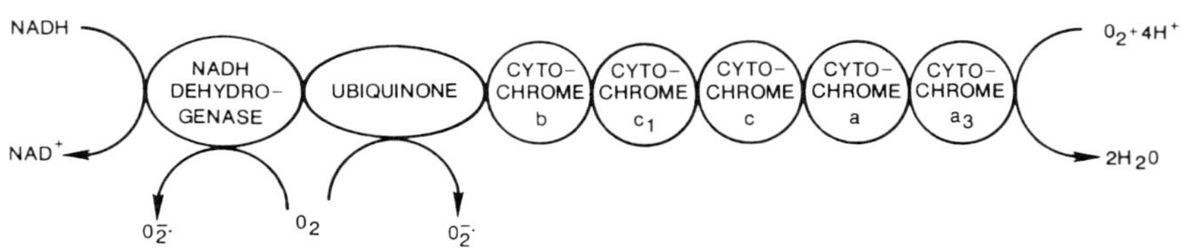

Figure 2 Sources of superoxide in the mitochondrial electron transport chain.

of the lungs and liver cells, where they participate in several metabolic and detoxification reactions. Turrens et al. (22) observed that the microsomal system accounted for 85% of the H_2O_2 produced in 100% O_2 by substrate-supplemented lung homogenates. Microsome production of H_2O_2 was 6.7 times that of mitochondria. Since individual cytochrome P450 isozymes can be induced by hyperoxia or suppressed by inflammatory mediators, the actual contribution of these microsomal enzymes to hyperoxic radical production in intact tissues is not known at the present time (24,25). H_2O_2 leaking from the mitochondria has the greatest potential for producing cell damage via OH· generated by the Fenton reaction. Therefore, the concentration of free Fe^{2+} ions in cells and extracellular spaces markedly influences the amount of damage caused by H_2O_2 released from cellular sources (17).

All major cell types found in lung tissue produce reactive oxygen metabolites under both basal and hyperoxic conditions. Cultured bovine endothelial cells secrete 0.03 nmol H_2O_2/min/10^6 cells into the extracellular spaces under basal conditions (26). However, the baseline secretion rate varies greatly with species (27,28), and sources of H_2O_2 production near the cell surface have been identified in addition to that derived from mitochondria and microsome electron transport enzymes (26). Endothelial H_2O_2 secretion from all sources increased linearly as O_2 was varied between 0 to 10% but reached a plateau at higher O_2 concentrations (29) and was increased by activation of protein kinase C, an increased intracellular Ca^{2+}, and bradykinin (30,31). $O_2\cdot^-$ secreted by endothelial cell $O_2\cdot^-$ increases vascular tone directly through action on smooth muscle or indirectly by reacting with and removing nitric oxide (NO·), the endothelium-derived relaxing factor (EDRF) (32). In rat lungs, the basal extracellular H_2O_2 production rates of endothelial cells, alveolar type II cells, and alveolar macrophages were 0.06, 0.07, and 3.1 nmol/min/mg protein, respectively (28,33), but hyperoxic exposure (95% O_2) of type II pneumocytes did not increase their rate of intracellular or extracellular H_2O_2 production (33). Guinea pig tracheal epithelial cells in primary culture produced H_2O_2 at a baseline rate of 0.044 nmol/min/mg protein only from their apical surfaces (34). H_2O_2 production was increased 4-fold with phorbol myristate acetate (PMA) and 2.3-fold with platelet activating factor (PAF) through activation of protein kinase C (PKC) (34,35). Lumenal secretion of $O_2\cdot^-$ by tracheal epithelial cells appears to be a defense mechanism against airborn bacteria.

Transition Metal Ions

Free iron can be released into the extracellular spaces by tissue damage, iron overload, or hemolysis (20). Since scavenger enzymes are only present in low concentrations in interstitial fluid, conditions favor OH· production by the Haber-Weiss reaction and subsequent lipid peroxidation, when parenchymal and inflammatory cells release $O_2\cdot^-$ and H_2O_2. Halliwell and Gutteridge (36) found that damaged tissues were more susceptible to oxidant injury than intact tissues because of metal ions released into extracellular fluids.

Xanthine Oxidase

Xanthine oxidase (XO) is one isozyme of a molybdo-pterin enzyme, which catalyzes the conversion of hypoxanthine to xanthine and xanthine to uric acid. When xanthine dehydrogenase (XD) is converted to XO by sulfhydryl oxidation (37,38), $O_2\cdot^-$ and H_2O_2 are produced during the formation of uric acid (9). Since ample purine substrate is normally available, conversion of the enzyme to the oxidase form is the rate-limiting step in $O_2\cdot^-$ production from this source. Although the XO reaction produces significant amounts of $O_2\cdot^-$ during ischemia-reperfusion injury, most studies indicate that this system does not contribute directly to hyperoxic injury. Rather, chemotactic factors are released, which recruit neutrophils to the lung and subsequently contribute to tissue damage. Hassoun et al. (39) found that XD/XO activity in endothelial cells was inversely related to O_2 tension and that activity was regulated at the transcriptional level. In contrast, vascular smooth muscle cells showed no XD/XO activity under normoxic conditions. Terada et al. (40) found that a variety of reactive O_2 metabolites produced either by the XD/XO reaction or neutrophils actually inactivated the XO in rat lungs and cultured endothelial cells. In other studies, endothelial cells supplemented with xanthine substrate or treated with allopurinol to inhibit XO activity showed no measurable differences in H_2O_2 production when exposed to hyperoxia (41). Panus et al. (42) observed a 98% decrease in XD/XO activity in endothelial cells after 48 hr of 95% O_2, and the enzyme was present only as XO. Therefore, XO-derived $O_2\cdot^-$ did not contribute to hyperoxic injury to endothelium in these studies. In contrast, XO did contribute significantly to oxidant production by cultured epithelial type II cells and also inhibited their surfactant production (43).

Xanthine Oxidase–Induced Chemotactic Factors

There is considerable evidence that XO-generated radicals contribute to neutrophil-induced injury during hyperoxia by activation of a neutrophil chemotactic factor (14,44). Moores et al. (45) and Bryan et al. (46) found that treatment of rats exposed to hyperoxia with either allopurinol or a tungsten diet to inhibit XO activity prevented the expected infiltration of neutrophils into alveolar spaces and lung tissue. Interestingly, lavage albumin concentration was even higher after allopurinol treatment, suggesting greater microvascular damage. The investigators proposed a scavenger effect of uric acid, neutrophil antioxidant enzymes, or induced tissue antioxidant enzymes to explain these findings. Indeed, allopurinol treatment of premature baboons subjected to hyperoxia resulted in enhanced levels of lung glutathione-pathway enzymes and SOD activity, a reduced neutrophil influx, and increased lung compliance (47). However, XO-generated radicals may also enhance neutrophil-induced tissue damage by protecting neutrophil elastases against inhibition by antiproteinases (48). Rats and endothelial layers fed tungsten to inactivate XO have reduced elastase-induced cell damage, and vascular permeability increases during hyperoxia.

Arachidonic Acid Metabolites

Arachidonic acid is particularly susceptible to peroxidation because of its four double bonds (10). Enzymatic oxidation of arachidonic acid by membrane cyclo-oxygenase generates arachidonate hydroperoxide (prostaglandin G_2) and hydroxy arachidonate (prostaglandin H_2), which can then produce $O_2\cdot^-$ by NADH oxidation (49). The cyclo-oxygenase pathway may be a minor source of $O2\cdot^-$, because normobaric hyperoxia did not increase prostaglandin or thromboxane production in rabbit lungs (50). Other types of alkoxyl and peroxyl radicals as well as malondialdehyde can be generated by nonenzymatic oxidation of arachidonate by ferrous iron or hemoglobin (9,51). The arachidonic acid bound to plasma or interstitial proteins is also thought to be a source of a chemotactic factor that promotes neutrophil infiltration into lung tissue during both ischemia/reperfusion (52) and hyperoxic injury (53,54). Wallace et al. (55) showed that this chemotactic factor cross-reacts with antibodies to leukotriene (LT) B_4, is inhibited by LTB_4 receptor antagonists, but differs from LTB_4 in chromatographic retention time. Thus, arachidonate could certainly contribute to hyperoxic injury by generation of oxygen radicals and producing chemotactic factors that cause neutrophil migration into lung tissues.

C. Mechanisms of Cellular Damage

Free radicals can produce injury at numerous sites in cells by oxidation of proteins, lipids, and carbohydrates (19). The site of the damage depends upon where the free radicals are generated and the location of compounds with unsaturated bonds that favor free-radical reactions. Damage to lipids and proteins in the plasma membrane has dramatic consequences for cell function. Disruption of the lipid bilayer increases membrane permeability, while amino acid oxidation and sulfide cross-linking of the membrane proteins disrupts their transport and enzymatic functions. These changes can cause ionic imbalances and ultimately lead to cell death (9,14).

Lipid Peroxidation

Lipid peroxidation of double bonds in cholesterol and fatty acids occurs when a hydrogen is lost to free radicals such as $OH\cdot$ and forms lipid alkyl radicals

(L·). These radicals are stabilized as conjugated dienes, lipid peroxyl radicals (LOO·), and hydroperoxides (LOOH) through a chain reaction within the cell membrane (9).

$$OH\cdot + LH \rightarrow H_2O + L\cdot \quad (8)$$

$$L\cdot + O_2 \rightarrow LOO\cdot \quad (9)$$

$$LOO\cdot + LH \rightarrow LOOH + L\cdot \quad (10)$$

Inclusion of these polar groups in the lipid bilayer can form blebs and potential leak sites in the plasma membrane (10). Membrane repair occurs through cleavage of the oxidized fatty acid from the membrane by phospholipase A_2, followed by reduction of the peroxide to an alcohol by the glutathione peroxidase system.

Protein Oxidation

The susceptibility of proteins to free-radical damage depends on their amino acid composition and the location of amino acids critical for maintaining conformation and enzymatic activity. Amino acids such as tryptophan, proline, and cysteine, which contain sulfur, or unsaturated groups can be oxidized by free radicals (19,56). Proteins such as albumin and collagen actually fragment when oxidized, while other proteins aggregate and undergo conformation changes by the formation of disulfide bridges (14,57). Many key enzymes that control vital cellular function are inhibited by free radicals, including ion-transport enzymes such as the membrane Ca^{2+}-Mg^{2+}-ATPase (58). Conformational changes in proteins may be corrected by heat-shock proteins (10), but mRNA for the production of the heat-shock protein HSP70 was only minimally induced by hyperoxia in rat lungs and rat lung fibroblasts (59). Although induction of large amounts of HSP70 with thermal stress did not protect against hyperoxic cytotoxicity (59), induction of heat-shock proteins protected cultured fibroblasts against H_2O_2-induced injury (60).

Nucleic Acid Damage

Free radicals produced by membrane oxidase systems near the nuclear membrane can disturb gene function by oxidation of bases and disassociation of DNA strands (19). Breaks in DNA strands and cell death increased in direct proportion to the dissolved oxygen concentration in cultured cells exposed to hyperoxia (61). Such DNA damage is critically dependent on free iron and the OH· generated by the Fenton reaction (62), with thymine and cytosine bases being particularly susceptible to oxidation (63,64).

A variety of enzymes exist to repair damaged portions of the DNA strand by excision and replacement of damaged segments and removal of oxidized bases (65). Poly(ADP-ribose) polymerase (PARP) cleaves nicotinamide from NAD to form ribose polymers, which are then available for repair of DNA strands (66). With low numbers of strand breaks, DNA repair can be quite rapid. However, with large numbers of DNA strand breaks, the cellular NAD is depleted to the extent that glycolysis is inhibited and cellular ATP stores are depleted (67). Spagg et al. (68) showed significant breakage of DNA strands within 15 min in the presence of only 50 μM H_2O_2, with endothelial cell lysis and ^{51}Cr release after 4 to 6 hr. These breaks in DNA strands were prevented by catalase but not SOD. Overactivation of PARP appears to be a mechanisms for cytotoxicity in some types of oxidant injury (66), because cell death was prevented by PARP inhibitors (67). This could be an intrinsic protective mechanism that sacrifices individual cells to prevent transmission of DNA errors. However, Christie et al. (69) concluded that depletion of the cellular protein and glutathione sulfhydryl pools, rather than PARP activation, was responsible for lysis of fetal distal airway epithelial cells, because PARP activity was depressed and cellular ATP content increased after exposure to 95% O_2 for 48 hr. Even DNAase activation of PARP was depressed during hyperoxia. These authors concluded that PARP activity was reduced by oxidation of critical sulfhydryl groups in the enzyme and that this mechanism was not responsible for cell death during hyperoxia.

D. Hyperoxic Cell Dysfunction

Endothelial Cells

An increase in permeability of the endothelial barrier to solutes and water in lungs is a characteristic feature of hyperoxic exposure and has been documented in several species (70). An increased microvascular permeability was indicated by increases in lung lymph flow and lymph protein and dextran clearances in unanesthetized sheep after 48 to 96 hr of breathing 100% O_2 (71–73). Both the increases in transcapillary clearance of large solutes and lung morphology indicate that large gaps form between capillary endothelial cells during hyperoxia (71). Both pulmonary endothelial and epithelial permeabilities increased simultaneously after 4 days exposure to 95% O_2 in hamsters (74) and after 48 hr of 100% O_2 in rats (75). In addition, Davis et al. (76) measured a significant increase in albumin concentration in lung lavage fluid obtained from human subjects after breathing 95% O_2 for only 17 hr. Transcapillary albumin clearance significantly increased at 48 hr in lungs of rats breathing 100% O_2 followed by edema formation and pleural effusion at 60 hr (75). Although structural change in the endothelium was not apparent in the lungs of rats exposed to 40 hr of 100% O_2 at 1 atmosphere (ata) (77), a depression of norepinephrine uptake was apparent after only 24 hr (78). Angiotensin-converting enzyme activity was depressed in dog lungs after 96 hr of hyperoxia (79), and active uptake of serotonin by cultured endothelial cells was inhibited at 18 hr of 95% O_2 exposure (80). These studies indicate that subtle changes in endothelial metabolism and junctional permeability may occur much earlier than morphologic changes and that susceptibility to injury varies between species. Moreover, hyperbaric and normobaric oxygen may produce cell toxicity by different mechanisms, because 1 ata O_2 for 48 hr inhibited serotonin uptake by pulmonary endothelial cells, while exposure to 100% O_2 for 11 hr at 2.5 ata failed to inhibit serotonin uptake (81).

Epithelial Cells

Paracellular Permeability

Junctional permeability of the alveolar epithelial barrier is normally more restrictive than that of the capillary endothelium, with an equivalent pore radius of only 0.8 nm (i.e., about 1/10 that of the capillary endothelium) (82,83). However, hyperoxia increases epithelial permeability in the lungs of several species. Alveolar ^{99m}Tc diethylenetriamine pentacetic acid (DTPA) clearance increases ninefold after 48 hr of 100% O_2 exposure in rats (75). In addition, alveolar-to-blood clearances of cyanocobalamin, cytochrome c, and albumin increase three to five times in rabbit lungs after 64 hr of 100% O_2 breathing (84), and transepithelial permeability–surface area (PS) products for sucrose and dextran 20 increased fivefold in hamster lungs after 4.5 days of 95% O_2 (85). Epithelial permeability returned to normal after 3 days for sucrose and 7 days for dextran, indicating restoration of the epithelial tight junctions after cessation of hyperoxic exposure (85). In contrast, recovery of the epithelial permeability in rat lungs occurred more slowly for small molecules than for albumin after hyperoxic exposure (86).

Fluid Clearance

Although the permeability of the paracellular pathway in alveolar epithelium is increased by hyperoxia, alveolar fluid accumulation is oppposed by an upregulation of active sodium transport, which increases fluid clearance from the alveoli (87–89). Increases in ouabain-sensitive Na^+ transport, Na^+, K^+-ATPase activity, Na^+, K^+-ATPase mRNA, and Na^+, K^+-ATPase protein have been demonstrated in alveolar epithelium of rat lungs following a 24-hr exposure to hyperoxia (86,90,91). Two types of apical Na^+ channels were also upregulated by hyperoxia on type II cells, and these Na^+ channels are thought to limit the rate of Na^+ movement across epithelia (92). Although less critical for fluid clearance, the epithelial Na^+-H^+ antiporter is also upregulated by hyperoxia (93). An increase in gene expression rather than increased numbers of type II cells appears to account for the increased transepithelial transport of Na^+ and airway fluid in these studies.

Surfactant

Surfactant production and turnover are generally reduced by hyperoxia (94,95). Impaired epithelial type II cell function occurs in rabbits exposed to 64 hr of

100% O_2, as indicated by a reduced phospholipid content and increased surface tension of surfactant (84). Interestingly, surfactant phospholipid rebounded to a level greater than control after returning the animals to room air for 8 days. The rabbits were protected against subsequent hyperoxic challenge, even though antioxidant enzymes were not significantly increased (96). Addition of exogenous calf surfactant also increased survival time and decreased the amount of lung damage in rabbits exposed to hyperoxia (97).

Type II cells in their early proliferative phase following injury do not secrete surfactants of normal composition. Exposure of baboons to 100% O_2 decreased the phophatidylcholine content and the ratio of phophatidylglycerol to phophatidylinositol in lung surfactant (95). In other baboons studies, 100% O_2 produced an obvious ventilation/perfusion mismatch, pulmonary edema, decreases in surfactant disaturated phophatidylcholine, and surfactant protein (SP-A) content at 96 hr of oxygen exposure (98). Exogenous surfactant failed to correct the impaired gas exchange, but the beneficial response to 10 cmH_2O of positive end-expiratory pressure (PEEP) was augmented. A selective control of individual surfactant components occurs at the transcription level during hyperoxia in hamsters, because mRNA for three types of surfactant related proteins (SP-A, SP-B, and SP-C) declined at different rates, while surfactant phospholipid actually increased (99). In addition, SP-B mRNA and protein increased in bronchial tissue but decreased in alveolar epithelium during hyperoxia in mice (100).

Surfactant function is also impaired by the plasma proteins in edema fluid formed during hyperoxia (101). In particular, fibrin monomers dramatically reduced hysteresis and increased surface tension of surfactant layers, whereas albumin had little effect on surfactant function (102).

E. Role of Neutrophils in Oxygen Toxicity

Alveolar edema, microvascular protein leak, and infiltration of granulocytes are a characteristic finding in lungs of animals exposed to 100% O_2 for 72 hr. (103). Lavage fluid in rats exposed to 64 hr of 100% O_2 has a marked increase in protein concentration and the numbers of neutrophils, lymphocytes, and red cells, but macrophage numbers are decreased (104). However, macrophages obtained from normal human subjects after breathing 50% O_2 for 44 hr produced increased amounts of LTB_4, a chemoattractant for neutrophils (105). In addition, neutrophils from lungs of hyperoxia-exposed rats are primed to increase their superoxide production (104). Although activated neutrophils are a rich source of oxygen free radicals and proteolytic granular enzymes, their contribution to tissue damage appears to be secondary to the initial hyperoxic tissue injury (44).

Neutrophils produce $O_2 \cdot^-$ by a membrane-associated NADPH oxidase that oxidizes NADPH to $NADP^+$, which is then recycled by the pentose monophosphate shunt pathway (9,18). H_2O_2 formed from $O_2 \cdot^-$ is then converted by neutrophil-derived myeloperoxidase into HOCl [Eq. (7)]. Myeloperoxidase constitutes some 5% of the neutrophil dry weight and is the substance that imparts the green color to pus draining from inflamed tissues (18). While a sufficient amount of HOCl can destroy cells, Weiss and Regiani (106) propose that the massive destruction of host cells, structural collagen, and elastin occurring in severe inflammatory reactions requires an interaction of oxidants with neutrophil elastase and proteinase inhibitors. Proteinase inhibitors such as α-macroglobulin and α-proteinase inhibitor are normally present in sufficient amounts to irreversibly bind all free elastase and prevent degradation of connective tissues. Oxidation of critical methionine residues inactivates the antiproteinase protective shield and leads to digestion of the extracellular matrix structures (18). Also, it is important to note that oxygen radicals are required to activate granular proteases (107).

A role for neutrophils in hyperoxic lung injury was suggested when Shasby et al. (103) observed an attenuation of the expected increase in lung weight and lavage albumin concentration after 40 hr of 100% oxygen exposure in rabbits rendered neutropenic by nitrogen mustard. However, many other animal studies have found no effect of leukopenia on hyperoxia-induced increases in lung edema or increases in endothelial or epithelial permeability (108–110). In isolated lung studies, hyperoxic damage preceded the addition of neutrophils and stimulated neutrophils to induce further tissue damage (111). Neutrophils added either with or without hyperoxia when not preceded by hyperoxic damage failed to produce additional lung injury (111). Further, Lin and Jamieson (112) observed no lung-protective effect of neutropenia in rats or mice subjected to 5.4 to 5.8 ata (550 to 585 kPa) oxygen. It is apparent that direct oxidant tissue injury causes the release of chemotactic factors, followed by a subsequent emigration of neutrophils, which then contribute to inflammation and lung damage (112).

Recent studies suggest that intercellular adhesion molecule-1 (ICAM-1) expression on endothelium and type I epithelial cells regulates neutrophil transmigration during hyperoxic lung injury. ICAM-1 is the ligand for B_2 integrins on the surface of neutrophils and controls transmigration through intracellular junctions (113). Kang et al. (114) found ICAM-1 concentrated around intercellular junctions between type I epithelial cells but only lightly dispersed on epithelial and endothelial surfaces in mouse lungs. 100% O_2 for 84 hr causes a loss of ICAM-1 at epithelial junctions but increases on type I and II epithelial cell surfaces—a change that facilitates neutrophil retention in the alveolar spaces. Weltz et al. (115) found a 56% increase in ICAM-1 mRNA at 48 hr of 95% O_2 and a fivefold increase in ICAM-1 protein after 96 hr, which was correlated with the neutrophil infiltration and lung injury in mice. Jensen et al. (116) found that mRNA for tumor necrosis factor (TNF)-α, interleukin (IL)-1α, and interleukin-6 increased in mouse lungs after 72 hr of hyperoxic exposure, and these cytokines are known to induce ICAM-1 expression in endothelial cells (117). Also, Wagner et al. (118) were able to block the neutrophil infiltration and lung injury with anti–ICAM-1 antibodies in mice exposed to hyperoxia. These findings suggest that increased expression and redistribution of ICAM-1 during hyperoxia facilitate emigration and retention of neutrophils and contribute to the inflammatory response.

II. Antioxidant Defenses

Substances that protect cells against free-radical damage constitute an antioxidant defense system. These compounds limit free-radical formation or propagation by donating an electron to inactivate the radical. These scavengers may be irreversibly degraded (sacrificial antioxidant) or regenerated by other antioxidants (119). Low-molecular-weight compounds that scavenge free radicals are present in both cellular and extracellular fluids and include ascorbic acid (vitamin C), α-tocopherol (vitamin E), β-carotene (vitamin A), uric acid, methionine, glutathione, cysteine, bilirubin, and glucose (9). Scavenger enzymes are strategically distributed primarily throughout the mitochondria and cytoplasm, where free radicals are normally generated and can reduce free radicals to less toxic compounds. The primary antioxidant enzymes are superoxide dismutase, catalase, and glutathione peroxidase (19). Also protective are the iron or copper chelating proteins ferritin and hemoglobin in the cells and transferrin, lactoferrin, ceruloplasmin, and albumin in extracellular fluid. These have antioxidant properties because they reduce the amount of transition metal ions available for the Haber-Weiss and Fenton reactions.

A. Low-Molecular-Weight Antioxidants

Vitamin E

Vitamin E consists of several isomers, with α-tocopherol being the most potent antioxidant (10) and the succinate ester of tocopherol its most active form (120). Due to its high lipid solubility, vitamin E is partitioned within plasma membranes, endoplasmic reticulum, and mitochondrial membranes and is a particularly important scavenger for terminating lipid peroxidation chain reactions (10). Dilley et al. (121) found that vitamin E protects polyunsaturated fatty acids in cell membranes of rat lungs, a major target for hyperoxic lipid peroxidation. Mitochondrial membrane lipids are protected with or without additional vitamin E, but dramatic decreases in microsomal membrane lipids occur when rats are made deficient in vitamin E. Knight et al. (122) observed that vitamin E levels are maintained at normal or above-normal levels even after 3 days of 95% O_2 exposure in newborn rabbit lungs, but on the fourth day a decrease in vitamin

E was accompanied by increased alveolar-capillary protein leak and decreased serotonin uptake. These studies indicate that vitamin E content in lung is maintained at near-normal levels during hyperoxia at the expense of depletion of liver stores (123).

There are conflicting results as to the effectiveness of exogenous administered vitamin E in preventing lung injury during hyperoxia (124). A deficiency of vitamin E predisposes rats to oxygen toxicity (125), but an excess amount does not necessarily protect animals against lung injury (126). Jacobson et al. (127) found that supplemental doses of vitamin E prevent lipid peroxidation, edema formation, and increased capillary permeability in lungs of rabbits exposed to 100% O_2 for 48 hr. Supplemental vitamin E prevented the loss of pulmonary vascular reactivity during hyperoxia (50) and reduced the hyperoxic inhibition of surfactant formation in newborn rabbits (51), but vitamin E failed to restore phophatidylcholine synthesis in hyperoxic cultured alveolar type II cells (128). These varying experimental results appear to relate to differences in the duration of hyperoxic exposure, vitamin E dose, and timing of its administration to exposed animals.

Vitamin C

Vitamin C (ascorbic acid) is a water-soluble compound that serves as a major antioxidant in the aqueous phase of tissues. Vitamin C accepts electrons from $O_2\cdot^-$, $OH\cdot$, and lipid radicals to inhibit lipid peroxidation. Ascorbate is preferentially consumed at the expense of other antioxidants and also serves to preserve and regenerate vitamin E in cellular membranes (129). This is an essential function to terminate the lipid peroxidation reaction, since vitamin E becomes a slowly reacting free radical after scavenging lipid peroxyl and alkoxyl radicals (10). In turn, reductase enzymes can regenerate ascorbate from dehydroascorbate through the glutathione and nicotinamide adenine dinucleotide (NADH) systems. Both vitamins E and C are present in extracellular fluids, including the alveolar lining fluid, and serve as a first line of defense against hyperoxia-derived oxidants in the alveolar spaces. Supplemental ascorbate decreases lung damage associated with hyperbaric hyperoxia (130), H_2O_2 production by lung tissue mitochondria in 50% O_2, lipid peroxidation of guinea pig lung tissues during hyperoxia (131), and both lipid peroxidation products and antielastase activity in lavage fluids from human volunteers (132). An energy-dependent ascorbate-sodium cotransporter found in alveolar type II cells and macrophages appears to also confer increased resistance to lung tissue damage in hyperoxic conditions (133). Vitamin C, glutathione, and dexamethasone attenuated surfactant abnormalities induced by hyperoxia in cultured rat alveolar type II cells (134). However, vitamin C can also have deleterious effects in the presence of excess iron, because it reduces Fe^{3+} to Fe^{2+}, so that Fe^{2+} becomes available for the Fenton reaction and leads to OH· induced nucleic acid strand breaks (135,136) and lipid peroxidation (10).

Vitamin A

Vitamin A (β-carotene) is also a superb antioxidant because it contains a long chain of conjugated double bonds (137). Carotenoids normally scavenge singlet oxygen and other free radicals, but they may also exhibit auto-oxidation and pro-oxidant properties at a P_{O_2} greater than 150 torr (19,138).

Glutathione

Reduced glutathione (GSH) is the major small-molecule antioxidant defense in the cytosol of cells. This sulfur-containing tripeptide (glutamine-cysteine-glycine) is the most abundant nonprotein thiol in cells. But the cellular content of reduced sulfhydryl groups located on proteins is ten times greater than that of the total glutathione pool (69). H_2O_2, $O_2{\cdot}^-$, OH·, lipid peroxides, ascorbate and α-tocopherol radicals are readily scavenged by glutathione peroxidase (GP) at the expense of GSH (Fig. 3) (9). Oxidized glutathione (GSSH) generated by

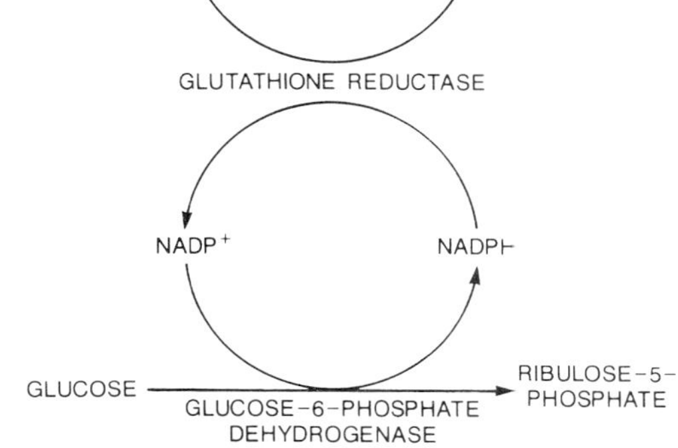

Figure 3 Diagram of antioxidant enzyme pathways for reduction of superoxide and hydrogen peroxide and recycling of reduced glutathione.

this reaction normally constitutes only ≈1% of the glutathione pool and is recycled to GSH by glutathione reductase, using the NADPH generated by the hexose shunt pathway (Fig. 3). Decreases in the ratio of GSH/GSSH are associated with lung damage during hyperoxia (139,140).

Reduced glutathione is the preferential pathway for reduction of low levels of H_2O_2 because the reaction has a lower Michaelis-Menton constant than does the H_2O_2-catalase reaction (141); its wide distribution and small size permit reactions with lipid hydroperoxides as well as H_2O_2 (20). Oxygen tolerance induced by sublethal hyperoxia is known to increase GP activity, cellular uptake of precursor amino acids, and the glutathione pool (142–144), but oxygen tolerance can also be inhanced by sparing the lung GSH pools through overexpression of SOD in lungs of transgenic mice (139), exogenous GSH administered to normal mice (145), and supplemental exogenous GSH and GSH precursor amino acids administered to cultured endothelial cells (146,147). Increased mortality and the sensitivity of rodents to lung damage and convulsions occur in both normobaric and hyperbaric (4 ata) hyperoxia when glutathione transcellular transport is inhibited (148), dietary cysteine is reduced (149), GSH is depleted using the GSH conjugator, dimethyl maleate (140,150), and selenium-dependent GP is inhibited by a selenium-deficient diet (151). However, the lung GSH pool is maintained during hyperoxia at the expense of the plasma and liver cysteine pools by enhanced cysteine uptake and GSH synthesis (139).

Uric Acid

Uric acid is now recognized as a significant scavenger of $O_2\cdot^-$ and $OH^\cdot$ and can also bind free iron and copper (10). This plentiful, endogenously produced antioxidant is present in both extracellular and intracellular fluid and spares other components of the small molecule antioxidant system, such as ascorbate (19). Uric acid reacts with $OH^\cdot$ at a rate that is similar to that of sulfhydryl compounds, but it is irreversibly degraded in the process (20). Genetic mutations in fruit flies that delete XO activity cause an increased susceptibility to oxidant stress, which suggests a vital antioxidant role for urate (152).

B. Scavenger Enzymes

Three enzymes—superoxide dismutase (SOD), catalase and glutathione peroxidase (GP)—reduce H_2O_2 and $O_2\cdot^-$ to water before they can be converted to more reactive oxygen species (see Fig. 4). Superoxide dismutase increases the spontaneous dismutation of $O_2\cdot^-$ to H_2O_2 [Eq. (1)] by approximately 10^4 times and is widely distributed throughout the body as three isoforms: (1) a copper-zinc enzyme (CuZnSOD) of 32 kDa comprising some 85% of total tissue SOD activity and is distributed in the cell cytosol and nucleus (153); (2) a manganese-based tetrameric enzyme (MnSOD) of 86 kDa comprising about 10% of total

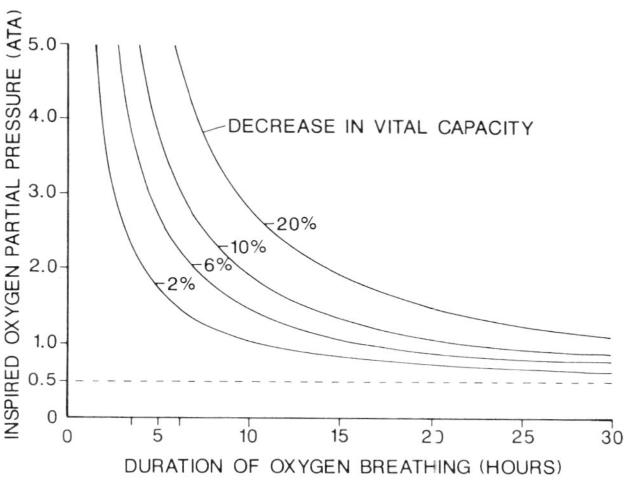

Figure 4 Predicted changes in vital capacity as a function of time and pressure for human subjects breathing 100% oxygen. (Adapted from Ref. 106.)

SOD activity and is present only in mitochondria (154); and (3) a 134-kDa copper-based SOD (CuSOD) comprising <5% of total SOD activity and is present in extracellular fluid, around matrix collagen, and in plasma and lymph (155).

Catalase and glutathione peroxidase (GP) are also widespread antioxidant enzymes that primarily scavenge H_2O_2. Catalase is a heme-containing homotetrameric enzyme of 240 kDa found in peroxisomes and cytosol, whereas glutathione peroxidase is found in cytosol and mitochondria. The glutathione peroxidase pool contains both selenium-based and selenium-independent forms and reduces H_2O_2 and organic peroxides at the expense of reduced glutathione (14) (Fig. 3). Catalase is confined primarily to peroxisomes and does not react readily with hydroperoxides larger than H_2O_2, such as lipid peroxides (141). The widespread availability of GP and cyclical regeneration of reduced GSH substrate makes this enzyme an essential scavenger system for prolonged scavenging of low levels of oxidants (141). Glucose-6-phosphate dehydrogenase and 6-phosphogluconate can also be considered antioxidant enzyme because they regenerate NADPH for the GSH redox cycle (156). Metallothionein, a low-molecular-weight, thiol-rich protein, has also been proposed as an expendable but renewable antioxidant (157).

In general, increased antioxidants enzyme levels attenuate hyperoxic damage, while inhibition of antioxidant enzymes augments damage; but isolating the function of a single enzyme system in vivo has been difficult. Early attempts to administer SOD in order to protect animals against hyperoxic injury were unsuccessful because the enzyme failed to enter cells (124). But when SOD and catalase were encapsulated in liposomes to enhance cellular entry, extended survival times of rats in 100% O_2 were obtained (158). Catalase but not SOD in infused liposomes also extended the time to convulsion of rats breathing 100% O_2 (159). In addition, the tracheal instillation of SOD and catalase bound to polyethylene glycol (PEG) significantly augmented antioxidant enzyme activity in alveolar type II cells, reduced alveolocapillary albumin leak, and prolonged survival of rats in hyperoxia (160,161). Both PEG-SOD and catalase are also effective when given by intraperitoneal injection in preventing increased lung permeability and increasing survival times of rabbits in 100% O_2 (127). However, PEG-SOD and PEG-catalase appear less protective than enzyme induction or liposome treatment in preventing hyperoxic damage (162). The effectiveness of catalase emphasizes the importance of scavenging H_2O_2 prior to formation of $OH^{\cdot}$ in the Fenton reaction.

C. Metal Chelator Proteins

As previously described, the transition metals Fe^{2+} and Cu^{2+} must be maintained at low levels in order to prevent the conversion of H_2O_2 and $O_2{\cdot}^-$ to OH·, a much more reactive species that catalyzes the formation of lipid peroxyl radicals (9). Free iron is normally maintained at low levels by binding to intracellular and circulating proteins (20). Iron bound to hemoglobin that is released by hemolysis of red cells is rapidly bound by haptoglobin (163). Ferritin is an intracellular protein with a high iron-storage capacity, so only a small pool of circulating free iron is normally available for chemical reactions (10). Free iron is maintained at low levels in extracellular fluids by binding to lactoferrin, transferrin, and ceruloplasmin (119,164). Transferrin transports iron in plasma and generally is present in amounts that are three times that of free iron, whereas lactoferrin is an iron-binding protein released by cells (20). Ceruloplasmin is a copper-containing glycoprotein that also has weak antioxidant properties. It can catalyze the oxidation of Fe^{2+} to Fe^{3+}, which then readily binds to transferrin (165). When the plasma iron stores become saturated or damaged cells release free iron, cellular resistance to oxidant-induced injury is greatly reduced because of the OH· production (20).

D. Lung Cell Antioxidant Capacity

Individual cell types found in the lung vary considerably in their antioxidant capacity. Suttorp et al. (166) examined the relative importance of various antioxidant systems when endothelial cells were exposed to hyperoxia (95% O_2). They found that inhibition of GSH synthesis with buthionine sulfoximine or inhibition of GP with selenium deficiency reduced cell survival, but catalase inhibition had no effect on survival time. Administration of exogenous sulfhydryl agents increased cell survival with or without increases in the GSH concentration. Thus, a functional GSH redox cycle, rather than the GSH levels or catalase activity, is primarily responsible for endothelial cell resistance to hyperoxia. In pleural mesothelial cells, glutathione cycling is also critical to scavenge exogenous H_2O_2, whereas catalase confers protection only at high levels of oxidant stresses (167). In contrast, freshly isolated rat alveolar type II cells preferentially scavenge exogenous H_2O_2 via a peroxisome catalase-dependent pathway, and inhibition of glutathione reductase produced only small effects (168,169). The greater resistance of alveolar type II cells to hyperoxia than alveolar type I or endothelial cells appears to be a function of their high catalase content and the large numbers of peroxisomes (170). Respective catalase activities were 59.3, 13.2, and 11.4 nmol O_2 produced per minute per milligram of protein in type II cells, alveolar macrophages, and endothelial cells (33).

Guinea pig tracheal epithelial cells possess a significant antioxidant capacity for scavenging exogenous H_2O_2, primarily at their apical surfaces (34). Of the H_2O_2 scavenging, 77% was attributed to catalase and glutathione, but moderate amounts of CuZnSOD are found throughout the cytoplasm and nucleus of airway epithelial cells and contribute to their antioxidant capacity. The increased amount of CuZnSOD may account for the higher oxidant resistance of upper airway epithelium as compared to that of the lower airways (171). In addition, increased mucin is released from tracheal epithelial cells challenged by oxidants and acts as an expendable scavenger molecule in fluid lining the airways (20).

Platelets and erythrocytes also have a significant antioxidant potential under hyperoxic conditions (20). Platelets adhere to endothelium within minutes of injury. They promote inflammation by release of thromboxane and serotonin, but in high concentrations they can inhibit neutrophil activation through release of adenine nucleotides, and scavenge a significant amount of $O_2 \cdot^-$ and H_2O_2 through the GSH pathway (172,173). In addition, red cells contain significant amounts of catalase, SOD, and components of the GSH cycle (20,77). Insufflation of red cells down the airways of rabbits prevented hyperoxic lung injury. Also, red cells aggregate in blood vessels during hyperoxia, where they may exert a scavenging effect (174).

III. Pulmonary Pathology of Oxygen Toxicity

The sequence of pathological changes that occur in lungs due to oxygen toxicity include a diffuse alveolitis and patchy edema that has been defined in three phases: (1) inflammatory, (2) proliferative-reparative, and (3) fibrotic (175). The morphological changes resulting from lethal and sublethal oxygen toxicity in rats have been elegantly described by Crapo et al. (77,176). In lethal hyperoxia (100% O_2 for 60 to 72 hr), few structural changes occur over the first 40 hr of exposure. Only mild interstitial edema with increased numbers of leukocytic cells, platelets aggregating within capillaries, and infrequent endothelial disruptions are seen at 46 hr. But from 60 hr of exposure until death, alveolar septa thicken by 56% and the number of endothelial cells decreases by 44%. Capillaries become narrowed and are packed with red cells, leukocytes, and platelets. Endothelial cells show patchy necrosis and swelling of intracellular organelles; they are separated from their basement membranes. However, no apparent structural changes are seen in epithelial cells or fibroblasts. In sublethal hyperoxia (85% O_2 for 14 days), platelet plugging occurs at 3 days and a moderate influx of neutrophils peaks at 5 days. By 7 days, endothelial cell numbers have decreased by 41% but have stabilized, their volumes are increased, and they contain more mitochondria and subcellular organelles. The number of type II epithelial cells and fibroblasts doubled by 7 days, and they contained increased numbers of mitochondria and lamellar bodies. Interstitial spaces thicken by an increase in matrix components and cell numbers, and the alveolar surface covered by type I cells slightly decreases.

Primates and humans develop similar lesions during exposure to hyperoxia but are more tolerant to 100% O_2 than rats and show a more vigorous proliferative phase (175). Monkeys will live for 13 days in 100% O_2, and type II epithelial cells almost completely cover the alveolar surfaces after 7 days of hyperoxia exposure (177). In baboons exposed to 60% O_2, type II cell numbers doubled at 14 days and septal interstitial and epithelial volumes increase after 8 weeks of recovery (176).

IV. Vascular and Airway Remodeling After Hyperoxic Injury

Injury and repair after hyperoxic exposure produce structural changes that can cause residual impairment of lung function. Necrosis of endothelial cells followed by hypertrophy and hyperplasia leads to extensive remodeling of the pulmonary vasculature (178). Obliteration of some vessels, encroachment of endothelium into the lumen of other microvessels, as well as muscularization of previously nonmuscular arterial segments (15 to 100 μm in diameter) result in pulmonary hypertension (179). Higher flow velocities through the remaining patent vessels and the higher vascular pressures produce secondary hypertrophy of medial and adventitial layers in larger pulmonary arteries (180). Although Coflesky et al. (181) found an increased medial and adventitial thickness in both large and small vessels in rat lungs exposed to hyperoxia, the maximal active tension induced by potassium chloride (KCl) was reduced. The threefold increase in pulmonary artery pressure was attributed to lower distensibility of the blood vessels and their smaller cross-sectional areas. Small postcapillary veins are also reduced in number and develop thicker muscular coats during hyperoxia (182). Contractile cells in small vessels are formed by fibroblasts recruited from the interstitium and intermediate cells, which align themselves in layers around the vessels, form elastic laminae, and develop contractile elements (183). Peaks in DNA synthesis occur in microvascular fibroblasts at 4 days in 87% O_2 and at 7 days for microvascular endothelium, with a recurrent peak at approximately 2 weeks after returning to air (184).

Significant remodeling also occurs in the airways of young rats after 8 days of exposure to 95% O_2 (185,186). These studies show a significant thickening of epithelial and smooth muscle layers of both small and large airways, which then become hyperresponsive to aerosol or intravenous methacholine. The hyperresponsiveness and increased wall thickness returns to control levels approximately 2 weeks after returning to air breathing (187). Hyperoxia-induced airway hyperresponsiveness has also been reported in response to serotonin in rats (188) and histamine and acetylcholine in guinea pigs (189) but not for histamine in sheep (73). Thus, these structural changes lead to residual increases in vascular and airway resistances that revert only slowly to pre-hyperoxia values.

A. Mechanisms of Cell Proliferation

The mechanisms that control cell proliferation and the repair phase of hyperoxic injury are under intensive investigation. Peptide growth factors in combination with cytokines produced by lung cells during hyperoxia induce cell division and proliferation. However, it is also known that growth of some cell types in culture is directly inhibited by high O_2 concentrations. In cultured rat lung type II cells and fibroblasts, cell proliferation is inversely related to the exposure time in 95% O_2. This occurs even though mRNA for cell cycle–linked gene products is sustained at high levels (190); it is postulated that free radicals inhibit protein translation. Proliferation of tracheal smooth muscle cells in culture is also inhibited by hyperoxia, even though protein synthesis in the cells has increased (191).

A likely stimulus for hyperoxia-induced cell proliferation is the release of platelet-derived growth factor (PDGF), which is a 30-kDa glycoprotein synthesized by platelets, macrophages, monocytes, and epithelial and endothelial cells (192). Platelet-derived growth factor is a mitogen for fibroblasts and smooth muscle cells and a chemoattractant for monocytes and neutrophils. Han et al. (193) reported a 1.4-fold increase in the mRNAs for PDGF-β and its receptor protein in rat lungs following 6 days of exposure to 85% O_2. These authors concluded that an increased transcription rate results in an increased release of PDGF-β by a subset of fibroblasts, which, in turn, stimulate other fibroblasts to proliferate. Fabisiak et al. (194) observed a 2.5-fold increase in PDGF-β mRNA after 3 days of exposure to hyperoxia. After 7 days, a significant increase in mRNA for both β and δ actin and muscle specific α-actin was present. These findings suggest that proliferation of smooth muscle and myofibroblasts occurs in response to PDGF-β release.

In other studies, mRNA for PDGF receptor proteins was released within hours in rats breathing 87% O_2, whereas peak mRNA responses for PDGF α and β chains occurred only after 12 to 18 hr and 3 days, respectively (195). These peak responses preceded proliferation of adventitial fibroblasts, epithelial cells, and precursor smooth muscle cells on day 4 of hyperoxia. While type II epithelial cells normally do not express PDGF receptors, receptor expression may be induced in injured epithelial cells (196). Epidermal growth factor (EGF) may also participate, since Powell et al. (197) have reported a 100-fold increase in mRNA levels of EGF and a heparin-binding type (HB-EGF) in rat lungs after 7 days of hyperoxia. These EGF peptides are also mitogenic for fibroblasts, smooth muscle, and epithelial cells and their appearance correlates with the hypertrophy and hyperplasia of microvessel walls. In situ hybridization experiments have localized the HB-EGF mRNA to eosinophils near microvessels.

In other rat lung studies, increases in mRNA for collagenase and tissue proteinase inhibitors peaked after 4 days, and that for type I collagen and transforming growth factor-beta (TGF-β) peaked at 14 days exposure to 85% O_2 (198). Increases in collagen, elastin, and tissue protein synthesis were observed after 7 days of 85% O_2 exposure secondary to TGF-β stimulation of fibroblasts (199). Thus, growth factors are elaborated by lung parenchymal and inflammatory cells during hyperoxia and initate cell proliferation to replace injured cells. However, increases in vascular and airway smooth muscle may result in pulmonary dysfunction. An increased production of connective tissue constituents replaces damaged structural proteins but can also lead to fibrosis.

V. Pulmonary Function and Hyperoxia

Although limits of exposure to high partial pressures of oxygen were originally defined in military diving situations using oxygen rebreathing apparatuses, more recent experimental studies show a detectable decrease in vital capacity and increase in microvascular permeability in lungs in humans after only 10 to 17 hours of breathing 100% O_2 (76,200). In addition, breathing pure oxygen for as little as 3 hr at 3 atm (304 kPa) can cause convulsions (1). In normal human subjects, the most sensitive indicators of oxygen toxicity are retrosternal pain, often preceded by a tickling sensation with a burning sensation on inspiration and dyspnea and/or cough (200,201). Montgomery et al. (202) compared measurements of lung and airway mechanics, Tc-DTPA clearance, carbon monoxide diffusion capacity (DL_{CO}), and enzyme markers of endothelial injury in normal human subjects breathing 21 to 100% O_2 for 17 hr. These functional measures did not change, but all subjects breathing 100% O_2 experienced chest pain. Visual signs of mucosal irritation appeared in the tracheal mucosa within only 6 hr breathing 100% O_2 (203).

Animals breathing high P_{O_2}'s eventually develop a decreased lung compliance and increased airway resistance (84,95,204,205), and changes in pulmonary function tests are seen in humans subjected to hyperoxic exposure at ambient pressures from 0.25 to 3.0 ata (200). A decreasing vital capacity (VC) has been the most useful pulmonary function index to monitor the progression of oxygen toxicity and to establish guidelines for using high oxygen partial pressures in diving conditions (200). Graded decreases in VC in humans are highly correlated with P_{O_2} levels and duration of exposure (see Fig. 4 on p. 53) (206). To establish a threshold P_{O_2} for injury, Clark and Lambertson (207) reviewed several human studies and concluded that an inspired P_{O_2} of 0.5 ata (50 kPa) can be breathed for extended periods of time without a decrement in pulmonary function. Since the severity of oxygen toxicity varies directly with both the O_2 partial pressure and the duration of exposure, curves were constructed from human data that predict the percent decrease in VC for 50% of subjects as a function of time and P_{O_2} levels (206). These hyperbolic curves are defined as:

$$P_{O_2}-0.5=bt^{m} \tag{11}$$

where P_{O_2} is the inspired P_{O_2} in ata, t is exposure duration in minutes, b is the intercept of the P_{O_2} axis at $t=1$, and m is a slope constant (m=−1.2 in Fig. 4). The percent decrease in vital capacity (% VC) for any exposure conditions can then be calculated using the following equation (208):

$$\%\Delta VC=0.011\ (P_{O_2}-0.5)\ t\ (\text{min}) \tag{12}$$

Since pressure exposures vary widely with depth and duration of dives, Bardin and Lambertsen (209) developed the concept of a unit pulmonary toxic dose (UPTD). This calculation normalized all oxygen exposures to an equivalent exposure time at 1.0 ata (101 kPa) P_{O_2}. Such an exposure time would produce a 4% decrease in VC in 50% of subjects with an 80% confidence limit of 1 to 12% and can be calculated using the following equation (208):

$$\text{UPTD}=t_x[(0.5/(P_x-0.5)]^{1/m} \tag{13}$$

where P_x is the P_{O_2} in ata, t_x is the exposure duration in minutes, and UPTD is in minutes. For example, UPTD units (minutes) are 615 min to produce a 2% decrease in VC, 824 min for a 4% VC decrease, 1425 min for a 10% VC decrease, and 2190 min for a 20% VC decrease. Table 1 shows the application of the above equations to pulmonary function data from Clark (206) for oxygen

Table 1 Effect of Hyperbaric Hyperoxic Exposure on Pulmonary Function Tests

ata	1.5	2.0	2.5	3.0
EXPOS. (min)	1062	540	342	204
UPTD[a] (min)	1892	1349	1085	780
%FVC	−20.4%	−19.1%	−13.8%	−11.8%
PRED. %FVC[b]	−11.7%	−8.9%	−7.5%	−5.6%
%FEF_{25-75}	2.9%	−29.2%	−30.8%	−11.8%
DLCO	−10.8%	−9.7%	−7.7%	−1.7%

[a] UPTD calculated from Eq. (13).
[b] PRED. %FVC = predicted decrease in FVC using Eq. (12).
Source: Modified from Ref. 206.

exposures at pressures of 1.5, 2.0, 2.5, and 3.0 ata (151, 202, 252, and 303 kPa). Using these data, the equations only slightly overestimate safe exposure periods while underestimating the decrease in pulmonary function. Although the UPTD unit system is very useful for evaluating permissible oxygen exposures at different times and depths in different diving conditions, individual responses can vary within a range of 30% of VC at exposure times >40 hr (208).

The cumulative hyperoxic exposure (CHE) used by Thorsen et al. (2) is a method for integrating the oxygen exposure pressure and time for P_{O_2} values in excess of 0.21 ata (21 kPa). This index is useful in considering pulmonary function tests other than VC and using P_{O_2} exposures <0.5 ata (51 kPa). It is used to evaluate the cumulative effects of P_{O_2} during working saturation dives, where

$$\mathrm{CHE} = \int [P_{O_2}(t) - 0.21]\, dt \tag{11}$$

Changes in airway mechanics appear to be more sensitive indicators of oxygen toxicity at great depths (>3.0 ata) than are decreases in VC. However, decreases in pulmonary function are not the limiting factor at these depths, because central nervous system effects predominate (201,210). In simulated descents to 3.0 ata (304 kPa) for 3.5 hr, Clark et al. (201) observed no statistical decrease in expired VC, even though the inspired VC was decreased by 3.6% and forced expiratory volume at one second (FEV_1) and mid-volume forced expiratory flow (FEF_{25-75}) were reduced by 5.9 and 11.8%, respectively. A reduced increase in the midexpiratory flow when a helium-oxygen mixture is being breathed suggests an increase in small-airway resistance. In a 28-day saturation dive to 2.48 ata (250 kPa) with oxygen pressures ranging from 0.4 ata (40 kPa) to 0.74 ata (75 kPa), no decrease in VC was observed, although FEF_{25-75} decreased (211). The expected decrease in VC at great depth may be masked by a training effect of breathing high-density gas or the emphysematous changes that are often observed in the lungs of professional divers (212).

The carbon monoxide diffusion capacity (DL_{CO}) appears to be the most sensitive indicator of oxygen toxicity, because DL_{CO} can be reduced at oxygen exposures below the minimal UPTD exposures predicted to decrease VC. In deep dives to 30.6 to 45.4 ata (3.1 to 4.6 MPa), DL_{CO} decreased, even though VC and closing volumes increased (201,213–215). Also, in dives to 30.6 ata (3.1 MPa) or greater, the decrease in DL_{CO} was proportional to cumulative hyperoxic exposure, even though P_{O_2} never exceeded 0.49 ata (49.5 kPa) (213,214). When Thorsen et al. (2) reviewed pulmonary function data from nine saturation dives ranging in depth from 1.5 ata (150 kPa) to 45.4 ata (4.6 MPa), they found that P_{O_2} exposures generally exceeded 0.4 ata only for short work periods. Significant correlations were obtained between the cumulative hyperoxic exposure [Eq. (11)] and decreases in DL_{CO} [0.02 %·kPa^{-1}·day^{-1}], closing volumes, and FEF_{25-75}. Total lung capacity and residual volume increase with cumulative pressure exposure, but neither hyperoxia or hyperbaric exposure correlate with VC changes.

In order to determine the mechanism responsible for producing the decrease in DL_{CO}, gas microemboli were monitored in peripheral veins and the pulmonary artery in three saturation dives using Doppler ultrasound. The observed decreases in DL_{CO}, also defined as a transfer factor (ΔTL_{CO}), significantly correlated with the accumulated bubble scores (Fig. 5). A significant decrease in DL_{CO} was observed after a dive to 5.5 ata for 25 min when air was used during decompression but not with oxygen decompression (187). DL_{CO} was also

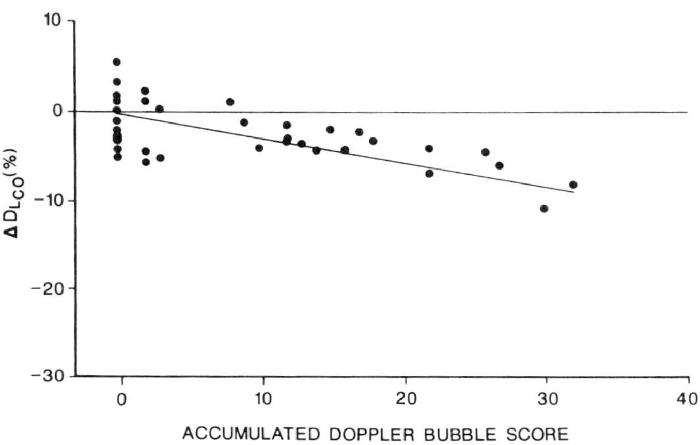

Figure 5 Relationship of carbon monoxide diffusion capacity in divers to the load of venous gas microemboli measured by Doppler ultrasound monitoring. (Adapted from Ref. 2.)

decreased during oxygen exposures of 1.5, 2.0, and 2.5 ata (151, 202, and 253 kPa) (Table 1), but not for a short exposure at 3.0 ata (304 kPa) (206). The decreased DL_{CO} may be secondary to capillary destruction by direct hyperoxic damage to endothelial cells (77) or vessel plugging and the subsequent inflammatory response associated with gas microemboli (216). Continuous infusion of gas emboli in sheep causes pulmonary hypertension and the loss of pulmonary capillaries (217); large gas emboli can actually derecruit entire vascular networks (218–220). When the DL_{CO} after hyperoxia is separated into its blood and membrane components, it is evident that loss of capillary volume is the mechanism responsible for this effect (221).

VI. Induction of Antioxidants and Oxygen Tolerance

A. Oxygen Tolerance in Experimental Animals

Increased tolerance to hyperoxic exposure is induced by low doses of endotoxin, cytokines, various oxidants, sublethal exposure to hyperoxia, or overexpression of antioxidant enzyme activity by gene transfection (14,19,20). Although the mechanisms that cause this increased O_2 tolerance are very complex, an increased expression of lung antioxidant enzyme activity appears to be a major factor. Increases of 30 to 150% in pulmonary SOD, catalase, and GP have been demonstrated (222,223). Frank et al. (224,225) found that rats pretreated with small doses of bacterial endotoxin were protected against a hyperoxic exposure that was always fatal to untreated rats. Increased activities of lung SOD, catalase, GP, and glutathione reductase were found after the pretreatment period (226,227). Cytokines such as interleukin 1 (IL-1) and tumor necrosis factor (TNF), which are released by endotoxin, may be involved with this protection, since both cytokines cause increased CuZn and MnSOD activities and protect the lungs against hyperoxia (228–230). However, Berg et al. (231) and Block et al. (78) found that both the serum of endotoxin-exposed rats and endotoxin itself protect rats and mice against hyperoxia even without increasing antioxidant enzymes. The authors proposed that the release of cytokines suppressed neutrophil activity, because TNF and IL-1 were increased in the protective sera (231). Altered function of the cytochrome P450 system (71,232,233), an increase in ceruloplasmin (234), increased prostacyclin production (235), and reductions in LTB_4, thromboxane B_2, and prostaglandin E_2 concentrations in alveolar fluid after endotoxin pretreatment indicate that these substances could also contribute to induced O_2 tolerance. Normal surfactant function is also a prerequisite for O_2 tolerance, because increases in exogenous or endogenous surfactant activity in rabbits prolonged survival times without increasing antioxidant enzymes (96).

Pretreatment with sublethal hyperoxia also protects against lethal O_2 exposure and provides increased lung antioxidant enzyme activity in rats (236) and guinea pigs (237). Pretreatment consists of a hyperoxic period followed by a normoxic "rest" period approximately one-quarter that of the exposure period. Extending the normoxic period to double the hyperoxic period (10:20 min) doubled the survival time of guinea pigs exposed to hyperoxia (238). Recently, Frank et al. (239) described a rest period of 24 hr on normoxic gas or 50 to 75% O_2 after an exposure of 48 hr at 95% O_2, which extended the survival of the rats in 95% O_2 by 3 to 7 days. Oxygen tolerance induced by sublethal O_2 exposure is not accompanied by a reduced mitochondrial $O_2 \cdot^-$ production, because Freeman et al. (240) found a linear increase in mitochondrial superoxide production (CN−-resistant respiration) in rat lungs that was proportional to the P_{O_2}. Mitochondrial $O_2 \cdot^-$ production was further increased after 7 days of hyperoxia, but the animals were more resistant to hyperoxic lung damage. In studying the greater O_2 tolerance of neonates as compared with adult rats (241), it was found that mitochondrial and microsomal fractions in adult rat lungs generated three to seven times more $O_2 \cdot^-$ than neonatal lung cell fractions. CuZnSOD is increased in neonatal rat lungs after O_2 exposure but not in adult lungs, such that the ratios of SOD to $O_2 \cdot^-$ production were two to three times higher in the lungs of neonates. The greater O_2 tolerance of neonates is obviously related to this favorable balance of scavenger enzymes relative to $O_2 \cdot^-$ production in oxidant stress.

Antioxidant enzyme levels can also be induced by exposure to many different oxidants, but the profile of antioxidant enzyme induction depends upon cell type, the type of oxidant challenge, and the animal's age (242). The greater hyperoxia tolerance of newborns as compared with adults is due to the rapid induction of SOD, catalase, and GP activities (243,244). Apparently, upregulation of mitochondrial MnSOD is sufficient for protection against hyperoxia (227), because endotoxin followed by hyperoxia increased both MnSOD mRNA production and MnSOD activity and conferred protection in adult rats. A 50% reduction in MnSOD activity by blocking G protein–mediated transcription resulted in lung edema and pleural effusion in rats breathing room air; this damage was prevented by hypoxia (245). Separate control of individual enzymes by specific oxidants is suggested because selective inhibition of CuZnSOD in endothelial cells resulted in a selective increase in CuZnSOD mRNA. Inhibition of other antioxidant enzymes did not cause the same effect on CuZnSOD mRNA (246). Clerch and Massaro (227) found that the mRNA for MnSOD, catalase, and GP were increased in rat lungs by either endotoxin or O_2 exposure, but enzyme activity was higher in rats with endotoxin-induced O_2 tolerance. They proposed that an increased stability of mRNAs for scavenger enzymes was crucial to the induced tolerance to hyperoxia. Hyperoxia also probably regulates enzyme induction by a direct oxidant effect on a catalase mRNA-binding protein, which increases mRNA stability (247). The increased O_2 tolerance produced by prenatal treatment with dexamethasone was also attributed to an enhanced increase in CuZnSOD and catalase (248), and the increase in catalase levels was controlled at the transcription level (249). Induced CuZnSod activity in rat lungs appears to be regulated at the pretranslation level in newborns and translational levels in adults, so both require increased production of mRNA (250). Jornot and Junod (251) observed a differential translational control of antioxidant enzyme production in studies of cultured human umbilical vein endothelial cells exposed to 5 days of 95% O_2 (Fig. 6). CuZnSOD and GP activities were increased but catalase activity decreased even though the mRNA levels increased for all of these enzymes. In other studies, a direct effect of specific oxidants on induction of certain enzymes may be inferred, since endothelial antioxidant enzyme levels were not altered by independently manipulating GSH content and the general redox state of the cells (252). Thus, mRNA for antioxidant enzymes is greatly increased by hyperoxia, and the ''rest'' period exposure apparently releases the inhibition of mRNA translation and allows synthesis of the antioxidant enzymes to proceed.

Augmentation of SOD activity by inserting additional gene copies also confers O_2 tolerance. When transgenic mice that overexpressed MnSOD or CuZnSOD in epithelial type II cells were exposed to 95% O_2, survival times were increased over those of transgene-negative litter mates (154,253). Bovine endothelial cells transfected to overexpress mouse MnSOD were also more resistant to hyperoxia (254), even though CuZnSOD appears to be preferentially induced in endothelial cells by hyperoxic challenges (251,255,256).

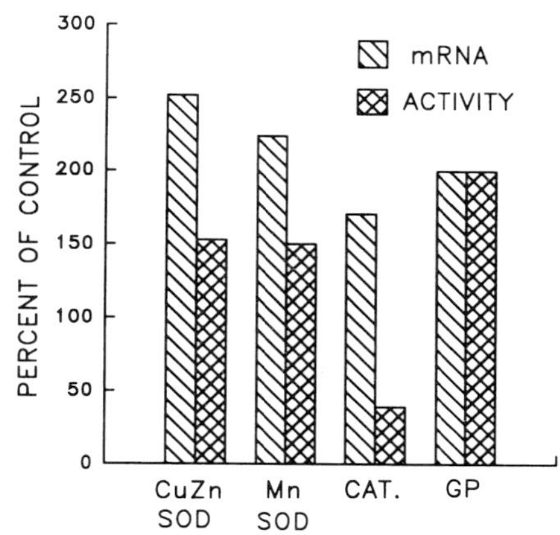

Figure 6 Increases relative to normoxic controls of mRNA and enzyme activities of copper-zinc superoxide dismutase (CuZnSOD), manganese SOD (MnSOD), catalase (CAT), and glutathione peroxidase (GP) in endothelial cells exposed to 95% O_2 for 3 days. (Data from Ref. 251.)

The susceptibility of upper airway epithelium in humans to O_2 injury is apparently related to the low constitutive levels of catalase and CuZnSOD and a failure of these enzymes to be upregulated when challenged by hyperoxia (257,258). Overexpression induced by transfection of human airway epithelium with human catalase cDNA increases the tolerance of the epithelial cells to hyperoxia (258).

Metallothionein, a cysteine-rich peptide that binds transitional metals, and tissue inhibitors of metalloproteinases are induced at the transcriptional level in lungs of mice exposed to 100% O_2 for 4 days. Increased mRNA and protein were measured in cells around arteries, airways, and lymphatics, particularly in the regions where edema and inflammation were present (259,260). Metallothionein content was increased 400 times in rat lungs after administration of a cadmium aerosol and bound 80% of the lung cadmium (157). But the role of metallothionein in inducing hyperoxic tolerance is uncertain.

B. Oxygen Tolerance in Humans

Although pharmacological means of extending O_2 tolerance have been successful in animal models, the only method that appears to have a reasonable application in humans is tolerance induced by preexposure to hyperoxia. Hendricks et al. (261) studied 6 subjects cycled between 2 ata of 100% O_2 for 20 min and 21% O_2 for 5 min (20:5) until a 10% decrease in VC was obtained. The cumulative exposure to 100% O_2 required to produce comparable decreases in VC using intermittent exposure was more than twice that for continuous O_2 breathing (Fig. 7). Subsequent studies with increased exposure and rest periods (60:15) or proportionally increased rest periods (30:30) did not markedly improve the O_2 tolerance (200). Extended saturation dives with hyperoxic work periods undoubtedly produces O_2 adaptation and enhancement of lung cellular antioxidant systems, but there are currently few data from human studies that demonstrate enzyme induction at levels similar to those observed in animals subjected to hyperoxia.

VII. Summary

During normoxic conditions, significant oxidative damage to the lung is prevented by a delicate balance between the oxygen-derived metabolites and antioxidant enzymes and small molecules that scavenge free radicals and oxidants. Hyperoxic damage to the lungs is caused by increased production of $O_2\cdot^-$ and H_2O_2 from oxidase and electron transport enzymes in subcellular organelles, which is a direct function of the ambient P_{O_2}. Whereas $O_2\cdot^-$ and H_2O_2 are relatively weak oxidants, their reaction with Fe^{2+} ions produces OH·, which initiates chain reactions of lipid peroxidation, inactivates crucial enzymes, and

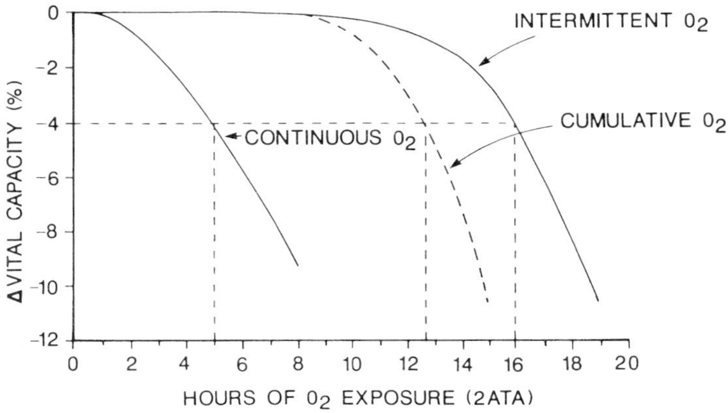

Figure 7 Percent decrease in vital capacity of human subjects breathing 100% O_2 at 2.0 ata, either continuously or intermittently. Dashed line show the cumulative exposure time after subtracting the rest periods in air. (Adapted from Ref. 261.)

damages vital nucleic acids. Chemotactic factors released from these damaged cells initiate an inflammatory response characterized by infiltration of neutrophils into the tissues, which compound the damage caused by the release of $O_2\cdot^-$ and protease enzymes. Impaired surfactant function can also lead to rapid changes in lung and airway mechanics. Tolerance to hyperoxia can be induced by sublethal exposures to oxidants, hyperoxia, or endotoxin primarily through an upregulation of antioxidant enzyme systems. Cell proliferation may also have a protective function but can result in remodeling, with residual airway and vascular dysfunction.

The incidence of hyperoxic exposure promises to increase in the future due to increasing clinical use of therapeutic hyperbaric oxygen and the increased duration and depth of military and commercial diving operations. Methods for enhancing oxygen tolerance in humans by pharmacological antioxidants or methods to enhance expression of endogenous antioxidant enzymes need to be determined in experimental studies. To that end, further research on the molecular pathways that control antioxidant enzyme induction will also be useful. Since exposure to high barometric pressures is accompanied by significant numbers of microembolic bubbles during decompression, improved indices for predicting safe hyperoxic exposure periods at great depths must be developed. Improved procedures will minimize damage to pulmonary capillaries and residual impairment of pulmonary function in divers and others exposed to hyperbaric O_2.

References

1. Kindwall EP. Uses of hyperbaric oxygen therapy in the 1990s. Cleve Clin J Med 1992; 59:517–528.
2. Thorsen E, Segadal K, Kambestad BK. Mechanisms of reduced pulmonary function after a saturation dive. Eur Respir J 1994; 7:4–10.
3. Tibbles PM, Perrotta PL. Treatment of carbon monoxide poisoning: A critical review of human outcome studies comparing normobaric oxygen with hyperbaric oxygen (see comments). Ann Emerg Med 1994; 24:269–276.
4. Hirn M. Hyperbaric oxygen in the treatment of gas gangrene and perineal necrotizing fasciitis: A clinical and experimental study. Eur J Surg Suppl 1993; 1–36.
5. McDermott JE. The diabetic foot: Evolving technologies. Instr Course Lect 1993; 42:169–171.
6. Magnant CM, Milzman DP, Dhindsa H. Hyperbaric medicine for outpatient wound care. Emerg Med Clin North Am 1992; 10:847–860.
7. Cianci P, Sato R. Adjunctive hyperbaric oxygen therapy in the treatment of thermal burns: A review. Burns 1994; 20:5–14.
8. Roth RN, Weiss LD. Hyperbaric oxygen and wound healing. Clin Dermatol 1994; 12:141–156.
9. Grisham MB. Reactive metabolites of oxygen and nitrogen in biology and medicine. Austin, TX: Landes, 1992:1–104.
10. Halliwell B, Gutteridge JMC. Free radicals in biology and medicine, 2d ed. Oxford, England: Clarendon Press, 1989:1–543.
11. Taylor AE, Matalon S, Ward P. Eds. Physiology of Oxygen Radicals, Bethesda, MD: Am Physiol Soc, 1986.
12. Sies H. Antioxidant activity in cells and organs. Am Rev Respir Dis 1987; 136: 478–480.
13. McCord JM, Fridovich I. Superoxide dismutase: An enzymatic function for erythrocuprein (hemocuprein). J Biol Chem 1969; 244:6049–6055.
14. Freeman BA, Crapo JD. Biology of disease: Free radicals and tissue injury. Lab Invest 1982; 47:412–426.
15. Rubbo H, Radi R, Trujillo M, et al. Nitric oxide regulation of superoxide and peroxynitrite-dependent lipid peroxidation. Formation of novel nitrogen-containing oxidized lipid derivatives. J Biol Chem 1994; 269:26066–26075.
16. Freeman B. Free radical chemistry of nitric oxide: Looking at the dark side. Chest 1994; 105:79S–84S.
17. Freeman BA, Crapo JD. Hyperoxia increases oxygen radical production in rat lungs and lung mitochondria. J Biol Chem 1981; 256:10986–10992.
18. Weiss SJ. Tissue destruction by neutrophils. N Engl J Med 1989; 320:365–376.
19. Yu BP. Cellular defenses against damage from reactive oxygen species. Physiol Rev 1994; 74:139–162.
20. Heffner JE, Repine JE. Pulmonary statogies of antioxidant defense. Am Rev Respir Dis 1989; 140:531–554.
21. Turrens JF, Freeman BA, Crapo JD. Hyperoxia increases H_2O_2 release by lung mitochondria and microsomes. Arch Biochem Biophys 1982; 217:411–421.

22. Turrens JF, Freeman BA, Levitt JG, Crapo JD. The effect of hyperoxia on superoxide production by lung submitochondrial particles. Arch Biochem Biophys 1982; 217:401–410.
23. Jamieson D, Chance B, Cadenas E, Boveris A. The relation of free radical production to hyperoxia. Annu Rev Physiol 1986; 48:703–719.
24. Okamoto T, Mitsuhashi M, Fujita I, et al. Induction of cytochrome P450 1A1 and 1A2 by hyperoxia. Biochem Biophys Res Commun 1993; 197:878–885.
25. Sakai H, Okamoto T, Yamamoto R, et al. Suppressive effect of interleukin-1 on pulmonary cytochrome P450 and superoxide anion production. Biochem Biophys Res Commun 1992; 185:1083–1090.
26. Kinnula VL, Whorton AR, Chang LY, Crapo JD. Regulation of hydrogen peroxide generation in cultured endothelial cells. Am J Respir Cell Mol Biol 1992; 6:175–182.
27. Panus PC, Radi R, Chumley PH, et al. Detection of H_2O_2 release from vascular endothelial cells. Free Radic Biol Med 1993; 14:217–223.
28. Kinnula VL, Everitt JI, Whorton AR, Crapo JD. Hydrogen peroxide production by alveolar type II cells, alveolar macrophages, and endothelial cells. Am J Physiol 1991; 261:L84–L91.
29. Kinnula VL, Mirza Z, Crapo JD, Whorton AR. Modulation of hydrogen peroxide release from vascular endothelial cells by oxygen. Am J Respir Cell Mol Biol 1993; 9:603–609.
30. Matsubara T, Ziff M. Superoxide release by human endothelial cells: Synergism between a phorbol ester and a calcium ionophore. J Cell Physiol 1986; 127:207–210.
31. Holland JA, Prichard KP, Pappola MA, et al. Bradykinin induces superoxide anion release from human endothelial cells. J Cell Physiol 1990; 143:21–25.
32. Katusic ZS, Vanhoutte PM. Superoxide is an endothelium derived contracting factor. Am J Physiol 1989; 257:H33–H37.
33. Kinnula VL, Chang LY, Ho YS, Crapo JD. Hydrogen peroxide release from alveolar macrophages and alveolar type II cells during adaptation to hyperoxia in vivo. Exp Lung Res 1992; 18:655–673.
34. Kinnula VL, Adler KB, Ackley NJ, Crapo JD. Release of reactive oxygen species by guinea pig tracheal epithelial cells in vitro. Am J Physiol 1992; 262:L708–L712.
35. Adler KB, Kinula VL, Akley N, et al. Inflammatory mediators and the generation and release of reactive oxygen species by airway epithelium in vitro. Chest 1992; 101:53S–54S.
36. Halliwell B, Gutteridge JMC. Oxygen free radicals and iron in relation to biology and medicine: Some problems and concepts. Arch Biochem Biophys 1986; 246: 501–514.
37. Engerson TD, McKelvey TG, Rhyne DB, et al. Conversion of xanthine dehydrogenase to oxidase in ischemic rat tissues. J Clin Invest 1987; 79:1564–1570.
38. Parks DA, Williams TK, Beckman JS. Conversion of xanthine dehydrogenase to oxidase in ischemic rat intestine: A reevaluation. Am J Physiol 1988; 254:G768.
39. Hassoun PM, Yu FS, Shedd AL, et al. Regulation of endothelial cell xanthine dehydrogenase xanthine oxidase gene expression by oxygen tension. Am J Physiol 1994; 266:L163–L171.

40. Terada LS, Beehler CJ, Banerjee A, et al. Hyperoxia and self or neutrophil generated O_2 metabolites inactivate xanthine oxidase. J Appl Physiol 1988; 65:2349–2353.
41. Paler-Martinez A, Panus PC, Chumley PH, et al. Endogenous xanthine oxidase does not significantly contribute to vascular endothelial production of reactive oxygen species. Arch Biochem Biophys 1994; 311:79–85.
42. Panus PC, Wright SA, Chumley PH, et al. The contribution of vascular endothelial xanthine dehydrogenase/oxidase to oxygen-mediated cell injury. Arch Biochem Biophys 1992; 294:695–702.
43. Freeman BA, Panus PC, Matalon S, et al. Oxidant injury to the alveolar epithelium: Biochemical and pharmacologic studies (discussion). Res Rep Health Eff Inst 1993; 54:1–30.
44. Repine JE, Cheronis JC, Rodell TC, et al. Pulmonary oxygen toxicity and ischemia-reperfusion injury: A mechanism in common involving xanthine oxidase and neutrophils. Am Rev Respir Dis 1987; 136:483–485.
45. Moores HK, Beehler CJ, Hanley ME, et al. Xanthine oxidase promotes neutrophil sequestration but not injury in hyperoxic lungs. J Appl Physiol 1994; 76:941–945.
46. Bryan CL, Lewis RE, Owens SL, et al. Allopurinol inhibition of neutrophilic alveolar response during hyperoxia. J Appl Physiol 1993; 75:357–363.
47. Jenkinson SG, Roberts RJ, deLemos RA, et al. Allopurinol-induced effects in premature baboons with respiratory distress syndrome. J Appl Physiol 1991; 70:1160–1167.
48. Rodell TC, Cheronis JC, Ohnemus CL, et al. Xanthine oxidase mediates elastase induced injury to isolated lungs and endothelium. J Appl Physiol 1987; 63:2159–2163.
49. Kukreja RC, Kontos HA, Hess ML, Ellis EF. PGH synthetase and lipoxygenase generate superoxide in the presence of NADH or NADPH. Circ Res 1986; 59:612–618.
50. Gurtner GH, Michael JR, Sciuto AM, Adkinson NF. Mechanism of hyperoxia induced vascular paralysis: Effect of antioxidant therapy. J Appl Physiol 1985; 59:953–958.
51. Ward JA, Roberts RJ. Vitamin E inhibition of the effects of hyperoxia on the pulmonary surfactant system of the newborn rabbit. Pediatr Res 1984; 18:329–334.
52. Zimmerman BJ, Grisham MB, Granger DN. Role of oxidants in ischemia/reperfusion induced granulocyte infiltration. Am J Physiol 1990; 258:G185–G190.
53. Fox RB, Hoidal JR, Brown DM, Repine JE. Pulmonary inflammation due to oxygen toxicity: Involvement of chemotactic factors and polymorphonuclear leukocytes. Am Rev Respir Dis 1981; 123:521–523.
54. Fox RB. Prevention of granulocyte mediated oxidant lung injury in rats by a hydroxyl radical scavenger, dimethylthiourea. J Clin Invest 1984; 74:1456–1464.
55. Wallace JL, Rioux KP, McKnight W, et al. Hemoprotein dependent production of a neutrophil activating factor from arachidonic acid. Am J Physiol 1992; 263:H1546–H1553.
56. Davies KJA. Protein damage and degradation by oxygen radicals: I. General aspects. J Biol Chem 1987; 262:9895–9901.
57. Davies KJA, Delsignore ME. Protein damage and degradation by oxygen radicals:

III. Modification of secondary and tertiary structure. J Biol Chem 1987; 262:9908–9918.
58. Sandu IS, Ware K, Grisham MB. Peroxyl radical mediated hemolysis: Role of lipid, protein and sulfhydryl oxidation. Free Radic Biol Med 1992; 16:111–122.
59. Strand C, Warshaw JB, Snow K, Jacobs HC. Heat shock does not induce tolerance to hyperoxia. Lung 1994; 172:79–89.
60. Spitz DR, Dewey WC, Li GC. Hydrogen peroxide or heat shock induces resistance to hydrogen peroxide in Chinese hamster fibroblasts. J Cell Biol 1987; 131:364–373.
61. Cacciuttolo MA, Trinh L, Lumpkin JA, Rao G. Hyperoxia induces DNA damage in mammalian cells. Free Radic Biol Med 1993; 14:267–276.
62. Imlay JA, Linn S. DNA damage and oxygen radical toxicity. Science 1988; 240: 1302–1309.
63. Brawn K, Fridovich I. DNA strand scission by enzymatically generated oxygen radicals. Arch Biochem Biophys 1981; 206:414–420.
64. Kuwabara M, Zhi-Yi Z, Yoshii G. ESR spin trapped radicals in aqueous solutions of pyrimidine nucleosides and nucleotides: Reactions of the hydroxyl radical. J Radiat Biol 1982; 41:241–1982.
65. Deng RY, Fridovich I. Formation of endonuclease III sensitive sites as a consequence of oxygen radical attack on DNA. Free Radic Biol Med 1989; 6:123–129.
66. Berger NA. Oxidant induced cytotoxicity: A challenge for metabolic modulation. Am J Respir Cell Mol Biol 1991; 4:1–3.
67. Schraufstatter IU, Hyslop DB, Hinshaw DB, et al. Hydrogen peroxide induced injury of cells and its prevention by inhibitors of poly(ADP-ribose) polymerase. Proc Natl Acad Sci USA 1986; 83:4908–4912.
68. Spragg RG. DNA strand break formation following exposure of bovine pulmonary artery and aortic endothelial cells to reactive oxygen products. Am J Respir Cell Mol Biol 1991; 4:4–10.
69. Christie NA, Slutsky AS, Freeman BA, Tanswell AK. A critical role for thiol, but not ATP, depletion in 95% O_2-mediated injury of preterm pneumocytes in vitro. Arch Biochem Biophys 1994; 313:131–138.
70. Taylor AE, Parker JC. The interstitial spaces and lymph flow. In: Fishman AP, Fisher AB, eds. Handbook of Physiology: Respiration, 4th ed. Vol. 4. Bethesda, MD: Am Physiol Soc 1985:167–230.
71. Hansen Flaschen JH, Lanken PN, Pietra GG, et al. Effect of 100% O_2 on passage of uncharged dextrans from blood to lung lymph. J Appl Physiol 1986; 60:1797–1809.
72. Bressack MA, McMillan DD, Bland RD. Pulmonary oxygen toxicity: Increased microvascular permeability to protein in unanesthetized sheep. Lymphology 1979; 12:133–139.
73. Fukushima M, King LS, Kang KH, et al. Lung mechanics and airway reactivity in sheep during development of oxygen toxicity. J Appl Physiol 1990; 69:1779–1785.
74. Wangensteen D, Piper R, Johnson JA, et al. Solute conductance of blood-gas barrier in hamsters exposed to hyperoxia. J Appl Physiol 1986; 60:1908–1916.
75. Royston BD, Webster NR, Nunn JF. Time course of changes in lung permeability

and edema in the rat exposed to 100% oxygen. J Appl Physiol 1990; 69:1532–1537.
76. Davis WB, Rennard SI, Bitterman PB, Crystal RG. Pulmonary oxygen toxicity: Early reversible changes in human alveolar structures induced by hyperoxia. N Engl J Med 1983; 309:878–883.
77. Crapo JD, Barry BE, Foscue HA, Shelburne J. Structure and biochemical changes in rat lungs occurring during exposures to lethal and adaptive doses of oxygen. Am Rev Respir Dis 1980; 122:123–143.
78. Block ER. Endotoxin protects angainst hyperoxic alterations in lung endothelial cell metabolism. J Appl Physiol 1983; 54:24–30.
79. Harabin AL, Homer LD, Bradley ME. Pulmonary oxygen toxicity in awake dogs: Metabolic and physiological effects. J Appl Physiol 1984; 57:1480–1488.
80. Block ER, Patel JM, Sheridan NP. Effects of oxygen and endotoxin on lactate dehydrogenase release, 5-hydroxytryptamine uptake and antioxidant enzyme activities in endothelial cells. J Cell Physiol 1985; 122 240–248.
81. Allen MC, Watt SJ. Effect of hyperbaric and normobaric oxygen on pulmonary endothelial cell function. Undersea Hyperb Med 1993; 20:39–48.
82. Taylor AE, Bishop VS, Guyton AC. Permeability of the alveolar membrane to solutes. Circ Res 1965; 16:353–362.
83. Egan EA, Nelson RM, Oliver RE. Lung inflation and alveolar permeability to non-electrolytes in the adult sheep. J Physiol Lond 1976; 260:409–424.
84. Holm BA, Notter RH, Siegle J, Matalon S. Pulmonary physiological and surfactant changes during injury and recovery from hyperoxia. J Appl Physiol 1985; 59:1402–1409.
85. Palazzo RM, Wangensteen OD, Niewoehner DE. Time course of functional repair of the alveolar epithelium after hyperoxic injury. J Appl Physiol 1992; 73:1881–1887.
86. Olivera W, Ridge K, Wood LD, Sznajder JI. Active sodium transport and alveolar epithelial Na-K-ATPase increase during subacute hyperoxia in rats. Am J Physiol 1994; 266:L577–L584.
87. Kennedy KA, Lane NL. Effect of in vivo hyperoxia on the glutathione system in neonatal rat lung. Exp Lung Res 1994; 20:73–83.
88. Carter EP, Duvick SE, Wendt CH, et al. Hyperoxia increases active alveolar Na+ resorption in vivo and type II cell Na,K-ATPase in vitro. Chest 1994; 105:75S–78S.
89. Khimenko PL, Barnard JW, Moore TM, et al. Vascular permeability and epithelial transport effects on lung edema formation in ischemia and reperfusion. J Appl Physiol 1994; 77:1116–1121.
90. Nici L, Dowin R, Gilmore Hebert M, et al. Upregulation of rat lung Na-K-ATPase during hyperoxic injury. Am J Physiol 1991; 261:L307–L314.
91. Sznajder JI, Olivera WG, Ridge KM, Rutschmen DH. Mechanism of lung liquid clearance during hyperoxia in isolated rat lungs. Am J Respir Crit Care Med 1995; 151:1519–1525.
92. Haskell JF, Yue G, Benos DJ, Matalon S. Upregulation of sodium conductive pathways in alveolar type II cells in sublethal hyperoxia. Am J Physiol 1994; 266:L30–L37.

93. Dreher D, Rochat T. Hyperoxia induces alkalinization and dome formation in MDCK epithelial cells. Am J Physiol 1992; 262:C358–C364.
94. Wright JR, Clements JA. Metabolism and turnover of lung surfactant. Am Rev Respir Dis 1987; 134:334–444.
95. King RJ, Coalson JJ, Seidenfeld JJ, et al. O2- and pneumonia-induced lung injury: II. Properties of pulmonary surfactant. J Appl Physiol 1989; 67:357–365.
96. Baker RR, Holm BA, Panus PC, Matalon S. Development of O_2 tolerance in rabbits with no increase in antioxidant enzymes. J Appl Physiol 1989; 66:1679–1684.
97. Loewen GM, Holm BA, Milanowski L, et al. Alveolar hyperoxic injury in rabbits receiving exogenous surfactant. J Appl Physiol 1989; 66:1087–1092.
98. Huang YC, Caminiti SP, Fawcett TA, et al. Natural surfactant and hyperoxic lung injury in primates: I. Physiology and biochemistry. J Appl Physiol 1994; 76:991–1001.
99. Minoo P, King RJ, Coalson JJ. Surfactant proteins and lipids are regulated independently during hyperoxia. Am J Physiol 1992; 263:L291–L298.
100. Wikenheiser KA, Wert SE, Wispe JR, et al. Distinct effects of oxygen on surfactant protein B expression in bronchiolar and alveolar epithelium. Am J Physiol 1992; 262:L32–L39.
101. Kobayashi T, Nitta K, Ganzuka M, et al. Inactivation of exogenous surfactant by pulmonary edema fluid. Pediatr Res 1991; 29:353–356.
102. Seeger W, Stohr G, Wolf HR, Neuhof H. Alteration of surfactant function due to protein leakage: Special interaction with fibrin monomer. J Appl Physiol 1985; 58:326–338.
103. Shasby DM, Fox RB, Harada RN, Repine JE. Reduction of the edema of acute hyperoxic lung injury by granulocyte depletion. J Appl Physiol 1982; 52:1237–1244.
104. Dedhia HV, Ma JY, Vallyathan V, et al. Exposure of rats to hyperoxia: Alteration of lavagate parameters and macrophage function. J Toxicol Environ Health 1993; 40:1–13.
105. Griffith DE, Garcia JG, James HL, et al. Hyperoxic exposure in humans: Effects of 50 percent oxygen on alveolar macrophage leukotriene B4 synthesis. Chest 1992; 101:392–397.
106. Weiss SJ, Regiani S. Neutrophils degrade subendothelial matrices in the presence of alpha-1-proteinase inhibitor: Cooperative use of lysosomal proteinases and oxygen metabolites. J Clin Invest 1984; 73:1297–1303.
107. Weiss SJ, Peppin G, Ortiz X, Ragsdale C. Oxidative autoactivation of latent collagenase by human neutrophils. Science 1985; 227:747–749.
108. Boyce NW, Campbell D, Holdsworth SR. Granulocyte independence of pulmonary oxygen toxicity in the rat. Exp Lung Res 1989; 15:491–498.
109. Laughlin MJ, Wild L, Nickerson PA, Matalon S. Effects of hyperoxia on alveolar permeability of neutropenic rabbits. J Appl Physiol 1986; 61:1126–1131.
110. Raj JU, Hazinski TA, Bland RD. Oxygen-induced lung microvascular injury in neutropenic rabbits and lambs. J Appl Physiol 1985; 58:921–927.
111. Krieger BP, Loomis WH, Czer GT, Spragg RG. Mechanisms of interaction between oxygen and granulocytes in hyperoxic lung injury. J Appl Physiol 1985; 58:1326–1330.

112. Lin Y, Jamieson D. Role of neutrophils in hyperbaric and normobaric oxygen toxicity. Pathophysiology 1995; 2:9–16.
113. Smith CW, Rothein BJ, Hughes MM, et al. Recognition of an endothelial determinant for CD18-dependent neutrophil adherence and transendothelial migration. J Clin Invest 1988; 82:1746–1756.
114. Kang BH, Crapo JD, Wegner CD, et al. Intercellular adhesion molecule-1 expression on the alveolar epithelium and its modification by hyperoxia. Am J Respir Cell Mol Biol 1993; 9:350–355.
115. Welty SE, Rivera JL, Elliston JF, et al. Increases in lung tissue expression of intercellular adhesion molecule-1 are associated with hyperoxic lung injury and inflammation in mice. Am J Respir Cell Mol Biol 1993; 9:393–400.
116. Jensen JC, Pogrebniak HW, Pass HI, et al. Role of tumor necrosis factor in oxygen toxicity. J Appl Physiol 1992; 72:1902–1907.
117. Dustin ML, Staunton DE, Springer TA. Supergene families meet in the immune system. Immunol Today 1988; 9:213–215.
118. Wegner CD, Wolyneic WW, LaPlante AM, et al. Intercellular adhesion molecule-1 contributes to pulmonary oxygen toxicity in mice: Role of leukocytes revised. Lung 1992; 170:267–279.
119. Halliwell B, Gutteridge JMC. The antioxidants of human extracellular fluids. Arch Biochem Biophys 1990; 280:1–8.
120. Fariss MW. Oxygen toxicity: Unique cytoprotective properties of vitamin E succinate in hepatocytes. Free Radic Biol Med 1990; 9:333–343.
121. Dilley ED, Jenkinson SG, Lawrence RA. Effects of hyperoxia and vitamin E on the fatty acid composition of rat lung microsomes and mitochondria. Am Rev Respir Dis 1989; 140:423–429.
122. Knight ME, McGehee CJ, Polak MJ, Andresen TL. Effect of hyperoxia on 5-hydroxytryptamine uptake by the neonatal rabbit lung. Pulm Pharmacol 1991; 4:151–157.
123. Kelly FJ, Cheeseman KH. Distribution of vitamin E between tissues during periods of hyperoxic and nutritional stress in the preterm guinea pig. Comp Biochem Physiol Comp Physiol 1993; 105:549–554.
124. Jamieson D. Oxygen toxicity and reactive oxygen metabolites in mammals. Free Radic Biol Med 1989; 7:87–108.
125. Frank L, Neriishi K. Endotoxin treatment protects vitamin E deficient rats from O_2 toxicity. Am J Physiol 1984; 247:R520–R526.
126. Hansen TE, Hazinski TA, Bland RD. Vitamin E does not prevent O_2 induced lung injury in newborn lambs. Pediatr Res 1982; 16:583–587.
127. Jacobson JM, Michael JR, Jafri MHJ, Gurtner GH. Antioxidants and antioxidant enzymes protect against pulmonary oxygen toxicity in the rabbit. J Appl Physiol 1990; 68:1252–1259.
128. Kennedy KA, Snyder JM, Stenzel W, et al. Vitamin E alters alveolar type II cell phospholipid synthesis in oxygen and air. Exp Lung Res 1990; 16:607–615.
129. Frei B, Stocker R, England L, Ames BN. Ascorbate: The most effective antioxidant in human blood plasma. Adv Exp Med Biol 1990; 264:155–163.
130. Jamieson D, van der Brenk HAS. The effects of antioxidants on high pressure oxygen toxicity. Biochem Pharmacol 1964; 13:159–164.

131. Wright JR, Colby HD, Miles PR. Lipid peroxidation in guinea pig lung microsomes. Biochim Biophys Acta 1980; 619:374–384.
132. Mohsenin V. Lipid peroxidation and antielastase activity in the lung under oxidant stress: Role of antioxidant defenses. J Appl Physiol 1991; 70:1456–1462.
133. Castranova V, Wright JR, Colby HD, Miles PR. Ascorbate uptake by isolated rat alveolar macrophages and type II cells. J Appl Physiol 1983; 54:208–214.
134. Loo CK, Smith GJ, Lykke AW. Effects of hyperoxia on surfactant morphology and cell viability in organotypic cultures of fetal rat lung. Exp Lung Res 1989; 15:597–617.
135. Gille JJ, Pasman P, van Berkel CG, Joenje H. Effect of antioxidants on hyperoxia-induced chromosomal breakage in Chinese hamster ovary cells: Protection by carnosine. Mutagenesis 1991; 6:313–318.
136. Herbert V, Shaw S, Jayatilleke E, Stopler-Kasdan T. Most free-radical injury is iron-related: It is promoted by iron, hemin, holoferritin and vitamin C, and inhibited by desferoxamine and apoferritin. Stem Cells (Dayt) 1994; 12:289–303.
137. Krinsky NI, Deneke SM. Interaction of oxygen and oxy-radicals with carotenoid. J Natl Cancer Inst 1982; 69:205–209.
138. Burton GW, Ingold KU. beta-carotene is an unusual type of lipid antioxidant. Science 1984; 224:569–573.
139. Rusakow LS, White CW, Stabler SP. O_2-induced changes in lung and storage pool thiols in mice: effect of superoxide dismutase. J Appl Physiol 1993; 74:989–997.
140. Langley SC, Kelly FJ. Depletion of pulmonary glutathione using diethylmaleic acid accelerates the development of oxygen-induced lung injury in term and preterm guinea-pig neonates. J Pharm Pharmacol 1994; 46:98–102.
141. Jones DP, Eklow L, Thor H, Orrenius S. Metabolism of hydrogen peroxide in isolated hepatocytes: Relative contributions of catalase and glutathione peroxidase in decomposition of endogenously generated H_2O_2. Arch Biochem Biophys 1981; 210:505–516.
142. Deneke SM, Fanburg BL. Regulation of cellular glutathione. Am J Physiol 1989; 257:L163–L173.
143. Deneke SM, Baxter DF, Phelps DT, Fanburg BL. Increase in endothelial cell glutathione and precursor amino acid uptake by diethyl maleate and hyperoxia. Am J Physiol 1989; 257:L265–L271.
144. Deneke SM, Steiger V, Fanburg BL. Effect of hyperoxia on glutathione levels and glutamic acid uptake in endothelial cells. J Appl Physiol 1987; 63:1966–1971.
145. Smith LJ, Anderson J, Shamsuddin M, Hsueh W. Effect of fasting on hyperoxic lung injury in mice. Am Rev Respir Dis 1990; 141:141–149.
146. Tsan MF, Philips PG. L-2-Oxothiazolidine-4-carboxylate protects cultured endothelial cells against hyperoxia induced injury. Inflammation 1988; 12:113–121.
147. Tsan MF, White JE, Rosano CL. Modulation of endothelial GSH concentrations: Effect of endogenous GSH and GSH monomethyl ester. J Appl Physiol 1989; 66: 1029–1034.
148. Peacock MD, Schenk DA, Lawrence RA, et al. Elimination of glutathione-induced protection from hyperbaric hyperoxia by acivicin. J Appl Physiol 1994; 76:1279–1284.

149. Deneke SM, Gershoff SN, Fanburg BL. Potentiation of oxygen toxicity in rats by dietary protein or amino acid deficiency. J Appl Physiol 1983; 54:147–151.
150. Weber CA, Duncan CA, Lyons MJ, Jenkinson SG. Depletion of tissue glutathione with diethyl maleate enhances hyperbaric oxygen toxicity. Am J Physiol 1990; 258:L308–L312.
151. Jenkinson SG, Jordan JM, Duncan CA. Effects of selenium deficiency on glutathione-induced protection from hyperbaric hyperoxia in rat. Am J Physiol 1989; 257:L393–L398.
152. Hilliker AJ, Duyf B, Evans D, Phillips JP. Urate-null rosy mutants of Drosophila melanogaster are hypersensitive to oxygen stress. Proc Natl Acad Sci USA 1992; 89:4343–4347.
153. Crapo JD, Oury T, Rabouille C, et al. Copper, zinc superoxide dismutase is primarily a cytosolic protein in human cells. Proc Natl Acad Sci USA 1992; 89: 10405–10409.
154. Wispe JR, Warner BB, Clark JC, et al. Human Mn-superoxide dismutase in pulmonary epithelial cells of transgenic mice confers protection from oxygen injury. J Biol Chem 1992; 267:23937–23941.
155. Oury TD, Chang LY, Marklund SL, et al. Immunocytochemical localization of extracellular superoxide dismutase in human lung. Lab Invest 1994; 70:889–898.
156. Jacob HS, Jandl JH. Effects of sulfhydryl inhibition on red cells: II. Glutathione in the regulation of the hexose monophosphate pathway. J Biol Chem 1966; 241: 4243–4250.
157. Hart BA, Voss GW, Shatos MA, Doherty J. Cross-tolerance to hyperoxia following cadmium aerosol pretreatment. Toxicol Appl Pharmacol 1990; 103:255–270.
158. Turrens JF, Crapo JD, Freeman BA. Protection against oxygen toxicity by intravenous injection of liposome entrapped catalase and superoxide dismutase. J Clin Invest 1984; 73:87–95.
159. Yusa T, Crapo JD, Freeman BA. Liposome-mediated augmentation of brain SOD and catalase inhibits CNS O_2 toxicity. J Appl Physiol 1984; 57:1674–1681.
160. Tang G, White JE, Gordon RJ, et al. Polyethylene glycol conjugated superoxide dismutase protects rats against oxygen toxicity. J Appl Physiol 1993; 74:1425–1431.
161. Walther FJ, Nunez FL, David CR, Hill KE. Mitigation of pulmonary oxygen toxicity in rats by intratracheal instillation of polyethylene glycol-conjugated antioxidant enzymes. Pediatr Res 1993; 33:332–335.
162. White CW, Jackson JH, Abuchowski A, et al. Polyethylene glycol-attached antioxidant enzymes decrease pulmonary oxygen toxicity in rats. J Appl Physiol 1989; 66:584–590.
163. Gutteridge JMC. The antioxidant activity of haptoglobin towards haemoglobin stimulated lipid peroxidation. Biochim Biophys Acta 1987; 917:219–223.
164. Gutteridge JMC. Antioxidant properties of the proteins caeruloplasmin, albumin, and transferrin: A study of their activity in serum and synovial fluid from patients with rheumatoid arthritis. Biochim Biophys Acta 1986; 869:119–127.
165. Chidambaram MV, Barnes G, Freiden E. Ceruloplasmin and the reactions forming diferric transferrin. FEBS Lett 1983; 159:137–140.

166. Suttorp N, Kastle S, Neuhof H. Glutathione redox cycle is an important defense system of endothelial cells against chronic hyperoxia. Lung 1991; 169:203–214.
167. Kinnula VL, Everitt JI, Mangum JB, et al. Antioxidant defense mechanisms in cultured pleural mesothelial cells. Am J Respir Cell Mol Biol 1992; 7:95–103.
168. Engstrom PC, Easterling L, Baker RR, Matalon S. Mechanisms of extracellular hydrogen peroxide clearance by alveolar type II pneumocytes. J Appl Physiol 1990; 69:2078–2084.
169. Kinnula VL, Chang L, Everitt JI, Crapo JD. Oxidants and antioxidants in alveolar epithelial type II cells: In situ, freshly isolated, and cultured cells. Am J Physiol 1992; 262:L69–L77.
170. Simon R, Edwards JA, Reza MM, Kundel RG. Injury of rat pulmonary alveolar epithelial cells by H_2O_2: Dependence of phenotype and catalase. Am J Physiol 1991; 260:L318–L325.
171. Kinnula VL, Yankaskas JR, Chang L, et al. Primary and immortalized (BEAS 2B) human bronchial epithelial cells have significant antioxidative capacity in vitro. Am J Respir Cell Mol Biol 1994; 11:568–576.
172. Heffner JE, Katz S, Halushka PV, Cook J. Human platelets attenuate oxidant injury in isolated rabbit lungs. J Appl Physiol 1988; 65:1258–1266.
173. McGarrity ST, Stephenson AH, Hyers TM, Webster RO. Inhibition of neutrophil superoxide anion generation by platelet products: Role of adenine nucleotides. J Leukocyte Biol 1988; 44:411–421.
174. Van Asbeck BS, Hoidal J, Vercellotti GM, et al. Protection against lethal hyperoxia by insufflation of erythrocytes: Role of red cell glutathione. Science 1985; 227:756–759.
175. Crapo JD. Morphologic changes in pulmonary oxygen toxicity. Annu Rev Physiol 1986; 48:721–731.
176. Crapo JD, Hayatdavoudi G, Knapp MJ, et al. Progressive alveolar septal injury in primates exposed to 60% oxygen for 14 days. Am J Physiol 1994; 267:L797–L806.
177. Kapanci Y, Weibel ER, Kaplan HP, Robinson FR. Pathogenesis and reversibility of the pulmonary lesions of oxygen toxicity in monkeys: II. Ultrastructural and morphometric studies. Lab Invest 1969; 20:101–117.
178. Reid LM. Vascular remodeling. In: Fishman AP, ed. The Pulmonary Circulation: Normal and Abnormal. Philadelphia: University of Pennsylvania Press, 1990:259–282.
179. Boxt LM, Katz J, Liebovitch LS, et al. Fractal analysis of pulmonary arteries: The fractal dimension is lower in pulmonary hypertension. J Thorac Imaging 1994; 9:8–13.
180. Jones R, Zapol WM, Reid L. Pulmonary artery remodeling and pulmonary hypertension after exposure to hyperoxia for 7 days: A morphometric and hemodynamic study. Am J Pathol 1984; 117:273–285.
181. Coflesky JT, Jones RC, Reid LM, Evans JN. Mechanical properties and structure of isolated pulmonary arteries remodeled by chronic hyperoxia. Am Rev Respir Dis 1987; 136:388–394.

182. Hu LM, Jones R. Injury and remodeling of pulmonary veins by high oxygen: A morphometric study. Am J Pathol 1989; 134:253–262.
183. Jones R. Ultrastructural analysis of contractile cell development in lung microvessels in hyperoxic pulmonary hypertension: Fibroblasts and intermediate cells selectively reorganize nonmuscular segments. Am J Pathol 1992; 141:1491–1505.
184. Jones R, Adler C, Farber F. Lung vascular cell proliferation in hyperoxic pulmonary hypertension and on return to air: Thymidine pulse-labeling of intimal, medial, and adventitial cells in microvessels and at the hilum. Am Rev Respir Dis 1989; 140:1471–1477.
185. Hershenson MB, Aghili S, Punjabi N, et al. Hyperoxia-induced airway hyperresponsiveness and remodeling in immature rats. Am J Physiol 1992; 262:L263–L269.
186. Hershenson MB, Garland A, Kelleher MD, et al. Hyperoxia-induced airway remodeling in immature rats: Correlation with airway responsiveness. Am Rev Respir Dis 1992; 146:1294–1300.
187. Hershenson MB, Abe MK, Kelleher MD, et al. Recovery of airway structure and function after hyperoxic exposure in immature rats. Am J Respir Crit Care Med 1994; 149:1663–1669.
188. Szarek JL. In vivo exposure to hyperoxia increases airway responsiveness in rats: Demonstration in vivo and in vitro. Am Rev Respir Dis 1989; 140:942–947.
189. Uyehara CF, Pichoff BE, Sim HH, et al. Hyperoxic exposure enhances airway reactivity of newborn guinea pigs. J Appl Physiol 1993; 74:2649–2654.
190. Clement A, Edeas M, Chadelat K, Brody JS. Inhibition of lung epithelial cell proliferation by hyperoxia: Posttranscriptional regulation of proliferation-related genes. J Clin Invest 1992; 90:1812–1818.
191. Absher M, Makrides W, Shapiro P, Evans JN. Hyperoxia inhibits proliferation of cultured rat tracheal smooth muscle cells. Am J Physiol 1994; 267:L101–L105.
192. Kelley J. Cytokines of the lung. Am Rev Respir Dis 1990; 141:765–788.
193. Han RN, Buch S, Freeman BA, et al. Platelet-derived growth factor and growth-related genes in rat lung: II. Effect of exposure to 85% O_2. Am J Physiol 1992; 262:L140–L146.
194. Fabisiak JP, Evans JN, Kelley J. Increased expression of PDGF-B (c-sis) mRNA in rat lung precedes DNA synthesis and tissue repair during chronic hyperoxia. Am J Respir Cell Mol Biol 1989; 1:181–189.
195. Powell PP, Wang CC, Jones R. Differential regulation of the genes encoding platelet-derived growth factor receptor and its ligand in rat lung during microvascular and alveolar wall remodeling in hyperoxia. Am J Respir Cell Mol Biol 1992; 7:278–285.
196. Antoniades HN, Galanopoulos T, Nieville-Golden J, et al. Injury induces in vivo expression of platelet derived growth factor (PDGF) and PDGF receptor mRNAs in skin epithelial cells and mRNA in connective tissue fibroblasts. Proc Natl Acad Sci USA 1991; 88:565–569.
197. Powell PP, Klagsbrun M, Abraham JA, Jones RC. Eosinophils expressing heparin-binding EGF-like growth factor mRNA localize around lung microvessels in pulmonary hypertension. Am J Pathol 1993; 143:784–793.

198. Moore AM, Buch S, Han RN, et al. Altered expression of type I collagen, TGF-beta 1, and related genes in rat lung exposed to 85% O_2. Am J Physiol 1995; 268: L78–L84.
199. Stirewalt WS, Coflesky JT, Young LH, Evans JN. Protein synthesis in pulmonary arteries from rats exposed to hyperoxia. Am J Physiol 1993; 264:L74–L79.
200. Clark JM. Oxygen toxicity. In: Bennett PB, Elliot DH, eds. The Physiology and Medicine of Diving, 2d ed. London: Baillie`re Tindall, 1992:121–169.
201. Clark JM, Jackson RM, Lambertsen CJ, et al. Pulmonary function in men after oxygen breathing at 3.0 ATA for 3.5 h. J Appl Physiol 1991; 71:878–885.
202. Montgomery AB, Luce JM, Murray JF. Retrosternal pain is and early indicator of oxygen toxicity. Am Rev Respir Dis 1989; 139:1548–1550.
203. Sackner MA, Landa J, Hirsch J, Zapata A. Pulmonary effects of oxygen breathing: A 6 hour study in normal men. Ann Intern Med 1975; 82:40–43.
204. Holm BA, Notter RH, Leary JF, Matalon S. Alveolar epithelial changes in rabbits after a 21-day exposure to 60% O_2. J Appl Physiol 1987; 62:2230–2236.
205. Matalon S, Holm BA, Notter RH. Mitigation of pulmonary hyperoxic injury by administration of exogenous surfactant. J Appl Physiol 1987; 62:756–761.
206. Clark JM. Pulmonary limits of oxygen tolerance in man. Exp Lung Res 1988; 14: 897–912.
207. Clark JM, Lambertsen CJ. Pulmonary oxygen tolerance in man and derivation of oxygen tolerance curves. In: Institute for Environmental Medicine Report. Philadelphia: University of Pennsylvania, 1970:1–70.
208. Harabin AL, Homer LD, Weathersby PK, Flynn ET. An analysis of decrements in vital capacity as an index of pulmonary oxygen toxicity. J Appl Physiol 1987; 63:1130–1135.
209. Bardin H, Lambertsen CJ. A quantitative method for calculating pulmonary toxicity: Use of the ''Unit Pulmonary Toxic Dose'' (UPTD). In: Institute for Environmental Medicine Report. Philadelphia: University of Pennsylvania, 1970.
210. Clark JM, Lambertsen CJ. Rate of development of pulmonary oxygen toxicity in man during oxygen breathing at 2.0 ATA. J Appl Physiol 1971; 30:739–752.
211. Thorsen E, Segadal K, Reed JW, et al. Contribution of hyperoxia to reduced pulmonary function after deep saturation dives. J Appl Physiol 1993; 75:657–662.
212. Calder IM, Sweetnham K, Chan KK, Williams MMR. Relation of alveolar size to forced vital capacity in professional divers. Br J Ind Med 1987; 44:467–469.
213. Suzuki S, Ikeda T, Hashimoto A. Decrease in the single-breath diffusing capacity after saturation dives. Undersea Biomed Res 1991; 18:103–109.
214. Cotes JE, Davey IS, Reed JW, Rooks M. Respiratory effects of a single saturation dive to 300 m. Br J Ind Med 1987; 44:76–82.
215. Thorsen E, Hjelle J, Segadal K, Gulsvik A. Exercise tolerance and pulmonary gas exchange after deep saturation dives. J Appl Physiol 1990; 68:1809–1814.
216. Bergh K, Hjelde A, Iversen OJ, Brubakk AO. Variability over time of complement activation induced by air bubbles in human and rabbit sera. J Appl Physiol 1993; 74:1811–1815.
217. Perkett EA, Brigham KL, Meyrick B. Continuous air embolism into sheep causes sustained pulmonary hypertension and increased pulmonary reactivity. Am J Pathol 1988; 132:444–454.

218. Dujic Z, Eterovic D, Denoble P, et al. Effect of a single air dive on pulmonary diffusing capacity in professional divers. J Appl Physiol 1993; 74:55–61.
219. Allison RC, Parker JC, Duncan CE, Taylor AE. Effect of air embolism on the measurement of extravascular lung thermal volume. J Appl Physiol 1983; 54:943–949.
220. Hlastala MP, Robertson HT, Ross BK. Gas exchange abnormalities produced by gas emboli. Respir Physiol 1979; 36:1–17.
221. Puy RJM, Hyde RW, Fisher AB, Clark JM. Alterations in the pulmonary capillary bed during early O2 toxicity in man. J Appl Physiol 1968; 24:537–543.
222. Frank L. Protection from O_2 toxicity by pre exposure to hypoxia: lung antioxidant enzyme role. J Appl Physiol 1982; 53:475–482.
223. Townsley MI, Taylor AE. Involvement of oxygen radicals in pulmonary edema. In: Miquel J, Quintanilha AT, Weber H, eds. CRC Handbook of Free Radicals and Antioxidants in Biomedicine. Vol. I. Boca Raton, FL: CRC Press, 1989:297–314.
224. Frank L, Yam J, Roberts RJ. The role of endotoxin in protection of adult rats from oxygen induced lung toxicity. J Clin Invest 1978; 61:269–275.
225. Frank L, Summerville J, Massaro D. Protection from oxygen toxicity with endotoxin. J Clin Invest 1980; 65:1104–1110.
226. Hamburg DC, Tonoki H, Welty SE, et al. Endotoxin induces glutathione reductase activity in lungs of mice. Pediatr Res 1994; 35:311–315.
227. Clerch LB, Massaro D. Tolerance of rats to hyperoxia: Lung antioxidant enzyme gene expression. J Clin Invest 1993; 91:499–508.
228. Tsan MF, Lee CY, White JE. Interleukin 1 protects rats against oxygen toxicity. J Appl Physiol 1991; 71:688–697.
229. Tsan MF, White JE, Santana TA, Lee CY. Tracheal insufflation of tumor necrosis factor protects rats against oxygen toxicity. J Appl Physiol 1990; 68:1211–1219.
230. Warner BB, Burhans MS, Clark JC, Wispe JR. Tumor necrosis factor-alpha increases Mn-SOD expression: Protection against oxidant injury. Am J Physiol 1991; 260:L296–L301.
231. Berg JT, Allison RC, Prasad VR, Taylor AE. Endotoxin protection of rats from pulmonary oxygen toxicity: Possible cytokine involvement. J Appl Physiol 1990; 68:549–553.
232. Mansour H, Levacher M, Azoulay Dupuis E, et al. Genetic differences in response to pulmonary cytochrome P-450 inducers and oxygen toxicity. J Appl Physiol 1988; 64:1376–1381.
233. Asson Batres MA, Stock MK, Hare JF, Metcalfe J. O_2 effect on composition of chick embryonic heart and brain. Respir Physiol 1989; 77:101–109.
234. Fleming RE, Whitman IP, Gitlin JD. Induction of ceruloplasmin gene expression in rat lung during inflammation and hyperoxia. Am J Physiol 1991; 260:L68–L74.
235. Holtzman RB, Zemaitis J, Adler L, et al. Role of eicosanoids in relative oxygen tolerance of newborn rabbits. Prostaglandins 1989; 37:481–491.
236. Crapo JD, Tierney DF. Superoxide dismutase and pulmonary oxygen toxicity. Am J Physiol 1978; 44:364–649.
237. Harabin AL, Braisted JC, Flynn ET. Response of antioxidant enzymes to intermittent and continuous hyperbaric oxygen. J Appl Physiol 1990; 69:328–335.

238. Harabin AL, Survanshi SS, Weathersby PK, et al. The modulation of oxygen toxicity by intermittent exposure. Toxicol Appl Pharmacol 1988; 93:293–311.
239. Frank L, Iqbal J, Hass M, Massaro D. New "rest period" protocol for inducing tolerance to high O_2 exposure in adult rats. Am J Physiol 1989; 257:L226–L231.
240. Freeman BA, Topolosky MK, Crapo JD. Hyperoxia increases oxygen radical production in rat lung homogenates. Arch Biochem Biophys 1982; 216:477–484.
241. Ischiropoulos H, Nadziejko CE, Kumae T, Kikkawa Y. Oxygen tolerance in neonatal rats: Role of subcellular superoxide generation. Am J Physiol 1989; 257: L411–L420.
242. Quinlan T, Spivack S, Mossman BT. Regulation of antioxidant enzymes in lung after oxidant injury. Environ Health Perspect 1994; 102 (suppl 2):79–87.
243. Keeney SE, Cress SE, Brown SE, Bidani A. The effect of hyperoxic exposure on antioxidant enzyme activities of alveolar type II cells in neonatal and adult rats. Pediatr Res 1992; 31:441–444.
244. Clerch LB, Massaro D. Rat lung antioxidant enzymes: Differences in perinatal gene expression and regulation. Am J Physiol 1992; 263:L466–L470.
245. Clerch LB, Neithardt G, Spencer U, et al. Pertussis toxin treatment alters manganese superoxide dismutase activity in lung: Evidence for lung oxygen toxicity in air-breathing rats. J Clin Invest 1994; 93:2482–2489.
246. Maitre B, Jornot L, Junod AF. Effects of inhibition of catalase and superoxide dismutase activity on antioxidant enzyme mRNA levels. Am J Physiol 1993; 265: L636–L643.
247. Clerch LB, Massaro D. Oxidation-reduction-sensitive binding of lung protein to rat catalase mRNA. J Biol Chem 1992; 267:2853–2855.
248. Keeney SE, Mathews MJ, Rassin DK. Antioxidant enzyme responses to hyperoxia in preterm and term rats after prenatal dexamethasone administration. Pediatr Res 1993; 33:177–180.
249. Clerch LB, Iqbal J, Massaro D. Perinatal rat lung catalase gene expression: Influence of corticosteroid and hyperoxia. Am J Physiol 1991; 260:L428–L433.
250. Hass MA, Iqbal J, Clerch LB, et al. Rat lung Cu, Zn superoxide dismutase: Isolation and sequence of a full-length cDNA and studies of enzyme induction. J Clin Invest 1989; 83:1241–1246.
251. Jornot L, Junod AF. Response of human endothelial cell antioxidant enzymes to hyperoxia. Am J Respir Cell Mol Biol 1992; 6:107–115.
252. Jornot L, Junod AF. Variable glutathione levels and expression of antioxidant enzymes in human endothelial cells. Am J Physiol 1993; 264:L482–L489.
253. White CW, Avraham KB, Shanley PF, Groner Y. Transgenic mice with expression of elevated levels of copper-zinc superoxide dismutase in the lungs are resistant to pulmonary oxygen toxicity. J Clin Invest 1991; 87:2162–2168.
254. Lindau Shepard B, Shaffer JB, Del Vecchio PJ. Overexpression of manganous superoxide dismutase (MnSOD) in pulmonary endothelial cells confers resistance to hyperoxia. J Cell Physiol 1994; 161:237–242.
255. Kong XJ, Lee SL, Lanzillo JJ, Fanburg BL. Cu,Zn superoxide dismutase in vascular cells: Changes during cell cycling and exposure to hyperoxia. Am J Physiol 1993; 264:L365–L375.

256. Das SK, Fanburg BL. Hyperoxia elevates Cu,Zn-superoxide dismutase of endothelial cells as detected by a sensitive ELISA. Enzyme 1992; 46:188–195.
257. Erzurum SC, Danel C, Gillissen A, et al. In vivo antioxidant gene expression in human airway epithelium of normal individuals exposed to 100% O_2. J Appl Physiol 1993; 75:1256–1262.
258. Yoo JH, Erzurum SC, Hay JG, et al. Vulnerability of the human airway epithelium to hyperoxia: Constitutive expression of the catalase gene in human bronchial epithelial cells despite oxidant stress. J Clin Invest 1994; 93:297–302.
259. Piedboeuf B, Johnston CJ, Watkins RH, et al. Increased expression of tissue inhibitor of metalloproteinases (TIMP-I) and metallothionein in murine lungs after hyperoxic exposure. Am J Respir Cell Mol Biol 1994; 10:123–132.
260. Horowitz S, Dafni N, Shapiro DL, et al. Hyperoxic exposure alters gene expression in the lung: Induction of the tissue inhibitor of metalloproteinases mRNA and other mRNAs. J Biol Chem 1989; 264:7092–7095.
261. Hendricks PL, Hall DA, Hunter WH, Haley PJ. Extension of pulmonary O_2 tolerance in man at 2 ata by intermittent O_2 exposure. J Appl Physiol 1977; 42:593–599.

6

Carbon Dioxide Retention

EDWARD H. LANPHIER

University of Wisconsin Medical School
Madison, Wisconsin

JOLIE BOOKSPAN

University of Pennsylvania
Philadelphia, Pennsylvania

I. Introduction

The term *carbon dioxide retention* can refer to any situation in which CO_2 produced by the body is retained in the body, causing internal CO_2 tensions to rise above normal levels. The circumstances can range from breath-holding (1) to clinical pulmonary disease. In diving physiology, the term has come to refer most commonly to *exertional hypoventilatory hypercapnia*. In simpler words, some divers fail to breathe adequately during exertion, although they are presumably capable of doing so.

This situation was perhaps first recognized at the U.S. Navy Experimental Diving Unit in the 1950s. Navy experimental divers developed high alveolar CO_2 tensions, especially during exercise, by failing to increase alveolar ventilation in proportion to the increase in CO_2 production. Attention was drawn to the resulting hypercapnia by an apparent increase in susceptibility to convulsive O_2 toxicity.

Carbon dioxide retention in diving was found to be aggravated by commonly encountered factors such as increased gas density; it complicated the development of techniques for safe use of O_2-enhanced N_2-O_2 breathing mixtures. After briefly attracting attention, CO_2 retention ultimately became an obscure curiosity of diving physiology.

Recently, a surge of interest in diving with nitrox mixtures has enhanced the potential importance of CO_2 retention. The development of increasingly practical "rebreathing" types of self-contained underwater breathing apparatus lends added importance to a normal respiratory response to CO_2.

II. Milestones

An understanding of CO_2 retention, its circumstances, and its consequences has developed gradually. A number of events and discoveries seem especially important.

1878: Paul Bert published his monumental work on the effects of barometric pressure (2). Bert described cerebral oxygen toxicity and demonstrated "auto-intoxication" of animals by their own CO_2. He was aware of a possible connection between CO_2 and O_2 toxicity.

1928: Forbes (3) and Wolff and Lennox (1930) (4) reported that CO_2 inhalation dilates pial arteries. In 1933, Sir Leonard Hill reported that CO_2 inhalation enhances O_2 toxicity in animals (5). In 1934, Shaw, Behnke, and Messer reported that CO_2 potentiates O_2 toxicity in humans (6). In 1935, Gibbs, Gibbs, and Lennox reported that raised alveolar CO_2 tension increases cerebral blood flow in humans (7).

1940: Samson Wright stated the prevalent view of the time: "Poisoning with CO_2 can never be inadvertent, because of the choking sensation aroused" (8).

1941: Case and Haldane concluded that CO_2 excess potentiates the effects of N_2 narcosis (9).

1942: Donald reported that Royal Navy torpedo O_2 divers suffered apparent cerebral oxygen toxicity at depths previously considered operational (10).

1944: Barlow and MacIntosh identified "Shallow water blackout"—unconsciousness under water in British World War II divers using O_2-rebreathing apparatus at shallow depths (0 to 20 fsw), some without warning or hyperpnea. This was confirmed as an effect of hypercapnia, and the problem largely subsided when CO_2 absorption canisters were improved (11).

1952 (published 1953): Cooperative Underwater Swimmers Project (CUSP). Lambertsen and associates observed that some divers swimming on a stationary underwater device were hypopneic. The data indicated hypoventilation in some divers and suggested CO_2 retention (12).

1955: Lambertsen et al. showed that CO_2 administration dramatically increases jugular venous P_{O2} (13).

1955: Lanphier reported on the theory of ''mixed gas'' diving and said that a given partial pressure of O_2 appeared to be more toxic when increased N_2 pressure was present (14).

1956: Lanphier et al. reported that some subjects retain CO_2 during moderate exertion, even with low-resistance breathing apparatus on dry land (15).

1958: Lanphier summarized 6 years of N_2-O_2 mixture physiology studies. The report culminated in two surprising recommendations: (1) Abandon use of high-O_2 N_2-O_2 mixtures due to unacceptably high levels of CO_2 and (2) Increase efforts to use He-O_2 mixtures for mixed-gas diving, as He mixtures did not produce increased PA_{CO_2}(16).

1959: Lambertsen et al. reported that CO_2 retention increases O_2 toxicity (17).

1965: Schaefer suggested that submarine escape tank instructors retain more CO_2 than the average untrained man. He posited a possible adaptation effect (18).

1974: Lally found that diver subjects exhibit higher PA_{CO_2} and lower $\dot{V}E$ than non-diver subjects (19).

1980: Kerem et al. reported that diver and nondiver subjects exhibit similar resting PA_{CO_2}, but during exercise PA_{CO_2} is higher in divers at the end of a breath-hold (20).

1980: MacDonald and Pilmanis found moderate, consistently elevated P_{CO_2} and characteristic hypoventilation in 10 of 10 male divers on open-circuit scuba during open-water dives (21).

III. The U.S. Navy Experience

In the autumn of 1951, one of the chapter authors, Edward H. Lanphier, M.D. (Lieutenant, Junior Grade, Medical Corps, U.S. Naval Reserve), reported for duty at the U.S. Navy Experimental Diving Unit (EDU), then located at the Naval Gun Factory (Navy Yard) in Washington, D.C. (now NEDU in Panama City, Florida). Lanphier had recently finished a research fellowship with Julius Comroe at the University of Pennsylvania. He enrolled in the Deep Sea Diving School, and on completing that course, began the medical officers' version of submarine school in New London (Groton) Connecticut. In the summer of 1952, Lanphier finished submarine school and returned to EDU as Assistant Medical Officer and physiologist.

The Experimental Diving Unit had not long before completed decompression procedures for hardhat He-O_2 diving. It was at about this time that a new option was receiving attention: use of self-contained underwater breathing apparatus, or SCUBA (scuba). By definition, scuba included O_2 and mixed-gas rebreathing units as well as open-circuit apparatus such as the Aqua-Lung. To most officers at EDU, self-contained diving was a (hopefully) passing fancy of whippersnappers. Lanphier was clearly one of these.

Of immediate concern was a plan, promoted by Dr. Christian J. Lambertsen of the University of Pennsylvania and certain personnel of the Office of Naval Research, to conduct the first specific study of the physiology of scuba diving. This was to be called the Cooperative Underwater Swimmer Project, or CUSP (12), and took place in late summer of 1952 in the hospitable waters of naval installations close to San Diego. To EDU, this sounded like an unnecessary exercise, but the organizers wanted Dr. Lanphier to be assigned.

The CUSP provided a focus for much of what followed, including the story of CO_2 retention. It also supplied the basis for useful techniques in related research. The report (12) is interesting reading in its own right, particularly considering what a pioneering effort CUSP really was. In addition to measurements of O_2 consumption and gas use in swimming, the first formal studies of foam neoprene wet suits were conducted there, and an early form of decompression computer was evaluated.

Upon returning to EDU, Lanphier found an able colleague in newly assigned EDU project officer Lieutenant Commander Jolly Dwyer, U.S.N. Dwyer was a graduate of the Naval Academy and had an additional year of study at MIT. Lanphier and Dwyer were given responsibility for several aspects of a recent EDU assignment: to work out a method of using mixed gas to reduce decompression requirements in diving for such practical applications as clearing mines from harbors.

The value of mixed gas hinges upon O_2 concentrations higher than the 21% O_2 in air. The partial pressure of N_2, potentially responsible for decompression illness, is correspondingly reduced. The theoretical background was thoroughly discussed in the EDU special report series of 1954 (22) 11 reports on self-contained diving prepared by Lanphier and Dwyer to become chapters in a new edition of *Submarine Medicine Practice* (23).

The decompression aspect of mixed-gas diving is rather readily handled by calculating the ''equivalent air depth'' of the mixture at a given depth and then using standard air decompression tables. Specifying suitable limits for exposure to O_2 presented a more complex problem. Oxygen partial pressure had to be relatively high in order to make mixed-gas diving worthwhile, but exceeding certain limits involved the risk of convulsive O_2 toxicity. This is not only all too often fatal when it occurs in open water but it can involve the death of a buddy attempting rescue.

One of the basic questions was how much O_2 a diver uses in a practical range of underwater swimming speeds. Lanphier and Dwyer had particular reasons for needing this information. They designed a study of O_2 consumption in swimming through set pathways in a swimming pool at specific speeds. For oxygen-rebreathing scuba, subjects used World War II Lambertsen Amphibious Respiratory Units (LARU). The investigators equipped these units with small, accurately calibrated gas cylinders and gauges so that changes in cylinder pressure could be converted to volumes of O_2 used (24).

IV. Early Encounters with Carbon Dioxide Retention

Three times during the O_2 consumption study, subjects swimming at higher speeds were observed to be swimming erratically, then seen not to be swimming at all, and finally found to be unconscious. These individuals experienced no hyperpnea or other warning. In one instance, Lanphier donned the LARU apparatus after an unconscious subject had been pulled out of the water. He purged the circuit correctly and began swimming. Within minutes, he had typical respiratory signs of CO_2 excess. Before he could get out of the water, he became confused and partially incapacitated. This was Lanphier's personal introduction to CO_2 toxicity in diving.

The only unifying link in these episodes was that in each case, the CO_2-absorbing Baralyme was either wet (and thus inactive) or exhausted (the indicator had changed color). The investigators realized that they were experiencing the same phenomenon earlier described by Barlow and MacIntosh (11), who studied this problem during the 1940s and demonstrated that it was due to CO_2 buildup. They called it *shallow water blackout.* (Later, other writers mistakenly applied that term to the entirely different mishap of hypoxic loss of consciousness upon ascent from breath-hold dives.)

Rendering the canisters as leakproof as possible and extending them to hold more CO_2 absorbent largely took care of the problem. The report (24) states, "These episodes suggest that insidious development of depressant levels of carbon dioxide, during work while breathing high concentrations of oxygen, is a serious potential problem in diving with rebreathing scuba."

V. Studies in Oxygen Tolerance

The EDU was aware of extensive oxygen tolerance studies by the Royal Navy (25), but there were persistent rumors that subjects had learned to simulate milder manifestations of oxygen toxicity (e.g., lip twitching) in order to avoid going all the way to convulsion. If true, this would have had the effect of producing unnecessarily conservative rules. In any event, the U.S. Navy needed O_2 tolerance data of its own.

Lanphier and Dwyer were convinced that deriving meaningful O_2 limits required exposing subjects to O_2 during significant work at depth. Depth would have to be simulated by increased pressure in one of EDU's "wet pots" (vertical pressure chambers containing water), and this meant that exertion would have to be accomplished in a rather small space.

Swimming with fins would provide the most relevant form of work. A simple and reliable device for stationary swimming had to be developed and calibrated in terms of the O_2 requirements already determined in free swimming. The EDU "trapeze" swim-ergometer was the result (26,27). The trapeze put the swimmer in a consistent but comfortable position and provided a steady but adjustable force that the subject had to oppose by swimming.

The EDU investigators first used 100% O_2 at various pressures to work out tolerance limits for O_2 itself (22,28). They initially established a tentative "limit curve" based upon presumably reliable data (Fig. 1). The actual tests were carried to 25% longer times than on the limit curve. No serious toxicity was observed "inside" the limit curve, so this was tentatively accepted as being safe.

It seemed rational to assume that the partial pressure of O_2 was the only crucial variable and on that basis to derive limits for mixtures. Instead, EDU tested actual mixtures under water at simulated depths. In doing so, they discovered what seemed to be a completely different picture. The first experiment produced a convulsion under conditions that they had assumed would be safe. Proceeding cautiously, they encountered no more convulsions, but problems suggestive of early O_2 poisoning or effects of CO_2 excess occurred where no difficulties had been expected (29).

It seemed clear at the time that dives with N_2-O_2 mixtures produced an unusual number of symptoms. The most plausible explanation of the findings

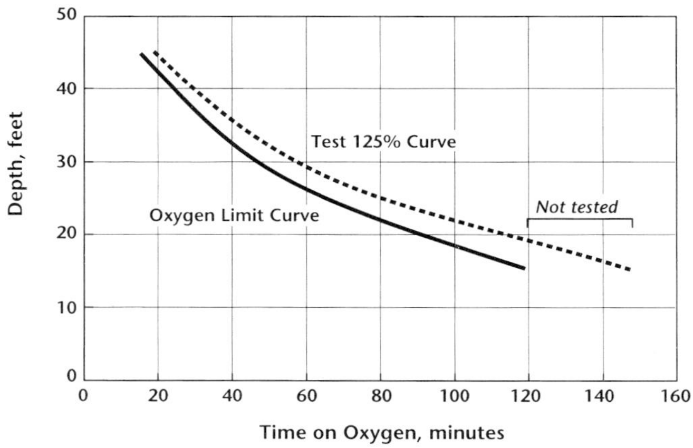

Figure 1 Proposed oxygen exposure limits (diving depth versus time) and test limits (125% of time) for an EDU O_2 tolerance study, 1953. (From Ref. 22.)

was abnormal presence of CO_2, but no source of CO_2 could be identified. One clue came from the CUSP study (12), where some subjects appeared to hypoventilate during exertion.

To follow this possible clue, EDU devised a method of measuring the volume of gas in the expiratory bubbles of divers swimming on the "trapeze" with open-circuit scuba (27). This showed that some of the divers did indeed breathe notably less than others. With many possible variables, this did not necessarily show that these men were retaining CO_2. The next step was to make arrangements to sample "end-tidal" gas for an estimate of levels of CO_2 in arterial blood. End-tidal P_{CO_2} was definitely high when N_2-O_2 mixtures were used during exertion at depth by certain individuals (Fig. 2).

The basic problem seemed to be that some divers did not increase their breathing sufficiently during exertion under any conditions, and factors such as increased gas density and higher P_{O_2} at depth exaggerated their tendency to retain CO_2 (29).

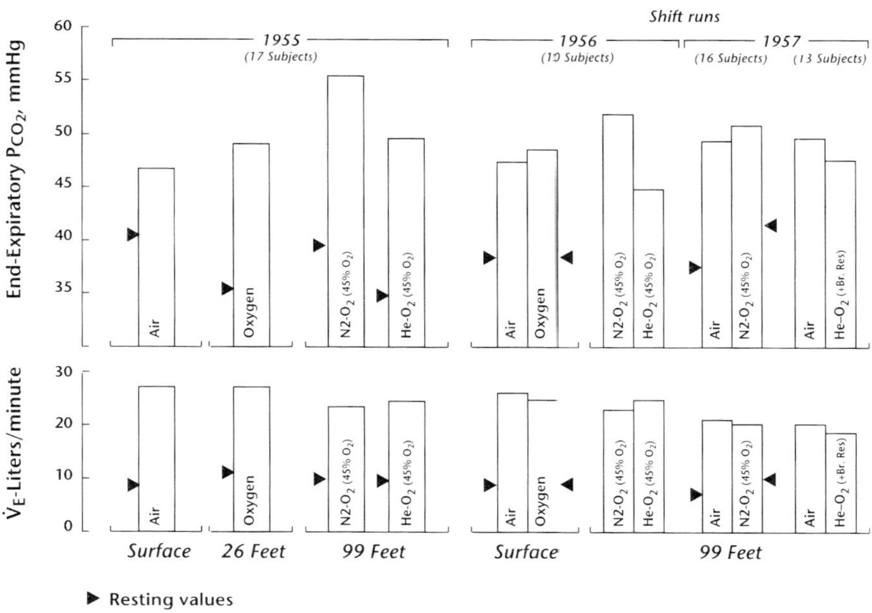

Figure 2 End-tidal CO_2 tensions (PET_{CO_2}), in millimeters of mercury, in working dives with different breathing gases and at pressures from 1 to 4 atm abs (resting values also indicated). 1955 series: a single breathing gas used throughout. Shift runs: a shift from one gas to another during the same dive. (From Ref. 16.)

Lanphier took several of the more extreme retainers to the University of Pennsylvania in Philadelphia to obtain blood-gas determinations in Lambertsen's laboratory (15). Lanphier, whose CO_2 levels were generally low, served as a would-be control. Simultaneous measurements by the EDU end-tidal method yielded what was considered satisfactory agreement with the arterial values, so use of the end-tidal procedure continued.

In 1956 and 1957, EDU investigators conducted further experiments like those reported earlier but with a potentially important difference: when two breathing media or procedures were being compared, instead of comparing results from separate experiments, a switch from one variable to the other was made during a single experiment (16). This approach confirmed that CO_2 levels rose with N_2-O_2 (nitrox) mixtures especially in some divers at depth, but remained close to normal with He-O_2 (heliox) mixtures (Fig. 2).

VI. Summarizing Concerns About Carbon Dioxide Retention

The 1958 EDU report on N_2-O_2 physiology (16) focused on CO_2 sensitivity and regulation under various diving conditions. This largely forgotten EDU report summarizes 6 years of research related to the use of N_2-O_2 mixtures to reduce decompression requirements. It also makes two surprising recommendations: (1) that attempts to utilize N_2-O_2 mixtures with elevated O_2 concentrations be abandoned and (2) that efforts to use He-O_2 mixtures in this way be intensified.

Increased susceptibility to central nervous system oxygen toxicity was the main concern. Specifically, divers breathing an N_2-O_2 mixture at depth developed higher CO_2 levels than when breathing 100% oxygen at the same P_{O_2} but at lesser depth. Presumably, because of his higher P_{CO_2} and its effect on cerebral blood flow, the diver breathing N_2-O_2 was more likely to have an oxygen convulsion. The importance of gas density in this phenomenon was suggested by the fact that the P_{CO_2} was elevated only slightly or not at all when helium was substituted for N_2 in the mixed gas inspired at depth. Divers differed greatly in the degree of their tendency to retain CO_2, but efforts to identify and protect the most pronounced "retainers" were not successful.

The conclusions from EDU research report 7-58 (16) are worth reproducing directly:

1. Retention of CO_2 during working dives at moderate depth is a definite reality.
2. Only when the breathing medium is an He-O_2 mixture is an increase in body CO_2 tension absent or small.
3. Nitrogen-oxygen mixtures, at least with an O_2 concentration close to 50%, produce somewhat higher CO_2 tension than does air under similar conditions. (The difference may not be statistically significant.)

4. Although increased breathing resistance and dead space both favor CO_2 retention, keeping these factors to a practical minimum does not eliminate the problem.
5. Some individuals are much more likely to develop high CO_2 tensions than others, but all individuals show a tendency in this direction, especially when breathing an N_2-O_2 mixture. There is no sharp dividing line between ''retainers'' and ''normals.''
6. There is a definite relationship between an individual's CO_2 levels during working dives and his respiratory response to inspired CO_2. However, there is insufficient correlation to provide clear justification for basing a selection (test) on this measurement.

''These preliminary conclusions lead to one major, final conclusion. The most effective method of minimizing the complications caused by carbon dioxide retention is to use helium-oxygen mixtures for mixed gas dives.''

VII. Enhancement of Inert Gas Narcosis by Carbon Dioxide

Nitrogen narcosis (30–32) is an inescapable feature of exposure to air or N_2 mixtures at depth. In addition to its effect on O_2 toxicity, elevation of P_{CO_2} can accentuate nitrogen narcosis when CO_2 retention coincides with exposure to a narcotic partial pressure of inert gas. Case and Haldane described this accentuation in 1941 (9), but Lanphier (32,33) was surprised to encounter it in an experience that might well have been lethal if it had occurred in open water.

Lanphier and a student assistant tested a newly constructed bicycle ergometer in a dry chamber at 7.8 atm abs. They breathed air from a demand-breathing circuit that included a recording gas meter and had been used successfully at lesser pressures. The test was to consist of 5 min of moderate work on the new ergometer.

It rapidly became obvious that the breathing circuit did not provide sufficient air, but both subjects were determined to complete the test. Both became comatose in a few minutes. Subsequent measurements indicated that they had achieved only about half of the alveolar ventilation needed to maintain normal $P_{A_{CO_2}}$. Dyspnea was extreme before loss of consciousness, and it became a terrifying sensation when consciousness started to return after exertion ceased.

Lanphier and the student were not CO_2 retainers, but it seems likely that the retention tendency would favor loss or impairment of consciousness under less arduous circumstances and might involve less warning of impending danger. Even nonretainers would presumably experience similar effects if narcosis were present along with failure or inadequacy of CO_2 absorption in closed- or semiclosed–circuit scuba. As has been noted elsewhere, consciousness is at risk when CO_2 absorption is inadequate in rebreathing scuba.

In 1966, Jarrett (34) reported a study of four fit men at dry-chamber pressures to 4 atm abs and at a range of work rates. End-tidal P_{CO_2} reached levels above 70 mmHg in some cases. The two subjects who had previous diving experience showed lower alveolar ventilation and higher levels of P_{CO_2} than the nondivers. Jarrett concluded that "tolerance to carbon dioxide is developed as an alternative to the increased work of respiration required to keep alveolar P_{CO_2} down to normal levels." His diver subjects, especially one of them, showed elevated end-tidal P_{CO_2} even at the lowest work rate at 1 atm abs. In this, they resembled subjects of the EDU studies.

In contrast to Jarrett (34), Lanphier and Camporesi (35) express a realistic but less relaxed view of CO_2 response in diving: "The ability to tolerate CO_2 exposure probably has enabled many divers to function exceptionally well in terms of work capacity, depth, and air requirements under some conditions. The same CO_2 tolerance under other conditions could make such divers the first to develop an O_2 convulsion, the most susceptible to N_2 narcosis, the most likely to lose consciousness from CO_2 itself, and perhaps the most prone to decompression illness."

Warkander et al. (36) described severe impairment of consciousness in two subjects exposed experimentally to high external breathing resistance during wet-chamber dives at 6.8 atm abs. In this case, the divers did not experience significant dyspnea. The authors conclude that "These incidents indicate that severe hypercapnia does not necessarily correlate with dyspnea and that severe disturbances in mental function due to hypercapnia can develop suddenly when high breathing resistance is encountered in diving." Based in part on such experience, Warkander et al. (37) proposed "physiologically acceptable" standards for breathing apparatus.

Sterba (38) reported a study of underwater bicycle ergometry with U.S. Navy divers in a pressure chamber. The subjects developed high end-tidal P_{CO_2} levels when breathing air at 190 ft and He-O_2 at 300 and 1000 ft. Above 65 mmHg, dizziness and headache occurred, while above 70 mmHg, severe confusion and amnesia developed. Individuals with values of 74 and 78 mmHg required rescue due to severe CO_2 narcosis.

Sterba concluded that $P_{ET_{CO_2}} = 70$ mmHg is a safe exposure limit for monitored diving and a termination criterion in evaluation of underwater breathing units. Lanphier (35) commented that even if such limits were acceptable, they would impose great responsibility on the accuracy of CO_2 monitoring.

The ability of CO_2 to accentuate narcosis had encouraged earlier attempts to explain depth narcosis entirely as a phenomenon of CO_2 excess (39,40). Answers to this suggestion include a study in which Hesser et al. (41) analyzed compressed-air narcosis into its CO_2 and N_2 components. They concluded that high N_2 and CO_2 pressures are simply additive in their effects on performance. Fothergill et al. (42) reported similar findings.

Bennett and Blenkarn (43) studied four resting subjects at 6.7 and 9.6 atm abs, alternating between air and He-O_2. Mental performance was clearly impaired during air breathing, but there was no evidence of hypoxemia or elevation of $P_{A_{CO_2}}$ under any of the experimental conditions.

Lanphier (44) proposed that impairment of consciousness from CO_2 retention was a major hazard of diving, especially through enhancement of inert-gas narcosis. Subsequent events did not appear to bear out this expectation, although such a mechanism would be impossible to rule out in many diving accidents (45).

Altered consciousness in diving was the main topic of an Undersea Medical Society workshop held in 1980 (46). Participants considered CO_2 retention and related abnormalities to be important among causes of impairment.

Morrison and coworkers (47) reported studies in two divers who had been rescued after losing consciousness at depth. Simulation of the circumstances in the laboratory induced high values of end-tidal P_{CO_2} in both men during exercise at 30 m (100 ft). When one was tested at 70 m (230 ft), he stopped work in less than 3 min because of severe dizziness. In their discussion Morrison et al. surmised that loss of consciousness in these divers probably reflected an interaction between hypercapnia and nitrogen narcosis. In the abstract of the same paper, however, they mentioned "reduced sensitivity to CO_2, perhaps caused by the interaction of hypercapnia and nitrogen narcosis." This rather casual suggestion brings up an important question that has proved difficult to answer: Can inert gas narcosis depress respiratory control as it does other central nervous system functions?

Lanphier (48) brought up the possibility that a vicious cycle might develop if narcosis depresses ventilation and if the resulting increase in $P_{A_{CO_2}}$ could, in turn, enhance narcosis. Lanphier's own experience indicated that severe narcosis does not abolish the respiratory drive or the experience of dyspnea (32,33), but the possibility of some depression of ventilation by narcosis has been difficult to rule out. For example, density and narcotic effects are essentially inseparable: if He is substituted for N_2 to avoid narcosis, the density is also greatly changed, and vice versa. There is some evidence, e.g., Giry et al. (49), that He narcosis inhibits ventilation.

With little change in density, NO in relatively low concentration (e.g. 30% at 1 atm abs) produces a narcotic effect subjectively indistinguishable from narcosis at depth. Bradley and Dickson (50) found that NO inhalation caused significant increases in $\dot{V}_E$ and respiratory frequency with decreases in tidal volume and $P_{A_{CO_2}}$ during both rest and work. These changes are the opposite of those seen with air at depth and were thought to reflect NO sensitization of the pulmonary stretch receptors. Webber (51) also reported an increase in frequency in a similar study; but his calculations indicated no net change in alveolar ventilation. Apparently, NO narcosis differs in significant ways from narcosis produced by N_2 at increased pressure.

Other attempts to distinguish the central nervous system effects of increased N_2 pressure from effects of increased gas density include those of Linnarsson and Hesser (52) and Hesser and Lind (53). Schaefer (54) reviewed earlier evidence that narcosis does not alter the basic CO_2 response. Gelfand et al. (55) analyzed the ventilatory responses of two male subjects over a wide range of pressure and gas density. The reduction of ventilatory response to CO_2 correlated with increased gas density but not with narcosis.

It seems very unlikely that narcosis, except perhaps with He, is responsible for CO_2 retention at depth. Whether pressure itself may have such an effect is unclear even in studies at great depth, such as those reported by Salzano et al. (56). Saltzman et al. (57) observed that resting $P_{A_{CO_2}}$ increased about 0.5 mmHg per atmosphere of increasing pressure. Tarasiuk and Grossman (58) support a direct effect of pressure on the respiratory center.

Carbon dioxide retention is most often caused by respiratory effects of increased gas density at depth or by any factor that increases the work of breathing, weakens respiratory drive, or decreases the efficiency of respiration. At the same time, there is no obvious explanation for the fact that some individuals retain CO_2 during exertion even when no complicating factors can be identified.

VIII. Respiratory Control in Exercise

The control of respiration in exercise has been characterized as a "continuing dilemma" (59). The remarkable precision of normal regulation of breathing in exercise has not been fully explained. Whipp (60) discussed the role of carotid chemoreceptors during exercise. The carotid bodies contribute to the normal $\dot{V}_E$ in air-breathing at moderate work rates but (perhaps paradoxically) $\dot{V}_E$ at 1 atm abs is essentially the same at steady states of moderate work, whether air or O_2 is breathed. A quite different situation exists with work above the anaerobic threshold: high concentrations of O_2 yield lower $\dot{V}_E$, even at maximum work. The carotid bodies in humans are the mediators of ventilatory response to acute metabolic acidosis (61), as associated with heavy work, and it appears that elevated O_2 pressure attenuates this response.

IX. Mechanisms of Carbon Dioxide Retention

Since no great change in P_{CO_2} ordinarily occurs during rest or exercise, alveolar ventilation generally remains proportional to CO_2 production. Circumstances that upset this relationship arise occasionally. Lanphier (35) attempted to evaluate factors apparently responsible for high end-expiratory P_{CO_2} values observed during work with N_2-O_2 mixtures at depth. In this effort, he utilized data from the 17 subjects primarily involved in the experiments conducted at EDU in 1955 (28). The P_{CO_2} values corrected for background gas effects in infrared gas analysis were derived from data presented in a subsequent report (Ref. 16, table 1).

In the present analysis, based on the same study (Fig. 3), we attempt to see how much several probable influences may have contributed to the elevation of P_{CO_2} above 40 mmHg. Most of the resting values (Fig. 2) were close to 40 mmHg; but exertion, even close to surface (at about 4 ft of depth in the pressure tank), yielded a mean P_{CO_2} of 46.7 mmHg. Whether this can be attributed entirely to a low ventilatory response to exertion or to breathing apparatus and related factors is not certain. Whatever the cause, this was actually the largest contributor to P_{CO_2} values above 40 mmHg at depth.

Breathing 100% O_2 at 26 ft was included because this reproduced the PI_{O_2} of 45% O_2 at 4 atm abs. It also involved an increase in pressure to 1.8 atm abs with the accompanying increase in gas density. The P_{CO_2} was elevated somewhat further, to 48.9 mmHg. Increased inspiratory O_2 pressure thus did not seem to be a large contributor to elevation of P_{CO_2}.

A major increase in P_{CO_2} to 55.1 mmHg, occurred with 45% O_2 in N_2 at 4 atm abs (99 fsw). Since the P_{O_2} had already been increased, this change could be attributed mainly to the increase in gas density in going from 1.8 to 4.0 atm abs. A partial check on this assumption was provided by the lower P_{CO_2} associated with 45% O_2 in He: 49.7 mmHg.

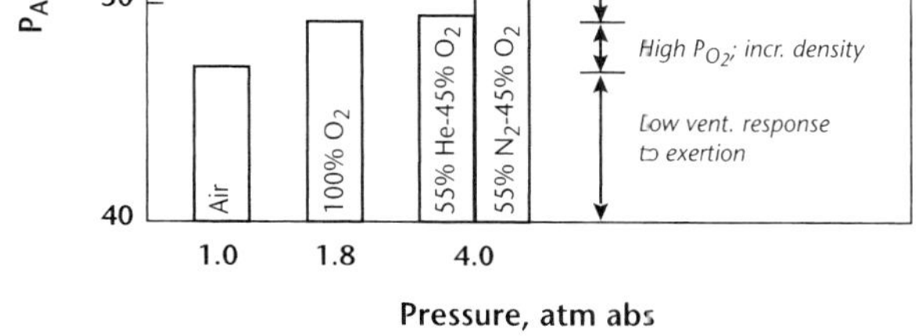

Figure 3 Carbon dioxide levels under different conditions and factors apparently responsible for elevation. The highest P_{CO_2} observed was with N_2O_2: 70 mmHg. (From Ref. 35.)

This series of experiments suggests the relative effects of work, P_{O_2}, and gas density. Further studies in 1956 and 1957 (Fig. 2) yielded less marked but otherwise similar changes (16). It is not surprising that one of the recommendations in the latter report was to abandon the use of high-O_2 N_2-O_2 mixtures in favor of mixtures of He and O_2. A number of convulsions occurred subsequently, but instead of following these recommendations, the allowable limits of P_{O_2} in nitrox diving were lowered progressively.

The potential importance of this matter justifies further discussion of the main factors apparently responsible for elevated values of P_{CO_2} during work at depth.

A. Inadequate Ventilatory Response to Exertion

Observations in the CUSP study (12) called attention to differences in ventilation among divers doing (presumably) very similar work at depth. Smaller volumes of ventilation suggest CO_2 retention. The explanation for such individual differences is, of course, uncertain. Inherited characteristics may be involved, as well as environmental and occupational influences. In a small group of men, Jarrett (34) found examples not only of the apparent influence of earlier diving experience but also of an abrupt change that might be attributed to a psychological influence.

B. Increased PI_{O_2}

High P_{O_2} decreases ventilation in some situations. Most of the emphasis in the summary and conclusions of the CUSP study (12) was on the fact that breathing O_2 instead of air markedly decreased ventilation and that ventilation (in surface terms) did not increase as much with greater depth, as has always been assumed. A diver doing the same amount of work has been expected, for example, to inspire twice as many gas molecules per unit time at 2 atm abs as at 1 atm abs. In practical terms, the duration of a given supply of compressed air in open-circuit scuba has thus been assumed to suffice for only half as much time at twice the absolute pressure. Of course, this need not be true if increased P_{O_2} or gas density simultaneously decreases the drive to breathe or the effectiveness of respiratory effort.

According to Cunningham (62) and Wasserman (63), a normal subject abruptly breathing 100% O_2 during air-breathing exercise will exhibit a fall in ventilation. Other authors find that at a given steady-state work rate below the anaerobic threshold, ventilation is not appreciably different between 100% O_2 breathing and air breathing.

Asmussen and Nielsen (64), Wasserman (63), Welch et al. (65), and Margaria et al. (66) found that ventilation is appreciably lessened while divers are breathing a high concentration of O_2 at work rates greater than the anaerobic threshold, up to maximal work. Since high inspired O_2 levels appear to attenuate or eliminate the carotid chemoreceptor response to lactic acid (67), this may help to explain CO_2 retention in working divers, assuming that many of them are at or above the anaerobic threshold.

Another effect may help to explain elevated P_{CO_2} in the presence of high $P_{I_{O_2}}$. When the $P_{I_{O_2}}$ is elevated, increased amounts of O_2 go into physical solution in the blood. The body utilizes dissolved O_2 before drawing upon O_2 carried by hemoglobin. Transport of CO_2 from the tissues normally depends in part upon combination of CO_2 with reduced hemoglobin. If the proportion of reduced hemoglobin is smaller than usual, CO_2 transport will be impaired, the CO_2 tension in blood and tissues must rise, and the H ion concentration will increase.

As explained by Lambertsen (68), these changes, affecting central respiratory control, would normally produce an increase in ventilation sufficient to lower arterial P_{CO_2} and thus cause some degree of cerebral vasoconstriction, reduce cerebral blood flow, and decrease the effective "dose" of O_2 to brain tissue. This potentially protective mechanism is readily derailed by CO_2 in the inspired gas or by increased work of breathing. It seems likely that a limited response to CO_2 would have a similar effect, leaving only impaired transport of CO_2 as a consequence of decreased availability of reduced hemoglobin.

C. Increased Work of Breathing

Increased work of breathing seems to account for much of the elevation of $P_{A_{CO_2}}$. High gas density at depth increases the work of moving gas through the diver's own airways as well as those of the breathing apparatus. The classical studies on the effects of added external resistance are those of Cain and Otis (69) and Zechman et al. (70). It is probably safe to assume that much the same effects would ensue from increased internal resistance. Both teams recognized effects upon CO_2 elimination. Cain and Otis (69) summarized the situation by saying, "The retention of CO_2 during resistance breathing indicates a compromise by the body. The body tolerates some rise in CO_2 tension in preference to expending the effort that would be required to keep it at the original level."

Fagraeus and Linnarsson (71) depicted a typical course of end-tidal P_{CO_2} in submaximal and maximal work on air at 1, 3, and 6 atm abs (Fig. 4). The subject was not a CO_2 retainer, as indicated by normal values in work at 100 W. The compensatory drop in $P_{A_{CO_2}}$ with a high workload occurred at 1 atm but was obscured at 3 atm and clearly absent at 6 atm abs. Increased gas density is almost certainly responsible for most of the differences seen here.

In a study of tolerance to various gases at extreme densities, Lambertsen et al. (72) found "a prominent reduction of total and alveolar ventilation." The response was unrelated to narcotic properties of the gases in question, demon-

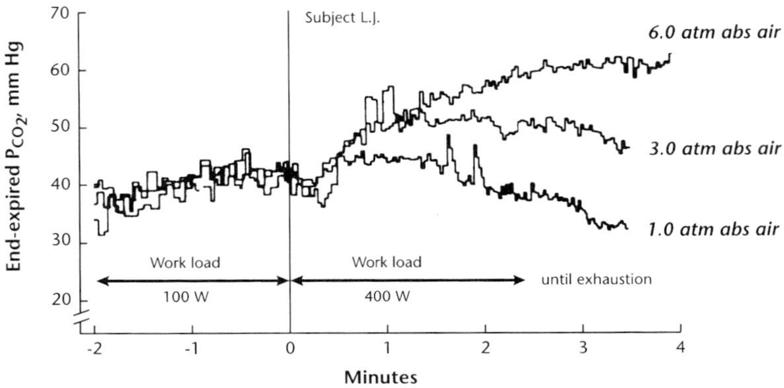

Figure 4 Typical time course of breath-by-breath end-expired P_{CO_2} during submaximal and maximal exercise breathing air at 1.0, 3.0, and 6.0 atm abs. (From Ref. 71.)

strating that ventilatory suppression was not a function of narcotic depression. Gas density and work of breathing limited pulmonary function.

X. Symptoms Reported by Divers

Low ventilation and high CO_2 levels are of concern in terms of the symptoms they may produce. Symptoms reported by diver subjects in the course of various simulated dives (29) are of some interest:

Transient dizziness early in a dive breathing 40% O_2 at 110 ft.
Severe headaches following dives of almost any kind.
Marked fatigue and dizziness after 16 min of breathing 40% O_2 at 110 ft and severe headache lasting several hours.
No symptoms except nausea after 23 min on 40% O_2 at 110 ft.
Grand mal convulsion after 20 min of 47% O_2 at 100 ft and nausea after 45 min on 50% O_2 at 90 ft.
Uncontrollable trembling (distinct from twitching and apparently not of emotional origin) after 4 min breathing 40% O_2 at 140 ft; headache and nausea after 35 min at 110 ft.
Unusual fatigue on first trapeze-swimming run (40% O_2 at 110 ft).
Severe nausea after 36 min of 40% O_2 at 110 ft.
Five subjects reported no symptoms.

It is impossible to derive a formal correlation between ventilation and symptomatology from these data, but subjects showing either consistent or episodic hypoventilation appeared much more likely to report symptoms than those who maintained relatively high ventilation. The amount of inter- and intraindividual variability was great.

XI. Carbon Dioxide Retention and Inspired Carbon Dioxide

The probable response of a CO_2 retainer to CO_2 in the inspired gas deserves consideration. The alveolar P_{CO_2} cannot be lower than the PI_{CO_2}. In practical terms (35), all that alveolar ventilation can do is to bring PA_{CO_2} down toward PI_{CO_2}. If the CO_2 response is weak, PA_{CO_2} may remain considerably higher than PI_{CO_2}.

A PI_{CO_2} of 10 mmHg is sometimes viewed as an acceptable level in air or gas supplied to a diver. An example will serve to illustrate what this implies. Doing moderate work with $\dot{V}_{CO_2}$ at 1.5 L/min STPD will require the $\dot{V}A$ to be about 32.4 L BTPS to maintain PA_{CO_2} at 40 mmHg if the inspired gas is free of CO_2 (35). In the same terms, if PI_{CO_2} is 10 mmHg, maintaining 40 mmHg would require $\dot{V}A$ to be 43.2 L/min. The increase is 33% of the normal $\dot{V}A$ and, especially in the absence of a normal ventilatory response to CO_2, would almost certainly not be achieved.

Increased $\dot{V}A$ and $\dot{V}E$ could become a considerable respiratory burden. At a higher work rate, with high gas density or with the limitations of breathing apparatus, an optimal increase would probably be impossible. Realistically, there would be a lesser increase in $\dot{V}E$ and an increase in PA_{CO_2}. Even rather small elevations can have serious implications under circumstances such as exposure to a near-toxic PI_{O_2}.

Investigators who have studied the implications of elevated PI_{CO_2} during exercise include Menn et al. (73). They used heavy exercise and found no difficulty in 30-min bouts at 15 mmHg PI_{CO_2}. At 30 mmHg, subjects completed 30 min of work despite dyspnea and intercostal pain with PA_{CO_2} values between 49 and 61 mmHg and an average $\dot{V}E$ of 103 L/min. In approaching maximum exertion, marked hypercapnia and acidosis were considered likely, with a PI_{CO_2} of 21 mmHg or more. Elliott et al. (74) concluded that a PI_{CO_2} of 15 mmHg results in severe acid-base disturbance at the limits of ventilatory capacity.

Clark and his associates (75,76) described acid-base, arterial gas, and ventilatory changes in work up to 80% of $\dot{V}_{O_2max}$ with PI_{CO_2} values up to 40 mmHg. The highest work rate at the highest PI_{CO_2} forced the subjects very close to maximum voluntary ventilation (MVV). The expected compensatory drop in PA_{CO_2} at higher work rates was seen in their subjects with a PI_{CO_2} of 0 or 10 mmHg but not with higher values.

XII. Why Carbon Dioxide Acclimatization?

Ordinarily, rising levels of CO_2 produce an increasingly uncomfortable desire to increase breathing. However, there is a great range of response. The main question behind CO_2 retention is: "Why do some subjects not increase ventilation to regulate their rising CO_2 levels?"

Some evidence suggests that the tendency to retain CO_2 increases with chronic exposure to high-CO_2 environments, such as those encountered during specific diving situations. In effect, the body becomes accustomed to higher levels, allowing them to occur without the usual autoregulation that would correct the situation.

In the first EDU studies (29), almost all of the subjects had been experienced suit-and-helmet ("hardhat") divers. The volumes of air needed for adequate ventilation of a helmet are very great, particularly at significant depth (35). Fully adequate ventilation of a helmet is unlikely, so acclimatization to CO_2 may have been an occupational necessity.

Divers sometimes had other reasons for elevation of their arterial P_{CO_2}, such as repeated deep breath-hold diving in submarine escape training. Schaefer (18) found that submarine escape tank instructors retained more CO_2 than the average untrained man. He suggested a possible adaptation effect. Kerem et al. (20) found that both diver and nondiver subjects exhibited similar resting arterial CO_2 levels; but when they were exercising, arterial CO_2 was higher in divers. They confirmed this in a later study of CO_2 retention during nitrox breathing (77).

MacDonald and Pilmanis (21) found a moderate, consistently elevated CO_2 level and characteristic hypoventilation in 10 of 10 male divers tested on open-circuit scuba during open-water dives.

Some sort of selection seems likely, where those who tolerate high CO_2 levels continue with their diving career while others drop out. That situation must be less prevalent today, so the number of CO_2-tolerant divers from that source may be considerably smaller. Perhaps some of the CO_2-retaining divers have sleep apnea and routinely experience high CO_2 levels during sleep.

In some cases, CO_2 retention occurs in subjects with no experience with high-CO_2 environments but who may be exposed in other ways. When scuba diving first became prevalent, "skip breathing" was often taught or popularized as a means of conserving the air supply in open-circuit scuba. Educational efforts to discourage skip breathing have had some effect, so fewer individuals have probably become CO_2-tolerant in this way.

Some CO_2 retainers lack any history of probable acclimatization. There are probably a few individuals who retain CO_2 with no suggestion that this is an adaptive response. A 1995 study by Clark et al. (78) found increased levels of arterial CO_2 with increasing exertion in normal subjects exposed to 2 atm of O_2 on dry land.

Dempsey et al. (59) conclude that significant, sustained CO_2 retention is "extremely rare in health even under the most extreme conditions of exercise intensity and flow limitation." However, Dempsey (personal communication, 1995) says that this does not necessarily apply to individuals who have become acclimatized to CO_2. At the same time, Dempsey says that in his years of attention to respiration in athletes, he has seen only one or two individuals who would qualify as CO_2 retainers according to our definition.

XIII. Identification of CO_2 Retainers

Various attempts have been made to identify CO_2 retainers in advance of critical exposures. Such people could be at unexpected risk of CO_2 blackout, unusual degrees of N_2 narcosis, or susceptibility to O_2 toxicity. Identification, for that reason, would be a helpful form of screening.

Early in the study cited (29,16), the main hope at EDU was that outstanding CO_2 retainers could be identified and kept from hazardous exposures. If so, others could take full advantage of the benefits of nitrox diving. A dry-land test of ventilatory response to various levels of inspired CO_2 was set up (16). There was a great spread of responses (Fig. 5), and these were compared with the CO_2 levels that the divers developed spontaneously at depth. In about 60% of cases, high CO_2 at depth corresponded to low response to inspired CO_2; but in the other 40%, such a relationship was not seen. The correlation was not good enough for a fair, reliable selection test.

In more recent work involving tethered swimming at a submaximal work rate, 11 of 19 subjects developed elevated CO_2 levels. A CO_2 rebreathing test did not clearly preidentify these people, leading to the conclusion that identification of CO_2 retainers may require a test with exercise (79). A tethered fin-swimming test is an example.

Elliott (80) has recommended that screening tests be developed for working divers doing heavy work on compressed air deeper than 120 ft who might be at risk of unconsciousness. The need for more accurate tests is evident.

XIV. Implications for Recreational Divers

The bulk of work in CO_2 retention has been in situations not characteristic of recreational diving. Might this population also expose themselves to conditions favoring CO_2 retention? Hashimoto's subjects (79) were 19 healthy recreational divers, many of whom reported low-air-use or dive-related headaches. One of the 19 had a history of impaired consciousness at depth on open-circuit scuba,

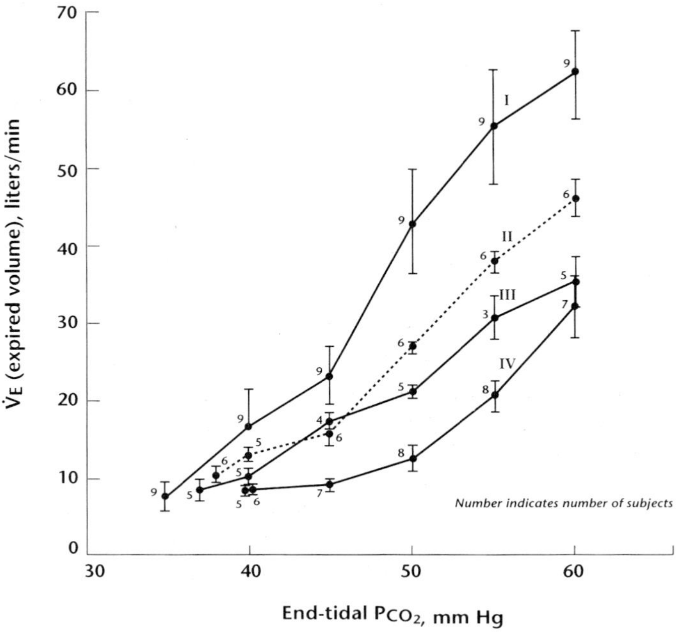

Figure 5 Expired volume versus end-expiratory P_{CO_2} in the EDU CO_2 response study of 1957. The subjects were classified into four groups according to their VE at P_{CO_2} = 50 mmHg. (From Ref. 16.)

with severe headache and nausea following dives. This subject was strongly encouraged to give up diving, which seemed to threaten his exceptional intellect if not his life. He took up other sports and is now an associate professor of physics at a university. Beyond what may seem obvious, the long-term effects of CO_2 retention are unknown.

As mentioned earlier, MacDonald and Pilmanis (21) reported elevated P_{CO_2} and hypoventilation in 10 of 10 male divers during open-water dives with open-circuit scuba. They compared PA_{CO_2} levels on land and under water during equivalent exercise and found greatly elevated CO_2 levels in some subjects during exercise under water. These values corresponded with decreased minute ventilation.

MacDonald and Pilmanis (21) attributed decreased ventilation to several possibilities, including "inhalation and exhalation resistance of the scuba regulator, restrictions of ventilatory movements by the wet suit and other diving equipment, increased respiratory work with a more dense breathing gas, pulmonary engorgement from body immersion, reduced alveolar CO_2 diffusion in a denser gas, and insensitive central chemoreceptors from increasing P_{O_2}.'' They also discussed the case study of a scuba-diver fatality, where an experienced diver using a borrowed regulator was found dead on the bottom with no sign of struggle and 1000 psi of air in his tank. The regulator was later bench-tested under simulated dive conditions and found to have extreme inhalation and exhalation pressures. High breathing resistance was cited as the cause of the accident.

XV. Avoiding Carbon Dioxide Retention

If the solution of the CO_2 retention problem does not lie in personnel selection, what other avenues are open? Avoidance of ''skip breathing'' and any other attempt to restrict ventilation to conserve air seems obvious; but this may be easier to recommend than to accomplish. Providing ventilatory assistance to divers may deserve investigation. An obvious solution would be to utilize He-O_2 mixtures instead of N_2-O_2. Previous studies (16,29) show that CO_2 retention is minimal or nonexistent when the breathing medium is an He-O_2 mixture. In the probable range of depths and times, He should not be much less desirable than N2-O_2 from the standpoint of decompression.

XVI. Conclusions

The present authors have little doubt that CO_2 retention occurs, that it reduces O_2 tolerance and enhances N_2 narcosis, and that it becomes a more significant problem as gas density increases. We believe, accordingly, that the allowable exposure to P_{O_2} should be cut back as depth increases—particularly in the use of N_2-O_2.

We are well aware that universal agreement on these points does not exist, and we ourselves do not pretend to know how large a practical problem CO_2 retention may be in present-day diving. Tending to confirm our basic premises, limits for O_2 exposure in practical diving have become progressively more conservative. Meanwhile, several potential causes of acclimatization to CO_2 have become less prevalent.

Not all investigators and authorities are in agreement with the findings and conclusions of the U.S. Navy EDU studies described here. Most notable among those with contrary opinions was the late Professor Kenneth Donald, whose contentions are embodied in his book *Oxygen and the Diver* (25). Especially in chap. 6, Donald takes issue with most observations and conclusions of EDU studies as reported by Lanphier (14–16,29). Donald's overall conclusion was that CO_2 retention and its alleged consequences remain unproven. In his chap. 7, Donald goes further to cast doubt upon studies elsewhere that support the idea of CO_2 retention and the need to restrict O_2 exposure as depth increases. Donald particularly distrusted end-tidal (end-expiratory) gas sampling and analysis as an index of CO_2 levels in the body.

Some of Donald's criticisms are admittedly well taken, and many of his contentions are difficult if not impossible to refute at this time. Overall, however, the only point on which the present authors can agree with Donald is the need for further study. Whether such investigations will ever be possible, only time will tell. We would urge that efforts be made instead to establish He-O_2 or ''trimix'' as breathing media for mixed-gas diving. Meanwhile, we urge that divers who use nitrox mixtures exercise caution with depth/time limits, reduce P_{O_2} limits—especially if CO_2 retention is suspected—and avoid ''skip breathing'' and other attempts to conserve gas.

References

1. Paulev PE, Naeraa N. Hypoxia and carbon dioxide retention following breath-hold diving. J Appl Physiol 1967; 22:436–440.
2. Bert P. La pression barometrique. Paris: Masson, 1878.
3. Forbes HS. Cerebral circulation: Observation and measurement of pial vessels. Arch Neurol Psychiatry 1928; 19:751–761.
4. Wolff HG, Lennox WG. The effects on pial vessels of variations in O_2 and CO_2 content of the blood. Arch Neurol Psychiatry 1930; 23:1097–1120.
5. Hill L. Influence of carbon dioxide in production of oxygen poisoning. Q J Exp Physiol 1933; 23:49–56.
6. Shaw LA, Behnke AR, Messer AC. The role of carbon dioxide in producing the symptoms of oxygen poisoning. Am J Physiol 1934; 108:652–661.
7. Gibbs EL, Gibbs FA, Lennox W. Regulation of cerebral carbon dioxide. Am J Physiol 1935; 111:557–566.
8. Wright S. Applied Physiology, 7th ed. New York: Oxford University Press, 1940.
9. Case EM, Haldane JBS. Human physiology under high pressure: I. Effects of nitrogen, carbon dioxide and cold. J Hygiene (Camb) 1941; 41:225–249.
10. Donald KW. Oxygen poisoning in man. Admiralty Experimental Diving Unit Report XVI, 1946.
11. Barlow HB, Macintosh FC. Shallow water blackout. U.P.S. 48(a). Royal Naval Personnel Committee 1944; 44/125.
12. National Research Council Committee on Amphibious Operations. Report of the Cooperative Underwater Swimmer Project (CUSP). Report NRC:CAO:0033, January 1953.
13. Lambertsen CJ, Ewing JH, Kough RH, et al. Oxygen toxicity: Arterial and internal jugular blood gas composition in man during inhalation of air, 100 percent O_2 and 2 percent CO_2 in O_2 at 3.5 atmospheres ambient pressure. J Appl Physiol 1955; 8: 255–263.

14. Lanphier EH. Use of nitrogen-oxygen mixtures in diving. In: Goff LG, ed. Proceedings of the 1st Symposium on Underwater Physiology. Publication no. 377. Washington, DC: National Academy of Sciences/National Research Council, 1955: 74–78.
15. Lanphier EH, Lambertsen CJ, Funderburk LR. Nitrogen-oxygen mixture physiology: Phase 3. End tidal gas-sampling system, carbon dioxide regulation in divers, carbon dioxide sensitivity tests. Research report 2-56. Washington, DC: U.S. Navy Experimental Diving Unit, 1956.
16. Lanphier, EH, Nitrogen-oxygen mixture physiology: Phases 4 and 6. Research Report 7-58. Washington, DC: U.S. Navy Experimental Diving Unit, 1958.
17. Lambertsen CJ, Owen SG, Wendel H, et al. Respiratory cerebral circulatory control during exercise at 0.21 and 2.0 atmospheres inspired P_{O_2}. J Appl Physiol 1959; 14: 966–982.
18. Schaefer KE. Adaptation to breath-hold diving. In: Rahn H, Yokoyama T, eds. Physiology of Breath-Hold Diving and the Ama of Japan. Publication no. 1341. Washington, DC: National Research Council/National Academy of Sciences 1965: 237–252.
19. Lally DA, Zechman FW, Tracy RA. Ventilatory responses to exercise in divers and non-divers. Resp Physiol 1974; 20:117–129.
20. Kerem D, Melamed Y, Moran A. Alveolar P_{CO_2} during rest and exercise in divers and non-divers breathing O_2 at 1 ATA. Undersea Biomed Res 1980; 7:17–26.
21. MacDonald JW, Pilmanis AA. Carbon dioxide retention with underwater work in the open ocean. In: Bachrach AJ, Matzen MM, eds. Proceedings of the 7th Symposium on Underwater Physiology. Bethesda, MD: Undersea Medical Society, 1981:197–207.
22. Lanphier EH, Dwyer JV Jr. Special Report Series, Diving with Self-Contained Underwater Breathing Apparatus. Washington, DC: U.S. Navy Experimental Diving Unit, 1954.
23. US Navy Bureau of Medicine and Surgery. Submarine Medicine Practice (NAVMED P-5054). Washington, DC: Navy Department, 1956.
24. Lanphier EH. Oxygen consumption in underwater swimming. Washington, DC: U.S. Navy Experimental Diving Unit Formal Report 14-54, 1954.
25. Donald, K. Oxygen and the Diver. Flagstaff, AZ: Best Publishing, 1993.
26. Lanphier EH, Dwyer JV, Walkowski AJ. A Trapeze Swim-Ergometer. Washington, DC: USN Experimental Diving Unit, Formal Report 1-55, 1955.
27. US Navy Bureau of Medicine and Surgery. Physiological considerations in the design and evaluation of breathing apparatus. In: Submarine Medicine Practice (NAVMED P-5054). Washington, DC: Navy Department, 1956:185–210.
28. U.S. Navy Bureau of Medicine and Surgery. Oxygen tolerance. In: Submarine Medicine Practice (NAVMED P-5054). Washington, DC: Navy Department, 1956:221–226.
29. Lanphier EH. Nitrogen-oxygen mixture physiology phases 1 and 2. Research report 7-55. Washington, DC: U.S. Navy Experimental Diving Unit, 1955.
30. Behnke AR. Inert gas narcosis. In: Fenn WO, Rahn H, eds. Handbook of Physiology, Sec 3. Respiration, Vol II. Washington, DC: American Physiological Society, 1965:1059–1065.

31. Bennett PB. Inert gas narcosis. In: Bennett PB, Elliott DE, eds. The Physiology and Medicine of Diving, 4th ed. London: Saunders, 1993:170–193.
32. Lanphier EH. Carbon dioxide poisoning. In: Waite CL, ed. Case Histories of Diving and Hyperbaric Accidents. Bethesda, MD: Undersea and Hyperbaric Medical Society, 1988:199–213.
33. Lanphier EH. Influence of increased ambient pressure upon alveolar ventilation. In: Lambertsen CJ, Greenbaum LJ Jr, eds. Second Symposium on Underwater Physiology. Washington, DC: National Academy of Sciences/National Research Council, 1963:124–133.
34. Jarrett AS. Alveolar carbon dioxide tension at increased ambient pressure. J Appl Physiol 1966; 21:158–162.
35. Lanphier EH, Camporesi EM. Respiration and exertion. In: Bennett PB, Elliott, DH, eds. The Physiology and Medicine of Diving, 4th ed. London: Saunders, 1993: 77–120.
36. Warkander DE, Norfleet WT, Nagasawa GK, Lundgren CEG. CO_2 retention with minimal symptoms but severe dysfunction during wet simulated dives to 6.8 atm abs. Undersea Biomed Res 1990; 17:515–523.
37. Warkander DE, Nagasawa GK, Norfleet WT, Lundgren CEG. Physiologically acceptable breathing resistance in divers' gear and external work of breathing (abstr). Undersea Biomed Res 1991; 18(suppl):99.
38. Sterba JA. Hypercapnia During Deep Air and Mixed Gas Diving. Report No. 12-90. Panama City, FL: Navy Experimental Diving Unit (NEDU), 1990.
39. Bean JW. Tensional changes of alveolar gas in reactions to rapid compression and decompression and question of nitrogen narcosis. Am J Physiol 1950; 16:417–425.
40. Seusing J, Drube HC. Die Bedeutung der Hypercapnie für das Auftreten des Tiefenrausches. (The significance of hypercapnia for the occurrence of depth-intoxication.) Klin Wachenschr 1960; 38:1088–1090.
41. Hesser CM, Adolfson J, Fagraeus L. Role of CO_2 in compressed-air narcosis. Aerospace Med 1971; 42:162–168.
42. Fothergill DM, Hedges D, Morrison JB. Effects of CO_2 and N_2 partial pressures on cognitive and psychomotor performance. Undersea Biomed Res 1991; 18:1–19.
43. Bennett PB, Blenkarn GD. Arterial blood gases in man during gas narcosis. J Appl Physiol 1974; 36:45–48.
44. Lanphier EH. Interactions of factors limiting performance at high pressures. In: Lambertsen CJ, ed. Proceedings of the Third Symposium on Underwater Physiology. Baltimore: Williams & Wilkins, 1967:375–385.
45. Childs CM. Unexplained loss of consciousness in divers. In: Smith G, ed. Proceedings of the 6th International Congress on Hyperbaric Medicine. Aberdeen, Scotland: Aberdeen University Press, 1979:373–376.
46. Lanphier EH, ed. The Unconscious Diver: Respiratory Control and Other Contributing Factors. 25th Undersea Medical Society Workshop, Madison, Wisconsin, September 18–20, 1980. Bethesda, MD: Undersea Medical Society, 1982.
47. Morrison JB, Florio JT, Butt WS. Observations after loss of consciousness under water. Undersea Biomed Res 1978; 5:179–187.

48. Lanphier EH Pulmonary function, In: Bennett PB, Elliott DE. The Physiology and Medicine of Diving and Compressed Air Work, 2d ed. London: Baillière Tindall, 1975:102–154.
49. Giry P, Battesti A, Hyacinthe R, Burnet H. Ventilatory tolerance to exercise during a hydrogen-helium-oxygen saturation dive (Hydra V). In: Brauer RW, ed. Hydrogen as a Diving Gas. Bethesda, MD: Undersea and Hyperbaric Medical Society, 1987: 179–196.
50. Bradley ME, Dickson JG Jr. The effects of nitrous oxide narcosis on the physiologic and psychologic performance of man at rest and during exercise. In: Lambertsen CJ, ed. Fifth Symposium on Underwater Physiology. Bethesda, MD: Federation of American Societies for Experimental Biology. 1975:617–626.
51. Webber JT. Respiratory effects of nitrous oxide narcosis. M.A. thesis, State University of New York at Buffalo, 1969.
52. Linnarsson D, Hesser CM. Dissociated ventilatory and central respiratory responses to CO_2 at raised N_2 pressure. J Appl Physiol 1978; 45:756–761.
53. Hesser CM, Lind F. Effects of exercise and hyperbaric air on ventilation and central inspiratory activity. In: Bachrach AJ, Matzen MM, eds. Proceedings of the Seventh Symposium on Underwater Physiology. Bethesda, MD: Undersea Medical Society, 1981:173–180.
54. Schaefer KE. Carbon dioxide effects under conditions of raised environmental pressure. In: Bennett PB, Elliott DE, eds. The Physiology and Medicine of Diving and Compressed Air Work. Baltimore: Williams & Wilkins, 1969:144–154.
55. Gelfand R, Lambertsen CJ, Peterson RE. Human respiratory control at high ambient pressures and inspired gas densities. J Appl Physiol 1980; 48:528–539.
56. Salzano JV, Camporesi EM, Stolp BW. Physiological responses to exercise at 47 and 66 ATA. J Appl Physiol Respir Environ Exerc Physiol 1984; 57:1055–1068.
57. Saltzman HA, Salzano JV, Blenkarn GD, Kylstra JA. Effects of pressure on ventilation and gas exchange in man. J Appl Physiol 1971; 30:443–449.
58. Tarasiuk A, Grossman Y. Respiratory-center activity under high pressure conditions. Proceedings of the Second International Meeting on High Pressure Biology, Paper No. 25, Toulon, France, 1990.
59. Dempsey JA, Forster HV, Ainsworth DM. Regulation of hyperpnea, hyperventilation, and respiratory muscle recruitment during exercise. In: Dempsey JA, Pack AI, eds. Regulation of Breathing, 2d ed. New York: Marcel Dekker, 1995:1065–1134.
60. Whipp BJ. Mechanics of ventilatory control during exercise. In: Lanphier EH, ed. The Unconscious Diver: Respiratory Control and other Contributing Factors. Bethesda, MD: Undersea Medical Society, 1982:49–61.
61. Wasserman K, Whipp BP, Koyal SN, Beaver WL. Effect of carotid body resection on ventilatory and acid-base control during exercise. J Appl Physiol 1975; 39:354–358.
62. Cunningham DJC. Integrative aspects of the regulation of breathing: A personal review. In: International Review of Science, Physiology. Series I. Respiratory Physiology, Vol II. London: Butterworths, 1974:345.
63. Wasserman K. Testing regulation of ventilation with exercise. Chest 1976; 70: 173S–178S.

64. Asmussen E, Nielsen M. Studies on the regulation of respiration in heavy work Acta Physiol Scand 1946; 12:171–178.
65. Welch HG, Mullin JP, Wilson GD, Lewis J. Effects of breathing O_2-enriched mixtures on metabolic rate during exercise. Med Sci Sports 1974; 6:26–32.
66. Margaria R, Camporesi E, Aghemo P, Sassi G. The effect of O_2 breathing on maximal aerobic power. Pflüger's Arch Physiol 1972; 336:225–235.
67. Whipp BJ, Ward SA. Coupling of ventilation to pulmonary gas exchange during exercise. In: Whipp BJ, Wasserman K, eds. Exercise: Pulmonary Physiology and Pathophysiology. New York: Marcel Dekker, 1991:271–307.
68. Lambertsen CJ. Respiratory and circulatory actions of high oxygen pressure. In: Goff LG, ed. Proceedings of the Underwater Physiology Symposium. Publication no. 377. Washington, DC: National Academy of Sciences/National Research Council, 1955:25–38.
69. Cain CC, Otis AB. Some physiological effects resulting from added resistance to respiration. J Aviat Med 1949; 20:149–160.
70. Zechman F, Hall FG, Hull WE. Effects of graded resistance to tracheal air flow in man. J Appl Physiol 1957; 10:356–362.
71. Fagraeus L, Linnarsson D. Maximal voluntary and exercise ventilation at high ambient air pressures. Forsvarmedicin 1973; 9:275–278.
72. Lambertsen CJ, Gelfand R, Peterson R, et al. Human tolerance to He, Ne, and N_2 at respiratory gas densities equivalent to He-O_2 breathing at depths to 1200, 2000, 3000, 4000, and 5000 feet of sea water (predictive studies III). Aviat Space Environ Med 1977; 48:843–855.
73. Menn SJ, Sinclair RD, Welch BE. Effect of inspired CO_2 up to 30 mmHg on response of normal man to exercise. J Appl Physiol 1970; 28:663–671.
74. Elliott JC, Finkelstein S, Roberts AP, Luft UC. Gas exchange and acid-base balance breathing low concentrations of CO_2 during exercise and recovery. In: Aerospace Medical Association Annual Scientific Meeting. Washington, DC: Aerospace Medical Association, 1970.
75. Clark JM. Tolerance and adaptation to acute and chronic hypercapnia in man. In: Proc Divers Gas Purity Symp. USN Supervisor of Diving, Rep 2-73, 1973: 1-1–1-20.
76. Clark JM, Sinclair RD, Lenox JB. Chemical and non-chemical components of ventilation during hypercapnic exercise in man. J Appl Physiol 1980; 48:1065–1076.
77. Kerem D, Daskalovic I, Arieli R, Shupak A. CO_2 retention during hyperbaric exercise while breathing 40/60 Nitrox. Undersea Hyperbaric Med 1995; 22:339–346.
78. Clark JM, Gelfand R, Lambertsen CJ, et al. Human tolerance and physiological responses to exercise while breathing oxygen at 2.0 ATA. Aviat Space Environ Med 1995; 66:336–345.
79. Hashimoto A, Daskalovic I, Reddan WG, Lanphier EH. Detection and modification of CO_2 retention in divers (abstr). Undersea Biomed Res 1981; 8(suppl):47.
80. Elliott DH. Loss of consciousness underwater. In: Diving Accident Management. Bethesda, MD: Undersea and Hyperbaric Medical Society, 1990: 301–310.

7

Gas Bubbles and the Lungs

ALF O. BRUBAKK and ANNE VIK

Norwegian University of Science and Technology
Trondheim, Norway

VALERIE FLOOK

University of Aberdeen
and Unimed Scientific Ltd.
Aberdeen, Scotland

I. Introduction

There is evidence from many studies that gas bubbles occur in the venous system during most decompressions (1–4). Data from the study of Eckenhoff et al. (5) indicate that once the sum of the partial pressures of all gases exceeds the environmental pressure, gas formation occurs in the venous system. The predominant theory about the growth of bubbles is that bubbles grow from preformed nuclei; the energy required to generate a bubble de novo is considerable, and high levels of supersaturation are needed to develop a gas phase in "pure solutions" (6). These nuclei may be composed of small (approximately 1 μm in diameter), stable gas bubbles (7).

Several studies have documented the relationship between the occurrence of many venous bubbles and the risk for clinical symptoms requiring treatment (1,8,9). This, together with the fact that bubbles are probably present in the venous system during most decompressions, suggests that a diver complaining of pain in a joint may be suffering from two different conditions—namely, tissue gas in and around the joint and pulmonary gas embolism.

It has been suggested that there is little relationship between gas bubbles detected in the pulmonary artery and clinical signs of decompression illness

(DCI). The main reason for this is that gas bubbles have been detected in the absence of symptoms (2). There seems, however, to be agreement that the risk of DCI increases with increasing number of bubbles. In our experience, having monitored many hundreds of air dives and numerous saturation dives, clinical symptoms do not occur in the absence of pulmonary artery gas bubbles. Nishi (2) points out that for air dives, decompression illness was always accompanied by vascular bubbles. Sawatzky (10), using the grading system developed by Spencer and Johanson (8), has shown that there is a 5 to 10% risk of decompression illness in individuals with a single observation of grade III to IV bubbles.

The term *silent bubbles* has been used to describe bubbles observed in the vascular system when there are no acute clinical symptoms of DCI (11). Normally all venous blood goes through the lung. If vascular gas bubbles are not truly silent—i.e., if they have any either short- or long-term effect on the organism—one would expect these effects to be observable in the lung.

A. The Nature of the Emboli

The lungs trap gas emboli just as they trap all emboli, but almost every aspect of the behavior of gas emboli in the lungs differs from the behavior of solid emboli. Much of our knowledge of the response of the lungs to embolization derives from studies concerning solid emboli—either blood clots or glass or plastic beads. Glass beads embolize the lower parts of the lungs, where blood flow is highest. Gas bubbles, being less dense than blood, will go mainly to the upper regions of the lungs, where blood flow is already lower than in the rest of the lung (12,13).

Gas emboli are easily deformable and, by changing shape, may move into smaller vessels than solid emboli would. Thus the size of vessels that may trap bubbles does not necessarily relate to the size of the bubbles entering the lungs.

Gas emboli are continually being absorbed, by solution in the blood and tissues and by diffusion into the gas phase of the alveoli; the size of the bubbles is static. Once the bubbles shrink to a certain minimum size, surface forces will cause more rapid collapse. A reduction in size will allow continuous forward movement into smaller vessels before final resolution. The time course for final disappearance of the bubbles depends on the total volume of gas emboli entering the lungs and the time period over which the embolization occurs (14).

Three forms of gas emboli have been used to study the effect on the lungs. These are:

A bolus of gas
Continuous infusion of gas bubbles

Bubbles resulting from decompression from one pressure to a lower pressure

Each of these techniques to introduce bubbles to the lungs has its own characteristics, which must be considered in the interpretation of experimental results.

Several animal species have been used to study the effects of venous gas emboli (VGE). The dog has been used most frequently, both in experiments using gas infusion or gas injection and after decompression (15–24). Studies of VGE have also been performed using sheep (25–28), pigs (29–31), goats (32), and smaller animals such as hamsters (33), rabbits (34), guinea pigs (35), and rats (36). Until the study of Bove et al. in dogs in 1974 (15), the measurement of physiological effects of VGE after decompression had been limited. Since then, studies have been made of the effects of VGE on the pulmonary and systemic circulations and on gas exchange in sheep (25,27), dogs (19–20,37), goats (32), and pigs (38).

Early experiments were mainly aimed at determining the lethal dose of venous injection of various gases in different animals (34,39). After the Second World War, measurements of several circulatory and respiratory variables were made during bolus injections of gas (40–42). During the last two decades, most of the studies have used continuous air infusion at a constant rate ($mL\cdot kg^{-1}\cdot min^{-1}$) to produce venous gas emboli (12,14,23,30,43–46). Gases other than air—such as helium, neon, nitrogen, carbon dioxide, and oxygen—have been used, and the effects on hemodynamic variables and on blood gases seem to depend partly on the physical properties of the gases within the bubbles and in the breathing gas (23,41,45–49). For example, carbon dioxide will induce less marked hemodynamic changes than nitrogen (23).

Gas injected as a bolus will be removed in a relatively short time. The effect on the lungs can be expected to depend on the size of the bolus and on how quickly it was injected. In contrast, a gas infusion lasts for a longer time and is usually injected at a smaller dose rate than a bolus, though a range of doses have been used. The effect on the lungs will depend on the rate at which the gas is introduced and on the total volume of gas used. Interpretation of experimental results from both bolus and infusion experiments is further complicated by the fact that the site of injection of gas will greatly influence the size of the gas bubbles that reach the lungs. There will be a redistribution of gases with the dissolved gases in the blood, to an extent depending on which gases are in the emboli. Gas injected peripherally has longer to exchange gas with the blood than does gas injected directly into the pulmonary artery. This is borne out by the work of Van Allen et al. as reported by Butler and Hills (44), which showed that the mortality rate in dogs was higher when air was injected into the central veins than when the injection was into peripheral veins. Furthermore, gas bubbles may be broken up into smaller bubbles on passage through the right ventricle and may emerge with a very close range of sizes (14,46). There may be a further breakdown at the bifurcations of the pulmonary artery system (50).

During and after decompression there will be a continuous release of gas bubbles to the pulmonary circulation, although the number of gas bubbles, and thus probably the volume of gas, will increase sharply and then decrease slowly following the dive (38,51). During decompression from saturation dives, venous bubbles may be present for many days. Decompression bubbles are even less well defined than injected bubbles, either for size or for the time course of arrival at the lungs. Hills and Butler (52) attempted to measure the diameter of decompression bubbles in the caval veins of dogs and found it to vary with time. At 5 min after the end of a simple decompression, the size range was 24 to 30 μm in one of their dogs, increasing to 50 to 160 μm between 25 and 35 min later. Figure 1 shows a comparison between the time course of bubble size change derived from Hills and Butler and the time course of the number of bubbles reaching the lungs following decompression; bubble counting was performed by ultrasonic scanning of the pulmonary artery (53). If bubbles are broken into a

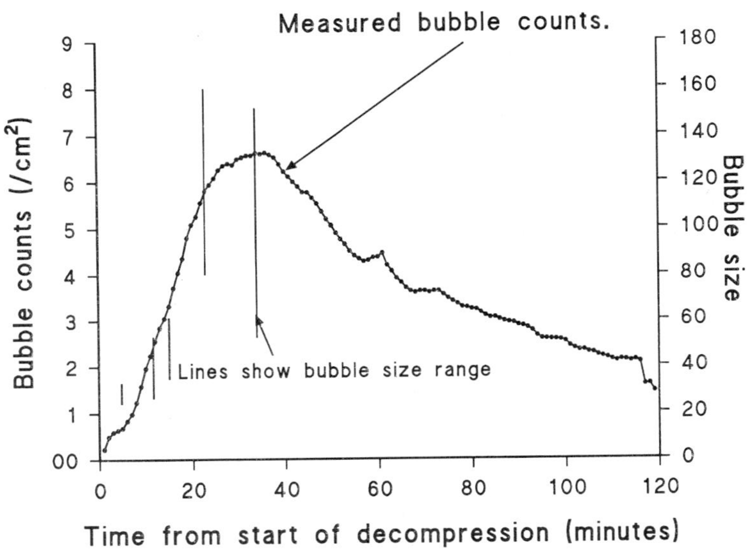

Figure 1 Comparison of the number of gas bubbles observed in the pulmonary artery after decompression and the relative size of bubbles. (From Refs. 52 and 53.)

greater number of smaller bubbles on passing through the right ventricle, this could explain the agreement shown. Assuming that the distribution of gas bubble sizes in the pulmonary artery is exponential (with considerably more small than large bubbles), as has been shown by Medwin for bubbles in seawater (54), this would indicate that most gas bubbles entering the pulmonary artery are small, probably well below 100 μm in diameter.

Gas emboli may block some parts of the pulmonary vascular bed, reducing or preventing blood flow through the regions of lung served by those vessels. Blockage of vessels is followed by a series of primary changes which are discussed in detail below:

1. Pulmonary arterial pressure and pulmonary vascular resistance will increase.
2. Parts of the lung downstream from the emboli will become areas of high ventilation–perfusion ratio ($\dot{V}/\dot{Q}$).
3. Blood will be diverted to other parts of the lung, creating areas of low $\dot{V}/\dot{Q}$.
4. Areas of high $\dot{V}/\dot{Q}$ (increased alveolar dead space), will increase alveolar oxygen ($P_{A_{O_2}}$) and lower alveolar carbon dioxide ($P_{A_{CO_2}}$) tensions.
5. Areas of low $\dot{V}/\dot{Q}$ (increased shunt or venous admixture), will reduce arterial oxygen (Pa_{O_2}) and increase arterial carbon dioxide (Pa_{CO_2}) tensions.
6. The increased range in $\dot{V}/\dot{Q}$ will change arterial to alveolar differences, $P(A\text{-}a)_{O_2}$, $P(a\text{-}A)_{CO_2}$, and $P(a\text{-}A)_{N_2}$.

Homeostatic mechanisms can be expected to minimize the changes in $\dot{V}/\dot{Q}$ and the blood-gas derangement. Though the presence of pulmonary gas emboli may cause the primary changes, the return to normal cannot be taken as evidence that the gas emboli have completely disappeared. Butler et al. (14) were able to demonstrate the continuing existence of emboli after pulmonary artery pressure, pulmonary vascular resistance, end-tidal carbon dioxide, and arterial carbon dioxide were all back to control levels.

II. Hemodynamic Effects of Gas Bubbles

A. Background

The hemodynamic effects of experimental VGE seem to vary depending both on the animal model and on the method of producing VGE. However, these differences probably influence only the magnitude of the responses. Generally, VGE leads to an initial rise in the pulmonary artery pressure (PAP) and pulmonary vascular resistance (PVR) and a decrease in arterial oxygen tension (Pa_{O_2}) (12,23,30,42,43,45). Central venous pressure usually increases and left atrial pressure may increase or decrease (41,42,55). Both arterial hypertension and hypotension have been reported, as have changes in cardiac output and systemic vascular resistance in both directions (12,21,23,26,30,41–43,45,56). Large doses of VGE are, however, always followed by a decrease in cardiac output ($\dot{Q}_T$), arterial hypotension, and death (30,41,57). Death may be caused by gas in the outflow tract of the right ventricle acting as a mechanical obstruction and preventing blood flow into the pulmonary circulation. An alternative mechanism could be failure of the right ventricle as a result of the increased PVR, arterial hypoxia, and hypercapnia. Studies that use spontaneously breathing animals may give different results from studies using mechanically ventilated animals (47), since the former animals may increase their ventilation and thereby are able to prevent an increase of carbon dioxide in the arterial blood.

There seems to be a relationship between infusion rate and the rate of increase in PAP (23,30). Maximal pressure attained seems also to be proportional to the infusion rate or to total dose injected until an upper limit is reached (43,44). In pigs, Vik et al. (30) found that infusion of air into the right ventricle produced a rate of increase in PAP that was dose-dependent, but the three doses used gave the same maximum value of PAP. The PAP increase slowed after the first few minutes of infusion and appeared to plateau at a level dependent upon the volume of gas introduced. When the dose was increased further, a fall in PAP appeared, probably caused partly by a failure of the right ventricle in the face of increased vascular resistance, hypoxia, and hypercapnia. Many workers consider the plateau as an indication that the rate of infusion is balanced by the rate of resolution of the gas bubbles (28,44,46). The plateau is often not very well defined even after 25 min of infusion in dogs (46) or 30 min of infusion in sheep (28), but it is well defined during 2 hr of infusion of 0.05 $mL \cdot kg^{-1} \cdot min^{-1}$ in sheep (58).

Evidence that the plateau in PAP results from a balance between the amount of gas infused and gas lost through the lungs comes from studies using different gases in the infusate. Verstappen et al. (23) infused dogs with gas bubbles containing He, Ne, O_2, or N_2 and found that the level of PAP was inversely proportional to the Krogh diffusion coefficient (the product of diffusion coefficient and solubility), which determines the rate of gas transport between intravascular bubbles and the alveolar space. The gases that reached a plateau within the 20 min of infusion were oxygen and helium, the two gases with the highest diffusion coefficients. This supports the idea that a plateau is reached when the diffusion of gas out of the bubbles is balanced by the infusion rate. The gases that diffuse less readily caused a greater and continuing rise in PAP. The relationship between PAP and the Krogh diffusion coefficient suggests that the gas leaves the lungs from bubbles lodged in precapillary vessels by movement through tissue to alveoli rather than directly into the alveoli from capillaries. Direct movement from capillary to alveoli would probably not be diffusion limited due to the very large surface area and short diffusion distances.

This would make the excretion of gas emboli independent of normal gas transfer routes.

Knisely et al. (59) demonstrated that bubbles were lodged in the pulmonary arterioles and were absorbed there, with only occasional bubbles reaching the capillaries. They concluded that the pathway for excretion of gas was in solution through the blood to the gas phase of the lungs. Using neon, they found that the gas appeared in the expired air after 2 min of infusion and reached a steady state after 10 min. As demonstrated by Vik et al. (38), the increase in PAP closely follows the change in the number of bubbles in the pulmonary artery. This can be seen from Fig. 2.

Following embolization with solid particles exceeding 200 μm in diameter, PAP and PVR do not increase until approximately 50% of the pulmonary vascular bed has been embolized (60). However, the changes in PAP recorded immediately following the start of gas infusion suggest that gas embolization has a much larger hemodynamic effect than a comparable infusion of solid emboli. For example, in the experiments described by Vik et al. (30), a 19% increase in PAP occurred within the first 2 min of the lowest infusion rate, when the pigs had received on average only 2.35 ml of gas. In another study (31), PAP increased to a maximum 3 min after a bolus injection of only 0.5 mL of gas bubbles less than 50 μm in diameter. Using much larger doses of air (1 $mL \cdot kg^{-1}$) injected as a bolus into the pulmonary artery in dogs, Berglund and Josephson (61) showed that PAP increased 140% within 20 sec.

The above suggests an increase in PVR before 50% of the vascular bed has been embolized. Malik (60) quotes work demonstrating that if the emboli

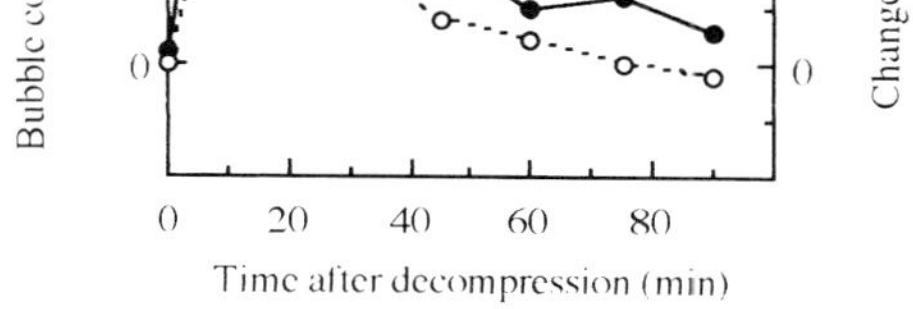

Figure 2 The relationship between increase in pulmonary artery pressure and number of bubbles in the pulmonary artery. The solid line depicts mean pulmonary artery pressure; the dotted line shows the number of bubbles in the pulmonary artery. (From Ref. 38.)

have a diameter smaller than 170 μm, considerably less than 50% of the vascular bed has to be occluded to get an increase in PAP. This indicates that it is the size of the emboli which is important. Fragmentation of gas emboli in the heart and at the bifurcations of the pulmonary artery system as well as resolution of the gas during passage to the lungs means that most bubbles are probably small. The increase in PAP seen from the very beginning of infusion probably results from vasoconstriction rather than simple mechanical obstruction.

Several studies (40,60,62,63) show evidence for vasoconstriction, which seems to be limited to smaller arteries and arterioles less than 100 to 200 μm in diameter. During air infusion, the bubble size at the infusion site is dependent on the internal diameter of the infusion catheter, which seems to vary between 0.4 and 1.6 mm in most studies (19,30,44,45,64). The bubble size in the lungs also depends on the flow at the infusion site and on any mixing in the ventricle (65). Albertine et al. (64) infused gas through a catheter with an internal diameter of 0.58 mm and found by histological examination that the air emboli were restricted to pulmonary vessels having a diameter of 100 to 1000 μm; most endothelial changes were observed in vessels smaller than 300 μm. In comparison, gas bubbles in the caval vein have been shown to have a diameter of 19 to 700 μm after decompression (52); in another study, numerous bubbles with a diameter of 4 μm were detected (66).

Vasoconstriction, by increasing PAP, increases the afterload of the right ventricle. If the vasoconstriction is confined to the precapillary vessels, the increased pressure will not be transmitted to the filtering microvessels (67). However, the fact that lymph and protein flow (see later) are increased despite a reduced surface area indicates that the filtering vessels are not totally protected from the increased PAP.

Josephson (63) compared the hemodynamic response to air embolization to that of complete vascular occlusion to determine the relative importance of mechanical obstruction and vasoconstriction in the increase of PAP and PVR following air embolism. The main results are summarized in Fig. 3. Mean values are shown; there was a considerable variation in response between animals. Pulmonary artery pressure was measured in the trunk of the pulmonary artery. The pulmonary artery in one lung was occluded by a balloon (A). This resulted in a 30% rise in PAP. Infusion of gas bubbles into the same artery gave a 98% rise (B), indicating that there is a vasoconstrictor effect in addition to the effect of the occlusion. There is probably some involvement in the contralateral lung, as infusion of gas into both lungs (E) resulted in only an additional 30% pressure increase. This effect may be humorally mediated. Occlusion of one lung while the other lung was infused with gas bubbles (C) resulted in a rise in PAP similar to the sum of the responses in A and B.

The result described in D, in which gas was infused into an artery after mechanical obstruction, resulted in an increase in PAP following obstruction in

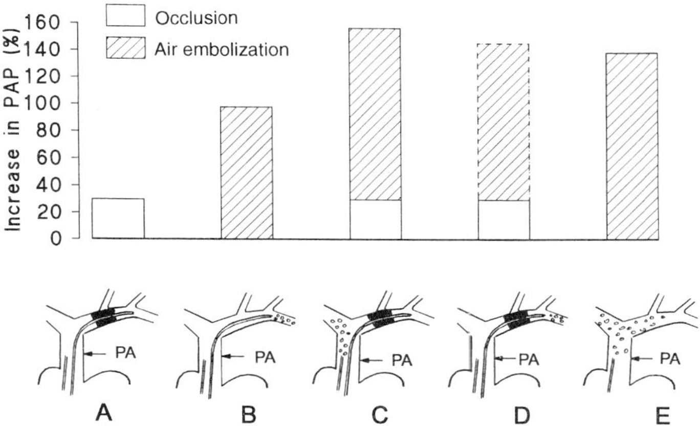

Figure 3 The effect of occlusion and air infusion on changes in pulmonary artery pressure. (A to E) Different experimental situations. The dotted lines around the box in D indicate that only 50% of the animals showed any response. (From Ref. 63.)

all animals, whereas half of the dogs did not respond to infusion of gas bubbles at all. An explanation for this may be that in the nonresponding dogs, there was not sufficient perfusion remaining in the lung to move the bubbles forward. In the dogs that did respond to infusion, the average increase in PAP was 116%, less than would be expected as the full response (A plus B). This result was taken to indicate that following mechanical obstruction, the blood flow was sufficient to move the bubbles forward and initiate local, humoral, and neurogenic responses but not to initiate humoral responses in the contralateral lung. The speed of response to infusion was different in the two situations, being 37 sec to maximum response following infusion (B,E) and 60 sec following mechanical obstruction and a greater and more rapid change arising from other effects, probably vasoconstriction.

There is disagreement about involvement of sympathetic mechanisms in mediating the increased PVR seen after microembolization (60). Some studies have shown that neither parasympathetic nor sympathetic blockade has any significant effect upon the hemodynamic response to air embolism (41,42). However, there are a number of studies indicating that humoral factors are responsible for vasoconstriction. The most likely humoral mediators of the pulmonary vasoconstrictor response after microembolization are thromboxane A_2, histamine, and serotonin (60). These mediators are released from platelets after aggregation, from mast cells, from intrapulmonary macrophages, and from leukocytes (see below). It is likely that mediator release or reflex mechanisms after microembolization can influence variables of the systemic circulation (56).

The changes in mean arterial pressure (MAP) and cardiac output ($\dot{Q}_T$) seem to be less predictable: A decrease in MAP has been observed in most studies (19,20,25,37), whereas an increase was observed in dogs (15) and pigs (38). A decrease in cardiac output was observed in sheep (27), but an increase seemed to occur in goats (32).

The effects of VGE after decompression seem to be comparable to those observed during gas infusion. During and after decompression experiments, the volume of gas in the venous circulation is unknown. The hemodynamic effects of decompression are dependent upon the number of bubbles in the pulmonary artery, which can be estimated using ultrasonic techniques (see below).

B. Species Differences

It is difficult to compare the results from different experimental animals with the use of different experimental preparations in different laboratories. However, species differences clearly exist. Air infusion rates of 0.30 to 0.35 ml/kg^{-1}·min^{-1} have been tolerated in dog experiments (18,22,44), whereas infusion rates of only 0.10 and 0.20 mL·kg^{-1}·min^{-1} induced cardiovascular collapse in pigs (30). The alveolar and capillary surface area relative to weight is smaller in the pig than in the dog (68–70). This can reduce the capacity for eliminating intravascular gas bubbles from the blood to the alveoli. Wolffe and Robertson concluded that the amount of intravenously infused air necessary to produce death in rabbits and dogs seemed to be directly proportional to the size of the pulmonary artery and its branches (34).

Many different species have been exposed to pressure and decompressed to study bubble formation. Small animals such as guinea pigs, cats, rats, mice, hamsters, frogs, and crabs have been used in experimental studies (33,71–73). Boycott et al. (74) argued that larger animals (e.g., goats) were preferable as models for humans, since both the uptake and elimination of gas, and therefore bubble formation, would be dependent on the relationship between cardiac output and weight.

The autonomic innervation of pulmonary vasculature varies in different species (75), which may explain differences in response. In addition, pigs and other animals such as sheep, goats, cows, and cats have intrapulmonary macrophages in the pulmonary circulation. These cells may release thromboxane A_2, a potent vasoconstrictor, when exposed to emboli in the pulmonary circulation (76). This fact could also contribute to the difference in response between dogs and pigs, since dogs have few intrapulmonary macrophages. Such cells have been observed in humans, although it appears that their number is relatively small in the normal lung (77).

III. Time Course of Bubble Resolution

The rate of bubble resolution is of importance both for the magnitude of the response and for the risk of breakthrough of gas to the arterial side (see below). For example, Mandelbaum and King (42) reported that a large air bolus caused longer-lasting changes in PAP in dogs than a smaller bolus. Berglund and Josephson (61) saw the changes in PAP and PVR reversed in 13 min following an air bolus; the changes lasted considerably longer if the emboli were plastic beads.

The disappearance of the bubbles depends on physical factors: the extent to which the gas in the bubble can enter into solution in the surrounding blood and tissue and the speed with which the gases can diffuse into the surroundings. Once the gas molecules from the bubbles have reached the gas phase within the alveoli, the level of ventilation will determine the rate of removal and therefore the gas levels in the tissue and blood. The excess pressure within the bubble, due to surface tension, influences gas removal, as does the presence of a "skin" of denatured protein, platelets, and leukocytes on the surface of the bubble (78).

Verstappen et al. (48) infused neon and measured the excretion of the gas through the lungs. The rate of excretion of neon from the lungs increased to the 10th min and thereafter equaled the rate of infusion. In the first phase, the pattern of ventilation influenced the rate of neon washout. There was no clear effect of ventilation on the washout of neon, which continued after infusion had stopped.

The bronchial circulation is a possible alternative route for gas exchange. This could be by transfer across the epithelium of the conducting airways or by the various types of anastomoses between bronchial and pulmonary circulation—for example, the Sperr arteries (60,79,80). Swenson et al. (81) conclude that these routes can account for up to 16% of any gas exchange by a diffusion-dependent route. These same routes have been implicated in the transfer of solid emboli across the lungs. They are difficult to identify in normal human lungs (75) but are present in lung disease and may be a source of species difference in the ability of the lungs to filter emboli.

Verstappen et al. (47,48) found that given volumes of oxygen, helium, neon, and air gave similar changes in PAP, whereas carbon dioxide produced very little increase in PAP. In these studies, the site of injection was the femoral vein, and it is possible that some of the gas was dissolved into the blood during transit. The larger capacity that the blood has for carbon dioxide could explain the apparent lack of effect. Spencer and Oyama (28) found smaller effects after injection of oxygen and carbon dioxide than of nitrogen on pulmonary and systemic circulation.

Melzer et al. (82) calculated the lifetime of bubbles in saturated and unsaturated liquids. The predicted lifetimes of bubbles of different sizes in ''saturated'' and ''unsaturated'' liquid are shown in Table 1.

These numbers show that the range for the lifetime of the bubbles depends on the degree of saturation of the liquid. The experimental results from Yang et al. (83) for both nitrogen and oxygen bubbles in plasma are very close to the tabulated predictions for bubbles in unsaturated solutions and suggest that the bubbles in the pulmonary capillaries are in a liquid that is unstirred. The diameter of the average pulmonary capillary is approximately 8 μm. If we ignore any change of shape of the bubble as it is exposed to the surrounding pressures and take the average transit time from pulmonary capillary to the left atrium as 2 sec, the results suggest that bubbles getting as far as the pulmonary capillaries will not survive long enough to reach the left atrium. This indicates that bubbles that actually do get through pass through larger vessels or shunts. However, gas may be pushed through the pulmonary vascular system if a continuous column of vascular gas is formed by the coalescence of bubbles, which is added to by incoming gas bubbles (30).

Butler et al. (14) amplified air bubbles in dogs by intermittently changing the breathing gas to N_2O and found bubbles in the pulmonary artery up to 43 min after air infusion. This time was considerably longer than that needed for the return of hemodynamic variables to preinfusion values. In infusion studies in which they used bubbles of He, N_2, or SF_6, Hlastala et al. (45) found that the recovery of PAP and expired P_{CO_2} depended on the gas, recovery from helium bubbles being fastest and from SF_6 bubbles slowest.

The hemodynamic effects of gas embolism and the time for bubble resolution may be influenced by changing the breathing gas. Following air embolism, Sergysels et al. (46) found that a switch to a breathing gas containing He and N_2O increased the hemodynamic response but had no effect on recovery time because the rate of recovery was also increased. When the switch was to a very much heavier gas mix, SF_6-O_2, the recovery was quicker and started as soon as the breathing gas was changed. Helium has a similar solubility in blood

Table 1 Bubble Lifetime in Liquids

	Bubble lifetime	
Bubble diameter	Saturated liquid	Unsaturated liquid
1 μm	5 msec	5 msec
8 μm	550 msec	190 msec
100 μm	1,000 sec (17 min)	50 sec
1,000 μm	1,000,000 sec (278 hr)	6,000 sec (1.7 hr)

Source: Ref. 82.

and tissues as nitrogen but can diffuse much more rapidly. This will cause an increase in PAP as gas bubbles increase in size following the gas switch. Nitrous oxide is more soluble than nitrogen in tissue and blood but has a similar rate of diffusion. The increased bubble size when nitrous oxide is used is probably due to easier movement of gas to the bubble. Because SF_6 is a very heavy molecule with a very low rate of diffusion, nitrogen moved out of the bubbles more rapidly than SF_6 moved in. A second gas switch to air from SF_6 reversed the recovery, presumably as the bubbles were amplified.

The effect of breathing gas on the resolution of bubbles suggests the possibility of using different breathing gases to remove bubbles more quickly from the lungs. Butler et al. (14) found a significant reduction in time to resolution of pulmonary gas bubbles in animals breathing oxygen. Sergysels et al. (46) suggest use of SF_6 to speed up the resolution of bubbles. However, they are careful to point out the problems of choosing the moment to return to air breathing, given that any remaining bubbles will be amplified by this switch.

Russell et al. (84) looked at the relative effects of treatment by pressure, oxygen breathing, and a combination of both on the removal of $^{15}N_2$ used in a bolus injection into dogs. Without treatment, 76% of the $^{15}N_2$ was recovered in 10 min, by which time PAP, systemic arterial pressure, and cardiac output had returned to control levels. Only the combined treatment increased the recovery of $^{15}N_2$ and speeded up the restoration of PAP and systemic changes to normal. We know from the work of Butler et al. (14) that this does not mean that all the gas bubbles have disappeared.

Biochemical processes may play a role in determining the lifetime of bubbles in the lungs and the passage of gas bubbles through the lungs. The presence of bubbles apparently leads to a reduction in surface tension of the blood (85,86). However, surfactant acts as a procoagulant and fibrinogen reduces the surface activities of the phospholipids, with a resultant increase in surface tension (87). The effect of surface tension on bubble transport through the lung is discussed in Sec. IV.C.

IV. Passage of Gas Bubbles Through the Lungs

The passage of gas bubbles through the lungs may be quite different from that of solid particles. While solid particles can only pass through channels with a diameter larger than the particle, gas bubbles may be deformed, can change their volume, and can coalesce into columns of gas. Thus the total volume of gas and its rate of arrival at the pulmonary vasculature may be more important than bubble size.

Gas bubbles in the arteries have been detected in divers after excursions (88), during decompression from saturation dives (89), and at autopsy after fatal accidents (90). Arterial gas bubbles have also been observed in both small and large animals during and after decompression (15,33,35,91,92). Thus, there is no doubt that arterial gas bubbles occur during or after some decompressions. Furthermore, during medical procedures, gas bubbles have been detected in the arteries of the systemic circulation after accidental VGE, both in patients without (93,94) and with extrapulmonary shunting (95,96).

In divers, there are several possible pathways by which venous bubbles may reach the arterial circulation. First, venous gas bubbles may travel through the pulmonary circulation and enter the pulmonary veins and left atrium, although the pulmonary circulation is usually considered to be a good filter for gas bubbles as well as for other emboli. Second, venous gas bubbles may pass through a patent foramen ovale (PFO) or other extraordinary connections in the heart to reach the left side of the heart. Third, if the lung has been overinflated during a rapid ascent, gas may escape directly into the pulmonary veins after alveolar rupture (97,98). It has been widely accepted that gas bubbles may occur in the cerebral circulation after such barotrauma. The diagnosis of arterial gas embolism seems until recently to have been confined to such cases (99,100). However, evidence of lung injury is seldom found during clinical or radiological investigation after arterial gas embolism following diving (97).

Finally, gas bubbles may form in the arterial circulation if the decompression rate is sufficiently fast, >0.3 to 1 fsw/sec (98,101). All gas nuclei in the blood will not be destroyed at compression and supersaturation of the arterial blood may occur during the rapid decompression. However, an experimental study using goats did not succeed in demonstrating such bubbles in the arterial circulation after a short hyperbaric exposure and a rapid decompression (102).

In animal studies, the occurrence of arterial gas bubbles has been monitored directly by inspection of the pulmonary veins, by collection of gas in a bubble trap connected to the aorta, or by the use of Doppler probes (24,26,28). Such Doppler probes have often been located on peripheral vessels. However, the transoesophageal (TEE)-transducer is probably a better tool to study the occurrence of arterial bubbles, as suggested by Furuya et al. (103). This technique provides an image of the left atrium and possibly also of the pulmonary veins close to the lungs. In addition, passage of gas bubbles through a PFO may be monitored. During the last decade, transoesophageal echocardiography has been used to detect gas bubbles in the left atrium or in the ascending aorta in air infusion studies (24,29–31,48,103–106) and in decompression studies (51).

A. Effects of Gas Volume

Paradoxical gas embolism has been studied experimentally by infusing air through a catheter into the venous circulation in dogs (16–18,21,22,24,30, 41,44,50), sheep (26,28), and pigs (30,107). The experimental work has usually aimed at studying transpulmonary passage of gas bubbles. Animals found to have an atrial septal defect have been excluded, at least for some of the studies. We may assume that animals with a PFO have also been excluded, although in their paper, Spencer and Oyama "excluded the existence of *obvious* right-to-left shunts in all animals" by postmortem investigation (28). It should be noted that PFOs may be as small as 1 mm in diameter and therefore can be difficult to detect even at autopsy (104).

The studies show that bubbles emerge into the arterial circulation if the animals receive gas at a sufficiently high rate during continuous infusion or at a sufficiently high dose during bolus injection. It therefore seems possible to overload the filtering capacity of the lungs. Studies in dogs anesthetized with pentobarbital (17,18,44) showed that filtering capacity was exceeded if the air infusion rate was 0.30 $mL \cdot kg^{-1} \cdot min^{-1}$ or higher, whereas arterial gas bubbles were detected at the nitrogen dose of 0.15 $mL \cdot kg^{-1} \cdot min^{-1}$ in unanesthetized sheep (28). With the use of pentobarbital anaesthesia in pigs, spillover to the left atrium occurred during infusion of air at a rate of 0.10 $mL \cdot kg^{-1} \cdot min^{-1}$ (30). These diverging results may indicate species differences, discussed below.

There seems to be a threshold dose of gas for transpulmonary passage of bubbles. Above this threshold, a dose dependency exists. The likelihood of transpulmonary passage increases if the infusion rate or the dose is further increased (18,24,30,44). In most studies, the spillover seemed to occur when the PAP was high (17,21,22,28,44). However, arterial gas bubbles have occurred in dogs (24) and pigs (30) during gas injection or gas infusion even at normal PAP values. The blood-bubble surface tension is one of the factors influencing the ease with which bubbles cross the lung (13,16,17).

The lung can be regarded as a filter where the risk of spillover is determined by the size of the emboli. For gas emboli, the situation is more complex, as gas is continuously eliminated through the lungs. Furthermore, gas bubbles can be deformed and coalesce to form a continuous gas phase within the vessels (30). The risk of spillover of gas will be dependent upon the relationship between gas elimination and the supply of gas.

Although the occurrence of arterial gas bubbles has been noticed in some decompression studies, transpulmonary spillover has not been studied systematically. Conclusions about transpulmonary passage during and after decompression seem to have been drawn without any account being taken of the fact that bubbles might have emerged through a PFO (15,33,35,91). However, the study of Brubakk et al. (88) in divers suggests that transpulmonary passage can occur in humans. Arterial bubbles were seen following 10 of 12 excursions from 300 to 250 msw. Although the incidence of PFO was not determined in these divers, an incidence of over 80% is unlikely, indicating that most of the arterial bubbles must have crossed the lungs.

The risk for spillover of gas will increase with increasing venous gas volume. During and after a decompression, the number of microbubbles in the venous circulation shows interindividual variation (3–5,38), observed both in divers and in experimental animals. In addition, it is difficult to estimate the volume of gas in bubbles (107,108). In one study (51), the arterial bubble count, as evaluated in a two-dimensional image using a TEE-transducer, showed the same time course as the venous bubble count in all pigs (with and without PFO) that had arterial gas bubbles. This could indicate a dose dependency for transpulmonary passage of microbubbles after decompression. As shown in Fig. 4, the breakthrough of gas will happen at a lower PAP when PFO is present than when it is not.

Some time will elapse between venous embolization and the appearance of bubbles in the pulmonary vein or the systemic circulation. Breakthrough will happen only when the filtering capacity of the lungs is overloaded. Spencer and Oyama (28) reported breakthrough of bubbles when the infused gas was oxygen or nitrogen but did not report the time of first appearance of bubbles. However, one figure in their paper shows evidence of the first appearance of bubbles in the brachiocephalic artery 20 min after the start of infusion. Butler and Hills (44) infused air into dogs for 30 min and found that the time to first appearance of bubbles in major arteries of the systemic circulation ranged from 18 to 90

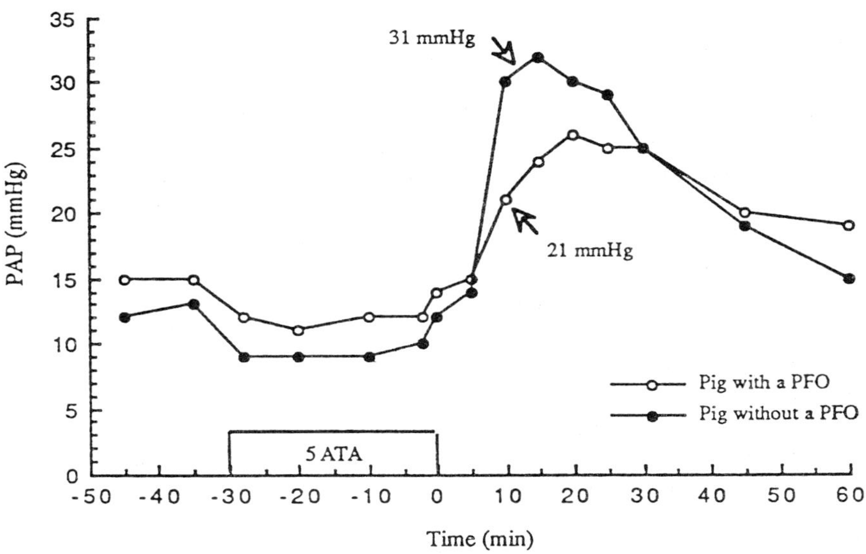

Figure 4 Changes in pulmonary artery pressure following 30 min exposure to 5 ata (500 kPa). The time of breakthrough for gas into the left side of the heart is indicated (arrows) in two pigs, one with and one without PFO. (From Ref. 51.)

min. In order for the bubbles to be present in the lung for such a long time, gas elimination must be reduced. Bubble-blood interactions—such as the development of a skin of plasma proteins, platelets and leukocytes or edema formation—might increase diffusion distances. This, however, is probably of minor importance; the more likely explanation for the delay is the time required to build up a column of gas within the vasculature until the leading edge is pushed through (30).

In their study in pigs, Vik et al. (30) found that breakthrough of bubbles occurred after 12 to 20 min in 4 of 6 animals during infusion of air at a rate of 0.1 $mL \cdot min^{-1} \cdot kg^{-1}$. However, if the animals had received a small infusion of air prior to the experiment, the time to breakthrough was increased to 29 min and only occurred in 1 out of 7 animals. We do not have any explanation for this. The data indicates an increased gas elimination following the second infusion, requiring more gas to be delivered before breakthrough occurred. An alternative explanation could be that parts of the circulation are blocked by columns of gas from the initial infusion (59).

B. Effects of Particle Size

If the lungs function as a sponge-type filter, the size of the bubbles may be important for any transpulmonary spillover to occur. Gas bubbles that are smaller than the capillaries may traverse the capillary bed to enter the pulmonary veins. It has been observed that microspheres with diameters below 8 μm readily passed through the pulmonary circuit in dogs, whereas only a few larger particles passed into the arterial circulation (109). However, it has been argued that bubbles as small as 8 μm, used as ultrasonic contrast, will totally dissolve in a shorter time than the pulmonary capillary-to-left atrial circulation time (82). (See also Sec. IV.C.)

The cutoff diameter for transpulmonary passage of gas bubbles may be larger than the 20 to 30 μm suggested by the data of Butler et al. (50) and by the theoretical analysis of Chang et al. (13); see Sec. IV.C. Injection of a foam of bubbles ($<$50 μm in diameter) into the right ventricle led to arterial bubbles in pigs (31). However, arteriovenous shunts or anastomoses in the pulmonary circulation may permit larger gas bubbles to escape filtration during certain conditions. The existence of such channels is still controversial (80). Some authors have postulated that there are arteriovenous anastomoses 390 to 500 μm in diameter (110–112), whereas others have argued that channels of such a size do not exist in normal lungs (59,113,114).

C. Effects of Surface Tension

Surface tension forces determine the pressure required to force bubbles through the lungs and this fact has been used by Butler and Katz (17) to determine the minimum vessel radius which allows passage of bubbles. In a different approach, Chang et al. (13) observed the pressure required to start and stop flow through a model system of tubes and used a theoretical analysis to extend their measurements to predict the minimum vessel which would allow bubbles to pass. The minimum bubble diameter derived by Butler and Katz (17) ranged from 11.3 to 29.8 μm; the theoretical diameter determined by Chang et al. (13) was 20 to 30 μm. However, in order to make the link between driving pressure and vessel size, it has been assumed that the contact angle for the bubble meniscus is zero. This implies a bubble with a hemispheric meniscus.

For a gas-liquid interface in a tube with an hydrophilic inner surface and having a circular cross-section with a radius r, the radius of the curvature of the meniscus, R, is

$$R = r/\cos\theta \tag{1}$$

where θ is the contact angle (115). A gas bubble within a tube has two menisci. Only when the bubble is stationary are the two menisci the same radius and the two contact angles the same. Figure 5a shows the general situation for a stationary bubble.

In Fig. 5, $R_1 = r/\cos\theta_1$ and $R_2 = r/\cos\theta_2$. For a stationary bubble (Fig. 5a), $R_1 = R_2$ and $\theta_1 = \theta_2$. For the bubble to move in the direction of the arrow (Fig. 5b), the pressure P_1 must exceed P_2. However, both must relate to the pressure inside the bubble, P_{in}, according to the equations

$$P_{in} - P_1 = 2\gamma\cos\theta_1/r \tag{2}$$

$$P_{in} - P_2 = 2\gamma\cos\theta_2/r \tag{3}$$

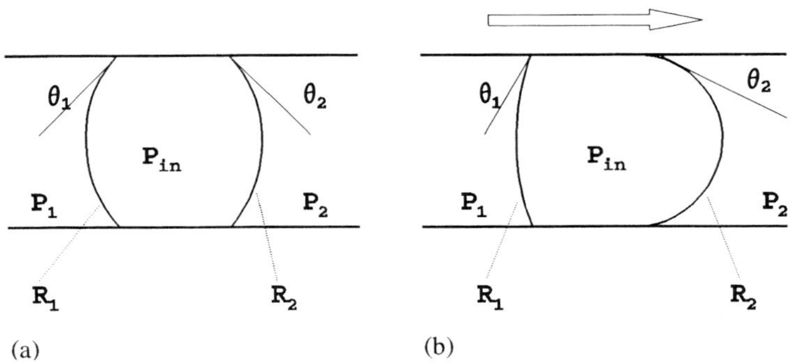

Figure 5 (a) A stationary bubble in a tube. (b) The bubble moving in the direction of the arrow. Contact angles are marked by θ and R indicates the radii of the menisci. Pressures inside the bubbles and on both side of the bubble are indicated by P.

where γ is the coefficient of surface tension. Thus the pressure difference across the bubble for movement to occur is

$$P_1 - P_2 = 2\ \gamma\ (\cos\ \theta_2 - \cos\ \theta_1)/r \tag{4}$$

To move the bubble forward, the pressure drop across the bubble causes θ_2 to decrease and θ_1 to increase, and the bubble takes the shape show in in Fig. 5b.

There are too many unknowns to solve the relationship for a tube radius of r. The extreme case is θ_2 equal to zero, where cos θ_2 will be 1. This leaves θ_1 able to take any value up to 180°, cos θ_1 equals -1, and $P_1 - P_2 = 4\gamma/r$. This value would double the values given by Butler and Katz (17) for the minimum vessel radius that can allow passage of bubbles.

Arterial gas bubbles have occurred in dogs and pigs during gas injection or infusion at normal PAP values (24,30). A reduction in surface tension could theoretically reduce the driving pressure necessary for transpulmonary passage. Pretreatment with hyperbaric oxygen seemed to permit 60-μm bubbles to escape pulmonary filtration in dogs, and the authors speculated about the possibility of increases in the concentration of surfactant molecules in the pulmonary blood after pretreatment with oxygen (16). However, the vasodilatory effect of oxygen may have contributed to these results.

Recruitment of surface-active molecules within the blood to the air-blood interface may reduce the surface tension of the blood-gas interface and thereby reduce the pressure needed for breakthrough according to the formula given above (52). Perry et al. (116) showed an attenuation of the PAP response after direct injection of surface-active substance before air infusion. The dogs had, however, received an air infusion pretreatment, and the reduced response could have been an example of the same tendency of a reduction in hemodynamic changes as observed in a study in pigs during the second infusion of air (30). When the same surface-active substance was infused in pigs in a dose able to reduce surface tension by about 15% (Hjelde, personal communication), there was no change in hemodynamic response except for a small increase in pulmonary vascular resistance, nor any change in spillover (105). Walder reported that in individuals with slightly lower surface tensions in blood (approximately 5%), the risk of DCI was significantly increased (117).

Since any reduction of the surface tension may influence both the resorption of gas—and thus the gas volume and the bubble size—as well as the direct transport of microbubbles through the narrow pulmonary vasculature, the ultimate effect on transpulmonary passage seems to be uncertain.

D. Effects of Different Gas Composition in the Bubble

If the risk of breakthrough of gas to the arterial side depends upon the ability of the lung to eliminate gas, one would expect helium bubbles to present a lower risk than nitrogen bubbles because of the higher diffusivity of helium. As mentioned above, helium bubbles do indeed result in a more rapid recovery of hemodynamic variables (45), but to our knowledge there are no studies on breakthrough where the two gases have been compared.

Spencer and Oyama (28) infused nitrogen, oxygen, and carbon dioxide at different rates in unanesthetized sheep. No arterial gas bubbles were observed during infusion of carbon dioxide, whereas 1 of 5 sheep receiving oxygen and 3 of 5 receiving nitrogen at a rate of 0.15 $mL \cdot kg^{-1} \cdot min^{-1}$ had arterial bubbles. These findings are as expected, considering the differences in blood capacity for these different gases.

E. Effects of Different Breathing Gases, Anesthesia, and Drugs

Nunn (118) found that air bubbles enlarged when placed in blood drawn from a patient who had been breathing nitrous oxide. The idea that air emboli might also enlarge in vivo when exposed to a soluble inspired gas was supported by Munson and Merrick, as evaluated by increased mortality in rabbits ventilated by nitrous oxide before embolization (119). Using microscopy in dogs, Presson et al. (120) observed that ventilation with helium or nitrous oxide enlarged the venous air emboli in the pulmonary vasculature. However, Losasso et al. (121) demonstrated no measurable effect on the incidence or severity of VGE when they were ventilating neurosurgical patients with 50% nitrous oxide if the ventilation with nitrous oxide was discontinued immediately upon Doppler detection of VGE. In a study by Butler et al. (18), the addition of nitrous oxide to halothane or pentobarbital anesthesia did not increase the incidence of spillover.

Yahagi and Furuya (24) have shown that it has been possible to reduce the threshold value for transpulmonary passage of gas in dogs by changing anesthesia from pentobarbital to halothane. The latter anesthetic may act as a vasodilator of the pulmonary circulation (122), but no difference in PVR was seen in the two groups. The authors suggest that effects on shunt flow may play a role. In a different study, arterial gas bubbles were detected at a much lower dose of air injected during halothane anesthesia than during ketamine or fentanyl anesthesia (106).

Similarly, aminophylline, another dilator of the pulmonary circulation, appeared to reduce the filtering capacity of calibrated air bubbles in dogs. Butler and Hills detected bubbles in the femoral arteries in all four aminophylline pretreated dogs after the injection of bubbles < 130 μm (50). Also, the effect of arterial gas bubbles was dramatic, resulting in arterial hypotension in the pretreated dogs. It has been suggested that vasodilators such as aminophylline and halothane reduce the filtering capacity of the lungs in dogs (24,50) because of the opening of arteriovenous shunts (24). In pigs, however, aminophylline did not seem to reduce the capacity to filter gas bubbles (31). It has also been suggested that a high PAP—for instance due to overloading with gas—can open such shunts (110,124).

F. Species Differences

Species differences probably exist in the effects of VGE on hemodynamics and gas exchange and on the filtering capacity of the lung (28,34,44). Extrapolation of the results to humans may therefore be questioned. For instance, the dog can be considered an ''athletic'' animal, whereas the human is grouped with the ''sedentary'' animals. The latter fact implies species differences in lung structure and function (68,69) according to the principle of symmorphosis (70). The higher threshold value for spillover in during air infusion in dogs compared with pigs could be due to the larger alveolar and capillary surface area in dogs and thus a larger capacity for gas exchange. Differences in filtering capacities could also be explained by differences in arteriovenous anastomoses in the pulmonary vasculature among the species. There seems to be no clear evidence for such anastomoses in any species, but the difference in response to aminophylline in dogs and pigs (31,50) could indicate that such anastomoses exist in the former species but not in the latter.

G. Passage of Gas Bubbles Through a Patent Foramen Ovale and Shunts

In as many as 20 to 34% of humans, dependent on age, the foramen ovale is patent after fetal life (124). Normally it is functionally closed, since the pressure in the left atrium is higher than the pressure in the right atrium and the septum primum functions as a valve. However, a spontaneous shunt, not dependent on a Valsalva maneuver or other factors to change the pressure gradient between the atria, is diagnosed in 5 to 6% of humans (125,126) by contrast echocardiography. False-negative results cannot be excluded with this method (127), giving an apparently lower incidence of PFOs than autopsy studies.

Studies by Moon and colleagues (128) and Wilmshurst and coworkers (129) demonstrated an increased risk of neurological decompression sickness in divers with a PFO compared to those without. Moon et al. showed that significantly more divers with neurological DCS had a right-to-left shunt than a control population (128). However, Cross et al. (130) showed that a PFO was detected in 31% of divers who never experienced decompression sickness. A number of these divers had performed dives that probably produced a significant number of venous gas bubbles, that resulting in an increase in PAP. An increase in PAP will lead to an increased transport of bubbles through a PFO (51). In air-infusion experiments in pigs with a surgically created atrial sepal defect, Black et al. (29) showed that arterial embolism occurred with only transient reversal of the normal left-to-right gradient in atrial pressure.

Although it is known that gas bubbles may pass through a naturally occurring PFO or other intracardial connections—e.g., during contrast echocardiography—few experimental studies have been designed to explore such passage of venous gas bubbles into the left side of the heart. Deal and colleagues collected 30 ml of air in a bubble trap placed across the arch of the aorta in a sheep that had a PFO, whereas little or no gas was collected in another sheep without a PFO (26). Vik et al. (104) found an increased risk of arterial gas bubbles after air infusion in pigs with a naturally occurring PFO versus the risk observed in pigs without a PFO.

The term *paradoxical gas embolism* (PGE) is used to describe arterial gas embolism after passage of venous gas bubbles either through the pulmonary circulation or via a PFO. Although both small and large animals have been used to study PGE after hyperbaric exposure, a distinction between animals with and without a PFO seems to have been made in only one study in pigs (51). The results showed that gas bubbles in the left atrium were also more likely to appear following hyperbaric exposure in pigs with a PFO. If a PFO is a risk factor for the occurrence of arterial gas emboli in divers during and after decompression, it may be advisable to select divers who do not have a PFO. However, Wilmshurst and Belder (131) argued recently that screening of divers for a PFO is not indicated, since there are several other etiological factors in decompression sickness. This conclusion is also supported by the study of Cross et al. (130). It must, however, be pointed out that we know little about the possible health effects of repeated arterial embolizations, and these recommendations may have to be reconsidered.

A recent study by Norfleet at al. (132) showed that no gas bubbles could be detected in the left ventricle in an individual with an open PFO (documented by echo-contrast) when grade IV bubbles could be seen in the right ventricle following hypobaric exposure. No explanation for this surprising finding was given, but perhaps the amount of gas in the pulmonary artery was insufficient to produce a right-to-left shunt. Butler et al. (133) recently showed that infusion of gas bubbles up to doses of 0.15 $ml/kg^{-1} \cdot min^{-1}$ in dogs, sufficient to double the PAP, did not cause a reversal of the normal right-to-left pressure gradients between the atria. This is in contrast to the study of Vik et al., who found arterial gas bubbles in the pig after a pressure increase of approximately 30% in the pulmonary artery (51).

V. Direct Effects of Bubbles on Lung Function

The main respiratory function of the lungs, to exchange oxygen and carbon dioxide and maintain normal blood gases, is achieved most efficiently when there is a minimum of wasted ventilation (dead space) and minimum volume of blood missing effective gas exchange (shunt or venous admixture). The distribution of effective ventilation must match the distribution of effective blood flow, $\dot{V}/\dot{Q}$. The changes in the lungs following embolization will have the effect of increasing the range of $\dot{V}/\dot{Q}$ ratios and of increasing alveolar dead space and venous admixture, possibly also increasing shunts. In this section we are mainly concerned with the changes occurring in the lungs; the consequential effect on blood gases is discussed in a later section. The reader is referred to Bouhuys (135) for a detailed discussion of these aspects of pulmonary physiology.

A. Distribution of Gas Bubbles in the Lungs

Chang et al. (12) measured perfusion index (local perfusion/total lung perfusion) in the different regions of the lungs following infusion of 0.1 $mL \cdot kg^{-1} \cdot min^{-1}$ of air into the femoral vein of dogs and found it to be higher in the lower part of the lungs. The gradient of perfusion index from top to bottom of the lungs became more marked the longer the infusion time. A short period of N_2O ventilation, which has the effect of amplifying bubble size, increased the gradient of perfusion index even further. These results are evidence that the gas bubbles distribute preferentially in the upper parts of the lungs.

Chang et al. (13) followed the experimental work with the development of a mechanical model and were able to demonstrate that, whenever there was a difference in height between two paths at a bifurcation, the majority of bubbles entered the higher limb.

The upper parts of the lungs are defined zones I and II (134) and are characterised by the fact that within these zones, alveolar pressure has an influence on blood vessel diameter. Glaizier et al. (136) have shown that in these zones, the red cells are deformed by alveolar pressure. It is reasonable to assume that gas bubbles would also be deformed, moving further into the vasculature. If bubbles are directly influenced by alveolar pressure, the pressure swings during ventilation could act as a "pump" to speed up absorption of the bubbles.

Knisely et al. (137) identified the final resting place of infused bubbles as the pulmonary arterioles, with a diameter 30 to 40 μm, and saw a change of shape of the bubbles to gas columns having lengths ranging from 200 to 300 μm. If these vessels are indeed the final resting place of bubbles, then movement of gas from them has to be by diffusion through the blood and tissue, as suggested by both Knisely et al. (59) and Verstappen et al. (48).

A consequence of gas bubbles moving mainly into the upper parts of the lungs is that blood is moved from areas that are already less well perfused to areas with higher perfusion. The lower parts of the lung have a relatively low $\dot{V}/\dot{Q}$, which is further reduced by this redistribution of blood.

B. Changes in the Ventilation/Perfusion Ratio

Pulmonary gas embolism may cause bronchoconstriction, probably mediated through the activation of thrombocytes, neutrophils, and macrophages (see later).

The magnitude of the shift in ventilation and the effect on blood gases as a consequence of bronchoconstriction may be species-dependent. One important factor is species-dependent differences in collateral ventilation pathways. These are known to be numerous in the dog and less numerous in the pig and sheep. In humans, there are few collateral pathways in young, healthy lungs but more in lungs of patients with chronic lung disease (138).

Khan et al. (139) showed changes in airway resistance and in dynamic compliance following bolus injection of gas in dogs and found that these changes were blocked by heparin, by making the animal thrombocytopenic, and by infusions of a serotonin antagonist. They concluded that the mechanism of airway constriction was related to serotonin release from platelets.

The alveoli served by an embolized section of the circulation will take a reduced part in gas exchange. If the emboli completely block the blood vessel, the alveoli will take no part in gas exchange. Whatever the degree of embolization, the carbon dioxide partial pressure will be low in these alveoli. Alveolar hypocapnia causes constriction of the peripheral airways—a mechanism that serves to minimize the derangement of arterial blood gases. Severinghaus et al. (140) showed that occlusion of a pulmonary artery resulted in bronchoconstriction, which was reversed by adding 8% carbon dioxide to the breathing gas. Levy et al. (141) also demonstrated that the shift in ventilation can be prevented by adding carbon dioxide to the breathing gas. The total blood flow through the lungs changes very little as a result of embolization, and this means that some parts of the lungs will receive increased blood flow. The alveoli in these areas of lung will contain a high partial pressure of carbon dioxide.

The redistribution of ventilation by hypocapnic constriction of the peripheral airways serves to offset the effects of embolization of small parts of the lungs. The overall effect of pulmonary embolization is that the balance between metabolically produced carbon dioxide and its removal from the lungs is changed transiently and a new equilibrium is achieved at a slightly higher arterial carbon dioxide level. This increase reflects the proportion of the blood flow that has been diverted from embolized vessels. Arterial hypercapnia acts on the central airways, causing them to constrict. This does not modify the distribution of incoming gas but might be expected to reduce ventilation. The magnitude of this effect depends on the degree of arterial hypercapnia. West (134) says that uncomplicated embolization does not usually give rise to impaired ventilation.

The time course of the redistribution of airflow appears to happen in two phases (141). An initial nonuniform bronchoconstriction seems to result from humoral and neural effects, can be largely blocked by heparin, and happens within two or three breaths. Later, localized bronchoconstriction results from the local hypocapnia. The initial effect cannot serve to redistribute gas because it happens in all regions. The local effect of hypocapnia is the important mechanism in terms of homeostasis.

The bronchoconstriction happens mainly in the small airways; therefore it is not possible to detect the effect as a change of airway resistance, as small airways make up only 10 to 20% of the total. However, because of the consequential changes in the areas of lung that are ventilated, it may be possible to detect a change of compliance by dynamic measurement techniques.

Some blood flow may continue to areas of lung with fully constricted airways, and this blood will form part of the increase in shunt flow seen after pulmonary embolization. The degree of shunt, manifest as arterial hypoxemia, can be reduced by positive end-expiratory pressure ventilation, which is assumed to open the closed airways (142). Deep breathing can also reverse hypoxemia after embolization, which again suggests the opening of previously closed airways and reduction in shunt fraction.

Venous admixture also comes from parts of the lung that have an increased proportion of the blood flow with a less than adequate increase of ventilation—in other words a low $\dot{V}/\dot{Q}$. In addition, shunt flow could arise through the arteriovenous shunts, which are implicated in the passage of large solid emboli but have not so far been identified in normal lungs.

Results from experimental work all indicate an increase in the range of $\dot{V}/\dot{Q}$ following gas embolization with development of a bimodal distribution. For example, Delcroix et al. (143), showed bimodal $\dot{V}/\dot{Q}$ distributions using a multiple inert gas elimination technique after embolization of dog lungs by autologous clots. Changes in physiological dead space following infusion have been reported by Levy et al. (141); changes in shunt fraction have been found by Verstappen et al. (47) in dogs and by Vik et al. (30) in pigs. Young et al (144), using glass beads, saw changes in $\dot{V}/\dot{Q}$ only when vessels greater than 150 μm were embolized.

Hlastala et al. (45) infused bubbles of He, N_2 or SF_6 at a rate of 0.2 $mL{\cdot}kg^{-1}{\cdot}min^{-1}$ into the femoral veins of dogs. Infusion at this site means that the bubbles reaching the lungs may be very small, having been to some extent absorbed during passage and broken into smaller bubbles in the heart. Hlastala et al. demonstrated a bimodal $\dot{V}/\dot{Q}$ distribution that was well established after 15 min of infusion. This change resulted from a shift of ventilation to regions of high $\dot{V}/\dot{Q}$ and of perfusion to regions of low $\dot{V}/\dot{Q}$. A marked increase in physiological dead space with a reduction in anatomical dead space was seen, which could mean that the increase in alveolar dead space was greater than might be expected from the change in physiological dead space. Hlastala et al. (45) conclude that increased alveolar dead space after gas embolization is due to areas of high $\dot{V}/\dot{Q}$ rather than pure dead space and that venous admixture from areas of low $\dot{V}/\dot{Q}$ is more important than shunt flow.

Neuman et al. (27) saw no evidence of $\dot{V}/\dot{Q}$ changes following mild decompressions in sheep that had Doppler-detectable bubbles. The PAP changes (+4 mmHg) were small, and an absence of blood gas changes suggest that mild decompressions, even though they produce bubbles, may not cause physiologically significant changes.

Flook et al. (145) report a significant reduction in anatomical dead space in pigs following decompressions that produced bubbles. Physiological dead space was increased and alveolar dead space increased to an extent directly proportional to the degree of bubbling detected by ultrasonic scanning of the pulmonary artery. Severinghaus and Stupfel (146) observed an increase in anatomical dead space following a bolus of air in artificially ventilated animals. Low arterial oxygen, as results from gas embolization of the lungs, can cause a centrally mediated effect on the volume of the large conducting airways of the lungs (147), which would cause a reduction in anatomical dead space. Arterial hypercapnia also causes changes in central airway caliber, but as arterial hypercapnia following embolization is less marked than arterial hypoxia; a low oxygen tension is the more likely cause of the reduction in anatomical dead space.

C. Changes in Lung Mechanics

Changes in the caliber of small airways cannot be detected by the usual methods of measuring airway resistance because the small airways make up less than 20% of total airway resistance. However one of the effects of changes in small airway caliber is to change the distribution of gas, and this is manifest as a change in compliance when dynamic techniques are used. The change in compliance occurs because the distribution of time constants in the lungs is widened and lung compliance becomes frequency-dependent.

Khan et al. (139) report a significant increase in airway resistance and reduction in lung compliance within 30 sec of an air bolus >0.2 ml/kg^{-1} injected into a peripheral vein in dogs. Similar results were obtained following an oxygen bolus; but after a nitrogen bolus, only the increase in resistance was seen. After carbon dioxide injection, there were no significant changes, and this is consistent with evidence from other workers, already discussed, that the carbon dioxide in the bolus was mostly dissolved into the blood before reaching the lungs. Gas boluses of He, Ne, Ar, and Xe gave no significant changes. The authors suggest that changes in the peripheral airways would not have been detected as an increase in airway resistance by their techniques and that therefore the changes in airway resistance they saw must reflect changes in more central airways. Inhalation of 3.5% carbon dioxide prevented the changes, presumably due to a bronchodilator effect.

Catron et al. (37) found reduced dynamic compliance in all except 1 of 19 dogs following a severe decompression. Airway resistance increases were seen only in those animals which did not survive 3 hr postdecompression—i.e., where the gas load was large enough to lead to cardiorespiratory failure.

D. Atelectasis and Surfactant

There is histological evidence of alveolar collapse (148) occurring about 1 hr after barium sulfate embolization. Alveolar ducts were the principal site of airway closure, but distal bronchioles were also involved. This may be a consequence of bronchoconstriction if the affected area of the lung continues to have some blood flow. That embolized vessels may still have some blood flow is corroborated by the finding that the increase in shunt fraction that can be measured following gas embolization reflects an increased venous admixture from parts of the lung having low $\dot{V}/\dot{Q}$ (45).

An alternative mechanism for airway closure is an increase in surface forces following a reduction in the surfactant lining of the lung. The reduction in shunt flow and restoration of arterial oxygen that follow deep breathing after embolization suggest a restoration of surfactant to the lung surface. Periodic increase in lung volume is one of the mechanisms by which the surfactant surface of the lungs is renewed. Deep breathing serves to pull new surfactant onto the surface.

Finley et al. (149) have measured the minimum value of surface tension in lung washings following ligation of the right pulmonary artery. The minimum surface tension was increased 2 hr after PA ligation, with big increases after 5 hr, 1 dyne$\cdot$cm^{-1} being the average value in the control lung and up to 17 dynes$\cdot$cm^{-1} in the ligated lung. These early increases in surface tension would lead to atelectasis. Their dogs still had atelectatic changes in the lungs after 24 hr; these abnormalities were reduced in dogs who survived to 35 days. Surface tension values returned to control levels after 100 days.

It seems likely that the reduction or absence of blood from affected areas of lung results in ischemic damage to type II cells, the alveolar epithelial cells that produce surfactant. Pulmonary arterial occlusion reduces the density of lamellar bodies in type II cells by 80%; as these are the storage sites for the surface-active phospholipids, this would considerably reduce the availability of surfactant.

Finley et al. (149) saw evidence of a rich collateral circulation in the lungs of dogs who were sacrificed 6 months after pulmonary ligation. This circulation may allow reestablishment of the surfactant system of the lungs. The links between the pulmonary and bronchial circulations are pathways by which some collateral circulation can develop, and the development of this circulation seems to parallel the restoration of pulmonary surfactant.

E. The Effect of Gas Bubbles on Blood Gases

Arterial hypoxemia, which develops within minutes of the start of gas infusion, is an immediate consequence of embolization of the lungs (30,45,46). This rapid change in arterial oxygen level and the fact that it does not depend on the development of pulmonary edema indicates that it does not arise as a result of increased diffusion distances. Following infusion with glass beads, there is a later, second stage of increased hypoxemia that does seem to depend on edema in that it does not happen if edema is prevented by heparin (139). Deep breathing can reverse hypoxemia following gas embolization, which suggests opening of closed alveoli, thus improving the oxygen exchange.

The basic changes in metabolic gas levels which happen following embolization are:

Reduction in end-tidal carbon dioxide
Increase in arterial carbon dioxide
Increase in alveolar oxygen
Decrease in arterial oxygen

The development of arterial-alveolar differences shows that these changes result from the increased range of $\dot{V}/\dot{Q}$ ratios within the lungs. The $P_{A\text{-}a_{O_2}}$ increases as the increase in alveolar dead space gives rise to the increased end-tidal oxygen and the increased venous admixture causes low arterial oxygen. The presence of areas of high $\dot{V}/\dot{Q}$ result in $Pa\text{-}A_{CO_2}$ changes that are usually smaller than the oxygen changes because of the difference in the shape of the dissociation curves and the very much larger storage capacity for carbon dioxide in the body than for oxygen. Areas of low $\dot{V}/\dot{Q}$ give rise to $Pa\text{-}A_{N_2}$, and the magnitude of this difference will be greater following embolization due to decompression—that is, during the period of nitrogen washout.

The magnitude of the changes may depend on whether the animal is breathing spontaneously or is ventilated. Vik et al. (107) showed smaller changes in arterial oxygen and carbon dioxide following infusion of gas if the animal were breathing spontaneously. This is as expected; mechanical ventilation imposes a fixed volume change and flow pattern on the lungs, whereas during spontaneous breathing, the breathing pattern is adjusted to optimize lung performance. Ventilation levels increased in the spontaneously breathing animals to offset the increase in dead space.

The changes in metabolic gas levels are well documented in the literature. For example, Sergysels et al. (46) report a drop end-tidal carbon dioxide as infusion of air continues, reaching a plateau after about 10 min. This returns rapidly to normal after the end of infusion. Arterial oxygen drops throughout the period of infusion and recovers during the first 10 min after the end of infusion. Arterial carbon dioxide continues to increase during infusion and recovery is slower than the recovery of arterial oxygen levels. These changes were magnified when the dogs were given nitrous oxide to breathe during the last 5 min of infusion. Nitrous oxide breathing after the end of infusion appeared to delay the recovery. This is as would be expected if nitrous oxide amplifies the gas bubbles.

When Hlastala et al. (45) infused He, N_2 and SF_6 bubbles, the magnitude of changes in blood oxygen and carbon dioxide depended on the gas; greater changes followed embolization with SF_6 than with helium or nitrogen. The difference between helium and nitrogen was small. Spencer and Oyama (28), using unanesthetized sheep, showed that nitrogen bubbles had a greater effect on arterial oxygen than oxygen bubbles; carbon dioxide bubbles had a statistically significant but small effect.

Neuman et al. (27) report no significant change in arterial oxygen in sheep following relatively mild decompression exposures despite a 60% increase in PVR. They explain the lack of change, which fits with the apparently unchanged $\dot{V}/\dot{Q}$ distribution in their sheep, as due to the fact that the gas bubbles must have lodged in very small vessels and were not affected the distribution of blood flow. Following more severe decompressions in dogs, Catron et al. (37) saw a reduction in arterial oxygen, which was greatest in those animals that failed to survive 3 hr postdecompression.

Flook et al. (53) report the effect of decompression bubbles in spontaneously breathing pigs. The degree of embolization varied widely between pigs, but there were significant increases in alveolar oxygen, arterial carbon dioxide, alveolar-arterial oxygen difference, and arterial-alveolar carbon dioxide difference and significant decreases in alveolar carbon dioxide and in arterial oxygen. There were significant correlations between bubble count and reduction in arterial oxygen, the increase in $P_{A}\text{-}a_{O_2}$, and the decrease in $P_{A}\text{-}a_{CO_2}$.

F. The Effect on Gas Exchange

Metabolic gas exchange will be influenced only marginally by gas embolism. Although the arterial carbon dioxide level increases and arterial oxygen drops due to the changed $\dot{V}/\dot{Q}$ after embolization, the levels stabilize—evidence that gas exchange is not reduced by more than the small changes in body gas stores consequent to the change in partial pressures.

The changes in $\dot{V}/\dot{Q}$ observed by Hlastala et al. (45) had little effect on inert gas washout. They used direct measurement of excretion of a range of gases and found that the presence of bubbles reduced the clearance of nitrogen from blood in a single passage through the lungs from 96 to 93%. From the relationship between gas solubility in blood and excretion, they suggest that the effect of decompression bubbles on the elimination of helium, the other commonly used diving gas, should be no more than that on nitrogen and perhaps less due to the more rapid diffusion of helium. If gas in bubbles mainly is eliminated through the capillary-alveolar route, we would have expected the large changes in $\dot{V}/\dot{Q}$ distribution to reduce gas elimination significantly. As this is not the case, it is reasonable to assume that gas from emboli mainly leaves by diffusion through blood and tissue at the level of the arterioles, as is also pointed out by Knisely et al. (59) and Verstappen et al. (48).

G. Changes in Lung Function Following Diving

Many aspects of diving affect lung function. Among these we may count the effect of prolonged periods of breathing gas mixtures of very high density, prolonged exposure to high levels of oxygen, and repeated episodes of venous gas emboli. It is not easy to determine the relative effect of each of these. The various groups studying lung function in commercial divers have tried to determine the cause by relating the changes to the diver's experience. However, this has usually been only in relation to the number of years the subject has been a diver, the maximum depth to which he has dived, or the proportion of time spent in saturation dives compared with surface-oriented air dives (150–152). To relate changes to the effect of decompression bubbles requires information about the number of decompressions experienced, and this is usually not available for any except the most recent years. No systematic studies have been performed on recreational divers.

In commercial diving, it is normal to use a slightly hyperoxic breathing mixture at depth. In addition, most decompression schedules use oxygen as a means of assisting inert gas washout, and it is therefore almost impossible to distinguish between the effects of pulmonary embolism and pulmonary oxygen toxicity.

The result of repeated exposure to gas emboli might be expected to be small airway disease following prolonged periods of bronchoconstriction (see Sec. V.C). This would be manifest as a reduction in carbon dioxide transfer factor. A reduction in gas transfer might also result from a reduced capillary gas-exchange area. Several groups of workers have concluded that divers have small-airway disease (151–153). The loss of elastic tissue that has been described is often attributed to the effect of prolonged breathing of dense gas, but it may perhaps also be due to prolonged bronchoconstriction.

Hyacinthe et al. (154) reported reduced carbon monoxide transfer factor per unit total ventilation 24 hr after a long dive to 470 m, with improvement at 2 weeks. The changes were reversed by 5 to 6 weeks. Gas bubbles and oxygen toxicity are equal contenders for the change. Likewise Cotes et al. (155) reported reduction in gas transfer factor following a single 300-m dive with incomplete recovery after 1 year, but they do not give any information about the diving undertaken by the subjects during that year. A similar decrease in transfer factor after a saturation dive was reported by Suzuki et al. (156).

Thorsen et al. (157) carried out a study of a large sample of Norwegian divers and found a reduced carbon monoxide transfer factor; they suggested that inflammatory change following gas embolism was a possible cause. The same authors have looked at the transfer factor and transfer per unit volume of alveolar ventilation following a single saturation dive (158) and found both to be lower than predive controls 1 to 3 days postdive and still slightly low after 4 to 6 weeks. They state that inflammatory changes arising from either oxygen toxicity or venous gas emboli could explain their findings. They suggest a thickening of the alveolar membrane or a reduction in capillary exchange area as the direct mechanism. Puy et al. (159) separated the effect of membrane and blood components on changes in transfer factor, concluding that changes in the capillary exchange area were the decisive influence.

The possible effects of oxygen toxicity are dealt with in the work of Dujic et al. (160), who studied divers following a single exposure to air at 45 m. Two different types of dives were performed: one used air during the decompression stop and the other oxygen. Following the air decompressions, arterial oxygen levels were reduced significantly, indicating the presence of an effective number of bubbles, which were confirmed by Doppler monitoring. Most divers showed no bubbles after the oxygen decompression, and arterial oxygen levels were as expected. The maximum drop in transfer factor was seen 20 min after surfacing, coinciding with the maximum bubble counts following the air decompressions. There was a significant correlation between reduction in transfer factor and bubble count. Following the dives using oxygen, there was a small but statistically insignificant reduction in transfer factor.

VI. Indirect Effects of Gas Bubbles on the Lungs

In considering the effects of gas embolism in the lung, it must be borne in mind that gas bubbles do not act only as mechanical emboli. When gas bubbles are formed, protein denaturation takes place at the blood-gas interface (161). This interface is a thin layer, approximately 20 nm thick, consisting of fibrin and gamma globulin (162–164). It acts as a foreign substance, activating formed elements of the blood and inducing biochemical changes such as complement activation (165). These mechanisms play a significant role in the response of the lung to venous gas emboli and are probably the basis for any long-term effects that may occur. At present, our understanding of the importance of these mechanisms is quite fragmentary. Much further work is needed to determine the relative influence of mechanical and biochemical effects of gas embolism. An understanding of these processes is necessary for development of a rational approach to treating or preventing lung injury caused by vascular bubbles.

The following sections deal with some of the consequences for the lung of activation of the complement system and the formed elements of the blood.

A. Effects of Bubbles on the Complement System

Gas bubbles activate the complement system in vitro (166,167). The degree of activation is dependent upon the amount of gas infused, varies considerably over time (several months), and is not dependent upon the gas composition of the bubble.

No relationship was seen between the degree of C5a activation in vitro and the level of C5a observed in vivo after air dives (168). The data indicates that gas bubbles may activate C5a receptors as well as C5a. This is supported by studies of Chenoweth et al. (169), who studied the activation of complement after cardiopulmonary bypass. They showed that an increase in C5a could not be observed in venous blood in vivo; however, an increase could be observed in vitro after incubation with membranes in serum but not in whole blood. This indicates that cells in the blood bind the C5a. Specific C5a receptors have been demonstrated on human leukocytes (170). Neutrophils that have been exposed to activation possess significantly fewer receptors for C5a (171). Recent data indicate that the binding process is reversible and that C5a can be released several hours and even days after they have been bound to neutrophils (172). Increased levels of C5a in blood have been demonstrated 14 hr after activation in divers (173); in patients undergoing heart surgery, activation has been demonstrated for even longer periods (174).

The activation of the complement system plays a significant role in inflammatory processes. The role played by complement activation in decompression injury in the lung is not clear. For instance, pretreatment with a C5 and C3 convertase–blocking agent did not reduce mortality from decompression in the rat (175). However, the data given above support the hypothesis that the complement system is activated by bubbles in the vasculature. Complement activation will lead to activation of neutrophils and could be the cause of the neutrophil activation that has been observed during decompression in humans (176) (see below). Complement activation can lead to the formation of multiple membrane attack complexes that will lead to destruction of nucleated cells (177). Furthermore, activation of C5a will lead to edema and promote infiltration of inflammatory cells (178). Another important effect of C5a activation is that it leads to vasoconstriction and a reduction in blood flow (179), thus further influencing distribution of perfusion in the lung. Complement activation seems to play a role in inducing pulmonary dysfunction after contact with artificial membranes (180). This mechanism is dependent upon the presence of leukocytes.

B. Effect of Bubbles on Blood Cells

Thrombocytes

Aggregation of thrombocytes may lead to the formation of blood clots, thus forming solid emboli, which may compound the effect of gas bubbles in the lung. Thorsen et al. (181) showed that gas bubbles lead to the aggregation of thrombocytes in vitro. Aggregation in vitro was strongest when the bubble diameter was between 40 and 120 μm. The degree of aggregation does not seem to be dependent upon the gas content of the bubble but only on its surface properties (182). Aggregation of thrombocytes by gas bubbles can be considerably enhanced by epinephrine (183). Both psychological and physical strain, as can be present in diving, will increase epinephrine levels (184).

Sequestered thrombocytes have been observed in the lung vasculature after air embolism (185). The presence of thrombin seems to be necessary for this and the release of thromboxane A_2 from platelets seems to be involved in the rise in PAP following embolization (186). Pretreatment with Indomethacin, a drug that inhibits thromboxane synthesis, abolished the dramatic PAP increase in pigs following infusion of an ultrasonic contrast medium containing bubbles (187). The magnitude of the change in PAP seen in this study, exceeding by far that observed in other air embolism studies, suggest that the denaturated protein layer coating the air bubbles amplified the hemodynamic effect of the emboli.

Several studies have demonstrated a reduction of thrombocyte numbers in circulating blood after dives (188,189). Other factors besides gas bubbles and decompression may contribute to this result, as activation of thrombocytes also occurs during the bottom phase of a saturation dive (Klausen, personal communication, 1995). A reduction in circulating thrombocytes has been reported in 10 out of 16 divers (63%) with vascular bubbles. An increased consumption of fibrinogen and a reduced platelet survival time were also observed. Only 1 of 18 divers (6%) having no bubbles showed these effects (190). In a study in rabbits where decompression was sufficiently severe to produce decompression sickness, the number of thrombocytes was decreased (191). The above data suggest that thrombocytes are activated by gas bubbles both in vitro and in vivo.

Leukocytes (Neutrophils)

Leukocytes are involved in many aspects of tissue injury and inflammation. Several studies have documented that leukocytes are activated by decompression. Philp et al. (192) showed that decompression led to a reduction in both thrombocytes and leukocytes. These reductions seem to be related to the presence of gas bubbles. During decompression from a saturation dive to 440 msw, where no gas bubbles could be detected, there was no reduction in leukocyte number (193). In a different study, Benestad et al. (194) showed that decompression led to activation of neutrophils. Contrary to what has been observed in thrombocytes, no activation of leukocytes seems to occur in vitro at pressure (Bjerkvik, personal communication, 1994).

A significant fall in neutrophils in the circulating blood was seen in sheep with respiratory decompression sickness (“chokes”). This reduction was seen immediately following decompression, while a drop in circulating platelets occurs later (25). No such reduction was seen in the pig following decompression with massive bubble formation, in spite of significant infiltration of leukocytes into the lung tissue (Brubakk et al., 1995, unpublished).

In a study in dogs, Moosavi et al. (195) showed that both neutrophils and platelets were sequestered in the lung after air embolization. They also observed gaps in the endothelial layer in the arterioles and activation of the clotting system. In sheep, Albertine et al. (64) demonstrated that neutrophils aggregate around the air bubbles and that the neutrophils seemed to be attached to the thin layer around the bubble. This can be seen in Fig. 6.

In this study, where air bubbles with a diameter of 1 mm were infused, gaps could be seen in the endothelial layer of pulmonary arterial microvessels with a diameter of less than 1 mm, half of these vessels being less than 300 μm. These changes could be seen after only one hour of infusion. Furthermore,

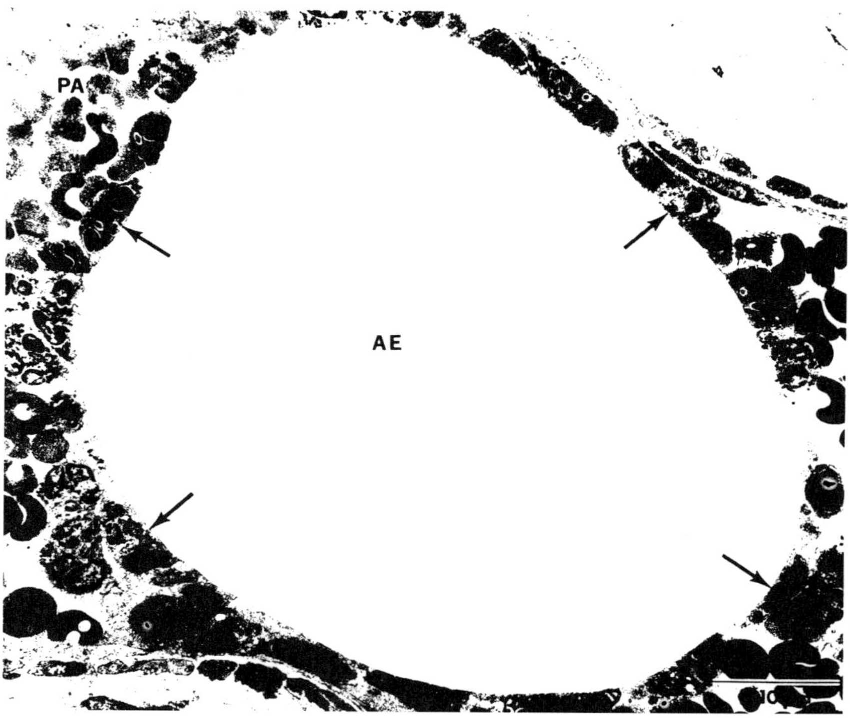

Figure 6 Adherence of leukocytes to the surface of a bubble marked AE. Arrows show leukocytes. PA = pulmonary artery. (From Ref. 64.)

thrombocytes did not seem to be involved in this process. The alveolar layer in the lung was intact, and the leukocytes were all located inside the vessels. This is a different observation from what we found in the pig after decompression (Fig. 7), where there were numerous leukocytes in the interalveolar space. Compared with the study of Albertine et al. (64), both fewer and smaller bubbles are probably involved.

Neutrophils may be sequestered in both the vessels and the lung parenchyma; the relative distribution may be a matter of degree of exposure to gas. Following 4 hr of air infusion in a dose sufficient to double the PAP, Staub et al. (196) showed that the number of neutrophils in the alveolar parenchyma doubled and the number in the pulmonary arterioles increased nearly seven times.

The studies indicate that damage to both arterioles and capillaries may occur after gas embolization and that neutrophils seem to be necessary for the induction of lung injury. In a study in sheep, Flick et al. (197) showed that removal of circulating leukocytes attenuated the increased permeability of the lung vessels seen after air embolization. Depletion of fibrinogen or platelets did not seem to have any effect (198,199). Other studies in rats also indicate that leukocyte activation plays a significant role in mediating the effects of air emboli (200); increased levels of both thromboxane B_2 and endothelin were seen, indicating their release and involvement in the increase in lung resistance.

The mechanism for activation of neutrophils is not known. It is probable that complement activation plays a significant role (201,202). Neutrophil activation is also exacerbated by the cytokine interleukin-8 (IL-8) (203). Neutrophil activation leads to the production of oxygen radicals (204); thus it is reasonable to assume that exposure to increased oxygen tensions may lead to similar changes and that increased oxygen tension and bubbles may have additive effects. This could have implications for the treatment of DCI.

Monocytes/Macrophages

Resident macrophages adhering to the endothelium (pulmonary intravascular macrophages, or PIM) have been identified in the lungs of several mammalian species (205). Such macrophages have been identified both in the baboon (206) and in humans (77), although they seem to be much less numerous than in other species like the pig or sheep. In sheep they occupy approximately 15% of the capillary blood volume, while they are found in only 2% of that volume in the baboon (206). However, PIMs may be induced by breathing high doses of oxygen (206) as well as other stimuli. The most important secretory product of these macrophages is thromboxane (207).

Even if humans have PIMs to a smaller degree than other species, circulating monocytes stay for a considerable time in the lung capillaries. The size

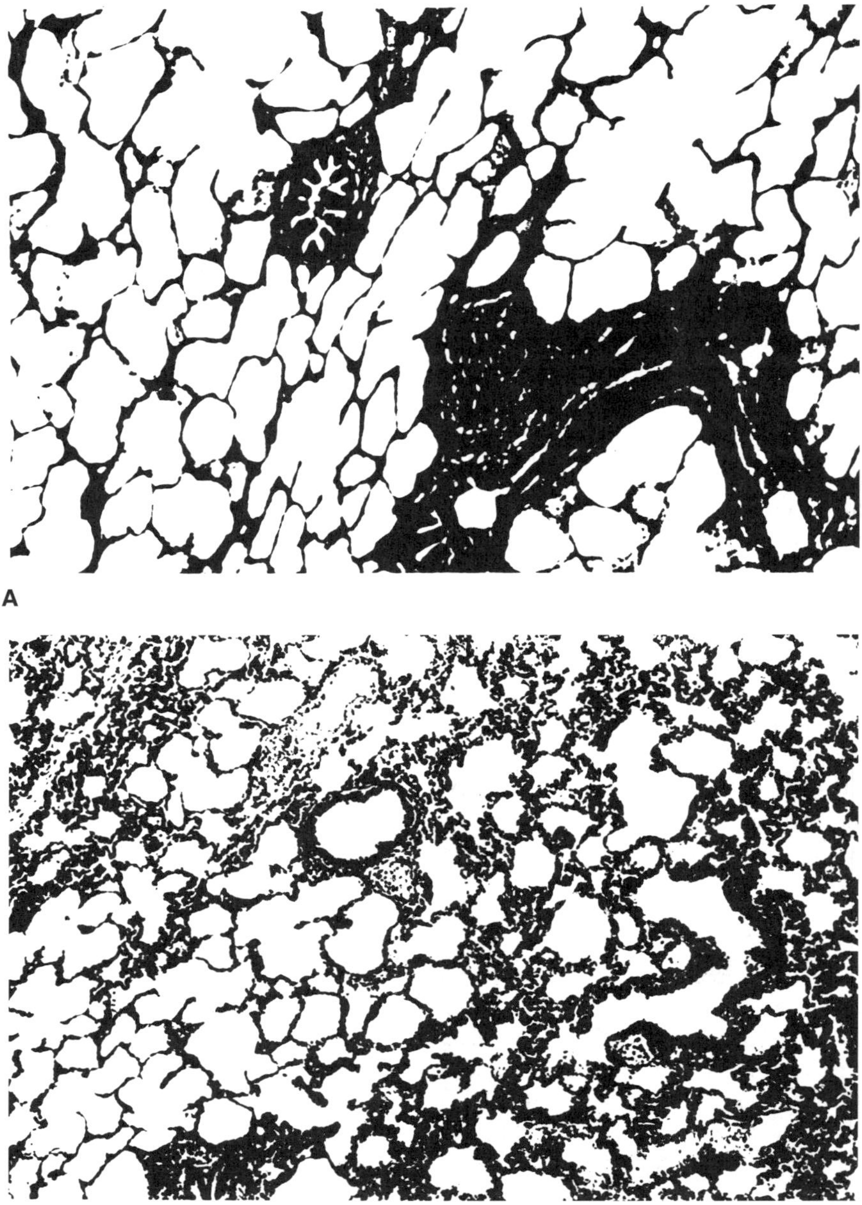

A

B

Figure 7 Histological picture of the lung of a pig exposed to gas bubbles (approximately grade III–IV) for 100 min (B) by comparison with the lung in an unexposed animal (A). H&E stain, 100×magnification.

of both neutrophils and monocytes is considerably larger than the size of the capillaries (8.5 versus 5.5 μm) (208–210); therefore the transport of these cells through the capillary is strongly dependent upon their deformability. Neutrophils traverse the lungs considerably more quickly than do monocytes (2 to 4 and 12 to 18 hr, respectively) (208). On activation, the deformability of leukocytes is reduced (211).

C. Effects of Bubbles on the Endothelium

As mentioned above, Albertine (64) found gaps in the endothelium of arterioles following air embolization. Moosavei et al. (195) saw the same and in addition gap formation occurring at the sites of embolic impact. They also reported degranulated platelets and neutrophils at the gap. There was a diffuse deposition of fibrin under the area of damage. In the bronchial venules, there was endothelium cell swelling and gap formation without damage to the membrane. They also reported that the alveolar epithelium was intact and that edema was present in the peribronchial region and in the adventitia of pulmonary arteries. The pattern of edema is similar to that seen by Catron et al. (37) in dogs following simulated dives to 300 fsw followed by a severe decompression. The edema was seen as cuffs around the pulmonary blood vessels and around the bronchi, more in the hilum than elsewhere. There was no alveolar edema.

In the study by Smith et al. (190), endothelial damage could be demonstrated in pigs exposed to severe decompressions. Endothelial damage has also been observed in several other studies, which showed that gas bubbles following decompression increased the permeability of the lung vasculature to Trypan blue (37,212–214). Those animals that had decompression bubbles were found at postmortem to have lungs filled with the dye. Animals that had dived but showed no evidence of bubble formation had the same staining pattern as control animals.

The exact mechanism for these endothelial changes is not clear but could be related to the activation of leukocytes (213). There is no conclusive evidence to distinguish between direct mechanical action and indirect humoral factors as the means of changing pulmonary vascular permeability. Sacks et al. (215) attributed the endothelial cell injury to release of oxygen radicals by activated intravascular granulocytes. Several other vasoactive substances have been demonstrated in the lung after severe decompression stress—for example, bradykinin (216) and smooth muscle acting factor (217), a substance capable of increasing vascular permeability and responsiveness to bradykinin. Histamine, serotonin, and bradykinin all induce separation of the intercellular junctions of the endothelium. (218).

The degree of damage to the endothelium can be evaluated by studying the transport of fluid over the vessel wall. Ohkuda et al. (78) infused air bubbles

300 μm in diameter into the pulmonary arteries of sheep, sufficient to increase PVR by between 60 and 300%. After an initial loading bolus, the infusion rate was adjusted to maintain a constant PVR at one of three levels within that range. They found a dose-dependent increase in lymph flow and lymph protein clearance with a negative lymph-to-plasma protein ratio for the two lowest doses but with a positive ratio at higher dose. The lower lymph-to-plasma protein ratio at the two lowest infusions is an indication that the pulmonary capillaries retain limited ability to sieve proteins at those infusion levels. Similar changes in lymph and protein flow were seen in sheep by Flick et al. (197) and by Pou et al. (58). The latter authors found no change in lymph/protein ratio despite using very low infusion doses of 0.05 $ml/kg^{-1}/min^{-1}$. The increase in lymph flow occurs despite the probable reduction in surface area available due to the embolization of some vessels. This suggests that the flow is from nonembolized vessels.

After the gas infusion is stopped, there is a further increase in lymph and protein flow despite the reduction in PAP (58,78,197). This is further evidence that the flow is from perfused vessels and the increase following cessation of infusion comes about as more and more vessels become open to flow following the absorption of gas bubbles that had blocked these vessels. This may indicate that changes in permeability last longer than the time for which bubbles are present. Figure 8 shows the time course of PAP and lymph flow.

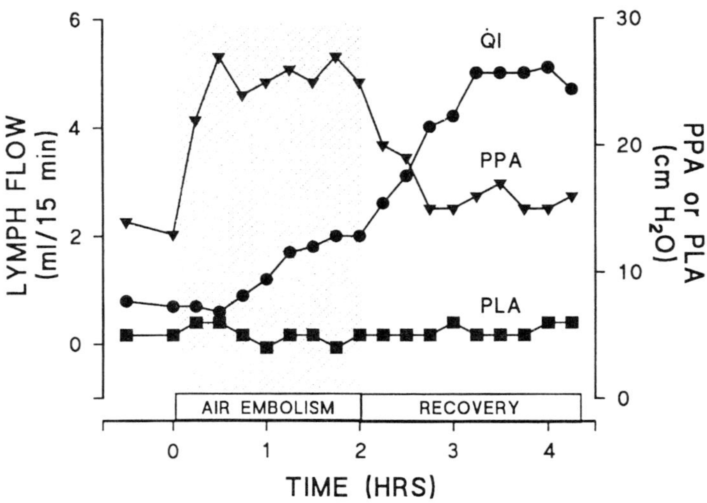

Figure 8 Relationship between PAP and lymph flow. Q̇I indicates lymph flow, PPA is pulmonary artery pressure, and PLA is pressure in the left atrium. (From Ref. 58.)

The relative importance of capillary and alveolar epithelium in determining the permeability properties of the alveolar-capillary membrane has been discussed by Schneeberger (219). Under most conditions, the pulmonary capillary endothelial junctions are impermeable to large molecules. They are, however, susceptible to stretching if the intravascular pressure is increased, leaving the alveolar epithelium as the final barrier to the movement of molecules between alveoli and capillaries.

VII. Diagnosis of Gas Bubble Embolism in the Lung

A. Clinical Diagnosis

The signs and symptoms of massive venous gas embolism (VGE) were described as early as 1885 by Senn (220): a ''millwheel'' murmur, gasping respiration, cyanosis, and cardiovascular collapse. The clinical signs of gas embolism in the lung following decompression will probably be quite minor. An increase in breathing frequency has been described; experimental studies have shown that this increase is proportional to the increase in right ventricular pressure (221). The authors demonstrated that the response is mediated through the vagal efferents. Heart rate also usually increases, but studies in dogs have demonstrated that this is a late phenomenon, occurring significantly later than changes in the electrocardiogram. The latter changes mostly consist of peaking of the P waves, which is also related to an increase in PAP (43). In the clinical literature, the typical millwheel murmur has been described (222–224), but that is usually a late sign and is heard mainly after circulatory detoriation (43).

In diving, the clinical symptoms of lung involvement is called ''chokes'' (11). This usually starts as a burning sensation in the substernal region, often associated with deep inspiration. The sensation is increased by increased ventilation and an uncontrollable cough develops. The time of onset is usually later than that of symptoms from joints and muscles. At autopsy, gas bubbles are seen in the interstitium, not in the vessels, and it was pointed out by Behnke (11) that ''*chokes may be a vascular reaction in the mucous membranes of the respiratory passage secondary to contiguous bubbles*.'' This indicates that the chokes are a manifestation of the inflammatory effects of the bubbles.

B. Ultrasound

Since the physiological effects of gas bubbles in the lung are related to the amount of gas in bubbles, quantification of the volume of gas entering the lung is of importance. Spencer and Oyama (28) asked in 1971 for ''techniques of determining the number and sizes of bubbles, as well as for computing the volume of gas passing through a given vascular channel.'' This goal has still not been reached.

When ultrasound is transmitted into the body, it is reflected from tissues having different acoustic properties. In vessels, the main reflector or scatterer, the red cells, is moving. It has been shown by Angelsen (225) that the scattering arises from fluctuations in the red cell concentration inside the sample volume of the ultrasonic transducer. The penetration of ultrasound is inversely proportional to the transmitted frequency. The most commonly used ultrasonic frequencies for studying the heart and the pulmonary circulation is 2 to 3 Mhz. If the transducer is placed in the esophagus (TEE probe), frequencies up to 7 Mhz can be used.

Bubbles are strong scatterers of ultrasound; thus ultrasonic systems can be used to detect bubbles in blood vessels. Traditionally, Doppler ultrasonic systems have been used; the equipment is cheap and easy to use even in remote locations (3). However, the Doppler systems have some disadvantages. Evaluation of the signals is very difficult and requires extensive training, in particular if few bubbles are present (226). The Doppler systems do not give any information about anatomical structures and their relation to the blood flow where the bubbles are detected. This relationship is of importance, particularly inside the heart, where complex flow behavior can be present and valves and heart walls give strong reflections that may be interpreted as gas bubbles.

When measurements in the pulmonary artery are made, the Doppler method, combined with information about the timing of the closure of the valves, can make it possible to estimate pulmonary artery pressure noninvasively (227). This is obviously of interest, as it is known that even apparently uneventful decompressions can lead to an increase in PAPs and pulmonary vascular resistance (27), suggesting the presence of bubbles.

The main effect of a gas phase is to increase the intensity of the reflected ultrasonic signal. Usually, the bubbles can be heard as separate ''chirps'' overriding the Doppler signal from the moving blood. Even when only a small number of bubbles is present, changes in the spectrum of the Doppler signal can be detected as an increase in both the low and high frequencies. (228). A recent study has shown that air emboli lead to an increase in the amplitude of the Doppler signal of 10 to 30 dB in the 200- to 2500-Hz range (229). Using data from Furness (230), it can be calculated that an aggregate of erythrocytes with a diameter of 120 μm will have approximately the same back-scattered intensity as a gas bubble with a diameter of 18 μm at 1 ata. Clarke et al. (231) stated that, in a standing ultrasonic field, a fat globule 200 μm in diameter resulted in the same signal as an air bubble 50 μm in diameter.

In most cases, bubbles have been detected by performing Doppler measurements in the pulmonary artery or the right ventricular outflow tract. Bubbles are quantified by subjective grading of the signals (2–4). This grading scale is nonlinear. It can often be difficult to distinguish between bubbles and the movement of valves and vessel walls, particularly if no high-pass filters are used.

Even though the ear is an excellent discriminator, this method is clearly unsatisfactory for quantitative evaluation of bubble content. Several methods for automatic counting have been proposed over the years (228,232–235). Generally it can be said that the automatic methods are of little use for evaluating the number of bubbles reaching the lungs, and subjective, aural bubble grading must still be considered the standard.

The use of ultrasonic scanners to detect gas bubbles is attractive as it enables distinction between gas bubbles occurring in the right or the left side of the vascular system. The occurrence of bubbles and their localization can be determined from the images. Ikeda et al. (236) proposed that the number of linear echoes per second could be used to evaluate the number of gas bubbles in M-mode images. Alternatively, the bubbles can be graded in the image or counted as the number of bubbles inside the sampled area of the vessel (bubbles per square centimeter) (237).

Figures 9A and 9B show images from an experimental study following decompression in pigs. Bubbles can be seen in both the aorta and the pulmonary artery. Note the difference in the intensity of bubbles in the two images; the stronger reflections in the aorta in Fig. 9B are larger bubbles transmitted through an open foramen ovale, while the less intense bright spots in Fig. 9A are bubbles that have been transported across the lung vasculature. This indicates that bubbles going through a PFO are larger than those moving across the lungs (see below).

In order to quantify the amount of separated gas, information is needed about both the number of gas bubbles and their size. The size of gas bubbles is not easily determined with an ultrasonic system. Lubbers and van der Berg (238) and Nishi (239) both demonstrated that the amplitude of the reflected ultrasonic signal is proportional to the size of the gas bubble as long as the bubbles are larger than the resonant size for the ultrasonic frequency used. Resonant frequency is inversely proportional to the radius of the gas bubble (54). For the ultrasonic frequencies commonly used in humans, resonant radii will be in the order of 1.5, 0.6, and 0.3 μm for ultrasonic frequencies of 2, 5, and 10 MHz, respectively. These values are valid at 1 ata. With increasing pressure, resonant size will increase due to the decreasing contribution of thermal and viscous losses. Thus the resonant peak in the scattering cross-section will increase (54), making assumptions about the relationship between bubble radius and reflected signal amplitude difficult. The bubble radius for resonance will be approximately ten times as high at 40 to 50 ata as at surface (6 μm for 5 MHz, 15 μm for 2 MHz). For bubbles around resonant size, the relationship between reflected intensity and size will be nonlinear, and the scattering cross-section will be larger than the geometrical cross-section (54). However, as was pointed out by Nishi (240), the use of several ultrasonic frequencies might still allow assumptions about bubble size. In a dive to 500 msw, we measured gas bubbles in the femoral

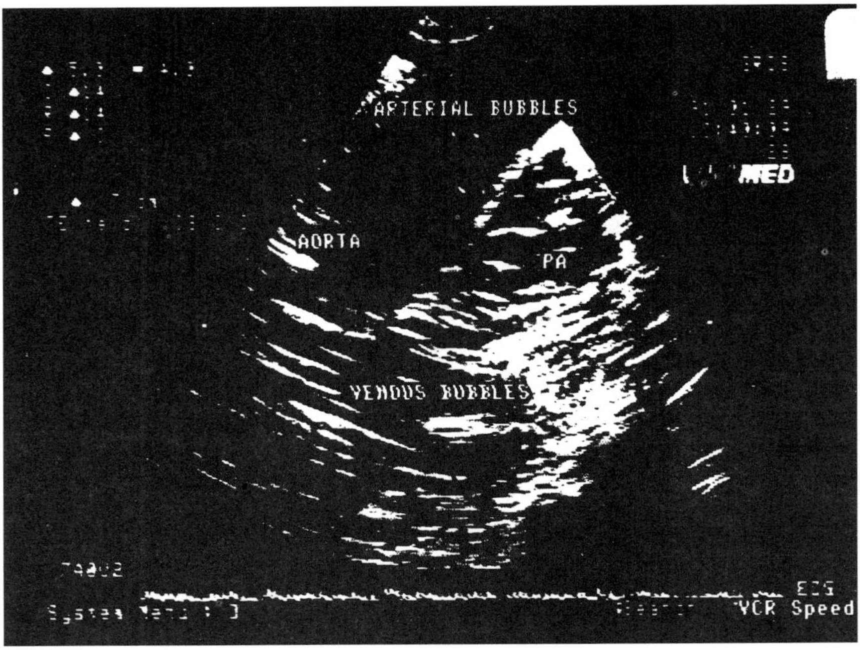
ARTERIAL BUBBLES
AORTA
PA
VENOUS BUBBLES
VCR Speed

A

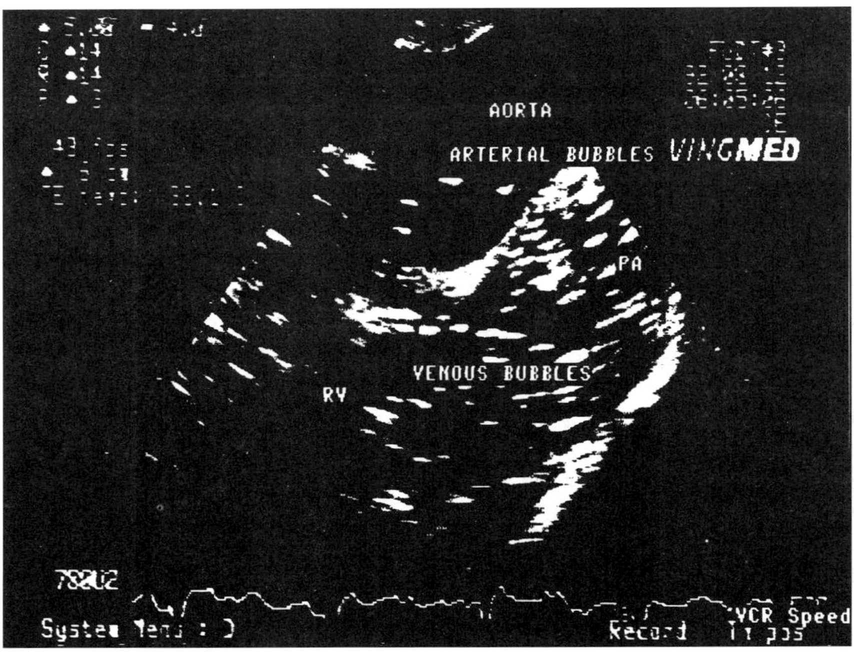
AORTA
ARTERIAL BUBBLES
VINGMED
PA
VENOUS BUBBLES
RV
VCR Speed
Record

B

vein simultaneously with 2- and 5-MHz transducers and a pulsed Doppler system. The method has been described previously (241,242). The number of bubbles detected with the 2-MHz system was about 70% of what was detected with the 5 MHz system, with a similar distribution of intensities. This would indicate that many bubbles were below 15 μm in size (235).

In practice, even given the theoretical relationship between bubbles size and reflected intensity, many problems exist. The most important are that the position of the bubble in the ultrasonic beam is not known and that most ultrasonic fields are heterogeneous (235). Even if absolute size cannot be determined, relative intensities can be evaluated, thus giving an indication about the relative size of bubbles in the right and left heart. Differences in intensity can be used to evaluate size difference in bubbles moving through the lung and bubbles moving through a PFO (see Fig. 9).

What is the smallest size of the bubble that can be detected with an ultrasonic system? This is a question that cannot easily be answered, as many factors relating to the properties of the ultrasonic system and to the organism are involved. In order to detect the bubble at all, the intensity of the reflected signal must be above a certain threshold and different from that of the surrounding tissue. Using a continuous-wave Doppler system with a frequency of 8 MHz, Butler and Hills (50) claim that bubbles down to 14 μm in diameter could be detected in the arterial system of dogs. A previous study with the same instrument showed similar results in vitro and also demonstrated that the threshold increased with decreasing flow velocity of the fluid (242). Our own experience is similar to this; we have been able to detect foam of bubbles with diameters between 10 and 50 μm with a 6-MHz transducer and a pulsed ultrasonic system in the pulmonary artery in pigs. It is however difficult to judge from this the ability of the system to identify single bubbles of the same size. Using the same system, single albumin-coated gas bubbles of a diameter of approximately 8 μm could not be detected. This is in no way conclusive, however, as these single particles may pass outside the sample volume. In a recent study based on the resonant properties of bubbles, Christman et al. showed that 4-μm bubbles could be detected in femoral veins of dogs decompressed from 100 msw (66).

In principle, a pulsed Doppler system will have a higher sensitivity than a continuous one, because the signal-to-noise ratio is better. The sensitivity of an ultrasonic imaging system will be at least as good. Gas bubble foam, where

---

Figure 9 Ultrasonic images from the right ventricle (RV), the pulmonary artery (PA), and the aorta in two pigs following decompression. The images were obtained with a 6-MHz ultrasonic transducer in the esophagus. (A) An animal with a closed atrial septum. (B) An image from an animal with a PFO. Bubbles can be seen as bright spots. Note the difference in intensity between the aortic bubbles in the two images, indicating that the bubbles in (A) are larger.

single bubbles have a diameter of 6 to 10 μm, is routinely used for contrast echocardiography, and Meltzer et al. (244) claim that microbubbles down to 10 μm can be detected using ultrasonic frequencies of 2 to 3 MHz. It must, however, be borne in mind that ''spontaneous ultrasonic contrast'' has been detected in the central venous system of perhaps up to 40% of patients studied (245,246). The occurrence of such high-intensity reflections inside the heart is dependent upon heart function and flow. It is likely that these contrast effects are caused by thrombi or perhaps erythrocyte aggregates, which probably cannot be differentiated from changes caused by gas bubbles. The detection threshold will decrease with increasing ultrasonic frequency and distance from transducer (247). Using ultrasonic frequencies of 20 MHz in an intravascular catheter–based scanning system, spontaneous ultrasonic contrast will be detected in the majority of individuals (Linker, personal communication).

Based on the above, it is impossible to make accurate general statements about the detection threshold and resolution of an ultrasonic system for bubble detection. However, it is probable that most Doppler and scanning systems, using frequencies between 2 and 10 MHz, are able to detect single bubbles with diameters above 20 to 50 μ. More sensitive systems are probably interesting only for experimental work, due to the occurrence of spontaneous contrast phenomena.

C. Indirect Methods

Changes in gas exchange in the lung can be used to measure the degree of air embolism. Reduction of end-tidal CO_2 seems to be a reliable measure of the degree of air embolization, as there is a quantitative correlation between the increase in pulmonary artery pressure and the reduction in carbon dioxide content (248). An increase in nitrogen content in the expired air can be detected following air embolism (249). Measurement of transcutaneous O_2 and CO_2 (250) as well as of airway pressure (251) has also been suggested. However it is important to remember that the return of these different variables to normal does not imply that the bubbles have all been resolved (14).

VIII. Conclusions

The occurrence of gas bubbles in the pulmonary artery following decompression has been noted for several decades. Most investigators have tended to focus on the relationship between bubbles and clinical symptoms of decompression illness, and little attention has been focused upon the possible effects of these bubbles on the lungs themselves.

Gas bubbles in the lungs elicit acute hemodynamic and ventilatory responses. Gas bubbles act as foreign surfaces and induce numerous biochemical and cellular changes in the blood vessels. Among these are activation of complement, thrombocytes, neutrophils, and monocytes. Changes in the endothelium are induced either by direct (mechanical) effects or more probably through the above activation. These changes lead to increased leakage of fluid into the extravascular space. Even minimal endothelial injury can give the endothelium procoagulant properties. This will induce activation of both biochemical and cellular responses, which could form the basis for injury to the lungs following decompression. All these changes are reversible, but some chronic damage may occur. The exact mechanism of many of these changes is not known and needs further study. Even after the acute effects of the gas emboli have disappeared, bubbles may still be present and the biochemical activity may persist.

The changes in lung function seen in divers, with a reduction in carbon monoxide transfer factor and reduction in compliance, may support the hypothesis that inflammatory processes in the lungs are a result of the decompression process.

The clinical implication of these changes is not clear and the extent of changes seen in individuals repeatedly exposed to small amounts of gas bubbles is not known. The data indicate, however, the importance of keeping the exposure to gas bubbles at the lowest possible level, thus making the development of decompression procedures that have a low level of vascular gas bubbles an important target.

References

1. Nishi RY. Doppler and ultrasonic bubble detection. In: Bennett PB, Elliott DH, eds. The Physiology and Medicine of Diving, 4th ed. London: Saunders, 1993:433–453.
2. Nishi RY. Doppler evaluation of decompression tables. In: Lin YC, Shida KK, eds. Man in the Sea. San Pedro, CA: Best Publishing, 1990:297–316.
3. Spencer MP. Decompression limits for compressed air determined by ultrasonically detected blood bubbles. J Appl Physiol 1976; 40:229–235.
4. Gardette B. Correlation between decompression sickness and circulating bubbles in 232 divers. Undersea Biomed Res 1979; 6:99–107.
5. Eckenhoff RG, Olstad CS, Carrod G. Human dose-response relationship for decompression and endogenous bubble formation. J Appl Physiol 1990; 69:914–918.
6. Hemmingsen EA. Nucleation of bubbles in vitro and in vivo. In: Brubakk AO, Kanwisher J, Sundnes G, eds. Diving in animals and man. Trondheim, Norway: Tapir Publishers, 1986:43–59.
7. Yount DE. Growth of bubbles from nuclei. In: Brubakk AO, Kanwisher J, Sundnes G, eds. Diving in animals and Man. Trondheim, Norway: Tapir Publishers, 1986: 131–164.
8. Spencer MP, Johanson DC. Investigation of new principles for human decompres-

sion schedules using the Doppler ultrasonic blood bubble detector: Technical Report. Seattle: Institute for Environmental Medicine and Physiology, 1974.

9. Nashimoto I, Gotoh Y. Relationship between precordial Doppler ultrasound records and decompression sickness. In: Shilling CW, Beckett MW, eds. Underwater Physiology: VI. Bethesda, MD: Undersea Medical Society, 1978:497–501.
10. Sawatzky KD. The relationship between intravascular Doppler-detected gas bubbles and decompression sickness after bounce diving in humans. Ph.D. thesis. York University, Toronto, 1991.
11. Behnke AR. Decompression sickness following exposure to high pressures. In: Fulton JF, ed. Decompression Sickness. Philadelphia: Saunders, 1951:53–89.
12. Chang HK, Delaunois L, Boileau R, Martin RR. Redistribution of pulmonary blood flow during experimental air embolism. J Appl Physiol 1981; 51:211–217.
13. Chang HK, Weber ME, Thomson J, Martin RR. Hydrodynamic features of pulmonary air embolism: A model study. J Appl Physiol 1981; 51:1002–1008.
14. Butler BD, Luehr S, Katz J. Venous gas embolism: Time course of residual pulmonary intravascular bubbles. Undersea Biomed Res 1989; 16:21–29.
15. Bove AA, Hallenbeck JM, Elliott DH. Circulatory responses to venous air embolism and decompression sickness in dogs. Undersea Biomed Res 1974; 1:207–220.
16. Butler BD, Hills BA. Effect of excessive oxygen upon the capability of the lungs to filter gas emboli. In: Bachrach AJ, Matzen MM, eds. Underwater Physiology: VII. Bethesda, MD: Undersea Medical Society, 1981:95–102.
17. Butler BD, Katz J. Vascular pressures and passage of gas emboli through the pulmonary circulation. Undersea Biomed Res 1988; 15:203–209.
18. Butler BD, Leiman BC, Katz J. Arterial air embolism of venous origin in dogs: Effect of nitrous oxide in combination with halothane and pentobarbitone. Can J Anaesth 1987; 34:570–575.
19. Catron PW, Thomas LB, Flynn ET, et al. Effects of He-O_2 breathing during experimental decompression sickness following air dives. Undersea Biomed Res 1987; 14:101–111.
20. Catron PW, Thomas LB, McDermott JJ, et al. Hormonal changes during decompression sickness. Undersea Biomed Res 1987; 14:331–341.
21. Gottdiener JS, Papademetriou V, Notargiacomo A, et al. Incidence and cardiac effects of systemic venous air embolism: Echocardiographic evidence of arterial embolization via noncardiac shunt. Arch Intern Med 1988; 148:795–800.
22. Katz J, Leiman BC, Butler BD. Effects of inhalation anaesthetics on filtration of venous gas emboli by the pulmonary vasculature. Br J Anaesth 1988; 61:200–205.
23. Verstappen FTJ, Bernards JA, Kreuzer F. Effects of pulmonary gas embolism on circulation and respiration in the dog: 1. Effects on circulation. Pflügers Arch 1977; 368:89–96.
24. Yahagi N, Furuya H. The effects of halothane and pentobartbital on the threshold of transpulmonary passage of venous air emboli in dogs. Anesthesiology 1987; 67: 905–909.
25. Atkins CE, Lehner CE, Beck KA, et al. Experimental respiratory decompression sickness in sheep. J Appl Physiol 1988; 65:1163–1171.

26. Deal CW, Fielden BP, Monk I. Hemodynamic effects of pulmonary air embolism. J Surg Res 1971; 11:533–538.
27. Neuman TS, Spragg RG, Wagner PD, Moser KM. Cardiopulmonary consequences of decompression stress. Respir Physiol 1980; 41:143–153.
28. Spencer MP, Oyama Y. Pulmonary capacity for dissipation of venous gas emboli. Aerospace Med 1971; 42:822–827.
29. Black S, Cucchiara RF, Nishimura RA, Michenfelder JD. Parameters affecting occurrence of paradoxical air embolism. Anesthesiology 1989; 71:235–241.
30. Vik A, Brubakk AO, Hennessy TR, et al. Venous air embolism in swine: Transport of gas bubbles through the pulmonary circulation. J Appl Physiol 1990; 69:237–244.
31. Vik A, Jenssen BM, Brubakk AO. Effect of aminophylline on transpulmonary passage of venous air emboli in pigs. J Appl Physiol 1991; 71:1780–1786.
32. D'Aoust BG, Swanson HT, White R, et al. Central venous bubbles and mixed venous nitrogen in goats following decompression. J Appl Physiol 1981; 51:1238–1244.
33. Lynch PR, Brigham M, Tuma R, Wiedeman MP. Origin and time course of gas bubbles following rapid decompression in the hamster. Undersea Biomed Res 1985; 12:105–114.
34. Wolffe JB, Robertson HF. Experimental air embolism. Ann Intern Med 1935; 9: 162–165.
35. Lever MJ, Miller KW, Paton WDM, Smith EB. Experiments on the genesis of bubbles as a result of rapid decompression. J Physiol 1966; 184:964–969.
36. Powell MR. Gas phase separation following decompression in asymptomatic rats: Visual and ultrasound monitoring. Aerospace Med 1972; 43:1240–1244.
37. Catron PW, Flynn ET, Yaffe L, et al. Morphological and physiological responses of the lungs of dogs to acute decompression. J Appl Physiol 1984; 57:467–474.
38. Vik A, Jenssen BM, Eftedal O, Brubakk AO. Relationship between venous bubbles and hemodynamic responses after decompression in pigs. Undersea Hyperbar Med 1993; 20:233–248.
39. Harkins HN, Harmon PH. Embolism by air and oxygen: Comparative studies. Proc Soc Exp Biol Med 1934; 32:178–181.
40. Gilbert JW, Berglund E, Dahlgren S, et al. Experimental pulmonary hypertension in the dog: A preparation involving repeated air embolism. J Thorac Cardiovasc Surg 1968; 55:565–571.
41. Holt EP, Webb WR, Cook WA, Unal MO. Air embolism: Hemodynamics and therapy. Ann Thorac Surg 1966; 2:551–559.
42. Mandlebaum I, King H. Pulmonary air embolism. Surg Forum. 1963; 14:236–238.
43. Adornato DC, Gildenberg PL, Ferrario CM, et al. Pathophysiology of intravenous air embolism in dogs. Anesthesiology 1978; 49:120–125.
44. Butler BD, Hills BA. Transpulmonary passage of venous air emboli. J Appl Physiol 1985; 59:543–547.
45. Hlastala MP, Robertson HT, Ross BK. Gas exchange abnormalities produced by venous gas emboli. Respir Physiol 1979; 36:1–17.

46. Sergysels R, Jasper N, Delaunois L, et al. Effect of ventilation with different gas mixtures on experimental lung air embolism. Respir Physiol 1978; 34:329–343.
47. Verstappen FTJ, Bernards JA, Kreuzer F. Effects of pulmonary gas embolism on circulation and respiration in the dog: II. Effects on respiration. Pflügers Arch 1977; 368:97–104.
48. Verstappen FTJ, Bernards JA, Kreuzer F. Effects of pulmonary gas embolism on circulation and respiration in the dog: III. Excretion of venous gas bubbles by the lung. Pflügers Arch 1977; 370:67–70.
49. Verstappen FTJ, Bernards JA, Kreuzer F. Effects of pulmonary gas embolism on circulation and respiration in the dog: IV. Origin of arterial hypoxemia during pulmonary gas embolism. Pflügers Arch 1977; 370:71–71.
50. Butler BD, Hills BA. The lung as a filter for microbubbles. J Appl Physiol 1979; 47:537–543.
51. Vik A, Jenssen BM, Brubakk AO. Arterial gas bubbles after decompression in pigs with patent foramen ovale. Undersea Hyperbar Med 1993; 20:121–132.
52. Hills BA, Butler BD. Size distribution of intravascular air emboli produced by decompression. Undersea Biomed Res 1981; 8:163–170.
53. Flook V, Brubakk AO, Eftedal O, et al. The effect of oxygen and of decompression bubbles on inert gas washout. SINTEF Report 1994, Trondheim. STF23 A94031.
54. Medwin H. Counting bubbles acoustically: A review. Ultrasonics 1977; 15:7–13.
55. Mehta M, Sokoll MD, Gergis SD. Effects of venous air embolism on the cardiovascular system and acid base balance in the presence and absence of nitrous oxide. Acta Anaesthesiol Scand 1984; 28:226–231.
56. Aibiki M, Ogura S, Seki K, et al. Role of vagal afferents in hypotension induced by venous air embolism. Am J Physiol 1994; 266:R790–R795.
57. Richardson HF, Coles BC, Hall GE. Experimental gas embolism: I. Intravenous air embolism. Can Med Assoc J 1937; 36:584–588.
58. Pou NA, Roselli RJ, Parker RE, Clanton JC. Effects of air embolism on sheep lung fluid volume. J Appl Physiol 1993; 75:986–993.
59. Knisely WH, Satterwhite WM, Wallace JM. An attempt to demonstrate pulmonary arteriovenous anastomoses in rabbits, cats and dogs, and discussion of literature pertaining to such shunts. Circulation 1956; 14:960–961.
60. Malik AB. Pulmonary microembolism. Physiol Rev 1983; 63:1114–1207.
61. Berglund E, Josephson S. Pulmonary air embolization in the dog: I. Hemodynamic changes on repeated embolizations. Scand J Clin Lab Invest 1970; 26:97–103.
62. Dalen JE, Haynes FW, Hoppin FG, et al. Cardiovascular responses to experimental pulmonary embolism. Am J Cardiol 1967; 20:3–9.
63. Josephson S. Pulmonary air embolization in the dog: II. Evidence and location of pulmonary vasoconstriction. Scand J Clin Lab Invest 1970; 26:113–123.
64. Albertine KH, Wiener-Kronish JP, et al. Quantification of damage by air emboli to lung microvessels in anesthetized sheep. J Appl Physiol 1984; 57:1360–1368.
65. Hills BA. Air embolism: Fission of microbubbles upon collision in plasma. Clin Sci Mol Med 1974; 46:629–634.
66. Christman CL, Catron PW, Flynn ET, Weathersby PK. In vivo microbubble detection in decompression sickness using a second harmonic resonant bubble detector. Undersea Biomed Res 1986; 13:1–18.

67. Whitteridge D. Multiple embolism of the lung and rapid shallow breathing. Physiol Rev 1950; 30:475–486.
68. Burri PH, Weibel ER. Ultrastructure and morphometry of the developing lung. In: Hodson WA, ed. Development of the Lung. (Lung Biol Health Dis Ser). New York: Marcel Dekker, 1977:215–268.
69. Weibel ER. Oxygen demand and the size of respiratory structures in mammals. In: Wood SC, Lenfant C, eds. Evolution of Respiratory Processes: A Comparative Approach. (Lung Biol Health Dis Ser). New York: Marcel Dekker, 1979:289–334.
70. Weibel ER. The Pathway for Oxygen. Cambridge, MA: Harvard University Press, 1984.
71. Blinks LR, Twitty VC, Whitaker DM. Animal experiments on bubble formation: Part II. Bubble formation in frogs and rats. In: Fulton JF, ed. Decompression Sickness. Philadelphia: Saunders, 1951:145–164.
72. Harvey EN. Animal experiments on bubble formation: Part I. Bubble formation in cats. In: Fulton JF, ed. Decompression Sickness. Philadelphia: Saunders, 1951:115–144.
73. McDonough PM, Hemmingsen EA. Bubble formation in crabs induced by limb motions after decompression. J Appl Physiol 1984; 57:117–122.
74. Boycott AE, Damant CC, Haldane JS. The prevention of compressed-air illness. J Hyg (Lond) 1908; 8:342–443.
75. Harris P, Heath D. The Human Pulmonary Circulation, 2d ed. Edinburgh: Churchill Livingstone, 1977.
76. Warner AE, Brain JD. The cell biology and pathogenic role of pulmonary intravascular macrophages. Am J Physiol 1990; 258(Lung Cell Mol Physiol 2):L1–12.
77. Dehring DJ, Wismar BL. Intravascular macrophages in pulmonary capillaries of humans. Am Rev Respir Dis 1989; 139:1027–1029.
78. Ohkuda K, Nakahara K, Bincher A, Staub NC. Venous air emboli in sheep: Reversible increase in lung microvascular permeability. J Appl Physiol 1981; 51:887–894.
79. Deffenbach ME, Charan NB, Lakshminarayan S, Butler J. The bronchial circulation: Small but vital attribute in the lung. Am Rev Respir Dis 1987; 135:463–481.
80. Nunn JF. Applied Respiratory Physiology. London: Butterworths, 1969.
81. Swenson ER, Robertson HT, Polissar NL, et al. Conducting airway gas exchange: Diffusion related differences in inert gas elimination. J Appl Physiol 1992; 72: 1581–1588.
82. Meltzer RS, Tickner EG, Popp RL. Why do the lungs clear utrasonic contrast? Ultrasound Med Biol 1980; 6:263–269.
83. Yang WJ, Echigo R, Wotten DR, Hwang JB. Experimental studies of the dissolution of gas bubbles in whole blood and plasma: I. Stationary bubbles. J Biomech 1971; 3:275–281.
84. Russell GB, Snider MT, Richard RB, Loomis JL. Venous air emboli with $^{15}N_2$: Pulmonary excretion and physiologic response in dogs. Undersea Biomed Res 1991; 18:37–45.
85. Hills BA, Butler BD. Migration of lung surfactant to pulmonary air emboli In: Bacharach AJ, Matzen MM, eds. Underwater Physiology: VII. Bethesda, MD: Undersea Medical Society, 1981:741–752.

86. Hills BA, Barrow RE. Air embolism: Possible role of surfactant on recompression. J Appl Physiol 1982; 52:119–123.
87. Taylor FB, Jr, Abrahams ME. Effect of surface active lipoprotein on clotting and fibrinolysis and of fibrinogen on surface tension of surface active lipoprotein: With a hypothesis on the pathophysiology of pulmonary atelactasis and hyaline membrane in respiratory distress syndrome of the newborn. Am J Med 1966; 40: 346–351.
88. Brubakk AO, Peterson R, Grip A, et al. Gas bubbles in the circulation of divers after ascending excursions from 300 to 250 msw. J Appl Physiol 1986; 60:45–51.
89. Hjelle JO, Eatock BC, Nordahl SH, Dick APK. Doppler monitoring during 3 dives to 360 msw. In Marroni A, Oriani G, eds. Proc EUBS 87 Diving and Hyperbaric Medicine, Palermo, Italy: European Undersea Biomedical Society, 1987:357–364.
90. Haymaker W, Johnston AD. Pathology of decompression sickness: A comparison of lesions in airmen with those in caisson workers and divers. Mil Med 1955; 117:285–306.
91. Spencer MP, Campbell SD. Development of bubbles in venous and arterial blood during hyperbaric decompression. Bull Mason Clin 1968; 22:26–32.
92. Wagner CE. Observation of gas bubbles in pial vessels of cats following rapid decompression from high pressure atmospheres. J Neurophysiol 1945; 8:29–32.
93. Black M, Calvin J, Chan KL, Walley VM. Paradoxic air embolism in the absence of an intracardiac defect. Chest 1991; 99:754–755.
94. Marquez J, Sladen A, Gendell H, et al. Paradoxical cerebral air embolism without an intracardiac septal defect. J Neurosurg 1981; 55:997–1000.
95. Gronert GA, Messick JM, Cucchiara RF, Michenfelder JD. Paradoxical air embolism from a patent foramen ovale. Anesthesiology 1979; 50:548–549.
96. Bedell EA, Berge KH, Losasso TJ. Paradoxic air embolism during venous air embolism: Transesophageal echocardiographic evidence of transpulmonary passage. Anesthesiology 1994; 80:947–950.
97. Gorman DF. Decompression sickness and arterial gas embolism in sports scuba divers. Sports Med 1989; 8:32–42.
98. Hills BA. Decompression Sickness. Vol. 1. Chichester, England: Wiley, 1977.
99. Neuman TS, Bove AA. Combined arterial gas embolism and decompression sickness following no-stop dives. Undersea Biomed Res 1990; 17:429–436.
100. Pearson RR. Clinical aspects of cerebral arterial gas embolism and decompression sickness with cerebral involvement. In: Francis TJR, Smith DJ, eds. Describing Decompression Illness. Bethesda, MD: Undersea and Hyperbaric Medical Society, 1991:55–60.
101. Kunkle TD, Beckman EC. Atraumatic air embolism in diving. Undersea Biomed Res 1981; 8:11–12.
102. Powell MR, Spencer MP, Smith MT. In situ arterial bubble formation and ''atraumatic air embolism.'' Undersea Biomed Res 1982; 9(suppl):10.
103. Furuya H, Okumura F. Detection of paradoxical air embolism by transesophageal echocardiography. Anesthesiology 1984; 60:374–377.
104. Vik A, Jenssen BM, Brubakk AO. Paradoxical air embolism in pigs with a patent foramen ovale. Undersea Biomed Res 1992; 19:361–374.

105. Jenssen BM, Vik A, Brubakk AO. Effects of treatment with Pluronic F-68 during continuous venous air embolism in swine. Undersea Hyperbaric Med 1993; 20: 17–26.
106. Yahagi M, Furuya H, Sai Y, Amkata Y. Effects of halothane, fentanyl and ketamine on the threshold for transpulmonary passage of venous air emboli in dogs. Anesth Analg 1992; 75:720–723.
107. Vik A, Jenssen BM, Brubakk AO. Comparison of haemodynamic effects during venous air infusion and after decompression in pigs. Eur J Appl Physiol 1994; 68:127–133.
108. Powell MR, Spencer MP, von Ramm O. Ultrasonic surveillance of decompression. In Bennett PB, Elliott DH, eds. The Physiology and Medicine of Diving, 3d ed. London: Baillière Tindall, 1982:404–434.
109. Ring GC, Blum AS, Kurbatov T, et al. Size of microspheres passing through pulmonary circuit in the dog. Am J Physiol 1961; 200:1191–1196.
110. Niden AH, Aviado DM. Effects of pulmonary embolism on the pulmonary circulation with special reference to arteriovenous shunts in the lungs. Circ Res 1956; 4:67–73.
111. Prinzmetal M, Ornitz EM, Simkin B, Bergman HC. Arterio-venous anastomoses in liver, spleen, and lungs. Am J Physiol 1948; 152:48–52.
112. Tobin CE, Zariquiey MO. Arteriovenous shunts in the human lung. Proc Soc Exp Biol Med 1950; 75:827–829.
113. Cheney FW, Pavlin J, Ferens J, Allen D. Effect of pulmonary microembolism on arteriovenous shunt flow. J Thorac Cardiovasc Surg 1978; 76:473–478.
114. Gordon DB, Flasher J, Drury DR. Size of the largest arterio-venous vessels in various organs. Am J Physiol 1953; 173:275–281.
115. Adam NK. The Physics and Chemistry of Surfaces, 2d ed. Oxford, England: Claredon Press, 1938.
116. Perry JC, Munson ES, Malgot MH, Shah DO. Venous air embolism prophylaxis with a surface active agent. Anesth Analg 1975; 54:792–799.
117. Walder DN. Serum surface tension and its relation to the decompression sickness of avaitors. J Physiol Lond 1948; 107:43–44.
118. Nunn JF. Controlled respiration in neurosurgical anesthesia. Anesthesia 1959; 14: 414–415.
119. Munson ES, Merrick HC. Effect of nitrous oxide on venous air embolism. Anesthesiology 1966; 27:783–787.
120. Presson RG, Kirk KR, Haselby KA, Wagner WW. Effect of ventilation with soluble and diffusible gases on the size of air emboli. J Appl Physiol 1991; 70:1068–1074.
121. Losasso TJ, Muzzi DA, Dietz NM, Cucchiara RF. Fifty percent nitrous oxide does not increase the risk of venous air embolism in neurosurgical patients operated upon the sitting position. Anesthesiology 1992; 77:21–30.
122. Drummond JC. Of venous air embolism, aminophylline, and volatile agents (letter). Anesthesiology 1984; 60:389.
123. Glenski JA, Cucchiara RF. Transcutaneous O_2 and CO_2 monitoring of neurosurgical patients: Detection of air embolism. Anesthesiology 1986; 64:546–550.
124. Hagen PT, Scholz DG, Edwards WD. Incidence and size of patent foramen ovale

during the first 10 decades of life: An autopsy study of 965 normal hearts. Mayo Clin Proc 1984; 59:17–20.

125. Guggiari M, Lechat Ph, Garen-Colonne C, et al. Early detection of patent foramen ovale by two-dimensional contrast echocardiography for prevention of paradoxical air embolism during sitting position. Anesth Analg 1988; 67:192–194.

126. Lynch JJ, Schuchard GH, Gross CM, Wann LS. Prevalence of right-to-left atrial shunting in a healthy population: Detection by Valsalva maneuver contrast echocardiography. Am J Cardiol 1984; 53:1478–1480.

127. Black S, Muzzi DA, Nishimura RA, Cucchiara RF. Preoperative and intraoperative echocardiography to detect right-to-left shunt in patients undergoing neurosurgical procedures in the sitting position. Anesthesiology 1990; 72:436–438.

128. Moon RE, Camporesi EM, Kisslo JA. Patent foramen ovale and decompression sickness in divers. Lancet 1989; 1:513–514.

129. Wilmshurst PT, Byrne JC, Webb-Peploe MM. Relation between interatrial shunts and decompression sickness in divers. Lancet 1989; 2:1302–1306.

130. Cross SJ, Evans SA, Thomson LF, et al. Safety of subaqua diving with a patent foramen ovale. Br Med J 1992; 304:481–482.

131. Wilmshurst PT, deBelder MA. Patent foramen ovale in adult life (editorial). Br Heart J 1994; 71:209–212.

132. Norfleet WT, Kumar VK, Butler BD. Patent foramen ovale and hypobaric decompression. Aviat Space Environ Med 1994; 65:273–275.

133. Butler BD, Robinson R, Sutton T, Kemper GB. Cardiovascular pressures with venous gas embolism and decompression. Aviat Space Environ Med 1995; 66: 408–414.

134. West J. Regional Differences in the Lung. New York: Academic Press, 1977.

135. Bouhuys A. The Physiology of Breathing. New York: Grune & Stratton, 1977.

136. Glazier JB, Hughes JMB, Maloney JE, West JB. Measurements of capillary dimensions and blood volume in rapidly frozen lungs. J Appl Physiol 1969; 26:65–76.

137. Knisely WH. Normal morphology and some defined pathologic conditions of fine vessels of mammalian alveoli. In: Winters W, Brest A, eds. Microcirculation. Springfield Ill: Charles C Thomas, 1969, chap. 13.

138. Macklem PT. Airway obstruction and collateral ventilation. Phys Rev 1971; 51: 368–436.

139. Khan MA, Alkalay I, Suetsugu S, Stein M. Acute changes in lung mechanics following pulmonary emboli of various gases in dogs. J Appl Physiol 1972; 33: 774–777.

140. Severinghaus JW, Swenson EW, Finley TN, et al. Unilateral hypoventilation produced in dogs by occluding one pulmonary artery. J Appl Physiol 1961; 16:53–60.

141. Levy SE, Simmons DH. Redistribution of alveolar ventilation following pulmonary thromboembolism in the dog. J Appl Physiol 1974; 36:60–68.

142. Caldini P. Pulmonary hemodynamics and arterial oxygen saturation in pulmonary embolism. J Appl Physiol 1965; 20:184–190.

143. Delcroix M, Mélot C, Vanderhoeft P, Naeje R. Embolus size affects gas exchange

in canine autologous blood clot pulmonary embolism. J Appl Phyiol 1993; 74: 1140–1148.
144. Young I, Mazzone RW, Wagner PD. Identification of functional lung unit in the dog by graded vascular embolization. J Appl Physiol 1980; 49:132–141.
145. Flook V, Koteng S, Holmen IM, Brubakk AO. The effect of decompression on pulmonary dead spaces. In: Cimsit M, ed. Proc EUBS 94 Diving and Hyperbaric Medicine. Istanbul: European Undersea Biomedical Society, 1994:271–276.
146. Severinghaus JW, Stupfel M. Alveolar dead space as an index of distribution of blood flow in pulmonary capillaries. J Appl Physiol 1957; 10:335–348.
147. de Burgh Daly M, Lambertsen CJ, Schweitzer A. The effects upon the bronchial musculature of altering the oxygen and carbon dioxide tension of the blood perfusing the brain. J Physiol 1953; 119:292–341.
148. Nadel JA, Colebatch HJH, Olsen CR. Location and mechanisms of airway constriction after barium sulphate microembolism. J Appl Physiol 1964; 19:387–396.
149. Finley TN, Tooley WH, Swenson EW, et al. Pulmonary surface tension in experimental atelectasis. Am Rev Respir Dis 1964; 89:372–378.
150. Çimsit M, Flook V. Pulmonary function in divers. In: Bachrach AJ, Matzen MM, eds. Underwater Physiology: VII. Bethesda, MD: Undersea Medical Society, 1981: 249–255.
151. Crosbie WA, Reed JW, Clarke MC. Functional characteristics of the large lungs found in commercial divers. J Appl Physiol 1979; 46–639–645.
152. Davey IS, Cotes JE, Reed JW. Relationship of ventilatory capacity to hyperbaric exposure in divers. J Appl Physiol 1984; 56:1655–1658.
153. Thorsen E, Segadal K, Kambestad B, Gulsvik A. Divers' lung function: Small airway disease? Br J Indust Med 1990; 47:519–523.
154. Hyacinthe R, Giry P, Brousolle B. Development of alterations in pulmonary diffusing capacity after a deep saturation dive with high oxygen level during decompression. In: Bachrach AJ, Matzen MM. eds. Underwater Physiology: VII. Bethesda, MD: Undersea Medical Society, 1991:75–83.
155. Cotes JE, Davey IS, Reed JW, Rooks M. Respiratory effects of a single saturation dive to 300 m. Br J Indust Med 1987; 44:76–82.
156. Suzuki S, Ikeda T, Hashimoto A. Decrease in the single-breath diffusing capacity after saturation dives. Undersea Biomed Res 1991; 18:103–109.
157. Thorsen E, Segadal K, Kambestad B. Characteristics of the response to exercise in professional saturation divers. Undersea Biomed Res 1991; 18:93–101.
158. Thorsen E, Segedal K, Myrseth E, et al. Pulmonary mechanical function and diffusion capacity after deep saturation dives. Br J Indust Med 1990; 47:242–247.
159. Puy RJM, Hyde RW, Fisher AB, et al. Alterations in the pulmonary capillary bed during early O_2 toxicity in man. J Appl Physiol 1968; 24:537–543.
160. Dujic Z, Eterovic D, Denoble P, et al. Effect of a single air dive on pulmonary diffusing capacity in professional divers. J Appl Physiol 1993; 74:55–61.
161. Lee WH, Hairston P. Structural effects on blood proteins at the gas-blood interface. Fed Proc Am Soc Exp Biol 1971; 30:1615–1622.
162. Lehto V-P, Kantola J, Tervo T, Laitinen LA. Ruthenium red staining of blood-bubble interface in acute decompression sickness in rat. Undersea Biomed Res 1981; 8:101–111.

163. Lehto V-P, Laitinen LA. Scanning and transmission electron microscopy of the blood-bubble interface in decompressed rats. Aviat Space Environ Med 1979; 50: 803–807.
164. Vroman L, Adams AL, Klings M. Interactions among human blood proteins at interfaces. Fed Proc 1971; 30:1494–1502.
165. Tamiya T, Yamasaki M, Maeo Y, et al. Complement activation in cardiopulmonary bypass, with special reference to anaphylatoxin production in membrane and bubble oxygenators. Ann Thorac Surg 1988; 46:47–57.
166. Ward CA, Koheil A, McCullough D, et al. Activation of complement at plasma-air or serum air interface of rabbits. J Appl Physiol 1986; 60:1651–1658.
167. Bergh K, Hjelde A, Iversen O-J, Brubakk AO. Variability over time of complement activation induced by air bubbles in human and rabbit sera. J Appl Physiol 1993; 74:1811–1815.
168. Hjelde A, Brubakk AO, Bergh K, Iversen O-J. Complement activation in divers following repeated air/heliox dives and its possible relevance to decompression sickness. J Appl Physiol 1995; 78:1140–1144.
169. Chenoweth DE, Cooper SW, Hugli TE, et al. Complement activation during cardiopulmonary bypass. N Eng J Med 1981; 304:497–503.
170. Chenoweth DE, Hugli TE. Demonstration of specific C5a receptor on intact human polymorponuclear leucocytes. Proc Natl Acad Sci USA 1978; 75:3943–3947.
171. Chenoweth DE, Hugli TE. Binding, internalization and degradation of human C5a by neutrophils (abstr). Fed Proc 1980; 39:1049.
172. Hetland G, Pfeifer PH, Hugli TE. Uptake of C5a by human polymorphonuclear leucocytes (PMN) *in vitro*: I: recovery of intact C5a from the cytosol. 11th Interdisiplinary World Congress on Antimicrobial and anticancer drugs (abstr). Genova, Italy: 1994:14.
173. Stevens DM, Gartner SL, Pearson RR. Complement activation during saturation diving. Undersea Hyperbaric Med 1993; 20:279–288.
174. Sellevold OT, Berg M, Rein KA. Heparin-coated circuit during cardiopulmonary bypass: A clinical study using closed circuit, centrifugal pump and reduced heparinization. Acta Anaesthesiol Scand 1994; 38:372–379.
175. Broome JR, Pearson RR, Dutka AJ. Failure to prevent decompression illness in rats by pretreatment with a soluble complement receptor. Undersea Hyperbaric Med 1994; 21:287–295.
176. Kilgore KS, Friedrichs GS, Homeister JW, Lucchesi BR. The complement system in myocardial ischemia/reperfusion injury. Cardiovasc Res 1994; 28:437–444.
177. Swerlick RA, Yancey KB, Lawry TJ. A direct in vivo comparison of the inflammatory properties of human C5a and C5a des arg in human skin. J Immunol 1988; 140:2376–2381.
178. Ward RA, Till GO, Kunkel R. Evidence for the role of hydroxyl radical in complement and neutrophil-dependent tissue injury. J Clin Invest 1983; 72:789–801.
179. Martin SE, Chenoweth DE, Engler RL, et al. C5a decreased regional coronary blood flow and myocardial function in pigs; implications for a granulocyte mechanism. Circ Res 1988; 63:483–491.
180. Craddock PR, Fehr J, Bribham KL, et al. Complement and leucocyte-mediated pulmonary dysfunction in hemodialysis. N Engl J Med 1977; 296:769–774.

181. Thorsen T, Brubakk A, Øvstedal T, et al. A method for production of N2 microbubbles in platelet-rich plasma in an aggregometer-like apparatus, and effect of platelet density in vitro. Undersea Biomed Res 1986; 13:271–288.
182. Thorsen T, Klausen H, Lie RT, Holmsen H. Bubble-induced, aggregation of platelets: Effects of gas species, proteins and decompression. Undersea Hyperbaric Med 1993; 20:101–120.
183. Thorsen T, Lie RT, Holmsen H. Induction of platelet aggregation in vitro by microbubbles of nitrogen. Undersea Biomed Res 1989; 16:453–464.
184. Opstad PK, Aakvaag A, Rognum TO. Altered hormonal response to short-term bicycle exercise in young men after prolonged physical strain, caloric deficit, and sleep deprivation. Eur J Appl Physiol 1980; 45:51–62.
185. McCandless BK, Kaplan JE, Cooper JA, Malik AB. Determinants of platelet kinetics: Effects of pulmonary microembolism. J Appl Physiol 1988; 65:1716–1722.
186. Garcia-Szabo RR, Minnear FL, Bizios R, et al. Role of thromboxane in the pulmonary response to pulmonary microembolism. Chest 1983; 83:768–788.
187. Østensen J, Hede R, Myreng Y, et al. Intravencus injection of Albunex microspheres causes thromboxane mediated pulmonary hypertension in pigs, but not in monkeys and rabbits. Acta Physiol Scand 1992; 144:307–315.
188. Philp RB, Freeman D, Francey I, Ackles KN. Changes in platelet function and other blood parameters following a shallow open-sea saturation dive. Aerosp Med 1974; 45:72–76.
189. Bernard EEP, Weathersby PK. Blood cell changes in asymptomatic divers. Undersea Biomed Res 1981; 8:187–198.
190. Smith KH, Stegall PJ, Harker LA, et al. Investigation of Hematologic and Pathologic Response to Decompression. Final report, Project #N00014-71-C-0273. Seattle: Virginia Mason Research Center, 1978.
191. Tanoue K, Mano Y, Kurroiwa K, et al. Consumption of platelets in decompression sickness of rabbits. J Appl Physiol 1987; 62:1772–1779.
192. Philp RB, Inwood MJ, Warren BA. Interaction between gas bubbles and components of the blood: Implications in decompression sickness. Aerospace Med 1972; 43:946–953.
193. Shinomiya N, Suzuki S, Hashimoto A, Oiwa H. Effects of deep saturation diving on the lymphocyte subsets of healthy divers. Undersea Hyperbar Med 1994; 21: 277–286.
194. Benestad HB, Hersleth IB, Hardersen H, Molvær OI. Functional capacity of neutrophil granulocytes in deep-sea divers. Scand J Clin Lab Invest 1990; 50:9–18.
195. Moosavi H, Utell MJ, Hyde RW, et al. Lung ultrastructure in noncardiogenic pulmonary edema induced by air embolization in dogs. Lab Invest 1981; 45:456–464.
196. Staub NC, Schultz EL, Albertine KH. Leucocytes and pulmonary microvascular injury. Ann NY Acad Sci 1982; 384:332–343.
197. Flick MR, Perel A, Staub NC. Leucocytes are required for increased lung microvascular permeability after microembolization in sheep. Circ Res 1981; 48:344–351.
198. Binder AS, Kageler W, Perel A, et al. Effct of platelet depletion on lung vascular permeability after microemboli in sheep. J Appl Physiol 1980; 48:414–420.

199. Binder AS, Nakahara K, Ohkuda K, et al. Effect of heparin and fibrinogen depletion on lung vascular permeability after emboli. J Appl Physiol 1979; 47:213–219.
200. Wang D, Li M-H, Hsu K, et al. Air embolism-induced lung injury in isolated rat lungs. J Appl Physiol 1992; 72:1235–1242.
201. Gardinali M, Cicardi M, Agostoni A, Hugli TE. Complement activation in extracorporeal circulation: Physiological and pathophysiological implications. Pathol Immunpathol Res 1986; 5:352–370.
202. Habbal MH, Carter H, Smith LJ, et al. Neutrophil activation in paediatric extracorporeal circuits: Effect of circulation and temperature variation. Cardiovasc Res 1995; 29:102–107.
203. Detmers PA, Lo SK, Olsen-Egbert E, et al. Neutrophil activating protein interleucin 8 stimulates the binding activity of the leucocyte adhesion receptor CD11b/CD18 on human neutrophils. J Exp Med 1990; 171:1155–1162.
204. Jacobson JM, Michael JR, Meyers RA, et al. Hyperbaric oxygen toxicity: Role of thromboxane. J Appl Physiol 1992; 72:416–422.
205. Staub NC. Pulmonary intravascular macrophages. Annu Rev Physiol 1994; 56:47–67.
206. Fracica PJ, Bertram T, Knapp M, Crapo JD. Pulmonary intravascular macrophages in normal and oxygen injured baboon lung tissue. Clin Res 1988; 36:A591.
207. Miyamoto K, Schultz E, Heath T, et al. Pulmonary intravascular macrophages and hemodynamic effects of liposomes in sheep. J Appl Physiol 1988; 64:143–152.
208. Downey GP, Doherty DE, Schwab B III, et al. Retention of leucocytes in capillaries: Role of cell size and deformability. J Appl Physiol 1990; 69:1767–1778.
209. Schmidt-Schonbein GW, Shih YY, Chien S. Morphometry of human leucocytes. Blood 1985; 56:866–876.
210. Guntheroth WG, Lachter DL, Kawabori I. Pulmonary microcirculation: Tubules rather than sheet and post. J Appl Physiol 1982; 53:510–515.
211. Sibille Y, Reynolds HY. Macrophages and polymorphonuclear neutrophils in lung defence and injury. Am Rev Respir Dis 1990; 141:471–501.
212. Levin LL, Stewart GJ, Lynch PR, Bove AA. Blood and blood vessel wall changes induced by decompression sickness in dogs. J Appl Physiol 1981; 50:944–949.
213. Stewart GJ, Ritchi WGM, Lynch PR. Venous endothelial damage caused by massive sticking and emigration of leukocytes. Am J Pathol 1974; 74:507–532.
214. Chrysanteou C, Springer M, Lipschitz S. Blood-brain and blood-lung barrier alterations by dysbaric exposure. Undersea Biomed Res 1977; 4:111–116.
215. Sacks T, Moldow CF, Craddock PR, et al. Oxygen radicals mediate endothelial cell damage by complement-stimulated granulocytes: An in vitro model of immune vascular damage. J Clin Invest 1978; 61:1161–1167.
216. Chryssanthou C, Kalberer J Jr, Kooperstein S, Antopol W. Studies on dysbarism: II. Influence of bradykinin and ''bradykinin antagonists'' on decompression sickness in mice. Aerospace Med 1964; 35:741–746.
217. Chryssanthou C, Theichner F, Goldstein G, et al. Studies on dysbarism: III. A smooth muscle-acting factor (SMAF) in mouse lungs and its increase in decompression sickness. Aerospace Med 1970; 41:43–48.

218. Fishman AP, Pietra GG. Permeability of pulmonary vascular endothelium. In: Lung Liquids. Ciba Foundation Symposium 1976; 38:29–28.
219. Schneeberger EE. Ultrastructural basis for alveolar-capillary permeability to protein. In: Lung Liquids. Ciba Foundation Symposium 1976; 38:3–21.
220. Senn N. An experimental and clinical study of air-embolism. Ann Surg 1885; 2: 198–214.
221. Lee BP, Lin YC, Chiang ST. Right ventricular pressure and ventilatory response to pulmonary gas embolism. Chinese J Physiol 1990; 33:145–160.
222. Marshall BM. Air embolus in neurosurgical anaesthesia: Its diagnosis and treatment. Can Anaesth Soc J 1965: 12:255–261.
223. Shivpuri DN, Viswanathan R, Sharma. Pre-symptomatic diagnostic sign of venous air embolism. J Indian Med Assoc 1959; 33:86–90.
224. Mischenfelder JD, Terry HR, Daw EF, Miller RH. Air embolism during neurosurgery. Anaesth Analg 1966; 45:390–395.
225. Angelsen BAJ. A theoretical study of the scattering of ultrasound from blood. IEEE Trans Biomed Eng 1980; 27:61–67.
226. Sawatzky KD, Nishi RY. Assessment of inter-rate agreement on the grading of intravascular bubble signals. Undersea Biomed Res 1991; 18:373–396.
227. Hatle L. Non-invasive methods of measuring pulmonary artery pressure and flow velocity. In: Chazov EJ, Sminov VN, Oganov RG, eds. Cardiology: An International Perspective. New York: Plenum Press, 1984:783–790.
228. Nishi RY, Livingstone SD. Intravascular changes associated with hyperbaric decompression: Theoretical considerations using ultrasound. Aerospace Med 1973; 44:179–183.
229. Koishi K, Sha M, Ohtaguro T, et al. Power spectrum of experimental gas embolism in dogs and a new device for its detection. Masui 1993; 42:1541–1547.
230. Furness A. Microbubble detection during extracorporeal circulation for open heart surgery. Ph.D. Thesis, University of Keele, 1977.
231. Clarke RE, Dietz DR, Miller JG. Continuous detection of microemboli during cardipulmonary bypass in animal and man. Circulation 1976; 54(suppl III):74–78.
232. Kisman K. Spectral analysis of Doppler ultrasonic data. Ultrasonics 1977; 15:105–110.
233. Belcher E. Quantification of bubbles formed in animals and man during decompression. IEEE Trans Biomed Eng 1980; 27:330–338.
234. Powell MR, Spencer WP. The pathophysiology of decompression sickness and the effects of Doppler detectable bubbles. Technical Report N00014-73-C-0094. Seattle: Institute of Applied Physiology and Medicine, 1980.
235. Brubakk AO. Ultrasonic methods for detection of gas bubbles. In: Brubakk AO, Hemmingsen BB, Sundnes G, eds. Supersaturation and Bubble Formation in Fluids and Organisms. Trondheim, Norway: Tapir Publishers, 1989:353–385.
236. Ikeda T, Suzuki S, Shimizu K, et al. M-mode ultrasonic detection of microbubbles following saturation diving: A case report and proposal for a new grading system. Aviat Space Environ Med 1989; 60:166–169.
237. Eftedal O, Brubakk AO. Detecting intravascular gas bubbles in ultrasonic images. Med Biol Eng Comput 1993; 31:627–633.

238. Lubbers J, van den Berg JW. An ultrasonic detector for microgas emboli in a blood flow line. Ultrasound Med Biol 1976; 2:301–310.
239. Nishi RY. Ultrasonic detection of bubbles with Doppler flow transducers. Ultrasonics 1972; 10:173–179.
240. Nishi RY. The scattering and absorption of sound waves by a gas bubble in a viscous liquid. Acoustica 1975; 33:65–74.
241. Brubakk AO, Torp H, Belcher E, Grip A. A possible method for estimating gas bubble size in the circulation. Undersea Biomed Res 1982; 9(suppl):9.
242. Brubakk AO, Torp H. Ultrasonic methods for monitoring decompression. In Nashimoto I, Lanphier EH, eds. Decompression in Surfaced-Based Diving. Bethesda, MD: Undersea and Hyperbaric Medical Society, 1987:107–114.
243. Hills BA, Grulke DC. Evaluation of ultrasonic bubble detectors in vitro using carefully calibrated microbubbles of selected velocities. Ultrasonics 1975; 13:181–184.
244. Meltzer RS, Tickner EG, Sahines TP, Popp RL. The source of ultrasonic contrast. J Cardiovasc Ultrasonogr 1980; 8:121.
245. Sigel B, Machi J, Beitler JC, et al. Variable ultrasound echogenicity in flowing blood. Science 1982; 218:1321–1323.
246. Arora RA, Teichholz LE, Meltzer RS. Spontaneous echocardiographic contrast in the inferior vena cava. J Cardiovasc Ultrasonogr 1984; 3:27–28.
247. Daniel WG, Nellessen U, Schroeder E, et al. Left atrial spontaneous echo contrast in mitral valve disease: An indicator for an increased thromboembolic risk. J Am Coll Cardiol 1988; 11:1204–1211.
248. Chang J-L, Albin MS, Bunegin L, Hung T-K. Analysis and comparison of venous air embolism detection methods. Neurosurgery 1980; 7:135–141.
249. Russel GB, Richard RB, Snider MT. Detection of venous air embolism in dogs by emission spectrometry. J Clin Monit 1990; 6:18–23.
250. Glenski JA, Cucchiara RF. transcutaneous O_2 and CO_2 monitoring of neurosurgical patients: Detection of air embolism. Anesthesiology 1986; 64:546–550.
251. Sloan TB, Kimovec MA. Detection of venous air embolism by airway pressure monitoring. Anesthesiology 1986; 64:645–647.

8

Pulmonary Barotrauma

T. JAMES R. FRANCIS

Naval Submarine Medical Research Laboratory
Groton, Connecticut

DAVID M. DENISON

Royal Brompton Hospital
and National Heart and Lung Institute
London, England

I. Introduction

Experiences in space travel, mountaineering, caisson work, and saturation diving show that people can be exposed to pressures ranging from 0.2 to 70 bar without serious harm to their lungs. However if they are exposed to *changes* in pressure as slight as 0.05 bar that are abrupt or unevenly applied, the lungs may rupture, with serious and sometimes fatal consequences.

This chapter concerns those accidents, assumed to be due to lung rupture, associated with diving. To make sense of these, it is necessary to review some anatomy, physics, and physiology and also to discuss similar phenomena that occur in clinical and aviation medicine or have been seen in experiments on other mammals.

Appended to the chapter are records of 16 cases of pulmonary barotrauma (PBT), drawn from some 250 we have seen that illustrate some of the discussion points and highlight the difficulties of establishing accurate histories and firm diagnoses relating to people who have suffered accidents under water. In some, barotrauma has become obvious only many hours after the last dive, when the diver's precise memories of critical details have faded. In others, events have been so dramatic and rapid that patients have been unable to recall whether they held their breath during ascent or not.

The only effective treatments for major lung barotrauma are the insertion of a chest drain to relieve a tension pneumothorax, the administration of fluids and oxygen, and recompression to ameliorate the neurological and other consequences of the condition. But facilities for such treatment are frequently distant from the dive site. It is therefore self-evident that, where possible, effective prevention is more important than delayed attempts at cure.

A. Some Relevant Anatomy

The anatomy of the lungs, pleural spaces, and mediastinum has been reviewed recently by a number of authors (1–4). Structural features relevant to lung rupture are as follows.

The bronchoalveolar tree consists of a branching system of tubes that divide more or less dichotomously over some 23 generations, terminating in grape-like clusters of alveoli that are about 0.3 mm in diameter. The tree is reinforced by a dense system of elastin and collagen fibers that originate in the larynx and travel through the walls of each branch, spreading over every alveolus and eventually burying themselves in the visceral pleura. The alveolar walls are covered by capillaries some 5 μm in diameter. The capillaries occupy about 95% of the wall surface and their contents can be regarded as a sheet of moving blood. Multiple studs or pillars of connective tissue, which spot-weld the walls of adjacent alveoli together, form the other 5%. The alveolar epithelium is less than 0.5 μm thick.

The pulmonary arterial tree lies directly alongside the bronchial tree, sharing a common capsule. The pulmonary venous tree lies between but separated from the arteriobronchial bundles. As the trees approach the hilum, the veins and airways come closer together. The central bulk of the lungs is vented by a centripetal tree of lymphatics that empty into the thoracic duct. The subpleural shells of the lungs are drained by a network of short centrifugal lymphatics that go into the subpleural interstitium. Most alveoli abut on each other, but some lie directly alongside the bronchoarterial bundles that penetrate the lung (Fig. 1). These "marginal" alveoli may be critical in some forms of lung rupture (5).

Mechanically, the airway can be thought of in three parts (Fig. 2):

1. The upper or *extrathoracic airway* that is not exposed to pleural pressure.
2. The next few generations of the bronchial tree, which are exposed to pleural pressure but are not attached to adjacent alveoli, form the *intrathoracic but extrapulmonary* airways.
3. The remaining many generations of bronchioles are intimately glued to surrounding alveoli and form the *intrapulmonary* airways.

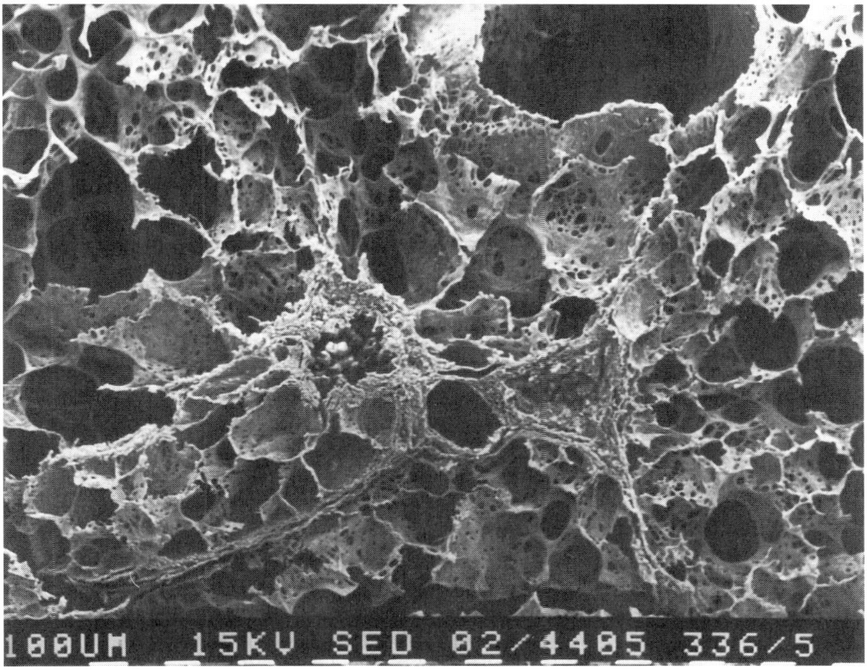

Figure 1 A scanning electron micrograph of an almost normal human lung. The horizontal scaling bars at the bottom of the scan are 100 μm long. The upper right part of the scan shows a respiratory bronchiole and the "marginal" alveoli that are immediately adjacent to it. All of the alveoli show minute fenestrae that probably represent the earliest stages of emphysema induced by smoking. (*Photograph kindly provided by Dr. Peter Jeffery, National Heart and Lung Institute, London, England.*)

The visceral pleura consists of single layer of mesothelial cells, about 1 μm thick, lying on a subpleural interstitium that is a few times thicker. It contains many circumferential elastin and collagen fibers, but the collagen/elastin ratio is much higher than in the lung (6). The visceral pleura is thinner at the lung's apex than at its base, and it merges into the parietal pleura at the hilum. It is fed by the bronchial arterial tree, but its blood drains via bronchial veins into the pulmonary venous tree. The underlying lymphatics do not penetrate the mesothelium and have no continuity with the pleural space. The healthy pleural cavity used to be thought of as a potential rather than actual space, but recent electron microscopic studies have shown it to be a continuous liquid film about 1 μm thick with a volume of a few milliliters (7).

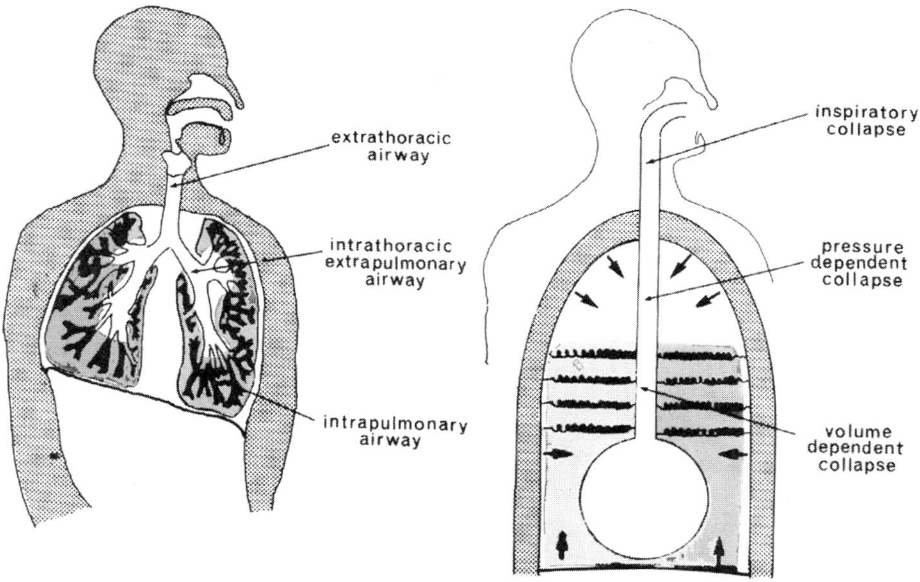

Figure 2 Sites of collapsible airflow limitation in the airways of a normal man. The extrathoracic airways collapse on inspiration, the intrathoracic extrapulmonary airways tend to collapse immediately on expiration (pressure-dependent collapse), and the intrapulmonary airways collapse progressively on expiration as the volume of the lung diminishes (volume-dependent collapse).

The parietal pleura is reflected from the hila to pass over the anterolateral surfaces of the mediastinum onto the inner surfaces of the chest wall and the upper surface of the diaphragm. In front of and above the heart the parietal pleurae of the two lungs meet and normally ensure that the right and left pleural spaces are separate. The parietal pleurae are fed and drained by the intercostal vessels and associated lymphatics. Some lymphatic vessels penetrate the mesothelium and are linked via stomata to the pleural space. In the past, it was considered that the parietal pleura was thinner at the thoracic apices than more caudally, but recent work suggests that its thickness does not vary with site.

The mediastinum—i.e., that volume lying between the medial aspects of the two parietal pleurae—is bounded by the thoracic inlet above, the spine and paravertebral gutters behind, the sternum in front, and the diaphragm below. It contains the heart and great vessels, the esophagus, vagi, phrenic and recurrent laryngeal nerves, ascending and descending lymphatics and sympathetic nerves. It includes various fascial planes that are very flimsy at birth but thicken somewhat with age. These are continuous with the tissue planes surrounding the trachea, larynx, esophagus, oropharynx, carotid and jugular vessels in the neck, the subclavian vessels and subcutaneous tissues of the chest wall and arms, the descending aorta and retroperitoneal space in the abdomen, and the broncho-vascular bundles extending from the hila deep into the lungs (8).

B. Some Relevant Physics

Physical factors involved in lung rupture vary from case to case, but the following influence many.

The pressure acting on us in air at sea level varies slightly with the weather but is very close to 1 bar. Ascending in air, the barometric pressure decreases exponentially, halving with every 18,000 ft of altitude (Fig. 3, Table 1). In air, the variation in ambient pressure from the uppermost to the lowermost parts of the body are trivial and ignored. Changes in pressure at one point in the open atmosphere dissipate through the system on an expanding spherical front at the speed of sound in air (335 $m.s^{-1}$ at sea level). That speed varies with the density of the gas and is slower at altitude than on the ground. Usual variations in

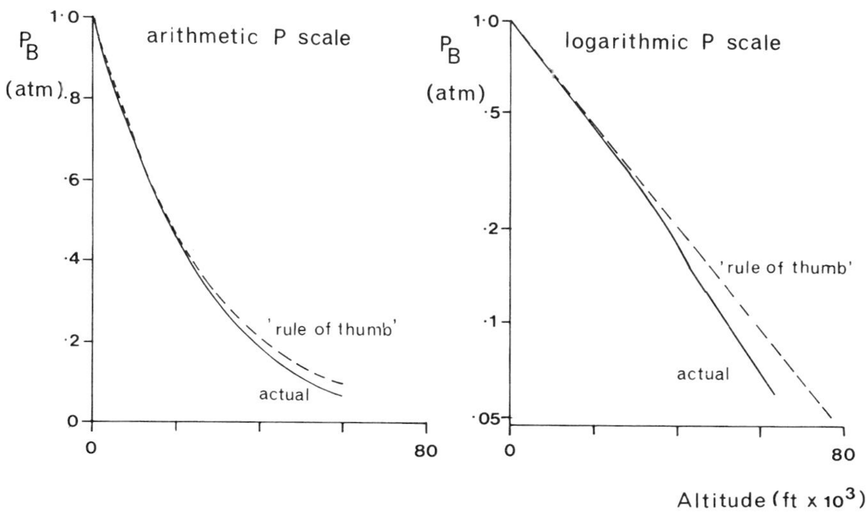

Figure 3 Arithmetic and logarithmic graphs of altitude in thousands of feet on the abscissa, against barometric pressure (in ata) on the ordinate. The rule-of-thumb curve in each graph is the pressure predicted by a strictly exponential decay, halving every 18,000 ft. The actual curves are those agreed for the Standard Atmosphere for aviation purposes, by the International Civil Aviation Organisation (ICAO) in 1964.

Table 1 Barometric Pressures[a]

Altitude (ft)	Pressure (mmHg)	Altitude (ft)	Pressure (mmHg)
0	760	20,000	349
2,000	707	25,000	282
4,000	656	30,000	226
6,000	609	40,000	141
8,000	564	50,000	87
10,000	523	60,000	54
15,000	429	70,000	37

[a]The barometric pressures agreed to exist at the given altitudes for the Standard Atmosphere of the International Civil Aviation Organisation (ICAO) in 1964.

barometric pressure due to weather disturbances are gradual and slight, on the order of 0.07 bar (i.e., +50 mmHg) at most, but are associated with changes in the incidence of pneumothoraces (9,10) and can provoke a spontaneous pneumomediastinum (Case 1). Some of these may be related to the raised incidence of allergen-induced asthma that precedes thunderstorms (11,12). Very abrupt changes in pressure (explosions), create waves of compression and rarefaction that pass through the body in a complex manner and can damage the lung extensively. In air, the pressure-time characteristic of the shock wave travels with the speed of sound in air (335 $m.s^{-1}$) and decays exponentially and quickly as it moves away from the detonation. As a result, even big explosions exert fatal effects only over short distances, but ensuing wind blasts can throw people about quite violently, with damaging effects (13).

Under water, shock waves are propagated more efficiently, over longer distances, at the faster speed of sound in water [1485 $m.s^{-1}$ (14)]. Peak pressures of 500 psi or more cause fatal lung injury, usually from rupture of pulmonary vessels. Although there is extensive tearing of alveolar walls and bleeding into the lung, pneumothoraces, pneumomediastinums, and surgical emphysema are rare, even in those survivors who continue to breathe spontaneously for long periods (13). Oddly, the same is true for blunt nonpenetrating injuries of the chest, unless ribs are fractured. [See Cases 2 and 3 and Stevens and Templeton (15)].

Descending in water, ambient pressure increases linearly with depth by 1 bar for each 10 m of descent. Thus, at a depth of 30 m, ambient pressures is 4 bar. Usual descent rates in diving are about 10 to 20 m/min, but in the compression phase of submarine escape, ambient pressure change accelerates exponentially, the pressure doubling every 4 sec. Preparing for an escape from

180 m, the submariner will have been compressed from 1 to 19 bar in about 20 sec (Fig. 4). Usual ascent rates in conventional diving are about 10 m/min. In submarine escape, they are about 3 m/sec, about twenty times normal.

Any object that includes gas in a compliant container will show vertical instability under water. There will be some depth at which it is neutrally buoyant. As it descends below that depth, it becomes heavier and heavier, accelerating to the bottom. As the object ascends above the depth of neutral buoyancy and the gas expands, the object becomes lighter and lighter, accelerating to the surface. Uncontrolled ascents of this sort frequently cause PBT, as in Cases 4 and 5.

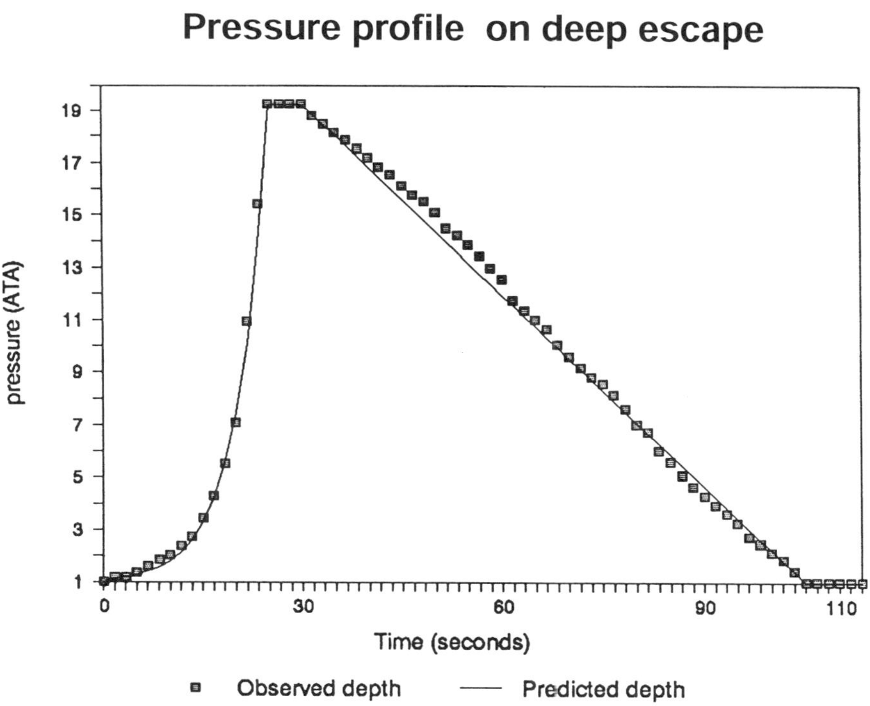

Figure 4 The pressure-time profile experienced by Royal Navy submariner H. A. Jones, escaping from a submarine submerged at a tower depth of 186 m, during the Royal Navy Deep Escape Exercise held off the coast of Norway in 1987. Note in his case that pressure is doubling every 5 sec, there is a 4-sec pause at escape depth while the tower hatch opens and he wriggles free, and a 52-sec linear ascent through the 186 m to the surface.

When there is a change in the pressure surrounding a vessel that communicates with the outside, it takes time for the vessel to regain pressure equilibrium with the surrounding fluid. During that time, the vessel is exposed to transmural pressures that may cause it to collapse or burst. In the case of a liquid-filled container of capacitance C emptying through a resistance R, the fluid level changes exponentially with a time constant proportional to the product CR (Fig. 5a). In a gas-filled vessel of volume V filling or emptying through an effective orifice of area A, the time course is complicated by changes in gas temperature and water-vapor content and is more nearly linear and proportional to V/cA, where c is the speed of sound in the gas at its pressure at any instant [see Fig. 5b and Haber and Clamman (16)].

In water, the variations in ambient pressure between the uppermost and lowermost parts of a submerged, water-filled sac, such as a lungless human body, are considerable but balanced by almost equal hydrostatic gradients within (17). In a gas-filled sac, such as the thorax, submerged to the same depth, the unitary gas pressure within is determined by the net force pressing on the asymmetrically shaped vessel from without. It is that pressure which would exist at the sac's centroid of pressure were it to be filled with water continuous with the water outside. Many experiments have shown that, for a typical adult male thorax, this point lies in the midsagittal plane some 19 cm below and some 7 cm behind the sternal notch (i.e., somewhere in the middle of the right atrium) (18) (Fig. 5c). Gas delivered to the lung at this pressure, when the chest wall is relaxed, will inflate it to its normal functional residual capacity. This eupneic pressure (''the pressure of good breathing'') is that at which the work of breathing under water is minimized.

Figure 6a shows an elastic, gas-filled balloon, modeling the lung, that empties through a floppy tube, modeling the airways when they are compressed by the syringe or thorax. When the plunger is advanced, the pressure immediately outside the balloon and tube rises. The pressure within the balloon is augmented by the elastic recoil pressure of the balloon at its volume at any instant. The pressure along the tube falls from the sum of $P_{syringe}$ and P_{recoil} at one end to $P_{ambient}$ at the other. It follows that at some point along the tube, the internal pressure will equal $P_{syringe}$. Proximal to that *equal pressure point*, the floppy tube will be inflated; distal to that point, it will be collapsed. In this system, the time constant of emptying lengthens the emptier the balloon becomes. The system is behaving as a Starling resistor.

If a balloon is inflated inside a variably compliant container, it will expand to follow the new shape of the enlarged container but burst if any part of the container wall is more compliant than the underlying part of the balloon.

Laplace's law ($P=2T/r$) relates the tension (T) in a vessel wall to the wall's radius of curvature (r) and pressure in the vessel's interior (P) (Fig. 6b). In principle, it determines the positive or negative pressures the chest wall can

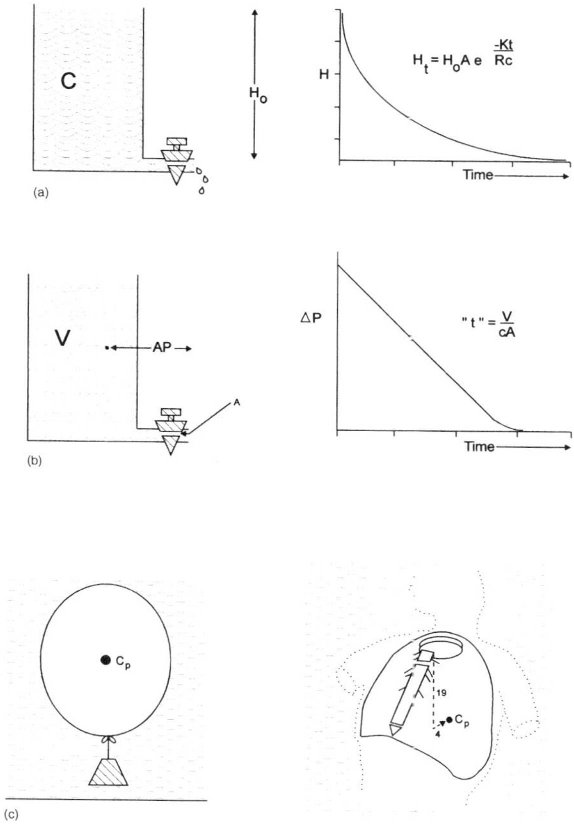

Figure 5 (a) The emptying under laminar-flow conditions of a vessel filled with liquid. The decay in the height (H) and therefore the pressure of liquid is strictly exponential, as indicated by the graph and equation on the right, where A is the constant converting height to pressure, R is the resistance of the tap, and C is the capacitance of the container. (b) The emptying of a gas-filled container under sonic flow conditions, which is more linear, where V is the volume of the container, A is the cross-sectional area of the orifice, and c is the speed of sound at the appropriate gas density. (c) The left-hand side of this panel shows the net pressure exerted on a submerged and tethered balloon, which would exist at its centroid of pressure (C_p). The right-hand side shows the same concept applied to the submerged chest wall.

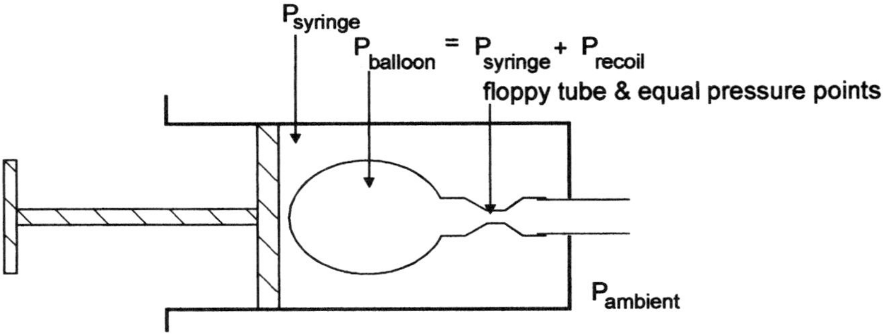

(a)

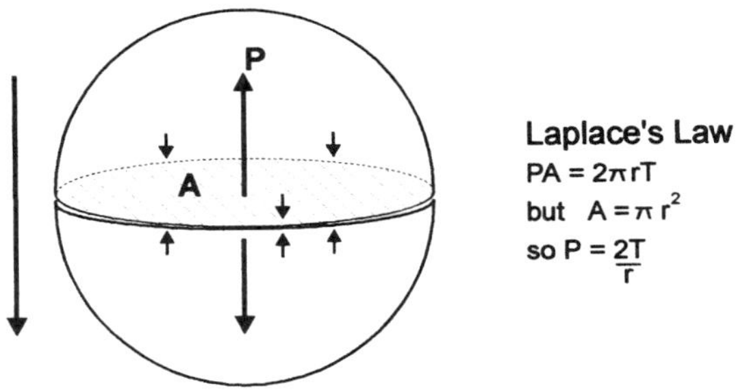

(b)

Figure 6 (a) A syringe containing a balloon emptying when compressed by the plunger, via a floppy tube, to the outside world. The tube collapses just beyond the equal pressure point, which becomes the flow-limiting segment. (b) A summary of Laplace's law relating the pressure (P) within a sphere of radius r to the tension per unit length (T) acting on its circumference. A = cross-sectional area of the sphere.

apply to the lung. It also determines the ease with which gas can escape from the lung into a moist but narrow cut surface and the ease with which gaseous emboli can travel down narrow fluid-filled tubes (19). It may underlie the frequency of pneumothoraces in the newborn (20) but does not explain at first sight why pneumothoraces should be some seven times more common in men than in women of the same age, whose thoracic cages are smaller but may be more compliant than those of men.

C. Some Relevant Physiology

If a hole is made in the chest wall, the underlying lung collapses and the chest wall springs outward, to its unrestrained resting position. Normally, surface tension holds the pleural surfaces of the lung and chest wall together, acting as the link between the two opposed springs, and the pair come to rest at an intermediate position at which the lung is roughly half full. The lung is then said to be at its functional residual capacity (FRC). The chest wall has to develop an inspiratory effort to make the lung bigger. On relaxing that effort, the system will return passively to FRC. To make the lung smaller, the thoracoabdominal wall has to produce an expiratory effort and, on releasing that drive, the system will return passively to FRC.

The graph in Fig. 7a shows the pressure-volume curve of the lung-chest wall combination, from the smallest lung volume that can be achieved voluntarily, (residual volume, or RV) to the greatest lung volume that normally can be reached (total lung capacity, or TLC). The curve is sigmoid, indicating that the system is most deformable (i.e., mechanically compliant) in the middle of its volume range. The chest wall becomes more rigid as it approaches RV and the lung stiffens markedly as it nears TLC.

The elastin fibers of the bronchoalveolar tree are the prime determinant of the system's compliance over most of its volume range, but the collagen

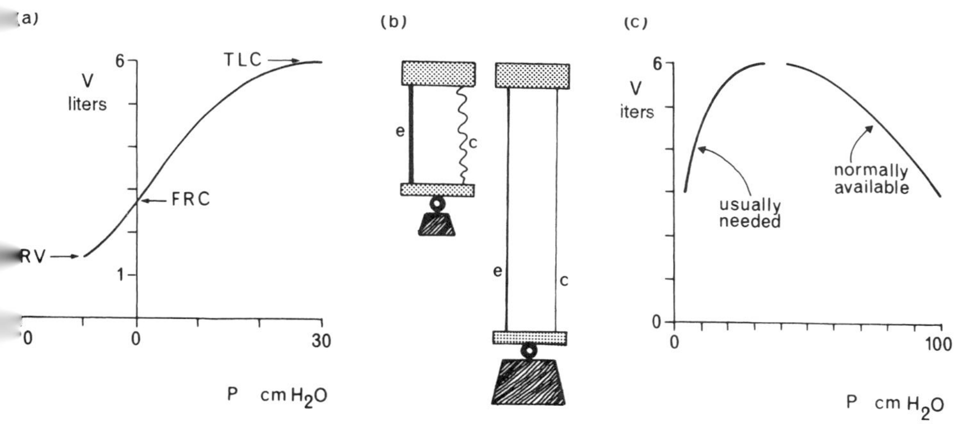

Figure 7 A summary of the factors influencing the pressure-volume characteristics of the lung in its upper volume register. (a) A plot of the inflation pressure (V) volume characteristic of the combined lung and chest wall of a normal adult male. (b) The relative contributions of elastin, e, and collagen, c, fibers. (c) Comparison of the upper part of the inflation pressure volume curve (usually needed), with the inspiratory pressures that the chest wall can develop (normally available) through the upper volume register.

fibers of the lung set the upper limit to its expansion, (21–23), as indicated by the diagram in Fig. 7b.

The graph in Fig. 7c shows two pressure-volume curves. The one labeled "usually needed" is simply that upper part of the curve on the left of the figure (a) which is most relevant to lung rupture. The other curve in Fig. 7c, labeled "normally available," shows the inspiratory transpulmonary pressures the chest wall is ordinarily capable of developing at given lung volumes. The two curves meet at TLC. Note that the lung itself can expand by a further 15% or so before it reaches its elastic limit. The healthy but unhindered human lung bursts at an inflation pressure of about 70 mmHg (see below).

As mentioned previously, the minimum gas volume of the lung that can be achieved by voluntary expiration is described as its residual volume. In children and adolescents it is set by the power of the expiratory muscles (mainly the abdominal wall), but if their chest walls are squeezed when they are at RV, more air can be heard to leave. In adults, RV is set by the collapsibility of the bronchial tree as bronchial closure precedes reaching the elastic limit of the chest wall. When their chests are squeezed at RV, no more air comes out, although some 1.5 L are still within.

At FRC, the fluid pressures in the pleural space average about -5 cmH_2O. The pressure in the film is lowest at the uppermost lung surface and greatest at its lowermost surface. The gradient of hydrostatic pressure in the film is usually between 0.3 and 0.5 cmH_2O per centimeter of descent. In essence, this is because the lung hangs from the uppermost parietal pleural surface and sometimes rests on the lowermost parietal pleural surface; that is to say, that the weight of the whole lung is concentrated at the apex of its upper surface (in any posture).

This is shown diagrammatically in Fig. 8A. The first drawing (a) shows an isotropic foam of alveoli and small airways filling a thoracic cage under weightless conditions, as in parabolic flight. Because there are no macroscopic gravitational forces of note acting on the foam, all its cells are the same size. The second drawing (b) shows the same foam exposed to normal gravity. Now the weight of the "lung" expands the upper cells, particularly where the stress is concentrated at the apex of the cage. The stress concentration that results is believed to favour the development of subpleural blebs of air that have escaped from alveoli which have fractured locally (24,25). The third drawing (c) introduces the exaggeration of this gradient by the weight of the heart and the abdominal viscera. The drawings in Fig. 8B illustrate the distribution of these effects, which depends on posture and also explains why the dependent blood vessels are more distended than those higher up, since the weight of contained fluid increases with descent down the lung.

The computed tomography (CT) scans in Fig. 8B, taken at full inspiration and again at full expiration, show that these gravitational variations are clearly visible in human lung and are more marked in expiration than inspiration. The upper lung is less dense because it has bigger alveoli and poorly distended blood

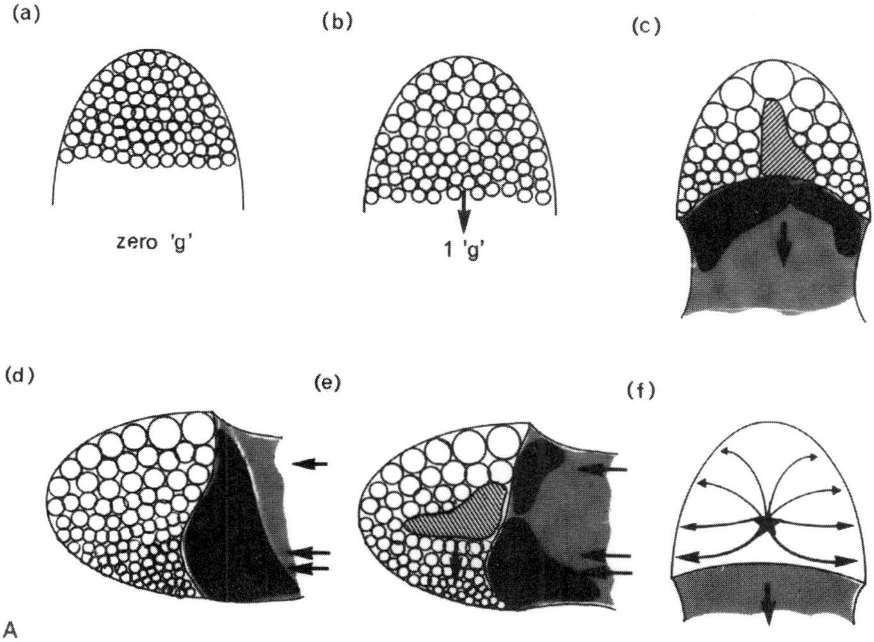

Figure 8A The effects of gravity upon the human lung. (a) A thoracic cage filled with an isotropic foam under zero gravity. All of the cells of the foam are the same size. (b) The same foam exposed to a gravitational force of 1 g. Now the uppermost alveoli and airways take the weight of the dependent parts of the lung and are larger than before. (c) This effect is exaggerated by introducing the weight of the heart and abdominal viscera, resting on and hanging from the diaphragm, respectively. (d and e) The situation in supine and lateral decubitus. (f) The distribution of microvascular size and blood flow in an upright lung.

vesels. The lower part of the lung is denser because it consists of smaller alveoli perfused by vessels that are better filled. On expiration, the effects become more obvious because the lung is more compliant and so more susceptible to gravity.

On inspiration, the expanding chest wall increases the negative pressure in the pleural film, expanding the intra- and extrapulmonary airways in the thorax, but the negative pressure conveyed to the gas in the airways is then transmitted to the extrathoracic airways, which tend to collapse. On expiration, the compressing chest wall raises the pleural pressure, causing the extrapulmonary, intrathoracic airways to collapse immediately (pressure-dependent collapse) and the intrapulmonary airways to collapse progressively as emptying proceeds (volume-dependent collapse), until, at RV, all routes to the mouth are closed somewhere along their length.

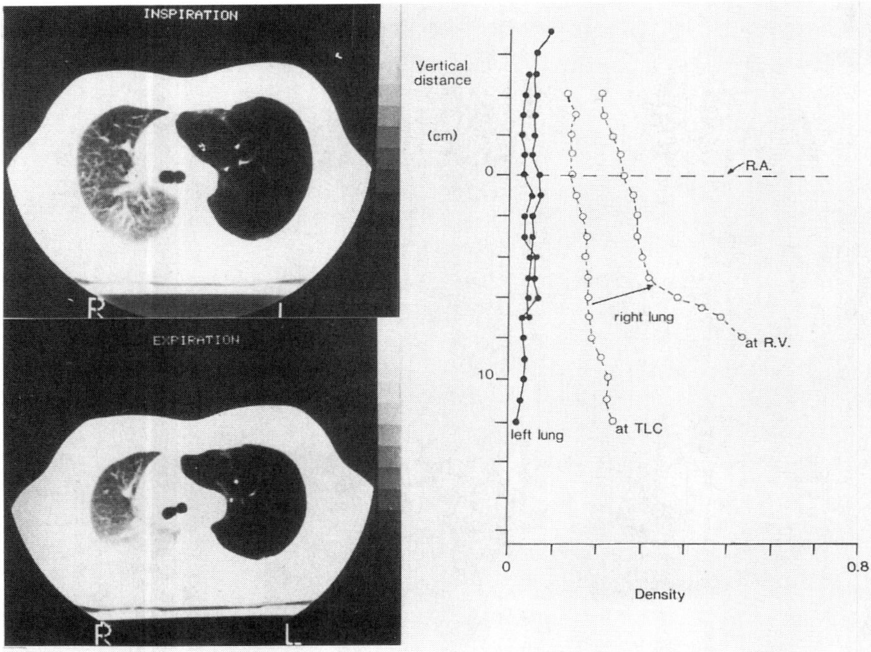

B

Figure 8B (B) The two CT scans show the actual density variations in the lungs of a patient with unilateral emphysema. The graph shows the variations in the normal (right) lung are much more marked in expiration (RV) than in inspiration (TLC).

These changes are responsible for the normal form of the maximal flow–volume loop of the healthy lung, shown in Fig. 9. The left-hand graph (a) displays simultaneous traces of esophageal pressure (the broken line) and respired flow (the continuous line) plotted against respired volume during a maximal flow volume–loop maneuver. Its axes are expiratory flow and positive esophageal pressure on the upper ordinate, inspiratory flow and negative esophageal pressure on the lower ordinate, and respired volume on the common abscissa.

The most leftward point of the loop represents the lung at TLC. The extreme right point of the loop represents the lung at RV. Subjects/patients are instructed to fill their lungs maximally "in their own time" and then to breathe out as fast and completely as they can and then to inspire to TLC as rapidly as possible.

At the start of the maximally forced expiration, when the lung is at TLC, esophageal pressure rises smartly to a fairly constant value that is sustained

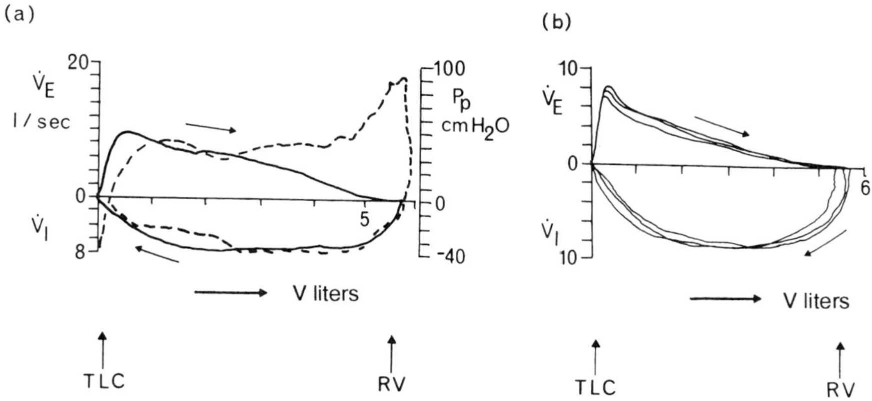

Figure 9 (a) Simultaneous recordings of respired flow, respired volume, and esophageal pressure (mean pleural pressure) during a maximal flow-volume loop maneuver in a healthy male subject. Note that expiratory flow falls continuously, although expiratory pressure is constant or rises as residual volume (RV) is approached. (b) The reproducibility of the maneuver in the same subject making three successive attempts at producing his maximal flow volume loop.

through expiration. However, expired flow falls continuously. This indicates that airway resistance is rising—i.e., airways are collapsing progressively. At the end of expiration, esophageal pressure rises somewhat even though expiratory flow has dropped to zero, implying that the bronchoalveolar tree is completely obstructed.

The form of the loop is highly reproducible within a normal subject and between normal subjects. At the start of the maneuver, expiratory flow rises rapidly to a maximum in about 0.2 sec, when about one-tenth of the vital capacity has been breathed out. Thereafter, expired flow decreases linearly with diminishing lung volume, to zero flow when RV is reached. On inspiration, the airways open rapidly and inspiratory flow follows a smooth and roughly semicircular return to the starting point of the curve, at TLC.

Typically, peak expiratory flows rise to two predicted FVC.sec^{-1}. After 1 sec, about 75% of the vital capacity has been exhaled. This volume, known as the forced expired volume in 1 sec, or FEV_1, is frequently compared with the FVC, and this FEV_1/FVC ratio is used as an index of airway obstruction in clinical practice. This is because, in ordinary expiration, the lung gets progressively smaller and, appropriately, the FEV_1/FVC ratio reflects the severity of the associated airway collapse.

However, in thinking of the liability to lung rupture during ascent in water, this measure is misleading. On sustained decompressions—e.g., continued ascents—expanding alveolar gas will hold the lung close to TLC, where airways are widely dilated, facilitating lung emptying. For this sort of emptying, peak expiratory flow (PEF) is a more relevant measure. The PEF indicates that the normal lung at TLC will vent a volume equal to one vital capacity in about 0.2 sec—i.e., the fully inflated respiratory system behaves as if it had an unimpeded time constant of emptying of no more than 0.3 sec. The experimental work of Haber and Clamann (16), referred to earlier, suggests that this figure will be almost independent of depth.

Vascular pressures in the pulmonary arterial tree average some 15 mmHg at the hilum of a resting lung and show a hydrostatic gradient of 1 cmH_2O per centimeter of descent. Venous pressures at the hila average 4 cmH_2O under the same resting conditions and show a hydrostatic gradient of 1 cmH_2O per centimeter of descent downward; above the hilum, however, positive alveolar pressures can compress pulmonary capillaries, temporarily breaking local venous returns.

Inspiration develops negative pressures in the alveoli and pleural spaces. These are transmitted to the heart and great vessels, drawing blood into the chest. Expiration raises the pressures in the alveoli and pleural spaces. These pressures compress the vessels, oppose the return of systemic venous blood, and expel blood from the thorax.

If the lung is forcibly inflated, events are different. Now the alveoli are expanding, but the vessels are being compressed. It is thought that this is one mechanism that may favor rupture of the walls of alveoli or small airways immediately adjacent to arterial bundles (5).

II. Pulmonary Barotrauma of Descent (Lung Squeeze)

During the descent phase of a breath-hold dive, the thoracic gas volume (TGV) will decrease in accordance with Boyle's law. Assuming that the lung was filled to total lung capacity (TLC) immediately prior to the dive, the depth at which this will be reduced to residual volume (RV) can be expressed as:

$$10*(TLC/RV-1)\text{msw}$$

For most people, this would occur at a depth of between 30 and 50 msw. If this depth were exceeded, the compliance of the lung and thoracic wall would increase, resulting in the generation of a relatively negative pressure in the airways, and barotrauma of descent (known as "lung squeeze") would result.

That the world record breath-hold dive, currently held by Pipin Ferreras, is to 127 msw, indicates that unless he has a TLC/RV ratio of 13.7, which is unlikely, the assumptions behind such a calculation are wrong. It has been suggested that the thoracic blood volume (TBV) increases during breath-hold dives and that, by reducing the residual volume, this effect would increase the theoretical maximum depth of such a dive (26). Evidence to support this idea was provided by Schaefer et al. (27), who carefully studied a series of breath-hold dives by Robert Croft to a maximum of 73 msw. With a TLC of 9.11 and an RV of 1.31, his theoretical maximum depth was 69.5 msw. They found that, depending upon the depth of the dive, the TBV increased by between 850 and 1047 ml. In the same report, they calculated that for Jaques Mayol (TLC 7.21; RV 1.881) to perform his (then) record dive to 70 msw, an increased TBV of 980 ml would have been required.

It seems that this effect explains the extraordinary depths to which breath-hold dives can be conducted without pulmonary injury and that factors other than lung squeeze limit the maximum depth that can be achieved by divers with normal lungs.

III. Barotrauma of Ascent

A. Definition

Vertical movement through a column of water is associated with substantial changes in pressure. Since the liquid and solid tissues of the body are effectively incompressible, such pressure changes are evenly distributed between these tissues and there is little alteration in their function. Indeed, very high pressures can be tolerated before there is any resultant tissue dysfunction (28).

The situation is different for tissues that contain or are adjacent to a gas phase, because this is liable to the constraints of Boyle's law. For some organ systems, such as the bowel, the contraction and expansion of its gaseous contents during increases and decreases in depth are normally of no consequence. This is because the bowel wall is highly compliant and, provided that no gas is introduced at depth, such changes in volume can normally be accommodated with the generation of only an insignificant pressure differential across its wall. However, where tissue compliance is limited, alterations in the volume of gas will be accompanied by the development of a more substantial pressure differential between the tissue and its adjacent gaseous phase. Furthermore, if gas is introduced into the space at depth, it will expand during ascent through the column of water. Unless this gas-containing space is allowed to vent freely with the ambient atmosphere, a pressure differential will develop between it and the surrounding tissue. It is this force that may result in tissue injury—known as barotrauma of ascent (29).

With respect to the lung, there is evidence that the degree of overpressure required to cause tissue injury is dependent on the extent to which the lung is splinted by its surrounding structures (30–32). More strictly, therefore, the tissue injury of PBT is caused by overstretching of the lung by a transmural pressure change rather than the change in volume of the intrathoracic gas.

B. Experience from Spontaneous Lung Rupture

Pneumothoraces

Pneumothoraces are unsatisfactorily classified into those caused by doctors (e.g., during transthoracic needle biopsy of the lung, transbronchial lung biopsy, or cardiothoracic surgery—called *iatrogenic* pneumothoraces), those that are due to penetrating or blunt chest trauma (*open* or *closed traumatic* pneumothoraces), or those that occur for other reasons (*spontaneous* pneumothoraces). The latter are *primary* if there is no obvious preexisting lung disease and *secondary* if such disease is manifest. Pneumothoraces have been excellently reviewed in detail by Voge and Anthracite (33) and by Light (34). Spontaneous pneumothoraces have a trimodal distribution with patients' age, affecting neonates with respiratory distress, young adults with no other apparent lung disorder, and patients over age 40, who commonly have extensive preexisting lung disease. It is those of the middle mode, comprising primary spontaneous pneumothoraces in young adults, that are of interest to diving.

Normally, pleural pressure is less than alveolar pressure throughout the respiratory cycle. It is also less than ambient (atmospheric) pressure throughout most of the resting respiratory cycle. Thus, if a hole is made in either the chest wall or the lung exterior, gas will be drawn into the pleural space. When gas enters this space, it allows the chest wall to spring out and the lung to collapse. As a rough guide, the lung collapse will account for three-quarters of the incoming volume of gas and expansion of the chest wall for the other quarter. If a pneumothorax is present and pleural pressure exceeds alveolar pressure throughout all or most of the cycle, gas will be pumped into the pleural space continuously, the ipsilateral chest wall will reach the elastic limit of its expansion, and the mediastinum will be driven to the contralateral side. When this happens, a tension pneumothorax exists. Nowadays it is most commonly caused by positive-pressure ventilation. The symptoms are of sudden respiratory distress, and the signs are those of a large pneumothorax coupled with a severe fall in arterial P_{O_2}. There may be some obstruction to systemic venous return, but most of the threat comes from the ventilation-perfusion mismatch that drops the P_{O_2} (35,36). The condition must be treated immediately.

The first peak in the age distribution of pneumothoraces occurs in the newly born, affecting between 1 and 2% of all live births. They develop during the first few attempts to expand the fluid-filled lung and are much more common in those born prematurely or inhaling meconium-stained liquor or other amniotic or birth canal debris. The infant lung is thought to tear at rather lower inflation pressures than the adult lung and infants' small chest walls are believed to exert disproportionately high tractions on the their lungs (Laplace's law). Curiously, pneumothoraces are much more common in male than female neonates.

The second peak in the distribution occurs in young adults. Up to the early 1930s, they were always attributed, without proof, to tuberculosis, but then Kjaergaard (37) showed that they were rarely accompanied by any underlying lung disease. Such primary spontaneous pneumothoraces may be caused by sudden but not necessarily forceful distortions of the chest wall, as in twisting to attach or find a seat belt; but most develop when subjects are at rest. Sixty percent are noticed in the first 3 hr of the waking day (38). They are much more frequent in young men than young women (in the ratio of 6 or 7 to 1), and they are very much more common in smokers than nonsmokers. In young men, ''light'' smoking increases the risk sevenfold, moderate smoking raises it some twentyfold, and heavy smoking about a hundredfold (34,39). Almost all are unilateral and affect the right and left lungs with equal frequency, but some 2% are bilateral, probably betraying a defect in the mesothelial barrier separating the two pleural spaces in the anterosuperior mediastinum. They rarely occur after age 40. Recurrence rates after recovery from a first spontaneous pneumothorax are high (about 50%), are more commonly ipsilateral than contralateral, but are very infrequent after an interval of 2 years or more (33,34,40).

Primary spontaneous pneumothoraces are believed to be due to the rupture of apical, subpleural blebs that have probably filled with alveolar air dissecting from splits in local small airways. The apices are the sites of stress concentrations in the upright lung [see Vawter et al. (24) and Fig. 8], and it is thought this explains the higher incidence in tall young men with tall, thin chests. Such blebs are also found at the sharp-edged apices of the lower lobes. The gravity-dependent density gradients seen in CT scans of healthy lobes suggest that, in the supine and prone postures at least, the major fissures act as shelves on which the uppermost lobe rests and from which the lowermost lobe hangs, so it is possible that there are important stress concentrations at these sites also (41,42).

Some ''spontaneous'' pneumothoraces are associated with forced inspiratory maneuvers such as hiccupping or the completion of functional tests of TLC or peak inspiratory pressures (Refs. 43 and 44 and Case 6). Such cases suggest that voluntary high inflations can stretch some parts of healthy lungs beyond their elastic limits.

The third peak in the incidence of spontaneous pneumothoraces with age appears in patients of age 40 or more. They are almost always secondary to preexisting lung disease—most commonly chronic obstructive airflow limitation—but are also seen in a wide variety of other obstructive and restrictive lung conditions. They equal the idiopathic form numerically but are more serious clinically because of the lack of pulmonary reserve.

Traumatic pneumothoraces are of two sorts. In the first, or closed form, a powerful blow to the rib cage causes a pneumothorax without puncturing the chest wall. Often, but by no means always, this is due to sharp ends of fractured ribs penetrating the underlying lung (Cases 2 and 3), but in some there is no evidence of rib fracture at all, and it is thought that a rapid concussion wave has torn the lung interior. In the second or open form of traumatic pneumothorax, the chest wall has been punctured and air is admitted directly from the atmosphere to the pleural space. If the area of the hole equals or exceeds that of the trachea there will be complete collapse of the underlying lung (Case 7).

More than half of all traumatic pneumothoraces are iatrogenic and usually due to transthoracic or transbronchial needle biopsies of the lung. Rates per procedure vary with the sensitivity of the detecting technique. Computed tomography scans suggest that almost all biopsies are accompanied by at least a small pneumothorax. Berquist et al. (45) reported a series of 430 patients who underwent transthoracic biopsies. Pneumothoraces were detectable in up to 57% by conventional chest radiography the following day. Miller et al. (46) completed a retrospective survey of 159 patients undergoing needle biopsy of whom 30% suffered pneumothoraces. These were more common in older patients with preexisting obstructive lung disease.

Apparent Lung Rupture Following Forced Expiratory Efforts

Other clinical experiences at sea level show that sudden and forceful expiratory efforts (e.g., ''Valsalva maneuvers'' as in childbirth, weight lifting, playing the trumpet, violent coughing against an expiratory resistance, or repeated attempts at producing a maximal expiratory pressure as a test of lung function) can force air through the walls of the respiratory tract, most probably at extrapulmonary or at extrathoracic levels (47–51).

Spontaneous Pneumomediastinum

Spontaneous pneumomediastinums are probably about 10 times rarer than spontaneous pneumothoraces. However, as many are asymptomatic (Cases 1 and 8) and only half are visible on a straight posteroanterior radiograph of the chest, their true incidence is unknown. They are said to be present in 5% of all children x-rayed for asthma (52,53). Often they are only suspected once dysphonia or cervical subcutaneous emphysema become obvious (54). Their natural history and management are reviewed extensively by Pierson (55). Recurrences are infrequent. The commonest presenting symptoms are retrosternal pain (88%), dyspnea (60%) and dysphagia (40%). Sixty percent also have cervical subcutaneous emphysema, and 12.5% have a concurrent pneumothorax (56).

Spontaneous mediastinum can sometimes cause mediastinal widening and mimic aortic rupture (57). In one retrospective study of 17 patients 12 years of age or more, 12 of the 17 gave a history of performing Valsalva maneuvers during the abuse of inhaled drugs (58). Recently, Fujiwara (59) reported spontaneous pneumomediastinum as a complication in 15% of patients with fibrotic lung disease, which may fit in with the observations of Colebatch (60,61) and of Brooks and Pethybridge (62) in diving.

As mentioned earlier, mediastinal gas may not come from the lung at all but from the upper respiratory tract, the oropharynx, or the esophagus (63). Identifying ruptures of the esophagus is important, since they can often be fatal unless dealt with very promptly (64).

C. Experience from Mechanical Ventilation

There are several forms of mechanical ventilation. In one, gas is supplied to the respiratory tract at higher than ambient pressure via an oronasal mask or an endotracheal tube (*positive-pressure ventilation*). In a second, all of the body but for the head and neck is surrounded by a rigid vessel (or ''iron lung''), which is cyclically decompressed while the airway is exposed to ambient air pressure (*negative-pressure ventilation*). In all but very minor details, these two forms of artificial ventilation have identical effects upon the lung and circulation. Both inflate the lungs but obstruct the circulation (65).

In a third form, the chest wall alone is surrounded by a rigid jerkin which is cyclically decompressed while the rest of the body remains exposed to ambient pressure (*cuirasse ventilation*). This form of ventilation inflates the lung and promotes the circulation (66).

As mentioned earlier, experiments on positive-pressure inflation of fresh human cadavers show that lungs expanding in an unsupported thorax burst at about 70 mmHg; but if the thorax is confined, they rupture in a different manner at pressures of about 110 mmHg (31,32). Many animal experiments have confirmed this (67,68).

In the early days of mechanical ventilation (e.g., with the Drinker negative-pressure iron lung) the technique was applied successfully for long periods of time at relatively low transthoracic pressures, about 30 cmH_2O, in patients with neurological disorders (usually polio) but healthy lungs. Since then, positive-pressure ventilation, often delivered by endotracheal tube, has been applied to very many people with damaged lungs (most frequently with neonatal or adult respiratory distress syndromes).

Not surprisingly, studies of such cases have shown that diseased lungs are more fragile than healthy ones. Diseased lungs often become stiff because of consolidation, loss of surfactant, fibrosis, and/or pulmonary interstitial emphysema. Stiff lungs need higher pressures to ventilate them (69). The pressure-volume curve of the diseased lung reflects the properties of the ventilateable part of the lung, as has been demonstrated by the use of CT (70). Mechanical ventilation leads to pulmonary capillary rupture and to pulmonary edema. These complications appear to be a function of lung volume rather than inflation pressure, so much so that Dreyfus et al. (71,72) have proposed that the term *barotrauma* should be replaced by *volutrauma*. As mentioned earlier, positive-pressure ventilation opposes systemic venous return, causing pulmonary vessels to collapse and increasing the transmural stress on neighbouring alveoli (5). Systemic hypovolemia compounds this and increases the risk of lung rupture (73).

Often a rise in pulmonary arterial pressure—i.e., upstream of the compressed intrapulmonary vessels—precedes a pneumomediastinum. Once the gas has escaped into the soft peripulmonary tissues (surgical emphysema), it can block cerebral venous return at the base of the neck (74). It can also escape from the soft tissues into systemic veins leading to paradoxical systemic venous gas embolism (75).

The most common sequences observed in mechanically ventilated patients in intensive care units are pulmonary interstitial emphysema (PIE) leading centripetally to pneumomediastinum and cervical emphysema and centrifugally to the appearance of subpleural pulmonary blebs. The appearance of blebs and/or surgical emphysema are ominous signs that a pneumothorax will soon follow. Sick patients tolerate pneumothoraces badly because they have little pulmonary reserve. In addition, most pneumothoraces on mechanically ventilated patients proceed to tension pneumothoraces (76,77). As pleural pressure rises, cardiac output falls (78).

Complication rates of mechanical ventilation vary widely from center to center because of many differences in case-mix severity and ventilatory practices. Zwillich et al. (79) reported a prospective audit of 354 consecutive patients given mechanical ventilation at one center of excellence. Of these, 30% suffered overprolonged attempts at intubation, 5 had massive gastric distention from a misplaced tube, and at least 34 had intubation of the right main-stem bronchus rather than the trachea. The latter error is serious because all of the ventilator output goes to one lung, which is therefore more likely to be overdistended and to rupture. In their series, this serious complication was often unrecognised for up to 24 hr. Gammon et al. (80) reported a series of 139 mechanically ventilated patients of whom 34 suffered PBT, 24 proceeded to a pneumomediastinum, and 10 of the 24 progressed to a pneumothorax. There are many other studies with similar findings, emphasizing the difficulties of intubating and ventilating fragile, diseased lungs. Occasionally, mechanical ventilation can lead to cerebral arterial gas embolism, which is difficult to diagnose but can be fatal (81).

In summary, many studies of lung damage during mechanical ventilation support the idea that the risk of rupture is rare at inflation pressures of 40 mmHg or less and substantial at pressures of 70 mmHg or more. Some show that respiratory gas can escape into the pulmonary arteries or capillaries and travel antidromically to fill the right heart with foam, or it can break into the pulmonary veins and travel orthodromically to the left heart and to the coronary, carotid, and cerebral circulations.

D. Experience from Aviation

Although the early work of Robert Boyle (82), Paul Bert (83), and others identified hypoxia and decompression illness as limitations to hypobaric decompression, it was not until the early twentieth century that strategies to overcome these problems—other than the provision of oxygen at ambient pressure—were developed. Haldane (84) realized that the maximum altitude to which men could go when breathing pure oxygen at ambient pressure would be about 40,000 ft. He also calculated that delivering oxygen at an overpressure of about 15 mmHg would enable them to fly a few thousand feet higher. In the years immediately before World War II, aviators were making brief excursion to 50,000 ft or slightly more, using a modified Siebe-Gorman diving dress to provide them with oxygen at a modest overpressure as suggested by Haldane. As the war proceeded, many unpressurized aircraft flew at 40,000 to 45,000 ft to gain a military advantage. To do this the aviators had to breathe pure oxygen at raised pressures of about 15 mmHg above ambient atmospheric pressure, and experience of mild prolonged positive-pressure breathing at altitude was gained.

Toward the end of World War II, the pressurized aircraft cabin was developed. This obviated the need for prolonged positive-pressure breathing and allowed aircraft to climb much higher, but it introduced two new problems: of rapid decompression and of the brief but profound positive-pressure breathing regimes that would be required to bring aircrew back safely if they lost cabin pressure suddenly at altitudes well above 45,000 ft. Thus air forces throughout the world embarked on a series of theoretical, animal and human studies on rapid decompression and brief but severe positive-pressure breathing. These have led to much of our current knowledge of PBT.

In essence, these studies have shown that the human lung can be decompressed very rapidly indeed without coming to harm provided that the glottis is kept open during the decompression. Heath (85) reported a series of 86,916 decompression runs to altitude that were without significant effects. These included 771 rapid decompressions. Hitchcock et al. (86) exposed 150 subjects to a total of 550 "explosive" decompressions. Holstrom (87) reported the safe outcomes of a large series of decompressions from an initial altitude of 10,000 ft to a final altitude of 40,000 ft in 1.6 to 2.3 sec. Bryan and Leach (88) did likewise for a series from 8000 to 40,000 ft (565 to 141 mmHg) in 2.5 sec. Ernsting et al. (89) safely completed six decompressions on each of three subjects, from 8000 ft to 40,000 ft in 1.6 sec. Holness et al. (90) successfully decompressed two subjects from 22,500 to 60,000 ft and from 45,000 to 80,000 ft.

While these studies were going on, other workers were looking at the physics of rapid decompression, appreciating that it was not the simple exponential affair that might have been expected, (16,91). Because of the wide range of the pressure swings and thus the severe cooling that occurs, because of the rapid evolution of water vapor into expanding gas in the lungs, and because the lungs are usually about half full and floppy at the moment of decompression, the gas in the lung tends to expand to fill the lungs first and then to vent through the trachea and glottis in a linearly decaying way with a time constant of about 0.5 sec. This fits in well with the conclusions drawn from the maximal flow–volume loop of the lungs at sea level, mentioned previously, and the experimental findings of Violette (92,93) and Luft and Bancroft (94).

Meanwhile, actual decompressions in flight were providing more evidence that the human lung could survive quite rapid decompressions. For example Achiary et al. (95) reported satisfactory outcomes to 15 abrupt decompressions with time constants of 0.1 to 3 sec in French high-performance aircraft, and Brooks (96) did likewise with 29 incidents of massive/explosive decompression in Canadian fighter aircraft over the 20-year period 1962 to 1982. In almost every case the crew were able to land their aircraft safely. This does not always happen. A graphic account of the realities of escaping from an aircraft breaking up in flight is given by Howard et al. (97). In 1982, Kolesari and Kindwall (98) described the case of a man who was accidentally decompressed from ground level to an altitude well in excess of 63,000 ft over 3 to 4 min, held there for 3 to 5 min, and then brought to ground level over another minute or so. The victim was profoundly unconscious on retrieval from the pressure vessel and was compressed to 6 bar 5½ hr later. Eventually, he was judged to show no neurological sequelae at all.

Running in parallel with the studies of experimental and accidental rapid decompressions were others intended to discover the positive-pressure breathing regimes that could be applied to bring air crew who had been rapidly decompressed to altitudes above 40,000 ft down below that threshold safely. Many of these are summarized by Ernsting (99,100), who designed the partial pressure suit assembly that is still used by the Royal Air Force today. In essence they show that 20 healthy young men could breathe at positive inflation pressures of 40 to 70 mmHg for 2 min without protection, but for longer periods it was essential to provide adequate counterpressure to the chest, the abdomen, and the legs. Inflation pressures of 30 mmHg can be accepted for 30 min or so before expiratory muscle fatigue sets in. Counterpressure must be applied to the chest wall to prevent dangerous expansion at higher pressures and must be simultaneously applied to the abdominal wall and hernial orifices to prevent excessive descent of the diaphragm. Counterpressure also has to be applied to the legs to combat the sequestration of blood and transudate in the thighs. At positive breathing pressures above 60 mmHg, distension of the neck, axillae, and arms becomes painful and has to be counteracted by adding sleeves and an appropriate helmet to the counter-pressure assembly.

As these studies proceeded, air forces were also exercised by another problem—the management of pneumothoraces in air crew. Several studies showed that pneumothoraces rarely occurred in decompression chamber runs or in flight (33,85,101–105), but as their recurrence rate was as high as 30 to 50% ipsilaterally and 10% contralaterally, it would be unsafe to allow affected air crew to return to flying, since an unsuspected recurrence would expand on ascent and might imperil the safety or completion of the mission (106). The current attitude is to offer affected air crew a bilateral pleurectomy soon after the first spontaneous pneumothorax and allow them to return to flying 3 months later. Some investigators are concerned that the risks of pleurectomy exceed those of a recurrence in flight and prefer to take air crew off flying duties for a year or more (107).

Although millions of passengers, many of whom have respiratory disease, travel commercially each year, PBT is rare in flight or in decompression chambers. In Cran and Rumball's series of 994 spontaneous pneumothoraces occurring in RAF personnel over a 22-year period (101), only 8 occurred in flight. This incidence was judged to be proportionate to the fraction of time spent in the air and was not thought to have been caused by the flights. Nonetheless, dramatic exceptions have been described in cases of preexisting lung disease (108,109). In contrast to decompression from depth, decompression to altitude rarely causes arterial gas embolism, and we have found only a single case report (110).

E. Experience from Diving and Escape from Submarines

A large proportion of cases of PBT occurs among inexperienced divers (111–114). In a large study of accidents arising from submarine escape training, the incidence of PBT among initial trainees is almost double that of requalifiers (115). In the diving setting, it is well recognized that a rapid ascent is a predisposing factor for PBT (116). This may occur, for example, as a result of panic following the loss or failure of a piece of equipment or running out of air. Should such panic result in involuntary closure of the glottis, PBT will be the consequence for all but the shallowest of ascents. Such crises are largely avoidable and panic is less likely to arise in experienced divers (117). Panic among the topside crew who unexpectedly surface the diver can also result in PBT (Case 9).

To avoid pulmonary overinflation, it is important to breathe out during a rapid ascent. This is not an intuitive action, particularly if the diver believes that he or she is out of air; it has to be learned. It is therefore not surprising that inexperienced divers are at greater risk of PBT than those who are more experienced. The reason why trainee submariners appear to be at greater risk than requalifiers is less clear. All submariners undertaking escape training are carefully trained and supervised in the water, with particular attention to adequate exhalation during ascent. The majority of trainees who have ''incidents on ascent'' return to submarine service 3 months later, so selective culling of the most vulnerable cannot be the explanation.

Most navies that train submariners in escape techniques do so infrequently, meaning that on each occasion these techniques need to be relearned. The most likely reason why initial trainees are more vulnerable is because they are more nervous than those undergoing repeat training, although how this translates into subsequent injury is unclear.

It is also apparent from submarine escape training that PBT may occur in personnel who have been witnessed to exhale, apparently adequately, throughout their ascent (118,119). Therefore, there are liable be other factors that may predispose an individual to PBT.

In the diving setting, attention has recently been focused on the possible role of breathing techniques in unexplained PBT. Lung rupture is commonly asymptomatic and is likely to occur frequently in normobaric life as a result of maneuvers such as coughing, sneezing, or taking and holding a deep breath (Case 6). A technique commonly employed by divers is ''skip'' breathing, in which the normal ventilatory pattern of inhale, exhale, and pause is replaced by inhale, pause, and exhale (117). It is likely that such a breathing pattern predisposes to lung rupture because the lung is repeatedly taken close to and maintained at its elastic limit. Under normobaric conditions, such a rupture may provoke the leakage of only small, asymptomatic amounts of gas into the mediastinum. However, if this were to occur at depth and the diver were then to surface, Boyle's law would cause the volume to increase in proportion to the depth at which the leakage occurred. In all but the most shallow of dives, such an expansion may be sufficient to provoke symptoms (Case 10). Another problem is that during the very rapid ascents of a submarine escape profile (Fig. 4), only a brief interruption to a controlled exhalation—caused by, for example, coughing, sneezing, or hiccuping—may be sufficient to provoke PBT. This is particularly so during the last few meters of an ascent when the rate of increase of thoracic gas volume is at its greatest.

F. Medical Factors That May Predispose to Pulmonary Barotrauma

It has been argued for many years that conditions causing airway obstruction predispose to PBT, and such arguments can be persuasive (120,121). Overdistention of the lung distal to the obstruction may occur as the diver ascends. In the case of reversible airway disease, support for this hypothesis has been provided by alarming anecdotal reports of asthmatics who have suffered from PBT (122). While there is little dispute that asthmatics who are symptomatic should not dive—both on the grounds of the risk of PBT and their reduced exercise tolerance—the situation with respect to asthmatics in remission is controversial (123).

As Edmonds observes (122), even if an asthmatic diver is asymptomatic upon entering the water, the underwater environment provides a number of potential triggers for an acute asthmatic attack:

1. Exertion (from overweighting, equipment drag, swimming against tides, etc.)
2. Inhalation of cold, dry air (adiabatic expansion of dehumidified, compressed air)
3. Inhalation of hypertonic saline through a faulty regulator
4. Breathing against a resistance (increased gas density, faulty regulator, low air supply)

As a result of such arguments, asthmatics have been excluded from military and commercial diving for many years and discouraged from sports diving. However, such exclusion is unenforceable in most jurisdictions. The consequence of this approach has been that there is no substantial data set from which an objective assessment of the risk of PBT in asthmatics as opposed to non-asthmatics can be determined (124,125). Recent attempts to gather such data have been criticized for poor study design (126–128) or are limited to small pilot studies (129). Nonetheless, they indicate that the risk of asthma provoking PBT may have been overstated in the past; until high-quality data are available, this issue will remain controversial (130).

The evidence for an association between chronic obstructive pulmonary disease (COPD) and PBT is also scant. This is for much the same reason as above. Also, unlike asthma, COPD is unusual in the generally young, fit population from which submariners and military, commercial, and the great majority of sports divers is drawn. There is radiological and autopsy evidence, albeit anecdotal, that bullous disease may predispose to PBT (118,131–133). However, small bullae and apical blebs are common and may avoid detection by routine radiography (Cases 11 and 12), and there is anecdotal evidence that diving may be possible with encysted pockets of intrathoracic, extrapulmonary gas (134). Furthermore, the autopsy evidence from cases of fatal PBT needs to be interpreted with caution, since pulmonary overinflation can cause blebs (Case 13), and careful histological examination is required to distinguish these from pre-existing disease (132).

Nonetheless, it can be argued intuitively that poorly communicating gas-filled spaces in the lung are liable to be vulnerable to barotrauma of ascent, particularly if the ascent is rapid. It is for this reason that Jenkins et al. (135) have recommended that patients with conditions that may predispose to bullae or subpleural blebs, such as Marfan's and Ehlers-Danlos syndromes, should be considered unfit to dive.

The complete obstruction of a small airway is unlikely to predispose to PBT, since the distal lung is likely to be atelectatic; even if it were not, the process of descent and ascent through a column of water is unlikely to result in a net increase in the volume of trapped gas, as in the bowel. However, incomplete obstruction could theoretically do so, as in bullous disease, by limiting the rate at which gas distal to the obstruction can leave the lung during ascent. Despite the attraction of this hypothesis, there is a dearth of compelling evidence to support it. Liebow et al. (131) reported a frequently quoted case of fatal PBT in a submariner undergoing escape training. At autopsy, an irregular calcified mass was found in the left main bronchus and a second in a superior segmental bronchus of the left lower lobe. The latter was associated with bronchiectasis, from which it can be surmised that there was substantial, chronic airway obstruction. Of interest, however, is that the extent of the PBT in this case was not confined to the left lower lobe or even the left lung, since a pneumothorax and substantial interstitial emphysema were found on the right side. Although the finding of interstitial emphysema associated with the bronchiectasis may be evidence that localized airway obstruction is a predisposing factor for PBT, the question as to whether the affected lung is more vulnerable than that served by normal airways is left open.

Unsworth (136) described a case of tension pneumothorax that arose following a session of hyperbaric oxygen therapy. The patient was subsequently found to have a neoplastic mass in the right middle lobe. The pneumothorax was effectively treated and there were consequently no acute autopsy findings. The attribution of the pneumothorax to airway obstruction due to the neoplasm must, therefore, be speculative. The same argument applies to the case reported by Calder (132), in which localized airway obstruction was implied by the finding of clinical and histological evidence of acute bronchiolitis. To further confound the role of involuntary airway obstruction, it now appears that indices of obstruction do not correlate with a risk of PBT. Benton et al. (115) studied the screening spirometry data of a population of healthy Royal Navy submarine escape trainees who had suffered unequivocal PBT. They confirmed the observation of Brooks et al. (62) that a lower than predicted FVC was associated with PBT rather than any measured index of obstruction.

These observations may provide supporting evidence for the hypothesis that reduced compliance is an important factor in the genesis of PBT, and this may apply both to the whole lung and to isolated segments (54,60,61). It can be envisaged that in a lung with patchy reduced compliance, two mechanisms may provoke PBT in circumstances of potential pulmonary overinflation:

1. The volumes of lung with reduced compliance will expand less than those with normal compliance and elastic structures in series with and adjacent to these volumes will be overstretched; therefore they will be vulnerable to rupture (60). (See Fig. 10, p. 197.)
2. Shearing forces will be generated at the junction between volumes of lung with differing compliance, which may be sufficient to cause lung rupture.

An extreme example of the former would be scarring of the lung parenchyma. However, Calder found, in a series of 13 cases, that the localization of lung rupture was inconsistently related to scarring (132). But see the discussion of mechanisms of lung rupture below.

The argument of reduced compliance may also apply to the observation of Benton et al. (115) that a low FVC, rather than indices of obstruction, appears to be associated with PBT in submarine escape trainees. As the lung reaches TLC, its compliance is reduced (Fig. 7), and, in a setting of potential pulmonary overinflation, it becomes more likely to rupture.

There can be little doubt that pleural scarring (32,131,132) can predispose to PBT, particularly pneumothorax. However, this is again a common condition and liable, if limited in extent, to be missed on a routine chest x-ray, which in any case may not be required for sports divers. Since it is likely that many thousands of uneventful dives have been conducted by personnel with pleural scarring, the magnitude of the risk of PBT associated with this is likely to be small.

G. Summary of the Circumstances for and Consequences of Lung Rupture

The diving population, being predominantly male and aged between the late teens and early forties, is vulnerable to spontaneous lung rupture in the absence of any significant mechanical stress. When this happens, it results in a primary pneumothorax or, more rarely, a pneumomediastinum. From a diving viewpoint, primary spontaneous pneumothoraces in the under-40 age group are unlikely to recur after an interval of 2 years. In the over-40 group, they are associated with preexisting lung disease and are more likely to proceed to a tension pneumothorax and to recur. Since the diving population is generally fit, secondary spontaneous pneumothoraces in the over-40 age group are not a common problem. Traumatic pneumothoraces in the absence of other lung disease heal naturally and do not recur.

We know from experiments and experience with ventilators that normal lungs will rupture at an inflation pressure above about 70 mmHg and that diseased lungs will do so at a lower pressure. Again, the common presentations are of pneumomediastinum and pneumothorax, and gas embolism is rare. Healthy lungs can be decompressed very rapidly to altitude over a pressure range of up to 0.5 bar without injury. If the lung is damaged, pneumothorax and pneumomediastinum are common and gas embolism is very rare.

In diving, the situation is different. Although very rapid ascents from great depth can be achieved without pulmonary injury (Fig. 4), lung rupture can occur from a dive as shallow as 1 msw (137) in which the overpressure generated, assuming a breath-holding ascent at TLC, cannot be much greater than about 70 mmHg. Although quantification is difficult, PBT in divers results in gas embolism far more commonly than in other circumstances, with pneumothorax being rare.

In divers, we have seen that skip breathing (inhaling to TLC and holding it prior to exhalation) may result in lung rupture. While normally of no clinical significance at sea level—causing a small, asymptomatic pneumomediastinum—this can provoke symptoms should it occur at depth, because the gas that has escaped from the lung expands as the diver surfaces.

We know that divers who fail to exhale during ascent or do so inadequately rupture their lungs. Although very occasionally cases are reported in the literature where a pulmonary lesion may have been the cause of the problem, there remains a group of divers and submarine escape trainees for whom, despite extensive investigation, no explanation for PBT can be found. This highlights, among other things, the limitations of even the most sophisticated investigative tools, which are frequently disadvantaged by being employed at some time after the accident. However, since only a very small lung defect is required for it to rupture, it is considered unlikely that even investigation shortly after the incident would prove more fruitful.

H. Mechanisms of Lung Rupture

Lung rupture cannot be studied experimentally in humans and experiments on other animals are of limited value because the geometry and mechanical properties of their lungs are different from ours. Hence the emphasis on epidemiology, the gradual accumulation of data from events that have occurred by chance, showing what the lung will tolerate and what it will not. Why are the patterns of lung rupture seen in aviation and mechanical ventilation so different

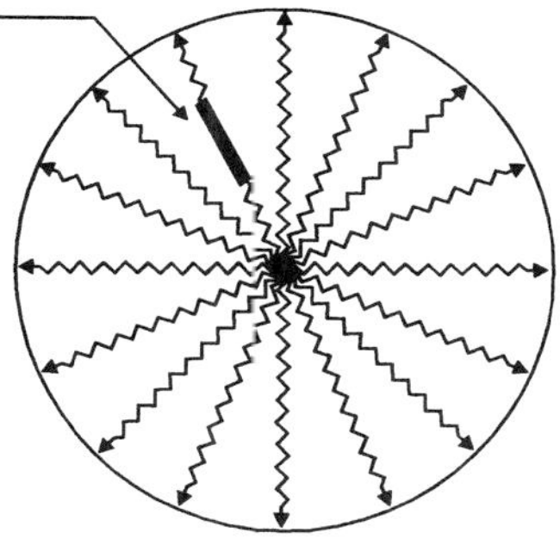

Figure 10 A diagram of an imaginary isotropic spherical lung with airways radiating from its center. The middle third of one of the airways is fibrosed. This strong scar concentrates abnormally high longitudinal stresses on the normal airway elements in series with it.

from those seen in diving? Why is it that pneumomediastinums and surgical emphysema are much more common than pneumothoraces in women giving birth, and why do they complicate such a small minority of births?

We have very little hard evidence to add to such discussion. The observations on skip-breathing and on pneumomediastinum following voluntary respiratory gymnastics suggest that apparently healthy lungs are close to their elastic limit when held at TLC. The tears in these instances must have occurred in the lung interior, otherwise they would have led to pneumothoraces, and they must have been close to bronchovascular bundles, otherwise gas would not have been able to reach the mediastinum. Why, as Colebatch and Brooks and Pethybridge proposed (60–62), is rupture of the lung during diving more likely to occur in small, stiff lungs than in large, obstructed ones? We note the Macklins' (5) elegant ideas on the particular vulnerability of "marginal" alveoli close to bronchovascular bundles and the possible compounding effect of hypovolemia. This, they argued, could increase the stress on the marginal alveoli if the cardiac output could not increase, thereby allowing the bronchovascular bundles to expand at a similar rate to the gas-containing elements of the lung. However, we wish to add two additional proposals:

1. Figure 10 shows an imaginary spherical and initially isotropic lung in which bronchovascular bundles and their associated collagen and elastin fibers radiate outward from the center of the sphere. As the "normal" lung is inflated, it expands isotropically, and stress is evenly distributed along each bundle with no one more liable to rupture than the others. Now introduce fibrosis into the middle third of one element

and inflate the lung again. The fibrosed part is stronger than the rest of the lung and therefore less liable to tear. But because it also cannot stretch, it puts additional stress on the normal elements in series with it, making them more liable than the rest of the bundles to rupture. This may explain Calder's observation that he could find no consistent association between the sites of lung rupture and pulmonary scarring (132).

2. It is also possible that, contrary to the Macklins' ideas, the displacement of blood into the thorax—which occurs with submersion, particularly during negative-pressure breathing (138,139)—causes a reduction in compliance which, rather like the lung close to TLC, makes it more liable to rupture.

The role of airway obstruction in PBT is now controversial, particularly with respect to asthma, and has probably been overemphasised in the past. Inspection of Fig. 6a shows that the forces causing airway closure during exhalation at sea level do not apply when the gas in the lung expands in accordance with Boyle's law, as the floppy "airway" will not obstruct the escaping gas. Only obstruction of a poorly flexible airway, such as a closed glottis, is liable to provoke lung rupture under these circumstances.

Under isobaric conditions, once the lung has torn, the gas will be pumped slowly by normal ventilatory movement toward the mediastinum and beyond, as summarized in Fig. 11. However, if the body is decompressed, the escaped gas will expand and explode into the compartments named as shown in Fig. 12 (140).

IV. The Distribution of Extrapulmonary Gas Following Pulmonary Barotrauma

Gas is normally found within the respiratory and gastrointestinal tracts. It is abnormal to find it elsewhere. The presence of aberrant air in the pleural, mediastinal, or adjacent subcutaneous spaces or in systemic arterial blood is usually accepted as evidence of lung rupture, but this is not necessarily so.

1. First, extensive ruptures of the lung interior from blast injury do not lead to the escape of much air unless the victim survives to make respiratory efforts (13,15,141–144).
2. Second, gas of nonpulmonary origin can appear in peripulmonary tissues (e.g., the pleural, pericardial, mediastinal, peritoneal, and retroperitoneal spaces, the soft tissues of the neck and chest wall, and the pulmonary and systemic vasculature) because:

   - It has been generated in situ by infecting organisms.
   - Swallowed air has been forcibly expelled from the gastrointestinal

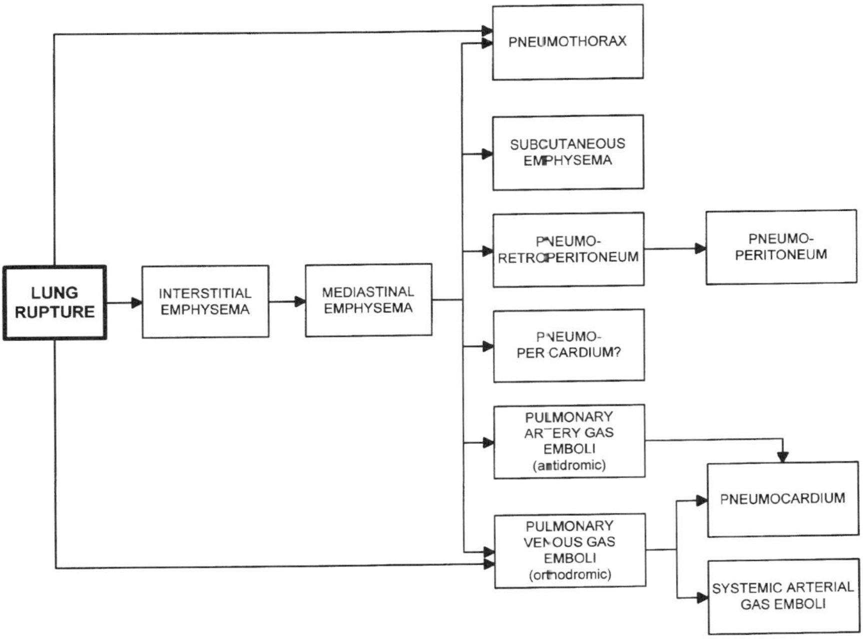

Figure 11 A summary of the routes that gas can take when escaping from a ruptured lung.

tract, as in the ruptured esophagus syndrome described by Boerhaave (145) and Agarwal and Miller (63).

- It has escaped from an extrapulmonary airway in the mouth, pharynx, larynx, trachea, or extrapulmonary bronchi and may have extended downward to the mediastinum or pericardium, burst through the thin hilar pleura to the pleural space, or been carried on down below the diaphragm (146,147).

3. Third, some penetrating injuries of the chest wall and much cardiothoracic surgery lead to an open traumatic pneumothorax with considerable or complete collapse of an intact lung. Closed heart bypass surgery can lead to the accidental introduction of gas emboli via bypass lines or oxygenators (bubble more than membrane oxygenators) (149–150).

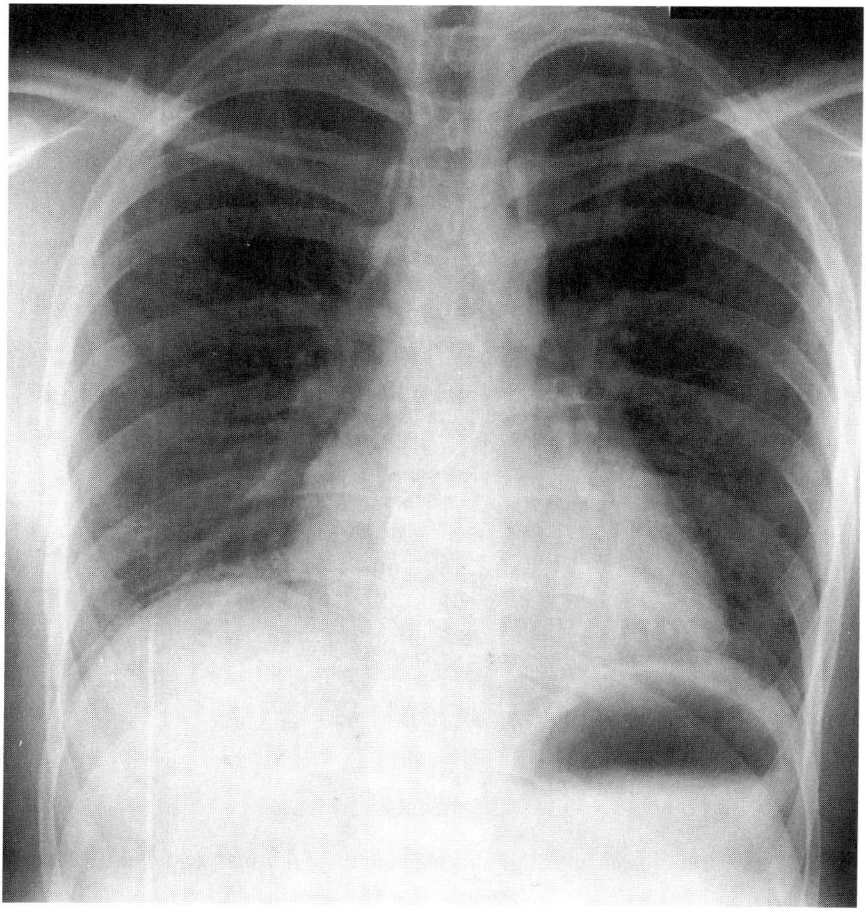

A

Figure 12A An example of a severe case of lung rupture in a young submariner. His normal chest radiograph immediately before his submarine escape training course.

4. Last, blood in the airways or in sputum often comes from broken vessels in the upper respiratory tract, especially the nose and perinasal sinuses. It is helpful to keep these reservations in mind when one is reading reports of presumed lung rupture.

Common forms of lung rupture occur under the following circumstances:

1. When pulmonary air has ruptured into the pleural space via the visceral pleura, from whence it may extend into the chest wall, partic-

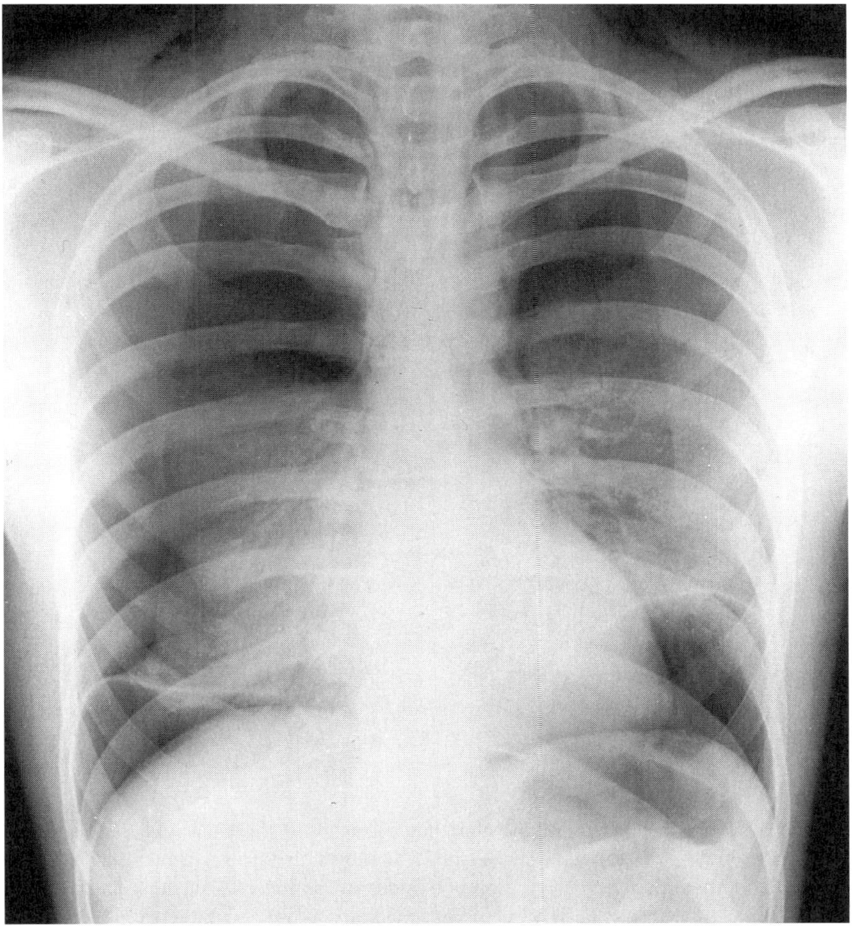

B

Figure 12B Submariner's chest radiograph following a bouyant ascent from 18 m. It shows bilateral pneumothoraces, a pneumomediastinum, and almost symmetrical extravasations of air from the mediastinum via the inferior pulmonary ligaments to lift the parietal pleura off the underlying muscle in both hemidiaphragms.

ularly if an inadequate drain is in place (spontaneous or closed traumatic pneumothorax).

2. When pulmonary air has been forced through the wall of a proximal airway, traveling centripetally along the bronchovascular bundles to reach the mediastinum (spontaneous pneumomediastinum/mediastinal

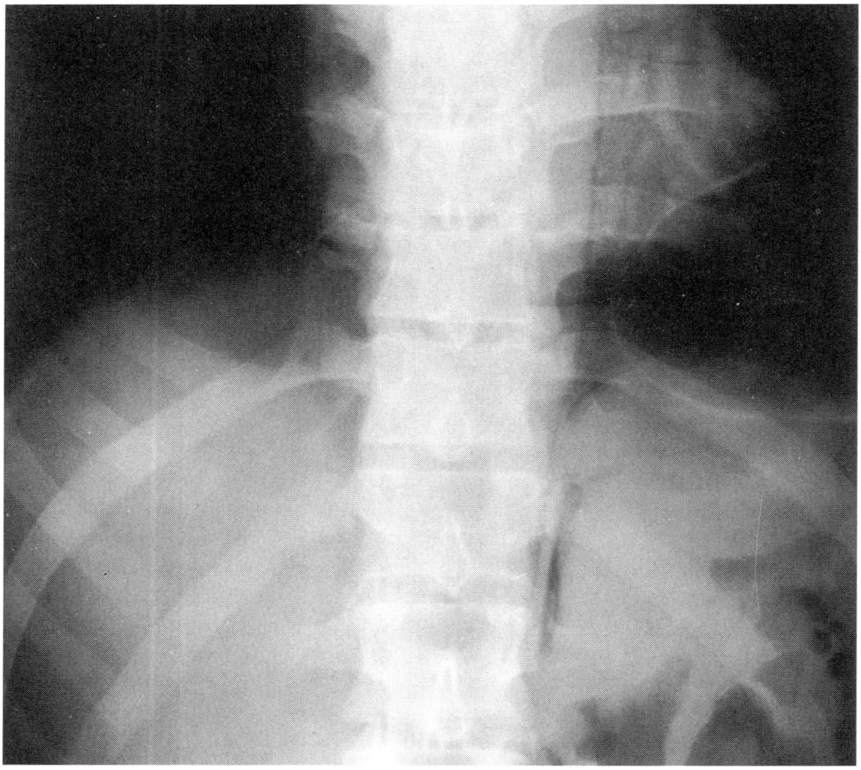

C

Figure 12C–E (C) A film of the abdomen taken in 70° head-down tilt after a delay of 20 min to allow intraperitoneal gas to rise. It shows air tracking down the side of the thoracic and abdominal aorta, lying on both sides of the left crus of the diaphragm, and a small collection below the left diaphragm medially as well as large subpleural suprephrenic collections. (D and E) CT scans of the latter and also small collections of air tracking down the sheaths of the great vessels close to the spine.

emphysema), from whence it can travel up into the neck (cervical emphysema), out along superficial fascial planes (subcutaneous emphysema), down into the pericardium or subdiaphragmatic spaces (pneumopericardium, pneumoretroperitoneum, pneumoperitoneum), or through the thin walls of the pulmonary arteries or veins, (pulmonary/systemic gas embolism).

3. When pulmonary air has escaped though the walls of usually many distal airways into the small bronchovascular bundles, splinting the

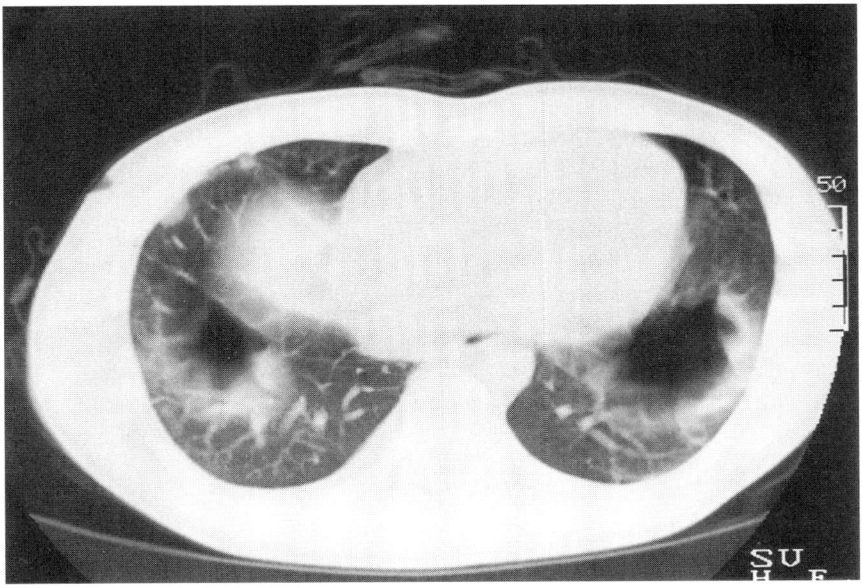

D

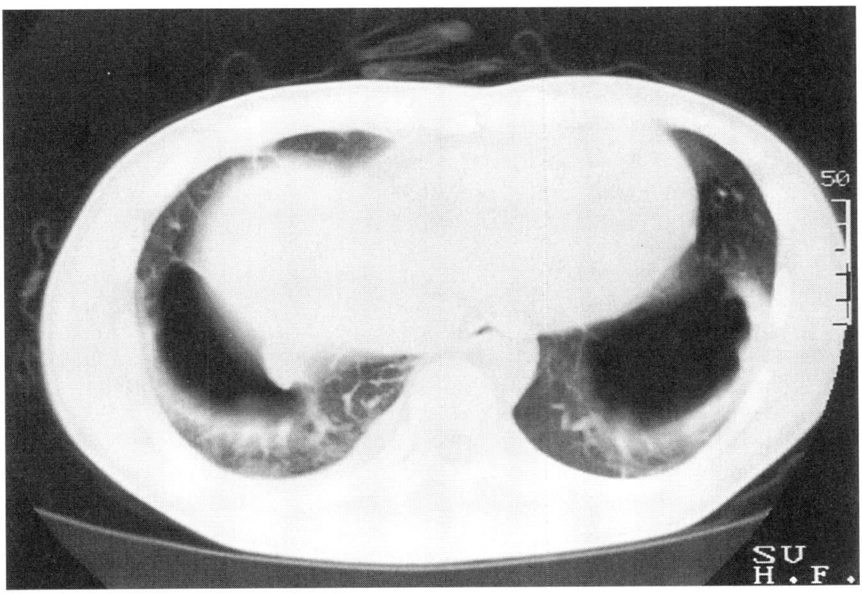

E

> lung as it travels centrally (pulmonary interstitial emphysema, or PIE). In this condition, it is increasingly difficult to breathe or to ventilate the lung artificially as the air-filled splints extend. A striking account of this condition, developing during spontaneous breathing, is given by Torry and Grosh (151), who cared for and reviewed a vast number of U.S. soldiers affected by the virulent influenza epidemic of 1918. They observed that many of these patients developed PIE, seen radiographically, that progressed to pneumomediastinum and cervical emphysema, often blocking venous return. Relief of the cervical obstruction was lifesaving [see also Coelho (74)].

Following lung rupture, the escaped gas may track in a number of directions, as shown diagrammatically in Fig. 11 (p. 199) and by conventional and CT radiographs of a severe case of pulmonary barotrauma in Fig. 12. The radiographs illustrate bilateral pneumothoraces, subcutaneous emphysema, subpleural gas at one lung base, and gas in the retroperitoneum.

In the case of hyperbaric decompression, it is difficult to assess the true frequency of the various manifestations of PBT for a number of reasons:

1. Not all cases are symptomatic. Even where gas embolism of the brain has occurred, the manifestations may be minor or transient and go unreported.
2. In all but the most trivial of hyperbaric exposures, it is impossible in most cases to determine with confidence whether neurological manifestations have arisen as a result of arterial gas embolism from PBT or as a result of bubbles formed in tissues supersaturated with gas (classical decompression sickness) (Case 14).
3. In many parts of the world, the collection of diving accident data is haphazard and therefore incomplete.

One specific circumstance where the latter two constraints do not apply is submarine escape training. Analysis of a series of 91 cases in which the diagnosis could be established with reasonable confidence (115) showed:

Pulmonary barotrauma only	9%
Neurological DCI only	69%
Pulmonary barotrauma and neurological DCI	22%

Pulmonary barotrauma in this series was defined as cases in which there was x-ray or clinical evidence of a pneumothorax or extra-alveolar gas in the lung parenchyma, mediastinum, or other site to which gas may track.

In a study of 140 cases of PBT in divers reported to the Institute of Naval Medicine over a period of 20 years (which suffers from all of the above constraints), Leitch and Green (119) described 78 cases that met similar diagnostic criteria. The distribution of these cases into the above categories was 10, 77, and 13% respectively. In a similarly constrained study of 64 diving casualties in Australia, Gorman (152) reported proportions of 66, 33, and 1% respectively. It can be seen that neurological manifestations, arising from the distribution of the escaped gas to the pulmonary venous circulation and subsequent cerebral arterial gas embolism, predominate.

Within the nonneurological categories of PBT, pneumothorax is uncommon, present in only 5% of cases in submarine escape trainees (153). Furthermore, in fatal cases, the finding of a pneumothorax at autopsy needs to be interpreted with caution as, in certain circumstances, it may be a consequence of postmortem events (Case 15). In the remainder, following the escape of gas into the interstitial tissues of the lung, its migration to the mediastinum may be continued, where sufficient gas has escaped cephalad to the subcutaneous tissues of the neck and head or caudally in the retropleural and retroperitoneal planes to form collections beneath the diaphragm, around the great vessels of the abdomen, and in the pelvis. Occasionally the radiological features may suggest a pneumopericardium, although close examination of the films commonly shows that such gas lies between the parietal pleura and pericardium (29). In particularly severe cases, a pneumocardium may be seen (154). It is assumed that gas in the left side of the heart has traveled orthodromically along the pulmonary veins and gas in the right side of the heart has traveled antidromically along the pulmonary arterial tree.

V. Clinical Features of Pulmonary Barotrauma

A. Generalized Symptoms of Lung Rupture

In the diving setting, the onset of PBT is commonly asymptomatic and the condition is only recognized an hour or more after the dive. In symptomatic cases, the onset is frequently associated with substernal pain and coughing, which is occasionally productive of pink, frothy sputum arising from alveolar hemorrhage (155). Dyspnea may accompany these symptoms. In only a small proportion of cases, this is due to the complication of a pneumothorax. In the majority of these cases, it is likely to be due to barotraumatic injury to the lung parenchyma.

Mediastinal Emphysema

As mentioned before, mediastinal emphysema may be asymptomatic. In a survey of 170 submariners undergoing submarine escape training, James (156) found radiological evidence of mediastinal emphysema in two, although both individuals involved were asymptomatic. Of symptomatic cases, the more severe tend to present within a few minutes of reaching the surface and less severe cases up to some hours after the provocative dive. The symptoms associated with mediastinal emphysema are of a sense of fullness in the chest or throat or a central, aching chest pain. In rare and severe cases, sufficient gas escapes into the mediastinum, particularly if this extends into the space between the pericardium and parietal pleura, to cause cardiac tamponade with its associated symptoms and signs. Precordial gas may be palpable and associated with crepitus synchronous with the pulse—Hamann's sign (157,158).

Subcutaneous Emphysema

Mediastinal gas commonly tracks cephalad into the neck, forming subcutaneous emphysema, which is detected by the characteristic crepitus on palpating the area. Commonly, the diver will notice this while showering or dressing after a dive. Others may notice the condition by a change in voice quality of the affected diver, which is generally raised in pitch and ''brassy'' in tone (Case 1). This has been attributed to injury of the recurrent laryngeal nerve, although a change to the frequency spectrum of the larynx, consequent upon it being surrounded by gas, is a more likely explanation in most cases.

Pneumothorax

The symptoms and signs of pneumothorax associated with PBT are the same as for any other cause. In the diving setting, they tend to be unilateral and incomplete, although exceptions are described (140,159). Large pneumothoraces are unusual and tension pneumothoraces are very rare. Before leaving this subject, it is worth highlighting the difficulty of diagnosing pneumothoraces in compression chambers (Case 15). Chambers are commonly poorly lit and cramped; consequently, observation is made more difficult than in a hospital examination room. The atmosphere in chambers is dense and commonly noisy; consequently percussion and auscultation of the chest is not easy. Because the patient is breathing a mixture containing a high partial pressure of oxygen, the onset of dyspnea and cyanosis, which can complicate bilateral or tension pneumothoraces, is delayed. Only a limited number of chambers have the capability for x-rays to be taken of patients inside them. Because of these difficulties, a high index of suspicion is required. Because pneumothoraces expand as the chamber is decompressed, this should be halted if there is any evidence of respiratory distress or tracheal deviation and the patient should be carefully examined for a pneumothorax.

Arterial Gas Embolism

Dutka (160) defined three clinical courses of arterial gas embolism (AGE) arising from submarine escape training. The first is a catastrophic presentation in which the victim experiences immediate collapse and is unresponsive to resuscitation measures and commonly dies before recompression can be undertaken. Such cases are characterized at autopsy by extensive gas embolism involving the circulation of the brain and heart. Cardiac arrest in such cases is due either to the direct effects of coronary artery occlusion or the consequences of brainstem embolism (161–163).

In the second presentation, the initial manifestations are more varied and may involve some of many neurological deficits of a generally cerebral distribution. These cases usually respond to prompt recompression but may demonstrate a relapsing pattern of recurrence and, commonly, worsening of the symptoms and signs (164). Although prompt and deep recompression has reduced the incidence of relapse, it has not eliminated it (113,165). The third presentation is distinguishable retrospectively from the latter by the generally good response to recompression therapy.

Although such a classification may be of some use in retrospective studies of gas embolism, it is of little help in the acute clinical setting. Indeed, the differential diagnosis of arterial gas embolism and decompression sickness involving the brain is now recognized as being very difficult except in isolated, specific circumstances where the inert gas burden acquired from a dive (the depth-time profile) is insignificant (166,167). In any case, the treatment of the two conditions is now similar, so the decision, even if arrived at, does not modify management.

The neurological manifestations that can arise from arterial gas embolism are protean, as shown in Table 2. Some cases show a multiplicity of presenting symptoms and signs, and a feature of all of the cases in Table 2 was an onset time of less than 8 min from reaching the surface, with many becoming symptomatic within 5 min. This is not surprising, as a latent interval of less than 10 min has traditionally been used as an absolute diagnostic criterion for AGE. Unfortunately, it is now recognized that a short latency is not exclusive to AGE and can occur in decompression sickness (DCS). In a study of 1070 severe human cases, 56% were found to have become symptomatic within 10 min (169).

Because the neurological manifestations described above are very similar to those that occur in DCS (170), the two conditions may coexist (171), and the approach to management has, in many centers, been harmonised (see below), attempts to discriminate between the two have largely been abandoned in favor of a unified diagnosis of acute neurological decompression illness (DCI) (172). Nonetheless, one feature of DCS that is exceptionally rare in cases where the only credible mechanism is AGE is involvement of the spinal cord. In none of the cases involving submarine escape trainees reviewed by Benton et al. (115) was there a pattern of neurological deficit consistent with injury to the cord.

Table 2 Symptoms and Signs in the Diagnosis of Arterial Gas Embolism[a]

Symptoms and signs	Percentage incidence	
	Submarine escape training	Diving
Coma with convulsions	7	18
Coma without convulsions	29	22
Stupor and confusion	14	24
Collapse	8	4
Vertigo	14	8
Visual disturbance	6	9
Headache	2	1
Unilateral motor changes	17	14
Unilateral sensory changes	10	8
Unilateral motor and sensory changes	6	1
Bilateral motor changes	1	8
Bilateral sensory changes	1	1

[a]Symptoms and signs diagnosed as arterial gas embolism arising from 114 submarine escape training and 74 diving accidents.
Source: Ref. 168.

This contrasts markedly with the pattern of disease seen in classical DCS (124,173).

There are, unfortunately, few routine investigations of value. There are two reasons for this:

1. The emphasis of management following a clinical diagnosis is rapid recompression rather than further investigation.
2. Few investigations have been found to be useful.

Only a summary is therefore provided below.

A plain radiograph of the chest may confirm the presence of extrapulmonary gas, and this may be indicative of PBT. However, it may be an incidental finding, as the neurological manifestations may have been caused by bubbles evolved as a consequence of inappropriate decompression. It can also serve to alert the physician to the presence of a pneumothorax, which may require specific management during recompression (see below). Yet unless the film can be obtained without delay, it is not considered worthwhile to postpone the definitive management of AGE for a chest x-ray. Computed tomography of the brain has been used in the assessment of acute neurological DCI *after* recompression, but a number of studies have shown that this is of little value, as the false negative rate is unacceptably high (174–176). For the same reason, magnetic resonance imaging, single-photon-emission tomography, and positron-emission tomography have proved to be disappointing investigative tools (177–180).

Electrophysiology has been used extensively in the investigation of acute neurological DCI, both as a means of assessing progress during recompression as well as subsequent rehabilitation (181). The results to date indicate that the various available techniques may be of some use in particularly severe cases, but the requirement for meticulous technique and the wide range of normal responses render them of little practical utility in the clinical setting (182–184).

VI. Management of Pulmonary Barotrauma and Sequelae

A. Mediastinal Emphysema

Most cases require no active intervention and resolve spontaneously over a period of hours or days even in severe cases. In cases where there is pain or respiratory distress, breathing normobaric oxygen at a concentration as close to 100% as possible (normally using a tight-fitting mask and demand valve) will ameliorate the symptoms rapidly.

B. Pneumothorax

The management of pneumothorax diagnosed once the diver is on the surface is along the same conventional lines as for spontaneous pneumothorax (185,186). Small pneumothoraces may occur asymptomatically and avoid detection or management. Where the diagnosis is made, these normally resolve spontaneously over a period of a few days, a process that can be accelerated by providing the patient with a high partial pressure of oxygen (187). As with mediastinal emphysema, this should be as close to 1.0 bar as possible and be delivered for 6 to 8 hr. Larger pneumothoraces that provoke dyspnea should be aspirated, with formal intercostal tube drainage resorted to only if aspiration is unsuccessful. The presence of a pneumothorax is not a contraindication to recompression if the patient also displays neurological manifestations, because the priority in such cases is to manage the injury to the nervous system. Since compression serves to reduce the volume of a pneumothorax and the provision of hyperbaric oxygen will greatly increase the rate of absorption of the extrapulmonary gas, it has been argued that recompression may be an alternative to thoracocentesis as a means of managing a pneumothorax while under pressure (188,189).

However, caution needs to be exercised during decompression. Occasionally, a pneumothorax generated by PBT continues to leak. In such circumstances, there may be little or no reduction in the volume of the pneumothorax during the recompression and bottom phases of a therapeutic table. During ascent, the volume of extrapulmonary gas will increase, generating a tension pneumothorax. Should any patient display signs of respiratory distress during decompression, whether or not a pneumothorax was diagnosed previously, a tension pneumothorax should be suspected and decompression halted. If it is confirmed by physical examination (which can be difficult in a chamber, particularly in the rare instances where bilateral pneumothoraces have been sustained), the chamber should then be compressed slowly to a depth at which the symptoms are relieved. The choice of subsequent management will depend upon the circumstances and may be limited to further periods of oxygen breathing or aspiration of the pneumothorax. In general, intercostal tube drainage of pneumothoraces in compression chambers should be avoided because aseptic conditions are difficult to achieve and aspiration is equally effective (189).

C. Arterial Gas Embolism

First Aid

The first aid management of neurological decompression illness—in addition to attention to maintaining the airway, breathing, and circulation—is the provision of 100% oxygen, rehydration, and arranging transportation to a recompression facility (114,190). Oxygen is beneficial in two ways: It will serve to reduce any arterial hypoxemia and, by reducing the partial pressure of inert gas in arterial blood and tissues, increase the rate of resorption of bubbles.

Divers with DCI display some dehydration. There are a number of reasons for this:

1. The effect of immersion and cold, which is a consequence of diving in all but the warmest of water, is to provoke a diuresis. Experienced divers using dry suits recognize this and may voluntarily dehydrate themselves prior to a dive.
2. Despite advice to the contrary, some recreational divers upset their fluid balance by drinking alcohol prior to diving.
3. Circulating bubbles are injurious to endothelium and provoke the extravasation of fluid through a number of mechanisms (191).

The choice of fluid and its route will depend upon the circumstances. In field conditions where intravenous rehydration is not possible, the oral route may be used when the patient has control of his or her airway. In other circumstances, the intravenous route is the one of choice. There is no clear evidence of an advantage of crystalloid over colloid solutions. However, the use of dextran has theoretical disadvantages on the grounds of occasional anaphylactic reactions and its association with a prolonged bleeding time, particularly where large doses are used. This may compound the punctate hemorrhages that are characteristically found in gas embolic injury to the brain (192) and is associated with a poor outcome. Isotonic solutions are preferable to hypotonic fluids on the grounds that they will tend to limit tissue edema, although the association between cerebral edema and brain function following AGE is not good (193). Finally, the use of glucose-containing solutions is not recommended, as there is experimental evidence that they may impair the outcome (194–196).

Transport

The victims of AGE have traditionally been nursed and transported in a 30° head-down posture. This was advocated on the theory that arterial bubbles would, through their buoyancy, tend to be distributed away from dependent structures. Experimental evidence to support this hypothesis was provided by Van Allen et al. (197), Atkinson (198), and Gorman et al. (199). However, it is now recognized that bubble embolization is but the first in a sequence of events that lead to endothelial injury, breakdown of the blood brain barrier (BBB), and perivascular edema (191,200). A head-down posture will raise intracranial pressure and potentially increase the rate of leakage across the injured BBB, and there is experimental evidence to suggest that the outcome from such a maneuver is poorer than if the patient is nursed horizontally (201). In addition to the theoretical disadvantages of a head-down posture, there are practical difficulties, such as the problem of maintaining it, the additional discomfort imposed on the patient, and the limitations imposed on resuscitation efforts. It is therefore generally accepted that conscious patients should be nursed and transported horizontally. Unconscious patients should be placed prone with the head turned to one side, (the recovery position).

Recompression

The primary treatments for the neurological sequelae of PBT are recompression and the administration of hyperbaric oxygen. The principles underlying these are as follows:

1. The reduction of bubble size (an effect of Boyle's law). It is important to recognize that the effect of pressure on the volume of a spherical bubble is greater than on its diameter (Fig. 13) and that the magnitude of this effect becomes progressively less with increasing pressure. However, there is evidence that, during their passage through the cerebral vasculature, the bubbles become progressively elongated as they traverse ever narrower vessels until the frictional resistance between the bubble and the vessel wall exceeds the driving arterial pressure and they arrest in the circulation (202). Although the response of the vessel is maximal vasodilatation (203,204), the process is repeated until either the bubble passes into the venous side of the circulation or arrests, sausage-shaped, in an arteriole. In such circumstances, the effect of pressure is, initially, to reduce the length of the bubble. The magnitude of this effect is in direct

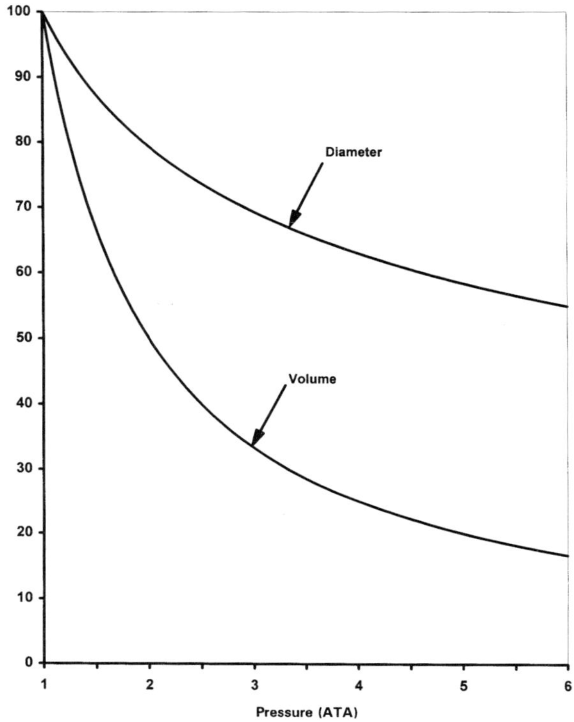

Figure 13 As the atmospheric pressure is increased, both the volume and diameter of a spherical bubble decreases, but the percentage decrease in volume is greater than in diameter.

proportion to the pressure applied and serves to reduce the frictional resistance and promote the clearance of the bubble.

2. To encourage the gaseous contents of the bubble to dissolve in surrounding tissues in accordance with Henry's law.

3. To promote the washout of inert gas from tissues and thereby provide an increased diffusion gradient for the inert gas constituents of the bubble into the surrounding tissues. It is recognized that the vasoconstriction induced by the administration of hyperbaric oxygen may slightly reduce this effect compared with the administration of 100% oxygen at sea level (205).

4. To enhance the oxygenation of hypoxic tissues. Because substantial amounts of oxygen can be carried in plasma under hyperbaric conditions, the oxygenation of tissues whose blood supply is compromised by the accumulation

of erythrocyte rouleaux (206) or aggregates of platelets (207) or leukocytes (208,209) may be improved.

5. Hyperbaric oxygen is a constrictor of cerebral vessels (210); therefore this effect may assist in reducing the perivascular edema consequent upon the breakdown of the BBB.

6. Hyperbaric oxygen has anti-inflammatory actions (210) that are likely to ameliorate the tissue reaction to injury provoked by the passage of bubbles through the cerebral circulation.

For many years it was thought that, of these two modalities, compression was the more important, and it was the practice in both the United States and British navies to select an initial treatment depth of 50 msw with the patient breathing either air or a mixture of 32½% oxygen/67½% nitrogen (U.S.N., Table 6A; R.N., Table 63—Fig. 14). These treatment tables were also extensively use by civilian authorities.

There are a number of practical difficulties and experimental observations that have increasingly served to raise doubts about the merit of this approach:

1. A treatment depth of 50 msw is normally achievable only in large, multiplace chambers. If only a small, monoplace chamber is available, an alternative strategy is required.
2. A principle of the use of this table is that the ascent from 50 to 18 msw should be undertaken only if the patient is asymptomatic. If not, then the therapeutic protocol is liable to become very protracted, lasting for as long as 3 days, which only well-equipped chambers can support.
3. If the chamber is compressed on air, as is commonly done, both the patient and the attendant are exposed to a narcotic concentration of nitrogen. This inevitably compromises the quality of the decision as to whether the patient is asymptomatic as well as other practical aspects of the management of the casualty.
4. Employing such a deep treatment depth means that both the patient and the attendant will absorb a substantial amount of inert gas and thereby incur a decompression obligation. This means that the chamber cannot be quickly surfaced in the event of an emergency without injury to the attendant and inflicting a further decompression insult on the casualty.
5. Decompression sickness has traditionally been treated at shallower depths in many centers. The U.S. and British navies have, for many years, used a short oxygen table with a maximum depth of 18 msw (Fig. 15) (211). Since it is now acknowledged that discriminating between DCS and AGE is, in most circumstances, very difficult or

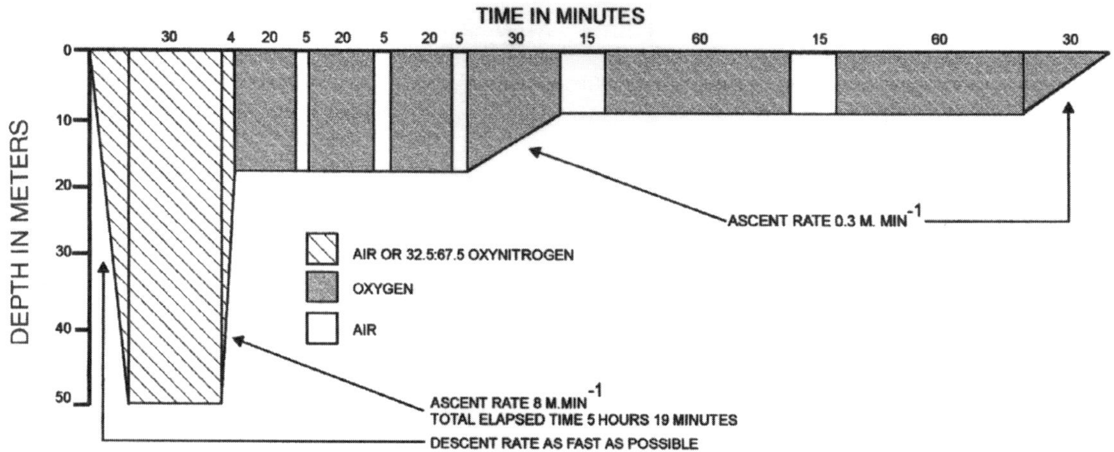

Figure 14 Royal Navy Treatment Table 63 (U.S.N. 6A). A treatment table that was designed specifically for the treatment of arterial gas embolism following pulmonary barotrauma. The initial compression is to 50 msw. If the patient is asymptomatic after a period of 25 min, ascent to 18 msw is followed by an identical pressure profile to R.N. Treatment Table 62 (Fig. 15). If there are persistent symptoms or signs, the R.N. protocol is for a 2-hr stay at 50 msw followed by a slow decompression on Table 64 (not shown), which takes a further 37 hr. It is important that both the chamber and available manpower be adequate to complete such long treatments.

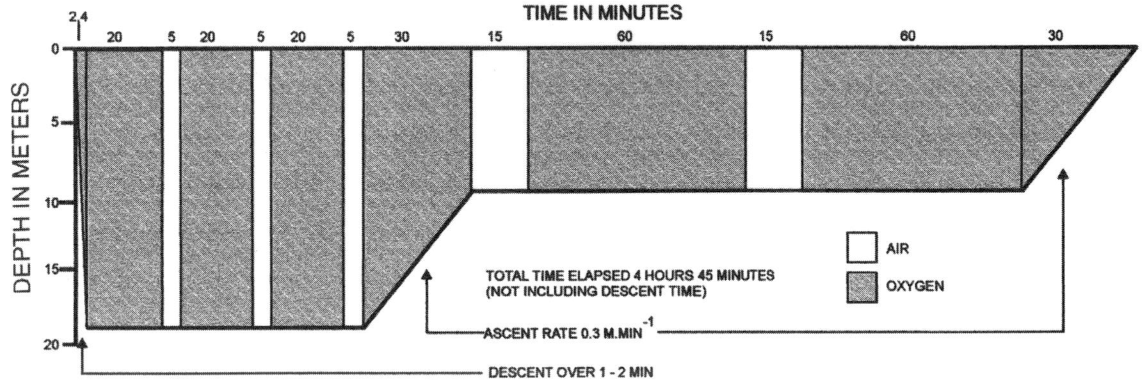

Figure 15 Royal Navy Treatment Table 62 (U.S.N. 6). This table is now widely used for the management of all forms of decompression illness. It can be used in a highly flexible manner, titrating the dosage of oxygen to the clinical status of the patient. This is achieved by extending the table with additional oxygen-breathing periods (and air breaks) at either 18 or 9 msw. The attendant(s) have to breathe oxygen for at least the final 30 min at 9 msw (1 hr for TT 63) and during the bleed to the surface. The duration of oxygen-breathing is determined by the number of extensions to the table.

impossible, the logic of selecting different treatment depths is highly questionable.

6. If a gas mixture of 32½/67½ oxynitrogen (as advocated by the Royal Navy) is not available, the $P_{I_{O_2}}$ at 50 msw is only 1.26 bar. This is far less than can be achieved using a shallow oxygen table.
7. There is experimental evidence that the great majority of gas that enters the cerebral circulation has only a short residence time (197,212). Since there is inevitably a delay in recompressing a casualty, it is probable that the effects of hyperbaric oxygen will predominate over those of compression.
8. A series of experimental studies has shown that there is no advantage to compression beyond 2.8 bar with respect to the clearance of bubbles from the cerebral circulation and functional outcome (212–216). There are also anecdotal reports in the literature in support of the authors' experience that acute neurological DCI can be satisfactorily managed using a short oxygen table, such as that shown in Fig. 15 (217,218).

Because of these arguments, there is a trend away from initiating treatment at 50 msw in favor of 18 msw, or 2.8 bar (219), leaving open the option of increasing the depth in very serious cases that continue to deteriorate. The maximum pressure at which the patient can breathe pure oxygen is 2.8 bar, and even at this pressure occasional episodes of central nervous system oxygen toxicity occur (220). If greater pressure is to be employed, the oxygen in the breathing mixture supplied to the patient has to be diluted with an inert gas. Because of its abundance, nitrogen has traditionally been used, although more recently interest has been shown in helium, and tables have been designed for its use (e.g. Fig. 16). One very practical benefit of using heliox is that nitrogen narcosis is avoided, which benefits the patient and attendant alike. Because the number of centers with the capability to provide heliox treatments is small, the experience of its use is limited. However, there is also some experimental and anecdotal evidence to suggest that this approach may be beneficial in decompression sickness (221–224), although there are no data to support the use of heliox in the management of purely embolic injuries. It will take well-controlled, randomized trials to establish the extent of any benefit, and it is unfortunate that, to date, such trials are notable only for their rarity in the field of hyperbaric medicine.

Adjunctive Treatments

There are few adjuncts to hyperbaric oxygen and fluid resuscitation that have been shown to be beneficial. Perhaps the most promising is lignocaine. A series of animal studies (225–228) and anecdotal case reports such as that by Drewry

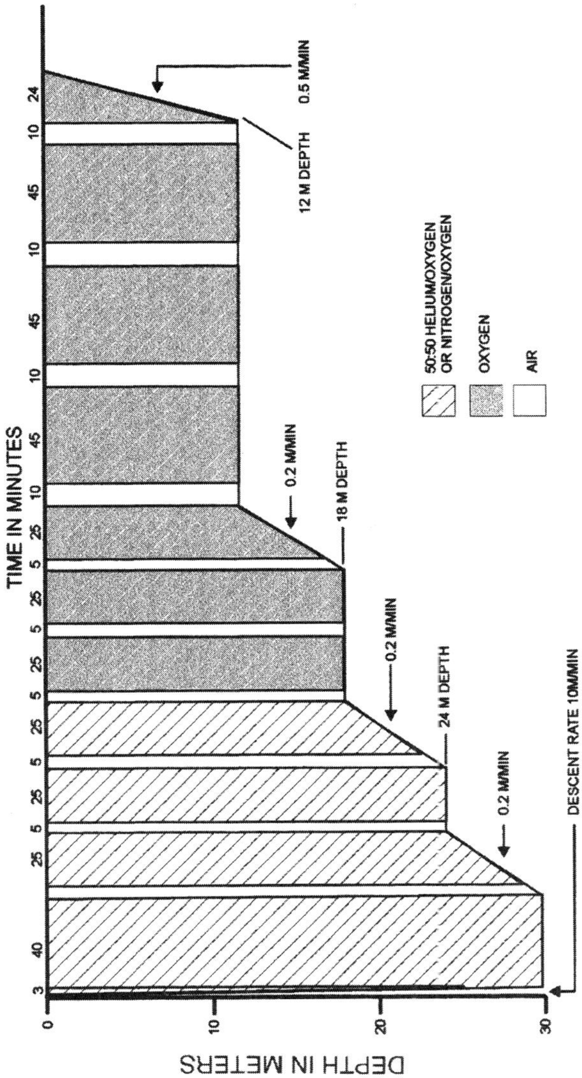

Figure 16 COMEX Table 30. This French table is used principally in commercial diving for the management of serious DCI. Although designed for use with 50:50 heliox, a 50:50 nitrox mixture can be used, as shown.

and Gorman (229) indicate that lignocaine promotes the recovery of brain function following gas embolism, and this effect is additive to that gained with hyperbaric oxygen. Unfortunately, no randomized trial of its use in humans has yet been undertaken. The other class of drug that has been used extensively in the management of gas embolism is that of the corticosteroids (29,119,164). However, despite early enthusiasm, there is little persuasive evidence that they are effective, in anti-inflammatory or larger doses, in an experimental model (230)—even when administered prior to the embolic insult—in humans (152,231).

VII. Summary

In the introduction to this chapter, we recognized that it is better to prevent pulmonary barotrauma than to rely on treatment that, for geographical reasons, may have to be delayed. However, a substantial proportion of cases occur for no apparent reason or for reasons that have been suggested only recently and have yet to be proved. The preventive measures in such circumstances should be aimed at avoiding situations liable to provoke the condition. Of these, training and experience are probably the most important. Military and most professional diving are subject to regulations designed to ensure this. Sports diving is not subject to such regulations, and it falls to diving clubs and associations to promote diving safety. The wearing of properly fitting equipment, the careful planning of dives and diving that plan, and avoiding emergency (panic) ascents and other hazardous underwater maneuvers are obvious precautions. The proper supervision of novices is another important preventive measure.

A more difficult area for prevention is the avoidance of diving with conditions that may predispose to PBT. The problem is that, up to now, the presence (or occasionally even history) of any pulmonary pathology has been considered a bar to diving. Consequently, there are no reliable data on which to base a risk assessment for each condition. When combined with the recognition that the precise mechanisms involved in pulmonary rupture are incompletely understood, defining rational pulmonary "fitness to dive" criteria is beyond mortal beings. It is hardly surprising that discussions on the subject all too readily degenerate into the airing of unsubstantiated, preconceived notions, anecdotes, and individual prejudice. Despite our personal experience and the work we have undertaken to prepare this review, we do not consider ourselves to be in a position to define hard and fast fitness criteria.

An obvious requirement is that pulmonary function must be adequate to sustain a sufficient level of aerobic activity for a diver to rescue him or herself or a buddy. The problem lies in defining that level and how it should be measured. It is possible to generate a list of conditions that may increase an individual's risk of developing PBT. The problems lie in defining how the condition is diagnosed—particularly as investigations become ever more sensitive, quantifying the risk, and determining what level of risk is acceptable.

We consider the way to overcome these problems is to expand the quantity and quality of available information. In addition to basic research into the mechanisms of lung rupture, we feel that a new approach to determining pulmonary fitness to dive is required. Rather than perpetuate a system of absolute and relative disqualifying criteria, we feel that these should be relaxed in gradual steps, but that this process should be undertaken only in conjunction with rigorous surveillance for and recording of diving accidents. Each step of relaxation being taken only if the incidence of PBT has not shown a statistically significant increase following the previous relaxation. Clearly, such an approach cannot be adopted by all diving populations, as it will require organization, resources, and, above all, time. However, without such an initiative, we feel that entry into the diving population will continue to be constrained by fitness criteria which, although well intentioned, are arbitrary and difficult to justify.

The situation with respect to treatment is little better. Neither the tables nor adjunctive medications have been subjected to controlled, randomized, blinded clinical trials. As a result, the optimal regimen for the management of acute neurological DCI remains a matter of opinion. A fundamental problem facing those who would like to remedy this situation is that few centers in the world deal with a sufficient number of cases each year to undertake such trials in a reasonable time frame. Thus, the difficulty of undertaking blinded trials in compression chambers is compounded by the necessity for multicenter and, almost certainly, international studies. It can therefore only be hoped that progress will be made in this direction, as it will take more than the persuading of individuals to undertake the necessary work.

Appendix: Case Reports

The 16 case records below come from some 250 divers and submariners with actual or suspected lung disorders whose clinical care was shared between the Institute of Naval Medicine in Alverstoke and the Royal Brompton Hospital in London. They illustrate the difficulties we experienced in diagnosing and treating pulmonary barotrauma and determining "fitness to dive" thereafter.

Case 1. A Trainee Naval Pilot, Age 19, on an Escape-and-Survival Course

Intellectually able, a good athlete and swimmer, taking part in an arduous survival course. This finished with a phase where he was "captured," interrogated, blindfolded, and left standing in the stress position (arms overhead leaning forward against a wall) for an hour or two. A bread roll was slammed into his mouth; he was then given half a glass of water but could not use his hands as he had to maintain the position. Five minutes later he experienced retrosternal discomfort.

When debriefed 11 hr later, the diver's voice was noted to sound ''funny'' and intermittently high-pitched. He had some soup and bread with no noticeable discomfort, but the rest of his team ''fell about laughing at his Mickey Mouse voice.'' He noted retrosternal pain on taking a deep breath and was seen by a Medical Officer, who diagnosed ''stress'' and arranged to see him again in 2 days. Later the same day he noticed crepitus over both shoulders, confirmed by another member of his team. His odd voice and bubbly skin persisted. Two days later, the Medical Officer noted subcutaneous emphysema and diagnosed a spontaneous pneumomediastinum.

Posteroanterior chest radiography confirmed the pneumomediastinum; no other pathology seen. Ear, nose, and throat review was negative. Ten days' sick leave was given. Repeat chest film showed resolution. Two weeks later, the diver's lung function and exercise tests were supernormal in all respects, as were contiguous CT scans of his lungs from apex to base in inspiration and again in expiration. We use the inspiratory scans to reveal abnormal opacities and defects of filling and the expiratory scans to reveal abnormal lucencies and defects of emptying. On the basis of these results and the absence of further signs and symptoms in the ensuing 3 months, the trainee returned to ''full flying and diving duties.''

Comment. Apart from indicating the extent to which the Armed Forces go to prepare their men for hostile interrogation, this case illustrates the difficulty of determining where the air in the mediastinum had come from. This man was not exposed to an important change in ambient pressure and extensive investigations failed to reveal any objective evidence of lung damage, yet he had a pneumomediastinum. In the circumstances it seemed reasonable to diagnose a traumatic pneumomediastinum, with a low recurrence rate, and find him fit to fly and dive after 3 months had elapsed.

Case 2. A 42-Year-Old Sports Diver with a Predive Traumatic Pneumothorax

This senior research technician in the pharmaceutical industry and moderate sportsman had no relevant medical history and had several years of problem-free sports diving experience, with some 350 dives to a maximum depth of 60 m.

On the third day of a diving holiday off the Sinai Peninsula, the diver completed a surface swim at 0830 hr and a 49-min dive to a maximum depth of 20 msw (with a slow ascent) at 1000 hr. Back on board the tender, he went for a surface swim at 1130 hr but slipped, falling heavily against the boat's rail and hitting his chest high on right side. It was very painful but there was no obvious bruising. At 1400 hr he made another surface swim, but was fairly sore and could not duck dive and snorkel as well as normally.

At 1500 hr the diver conducted his second dive, this time to 30 msw, ascending to 15 msw with 8 to 9 min of nonstop time in hand. He left 15 msw and became acutely dyspneic at 8 msw but made a controlled ascent, stopping for 1 min at 6 msw. On arrival at the surface he was in severe respiratory distress. An immediate diagnosis of right pneumothorax was made (was on a vessel full of medical students and nurses). He was given oxygen, but from a demand valve that was painful to draw on. Free-flow attempts wasted too much gas (and might have aggravated his lesion). Subcutaneous emphysema was also present, but no obvious neurological symptoms or signs. Four hours later, he arrived at a compression chamber, where the diagnosis of traumatic pneumothorax not requiring compression was made. The tension pneumothorax was relieved by a chest drain. A chest film showed a fracture of the right second rib. He made an uneventful recovery.

Seen several months later, the fracture had healed and the pneumothorax completely resorbed. As more than three incident-free months had elapsed, he was declared fit to dive.

Comment. This case shows the importance of *not* diving after even a modest blunt chest injury. After such injuries, divers should wait for 3 days to see if traumatic pneumothorax appears. Simple closed traumatic pneumothoraces heal quickly and rarely recur. Hence such divers are generally fit to dive after 3 months.

Case 3. Traumatic Pneumothorax During Dive in a 27-Year-Old Commercial Diver

This mentally and physically robust commercial diver played rugby to county standards, preferred contact sports to less brutal forms of physical endeavor, joined the Navy at age 16 for excitement but, despite being on the Field Gun Display Team, was disappointed and transferred to the Marines and then to commercial diving, where he undertook mainly coastal work, on air, to 50 msw. No previous chest disease or diving accidents. Assisted with the laying of a major storm drain off the Irish Coast.

The drain was 1½ to 2 m in diameter and 350 m long, with the landward end sealed by a metal grid and the upturned and flanged distal end by a heavy plate kept in place by 32 bolts. Tap valves in center of the plate allowed air to be vented from the drain before the plate was removed. The diver was told that the drain was full of water and he was required to unbolt the plate and attach it to the hook and chain of a barge crane. To do this, he stood about waist high in an annular concrete collar some 1½ m wider than the pipe and flange. On completion of this task, the crane lifted the plate, but the pipe was still full of air. Water rushed in and he was angled over the pipe and swept along it, tumbling all the way until, some 50 m into the pipe, he was halted by his air line. His lifeline and communication link had been severed. Although severely injured and disoriented, he reasoned correctly that his air line would lead him to the open end of the drain, where he would be met the standby diver. As they ascended, his chest pain got markedly worse. On the barge, his suit was cut away, revealing gross surgical emphysema extending from his neck over the right hemithorax and arm and onto the abdomen. He was given 100% oxygen and arrived at the local hospital 45 min later. Good air entry on left, poor on right, neck veins distended—a right tension pneumothorax was diagnosed. A chest drain was inserted prior to x-ray. Films revealed fractures of eighth, ninth, and possibly seventh ribs; no bony injury to the pelvis. Over the next few days his surgical emphysema spread and his pneumothorax slowly resorbed (on continuous drainage). He left the hospital with some patchy shadowing at right base to return to the United Kingdom (by boat, not air).

Ten weeks later the diver's lung function had returned to superfit premorbid values, but a plain chest film showed the rib fractures to be unhealed, the transverse fissure prominent, and considerable opacity over the right lower zone. Computed tomography displayed substantial unloculated right-sided effusion spreading into the transverse fissure, with some slight folding of the right upper lobe but no other signs of lung damage. The unhealed ends of the ribs were probably responsible for persistent effusion, which was probably sanguineous and likely to become organized/infected. The patient went for surgery and made a gradual recovery but was then rated permanently unfit to dive.

Comment. This patient had a classic tension pneumothorax and continuously developing subcutaneous emphysema, although there was no mention of a pneumomediastinum in any of the radiological reports. There is no way of knowing which preceded what. The diver's life was saved by his own professionalism and first-class care in the local hospital.

Cases 4 and 5. Fatal and Near-Fatal Barotrauma in Two Inexperienced Divers

These cases concern a young man and his best friend's bride. The man had learnt to scuba dive over a period of a couple of years by means of about 10 dives in a gravel pit, using borrowed equipment and instructed by his father. The girl had made about 10 dives in a local swimming pool as a student. The girl married the man's best friend and, very soon after, the couple invited the man to join them to dive on holiday off the coast of South Wales. The man and the girl met for the first time early one afternoon on the beach. The man had borrowed a wet suit and weight belt from another friend who was substantially larger than he. About 4 p.m., not realizing that dusk comes early to the sea, the man and the girl decided to go in search of fish for tea. The friend/husband stayed on the beach. Neither diver had dived in the sea before. They followed the gently sloping, sandy bottom to a maximum depth of 27 feet. The man, whose suit was too large and whose borrowed weight belt was too heavy, bumped his way along the bottom throwing up clouds of sand, which added to the sense of a darkening, sinister gloom. He panicked and signaled to the girl that he was going up. They arrived at the surface together. She died instantly; he lost consciousness a minute or two later. Upon being seen from the beach, they were dragged from the water and he was taken to the local hospital, which wisely refused him entry and sent him directly to the local naval chamber, where he regained consciousness.

Subsequent lung-function tests revealed a mild obstructive defect probably related to the young man's previous smoking habit. Computed tomography showed a healed tear in one lung. He was deemed permanently unfit to dive.

Comment. Needless death and injury from diving in dark, open water using unfamiliar kit, without proper training. Panic is one of the commonest causes of death from diving. Proper training is lifesaving; prevention is much more effective than necessarily late attempts at cure.

Case 6. A 24-Year-Old Submariner Referred Because of a Low Forced Vital Capacity

This man had been a submariner for 7 years, having passed two submarine escape training courses without incident and no symptoms whatsoever. He was referred immediately before his third escape course because of the findings by Brooks and Pethybridge (62) that small lungs for body size predisposed divers and submariners to lung rupture.

A full set of routine lung-function tests showed that the diver's FVC, TLC, and RV were below the lower limits for healthy men of his age, but his carbon monoxide transfer per liter of accessible gas volume (KCO) was slightly raised. This suggested that lung expansion was limited from without rather than within the lung (232). Pulmonary compliance was normal at 0.21 L/cmH_2O. Contiguous CT scans of lungs from apex to base during full inspiration showed patchy pleural thickening over the whole of the right lung plus bilateral tenting of the diaphragm and a medial right pleural invagination. Late in the course of these inspiratory scans, the diver developed a wholly asymptomatic pneumomediastinum, which was obvious on the expiratory scans that followed (Fig. 17). It extended up the aortic sheath to the carotids and down the sheath into the abdomen. Repeat lung function tests and chest radiograph were unchanged the following morning.

The diver was discharged with the recommendation that he be fit for submarine duty but not for further escape training until at least 3 incident-free months had elapsed and his case had been discussed in detail.

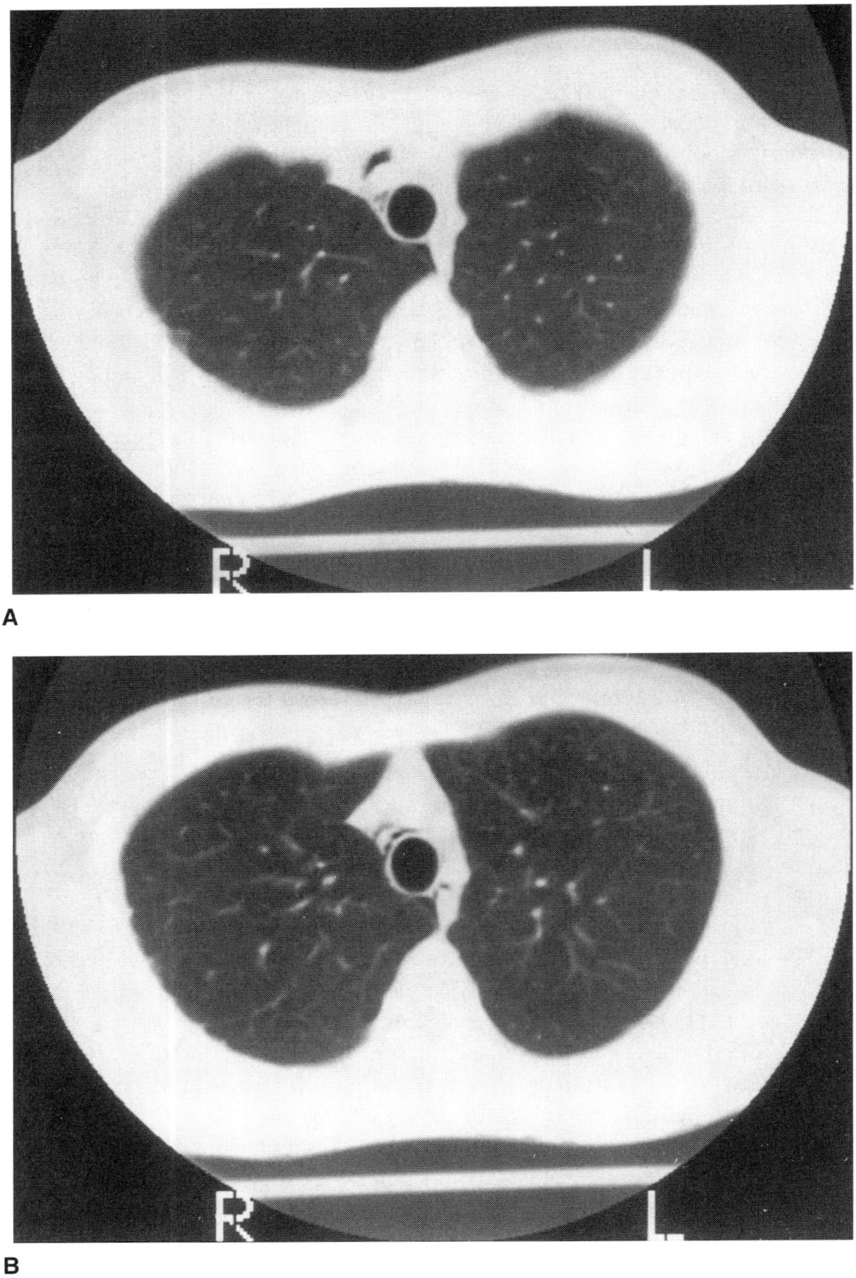

A

B

Figure 17 CT scan of mediastinal emphysema (Case 6). These cross-sectional views of the upper thorax show a pneumomediastinum initiated by deep inspirations on the scanning table. Both views show air surrounding the trachea. The upper view also shows a substantial pocket of air in front of the brachiocephalic vein.

Comment. This case supports the views of Colebatch (60,61) and of Brooks and Pethybridge (62) that lungs which are small for body size are liable to rupture. It also shows that simply taking deep breaths in the absence of any change in ambient pressure can provoke this. It prompted us to review the CT scans of some 200 other divers, which revealed one other who developed a small pneumomediastinum on the scanning table.

Case 7. Traumatic Pneumothorax in a 25-Year-Old Commercial Diver

The diver grew up and trained as a commercial diver in Kenya, New Zealand, and the United States. He returned to work in Uganda. A wholly innocent victim, he was hit from behind by three bullets in crossfire between police and a local drug gang. He drove 2 mi with one hand, lying crouched on the front seat and being mistakenly pursued and shot at by police. He arrived at the hospital almost exsanguinated. Radiographs showed one bullet lodged in the lumbar spine; the second destroyed the right kidney and splintered into the liver; while the third was deflected upward, bouncing up the right rib cage, and finishing about 1 cm deep in the right lung. Complete collapse of right lung meant that this was seen only when the lung reflated. He underwent immediate surgery and transfusion and made a slow recovery.

Several months later, when the diver's lung function was supranormal, a CT scan showed that the third bullet lay in the medial segment of the right middle lobe, with no obvious track through adjacent lung. There was no pneumothorax but some pleural thickening in the transverse fissure and at the right base, consistent with the previous right hemothorax as well as some distortion of subpleural lung in right lower lobe. The surgical consensus was that despite the proximity to the heart and great vessels, the third bullet was best left in situ.

Comment. This traumatic pneumothorax was associated with substantial pleural and some lung damage, rendering the patient permanently unfit to dive.

Case 8. A 23-Year-Old Submariner

Born and raised in the countryside, this diver had a healthy childhood but for slight eczema. He was not considered ''chesty'' and there was no mention of asthma. A reasonable sportsman, cross-country runner, and good swimmer, he joined the Navy as a medical assistant at age 19. In the Submarine Service, 18 months later, his spirometry was normal and he passed the submarine escape training course, which includes rapid ascents from 28 msw, without incident.

Seventeen months later, the diver was aboard a moored submarine undergoing a routine leak test in which the compartment pressure dropped quite slowly by some 50 mmHg. It was held at that slightly subatmospheric pressure for 30 min and then equalized with outside pressure over 10 to 15 sec. The diver noted nothing abnormal through the test, cycled the 7 m home at speed, enjoyed an active but not overvigorous night, and cycled back to the submarine the next morning. At 10 a.m. he noticed a definite precordial pain, and at 3 p.m. he observed that deep breathing caused a sharp right basal and left apical chest pain that was aggravated by swallowing. A medical officer diagnosed esophagitis, but ordered a chest radiograph to exclude the remote possibility of pneumomediastinum. Feeling it was too late to get a chest x-ray that day, the patient cycled home at speed with similar symptoms as before, complicated by some worsening of the pain on swallowing. The next morning, feeling somewhat better, he got a lift to the boat with a friend and began work. Some hours later he remembered to have the chest film taken. It showed a pneumomediastinum extending along the heart borders and up above the aortic arch. It resolved without treatment over the next few days.

Five weeks later a full set of lung function tests (maximal flow–volume loop, whole-body plethysmography, and carbon monoxide transfer) were normal or supernormal, as were contiguous CT scans of his lungs from apex to base in full inspiration and full expiration. Esophagoscopy revealed nothing abnormal, but esophageal function tests showed a sustained acidity and some reduction in motility of the middle segment.

Comment. The pressure drop in the leak test on the submarine was equivalent to taking several minutes to ascend through the top 2 ft of seawater while breathing freely: recompression at the end of test was equivalent to the first several seconds of a very lazy duck dive. Spontaneous pneumomediastinums are frequently asymptomatic and therefore underdiagnosed. They often, as here, take many hours to develop. In the absence of pathology, they rarely recur. This man was found medically fit to fly and dive after an incident-free interval of 3 months.

Case 9. A 34-Year-Old Commercial Diver Who Was Pulled up Too Fast

An intelligent, well-balanced underwater welder, this diver was working off the Indian coast to a maximum depth of 180 msw. He had had normal childhood illnesses plus chickenpox at the age of 16 years. He was repairing the interior of an underwater habitat at a depth of 26 msw when, a few minutes into the dive, his surface demand supply flew off. He had to take his helmet off to get at his scuba reserve, so he took a good look around to memorize his escape route before doing so. Helmet off and effectively blind, he found that the pillar valve of the scuba set had jammed. By then, however, his buddy outside the habitat had spotted the escaping surface-supplied air. They buddy-breathed to the bottom of the shot line and alerted topside that the diver was in trouble and was coming up. Suddenly the victim realized that he was being pulled up very fast, attributed it to a known troublesome manta ray, and struggled to breathe out continuously. At the surface, he found that topside had panicked and pulled him up at speed. Ten minutes later he was instructed to go back down and finish the job. He did so, working on the habitat for 2 hr. He then made a controlled ascent, but, stopping at 6 msw, felt that he was drowning. He could not tell topside, who were using RT to talk to another diver. At the surface, he coughed up half a cupful of blood, to which the supervisor is said to have responded "Ah, you have been taking aspirin again!" He was given a surface decompression (not therapeutic) profile starting at 12 msw on intermittent oxygen. Although he demanded a therapeutic table, he was told it was not necessary. On leaving the chamber he was examined by a medical attendant, who thought he had some fluid on the lung, having probably inhaled water. He was kept at sea level for 1 week before flying back to the United Kingdom.

When the diver was seen 14 months later, plain films showed calcific shadows but nothing else. A full set of routine lung function tests proved normal, as did perfusion and ventilation records obtained from each lobe during fiberoptic bronchoscopy. More than three incident-free months had passed, so he was deemed fit to dive.

Comment. Uncontrolled ascents can come from unintended suit or buoyancy-compensator inflation, overrapid bell ascents (see Case 16), pressure vessel failures (233), or, as here, topside panic. The diver's responses were exemplary and highly professional. Those of the people at sea level were not. As before, proper training is vital and prevention is much better than attempted cure.

Case 10. One of Several Divers "Skip Breathing" but Ascending Normally

We have seen at least five trainee naval divers who have given virtually identical histories, thus questioning the safety of the widespread technique of skip breathing. Early in the naval diving course, participants spend several hours a day under water, completing endurance swims, following a jackstay laid on the horizontal concrete base of an old torpedo testing range at a maximum depth of 9 msw. Current culture demands that they stay down as long as possible on the self-contained air supply provided; coming up early is considered "wimpish." To conserve air, most men take occasional very deep breaths and hold themselves at TLC for as long as possible at every breath. Each swim lasts 50 to 60 min and is terminated before the gas supply runs out completely by a controlled ascent.

This case concerns a 22-year-old naval officer who, on the day in question, completed six jackstay swims as described above. All the dives were unremarkable. There were no rapid or uncontrolled ascents, and each time he made sure to breathe out continuously as he slowly came to the surface.

After the third dive, the trainee noted mild central pain on inspiration. There was no radiation or shortness of breath. He continued to dive and noticed that these symptoms resolved at depth and returned on ascent. There were no neurological symptoms. He experienced mild dysphagia at home that evening but did not report it. He awoke the next morning with surgical emphysema of the neck and upper chest plus a pneumomediastinum on chest x-ray. These resolved without treatment over the next few days.

When the diver was seen 3 months later, a full set of routine lung-function tests were normal. Computed tomography at full inspiration from apex to base was normal, but the expiratory scans revealed a small subpleural bleb on the phrenic surface of the right lung plus, possibly, some air around the descending thoracic aorta. Repeat scans 1 month later showed that the bleb was still present but the para-aortic air had gone. He was deemed medically unfit to dive.

Comment. This case and several others like it have drawn attention to the vital importance of avoiding taking really deep breaths before or during a dive. In most cases of subcutaneous emphysema (implicitly accompanied by a minor and asymptomatic pneumomediastinum), we would declare the patient fit to dive 3 incident-free months later. Subpleural blebs away from the sharp edges of the phrenic surface of the lung are uncommon and are associated with previous hyperinflation, especially in infants. In this case the presence of the bleb swung the decision the other way, although objective evidence to support this decision is lacking.

Case 11. A 32-Year-Old Diver with Pleurectomy and Oversewn Apical Bullae

This man was exceptionally fit and a keen sport diver. At age 29, he developed a large, spontaneous left tension pneumothorax. He proceeded to pleurectomy and oversewing of apical bullae ''because he was a keen sub-aqua devotee.'' Surgical entry via the sixth rib (not resected), pleura resected to level of hilum all round and removed. Full recovery within 1 month but for residual elevation of left hemidiaphragm with some pleural thickening.

The man resumed diving 15 months later and has made very many dives since, including several rapid ascents. He was a U.K. diving instructor and had equivalent qualifications from German and French diving associations. Three years later, on the occasion of his diving medical, he was referred because of his history. His lung-function results were normal in all measured respects. Chest x-ray, read by the then Director of Radiology at the Royal Brompton National Heart and Lung Hospital, was ''normal but for little basal thickening. No evidence of air trapping or other features of significance.'' Computed tomography at the same time showed cystic area in *left* upper zone, which did not empty completely on expiration, with similar findings at the right apex and possibly the left base. Eventually, he was found fit to dive.

Comment. A very difficult case raising an important precedent. Without the CT scan, the diver would be judged, on the basis of the best lung function and chest radiology available, to be fit to dive. The scan showed information we would not have had before, revealing that the surgery on the left lung had left him with trapped gas anteriorly, which could not be seen in posteroanterior or lateral views. Taking account of these would open the floodgates to a quite impractical need for CT scans on all divers, even if they had normal lung function and chest radiographs. This would impose unacceptable costs and radiation burdens. If no account were taken of the scans, we could be accused of knowingly allowing men to dive with abnormal lungs, but this diver had dived successfully with these very same lungs for 3 or 4 years and had made some rapid ascents with them. Should we have acted on clinical suspicion and perhaps poorly documented folklore or the evidence of the diver's uneventful experience? The latter view prevailed, hence fit to dive.

Case 12. A 33 Year-Old Trainee Submariner with Bilateral Apical Disease

A 33-year old trainee submariner who transferred from another branch, this man had had normal childhood illnesses and nothing else, specifically no history of tuberculosis. He had been a keen sportsman since boyhood. His inspiratory and expiratory chest radiographs immediately prior to escape training were considered normal in all respects. During escape training, he completed two ascents from 9 m with no problems. On leaving the water after an 18-m ascent, he stumbled on the ladder, felt unwell, and slowly developed a right hemiparesis. He was immediately recompressed to 50 msw with a rapid reversal of symptoms and signs but for hyperreflexia and bilateral ankle clonus, which has persisted since and may have been present before. An HMPAO-SPECT brain scan on the same day was interpreted as demonstrating a left-sided abnormality, in keeping with his right-sided hemiparesis.

The diver was investigated one week later to discover whether there was a contributory pulmonary cause. Routine lung-function tests were normal in all respects for an ex-smoker. Conventional inspiratory, expiratory, and apical radiographs of the chest were also normal. The CT scans of his chest showed bilateral pleural fibrosis and several small bullae at each apex which, even in retrospect, could not be seen on the plain films. The fibrosis must certainly have been present before the incident. We think the bullae, which were intact and thin-walled, must also have been present before. No abnormality was detected in cerebral CT scans. It was recommended that he be rated unfit for diving or submarine escape training.

Comment. Scanning by HMPAO was in its infancy at this time and capable of being overinterpreted, which is a serious problem with novel and increasingly sensitive imaging techniques, as is true of CT scanning here. Many more people have apical bullae than ever have spontaneous pneumothoraces.

Epidemiological data are badly needed. This diver's pleural fibrosis swung the ''unfit'' decision.

Case 13. A 42-Year-Old Submarine Escape Training Officer

This diver had had normal childhood illnesses. He joined the Navy at age 15 and had pneumonia 1 year later, nothing else. He joined the submarine service at age 19 and became a Ship's Diver and Escape Training Instructor. He undertook many free ascents from 9, 18, and 28 msw each week while training others and had undertaken four previous deep escapes, all successfully.

In 1987 the diver took part in ''world record'' deep escape trials off Norway, making successful, incident-free escapes from 30, 90, 120, and 150 msw. Two days later made an ascent from 180 msw. During the compression phase, he noticed that his hood had collapsed slightly, so he delayed his exit from the tower briefly to inflate it (otherwise he would have come out ''vacuum-wrapped,'' with insufficient buoyancy). His total bottom time was 31.7 sec, which was 1.7 sec over the limit according to Navy tables. He experienced some gut pain at 30 m, which was relieved at the surface by belching. He had no other symptoms until 10 min later, when he developed left facial paresthesia and paresis and a staggering gait. He was immediately recompressed to 50 msw with complete resolution of his symptoms and has remained well subsequently.

The diver was referred for lung-function and CT studies to help determine the cause. Was it arterial gas embolism or decompression sickness? His spirometry was normal or better, but there was evidence of some gas trapping (shortfall of VA on TLC) and a high KCO, suggestive of slight bleeding into the lung. Computed tomography in inspiration and expiration showed small but definite cysts on the phrenic surface of the right lower lobe, which did not empty on expiration. Because of this finding, it was concluded that barotrauma was a more likely diagnosis than decompression sickness. Repeat tests 6 months later were identical suggesting that the carbon monoxide transfer was not reflecting recent hemorrhage. Therefore the man was rated fit to dive.

Comment. Difficult decision affecting the life of a brave man. We are still unsure whether it was right or not. This emphasizes the lack of hard evidence in this field. Good multicenter epidemiological studies to common standards are needed because no one country has enough data.

Case 14. A 41-Year-Old Submarine Escape Training Instructor

This man had had normal childhood illnesses, and nothing else. He joined the Navy at age 15 and the Submarine Service at 18. He served at sea until age 22. But for a 2-year break at sea, he had been an Escape Training Instructor for the following 19 years, making several ascents a week from 9, 18, and 28 m. He also took part in five deep escape trials. In the last of these, after successful escapes from 30 msw, he proceeded to one from 90 m. Midway through the ascent, he noted a transient sharp pain in the right mid-axillary line rising to the axilla. It disappeared soon after he reached the surface. Conventional chest films from several angles, taken at Bergen Hospital, were all normal. He returned to full-time escape instructing.

Seven months later this man took 10 others through the 9-m lock and was at that pressure for about 15 min. The following day he made three open bell dives to 27 m to pick up some heavy (40-lb) metal plates from the floor of the tower. His total dive time was 18 min. During the last bell ascent, breathing freely from the bell air, he coughed slightly from irritation of cold vapor (adiabatic cooling), which was quite normal. Some 20 min later noted left-sided paresthesia and incoordination spreading up from the leg to the head. He was quickly recompressed on RN Table 63. His symptoms disappeared at 20 msw. No memory of breath-holding or of any chest symptoms during the ascent (Bell ascents take about 30 sec from 28 m, compared with 10 sec for a hooded ascent and 100 sec for an unassisted free ascent).

Six weeks later, routine lung function tests were normal in all respects but CT scans of the diver's lungs showed the right apex traversed by a line of solid tissue, almost certainly a shallow pleural fold separating a small posteromedial part of the apex from the rest. The separated part appeared normally aerated and vascularized; it was therefore not a bullus but possibly a frustrated representation of an azygous lobe. Expiratory scans showed that the separated part emptied normally, but a volume of about 10 ml at the apex of the right lower lobe and a smaller spherical volume in the right costophrenic recess did not. It was recommended that he be rated unfit for diving or escape instructing.

Comment. The development of DCS after a total dive time of 18 min—fragmented into three dives at a maximum depth of 28 m—is unusual. The delay of 15 to 20 min in the development of symptoms from lung rupture is also unusual. It is possible that a small, asymptomatic air embolism from lung rupture during ascent could expand to symptomatic size by absorbing dissolved gas from cerebral tissue subsequently, and that might be the explanation. The balance of probabilities favors an event in the right lung, conceivably consequent on some damage during a deep escape trial and the straining breath holds required to lift 40-lb plates at 28 m; hence the rating unfit to dive. This case illustrates, again, difficulties of diagnosis and "disposal."

Case 15. A 24-Year-Old Submarine Escape Trainee

This fit young man was undertaking escape training for the third time in his career in submarines. Having had no breakfast, he attended the training tank at 0830 hours and declared that he had been well since his screening medical examination 3 weeks before. The first part of his training was to duck his head under water and breathe out in a steady blow. However, he had difficulty with this and delayed the other trainees while he perfected his technique. Having satisfied the instructor, he took the lift to the ground floor of the tank, changed into an escape suit, and was briefed on what to do when he made his escape from 28 msw. His ascent through the water was uneventful but, on arriving at the surface, he emitted a high-pitched expiratory gasp. Almost immediately, he collapsed unconscious into the water, was removed to a stretcher, and quickly compressed in a chamber to 18 msw. After 20 min, he remained deeply unconscious in a decerebrate posture although he was breathing spontaneously. There was no clinical evidence of a pneumothorax, although subcutaneous emphysema was palpable in the neck. The decision was made to compress to 50 msw. Some 30 min later he suffered cardiac and respiratory arrest and, despite a vigorous resuscitative effort, died.

The body was decompressed in the man lock and taken to the local hospital, where the chest was x-rayed before the body was placed in the mortuary. At autopsy the following morning, the chest was opened under water and large volumes of gas escaped as each pleural space was opened. Both lungs were collapsed and bilateral tension pneumothoraces were diagnosed. Examination of the postmortem chest film, however, showed that no pneumothorax was present immediately after the body was decompressed. It was concluded that much of the inert gas that had been absorbed while the patient had been alive in the compression chamber had ''off-gassed'' into the thoracic cavity while in the mortuary and that bilateral tension pneumothoraces were not the cause of death.

Comment. This case demonstrates that PBT can occur for no apparent reason and that, despite prompt recompression therapy, the acute neurological insult of gas embolism can be fatal. From a forensic point of view, this case demonstrates the value of x-raying the body shortly after death. Without that evidence and recognizing the considerable difficulty in diagnosing bilateral pneumothoraces inside a compression chamber, an incorrect conclusion as to the cause of death could have been reached.

Case 16. A 41-Year-Old Commercial Diver Blown Upward Rapidly

This underwater welder was one of a team of three repairing a pipeline off the Indian coast. They had been in saturation, working from a pressure chamber on a diving support vessel held at 7 ata, for many days. Each day they descended in a bell to 60 m, two men leaving the bell on 50-m umbilicals to work on the bottom (70 m) while the third man stayed within, tending their lines. They took turns at being ''bell man.''

On this occasion one of the divers worked on the sea bed while the other (the patient) was asked to inflate lifting bags on the roof of a 60-ton underwater welding habitat. This is about the size and shape of a floorless bungalow; it is dropped over the pipeline and filled with "air" at ambient pressure to enable the men to weld in a gaseous environment rather than in water. The habitat was too heavy for the unusually soft sea bed surrounding the stretch of pipeline in question.

As the patient inflated the bags under instructions from "topside," the habitat suddenly became positively buoyant and swept upward, pinning the man to the upper deck and snapping his lifeline and communications link, until his gas line became taut at a depth of about 7 m. By this time he had been pulled into a narrow metal gulley on the side of the habitat and was about to be drawn through it. The gas line encircled his chest caused great pain. The patient, who was a physical fitness fanatic, was able to squat thrust his way out of the gulley at about 7 m. The habitat raced upward, striking the support vessel, rupturing one lifting bag, turning turtle, filling with water, and accelerating back to the bottom, just missing the bell and the other diver, to sink some 3½ m into the sea bed below.

The patient, in respiratory distress, was able to pull himself down his taut gas line and return to the tilted bell with the other diver. They secured a seal on the bell and returned to the diving support vessel, where they stayed in saturation and decanted gradually to 1 ata over the next 8 days. The patient spat blood on returning to the bell and suffered considerable chest pain, but he did not show any surgical emphysema, dysphonia (difficult to judge on a heliox mix at that pressure), or gross neurological signs. A chest x-ray taken several days later, after arrival at the surface, showed normal lung fields but a compression fracture of T4.

At present, many months later, his vital capacity and total lung capacity are still much smaller than before the incident. He is presumed to have ruptured his lung and is still considered temporarily unfit to dive.

Comment. This last case is included to illustrate the problems of vertical instability that can sweep a diver to the surface very rapidly. As the habitat ascended, the gas in its interior and in the lifting bags expanded, making the structure more and more buoyant as it rose. The patient had no control over his ascent, during which he was obliged to hold his breath and "squat thrust" to avoid further injury. This may well have caused lung injury but, many days later, objective evidence of this event, apart from the drop in lung volume, had disappeared, showing again the difficulties of diagnosing pulmonary barotrauma.

Acknowledgments

We are most grateful to Dr Stuart Mitchell of the Defence Research Agency Centre for Human Sciences, Farnborough, for so generously allowing us access to his extensive collection of references on decompression to altitude. To Dr.

David Hansell, Director of Imaging at the Royal Brompton Hospital, London, we extend our gratitude for freely giving of his substantial expertise to interpret the x-rays and scans of all 250 patients from which the illustrative cases were drawn. We would also like to extend our thanks Allison Harvey of the Institute of Naval Medicine, Alverstoke, for her great skill in producing many of the graphic images we have used.

References

1. Chretien J, Bignon J, Hirsch A, eds. The Pleura in Health and Disease. New York: Marcel Dekker, 1985.
2. Bannister LH. Respiratory system. In: Williams PL, ed. Gray's Anatomy, 38th ed. Edinburgh: Churchill Livingstone, 1995:1627–1682.
3. Pierson DJ. Disorders of the mediastinum. In: Murray JF, Nadel JA, eds. Textbook of Respiratory Medicine, 2d ed. Philadelphia: Saunders, 1994:2235–2249.
4. Broaddus VC, Light RW. Disorders of the pleura: general principles and diagnostic approach, In: Murray JF, Nadel JA, eds. Textbook of Respiratory Medicine, 2d ed. Philadelphia: Saunders, 1994:2145–2163.
5. Macklin MT, Macklin CC. Malignant interstitial emphysema of the lungs and mediastinum as an important occult complication in many respiratory diseases and other conditions: An interpretation of the clinical literature in the light of laboratory experiments. Medicine (Baltimore) 1944; 23:281–358.
6. Staub NC, Wiener-Kronish JP, Albertine KH. Transport through the pleura. In Chretien J, Bignon J, Hirsch A, eds. The Pleura in Health and Disease. New York: Marcel Dekker, 1985:174–175.
7. Albertini KH, Wiener-Kronish JP, Bastacky J, Staub NC. No evidence for mesothelial cell contact across the costal pleural space of sheep. J Appl Physiol 1991; 90:123–134.
8. Marchand P. The anatomy and applied anatomy of the mediastinal fascia. Thorax 1951; 6:359–368.
9. Accard JL, Patte F, Combes F, et al. Pneumothorax spontanée: Etude cliniques, correlation meteorologiques, evaluation et traitement. Rev Tuberc Pneumol (Paris) 1972; 36:431–446.
10. Bense L. Spontaneous pneumothorax related to falls in atmospheric pressure. Eur J Respir Dis 1984; 65:544–546.
11. Celenza A, Fothergill J, Kupek E, Shaw RJ. Thunderstorm associated asthma: A detailed analysis of environmental factors. Br Med J 1996; 312:604–608.
12. Davidson AC, Emberlin J, Cook AD, Venables KM. A major outbreak of asthma associated with a thunderstorm: Experiences of accident and emergency departments and patients' characteristics. Br Med J 1996; 312:601–604.
13. Clemedson C-J. Blast injury. Physiol Rev 1956; 36:336–354.
14. Shilling CW. Blast. In: Shilling CW, Carlston CB, Mathias RA, eds. Physician's Guide to Diving Medicine. New York: Plenum Press, 1984:421–426.
15. Stevens E, Templeton AW. Traumatic nonpenetrating lung contusion. Radiology 1965; 85:247–252.

16. Haber F, Clamann HG. Physics and Engineering of Rapid Decompression: A general theory of rapid decompression. Report 3. Randolph Field, TX: U.S. Air Force School of Aviation Medicine, 1953.
17. Howard P, Ernsting J, Denison DM, et al. The effects of simulated weightlessness upon the cardiovascular system. IAM report 368. London: Ministry of Defence (Air), 1966.
18. Lanphier EH, Camporesi EM. Respiration and exertion. In: Bennett PB, Elliott DH, eds. The Physiology and Medicine of Diving, 4th ed. Edinburgh: Churchill Livingstone, 1993:110.
19. Hills BA. The Biology of Surfactant. Cambridge, England: Cambridge University Press, 1988.
20. Greenhough A, Wood S, Mosley CJ, Davis CA. Pancuronium prevents pneumothoraces in ventilated premature babies who actively inspire against positive pressure inflation. Lancet 1984; 1:1–3.
21. de Troyer A, Yernault JC. Inspiratory muscle force in normal subjects and patients with interstitial lung disease. Thorax 1980; 35:92–100.
22. Denison DM. Physiology. In: Clark TJH, ed. Clinical Investigation of Respiratory Disease. London: Chapman & Hall, 1981:33–94.
23. Denison DM, Pierce RJ, Waller JF. Does the lung work? How big are the lungs? Br J Dis Chest 1981; 75:371–385.
24. Vawter DL, Matthews FL, West JB. Effect of shape and size of lung and chest wall on stresses in the lung. J Appl Physiol 1975; 39:9–17.
25. West JB. Regional Differences in the Lung. London: Blackwell, 1974.
26. Rahn H: The physiological stresses of the Ama. In: Rahn H, Yokoyama T, eds. Physiology of Breath-Hold Diving and the Ama of Japan. Publication 1341. Washington, DC: National Academy of Sciences, National Research Council, 1965:113–117.
27. Schaefer KC, Allison RD, Dougherty JH, Pulmonary and circulatory adjustments determining the limits of depths in breath-hold diving. Science 1968; 162:1020–1023.
28. Brauer RW, Beaver RW, Hogue CD, et al. Intra- and interspecies variability of vertebrate high pressure neurological syndrome. J Appl Physiol 1974; 37:844–851.
29. Pearson RR. The aetiology, pathophysiology, presentation and therapy of pulmonary barotrauma and arterial gas embolism resulting from submarine escape training and diving. MD thesis. University of Newcastle upon Tyne, 1981.
30. Polak B, Adams H. Traumatic air embolism in submarine escape training. USN Med Bull 1932; 30:165–176.
31. Malhotra MS, Wright HC. Arterial air embolism during decompression and its prevention. Proc R Soc Lond B 1960; 154:418–427.
32. Malhotra MS, Wright HC. The effects of a raised intrapulmonary pressure on the lungs of fresh unchilled cadavers. J Pathol Bacteriol 1961; 82:198–202.
33. Voge VM, Anthracite R. Spontaneous pneumothorax in the USAF aircrew population: A retrospective study. Aviat Space Environ Med 1986; 57:939–949.
34. Light RW. Pneumothorax. In: Murray JF, Nadel JA, eds. Textbook of Respiratory Medicine, 2d ed. Philadelphia: Saunders, 1994:2193–2210.

35. Rutherford RB, Hurt HH, Brickman RD, Tubbs JM. The pathophysiology of progressive tension pneumothorax. J Trauma 1968; 8:212–217.
36. Gustman P, Yerger L, Wanner A. Immediate cardiovascular effects of tension pneumothorax. Am Rev Respir Dis 1983; 127:171–174.
37. Kjaergaard P. Spontaneous pneumothorax in the apparently healthy. Acta Med Scand 1932; 43:1–159.
38. Bense L, Lars-Gosta W, Hedenstierna G. Onset of symptoms in spontaneous pneumothorax: Correlations to physical activity. Eur J Respir Dis 1987; 71:181–186.
39. Bense L, Ecklung G, Wimun LG. Smoking and the increased risk of contracting spontaneous pneumothorax. Chest 1987; 92:1009–1012.
40. Abolnik IZ, Lossos IS, Gillis D, Breuer R. Primary spontaneous pneumothorax in men. Am J Med Sci 1993; 305:297–303.
41. Millar AB, Denison DM. Vertical gradients of lung density in healthy supine men. Thorax 1989; 44:485–490.
42. Millar AB, Denison DM. Vertical gradients of lung density in supine subjects with fibrosing alveolitis or pulmonary emphysema. Thorax 1990; 45:602–605.
43. Bayne CG, Wurzbacher T. Can pulmonary barotrauma cause cerebral air embolism in a non-diver? Chest 1982; 81:648–651.
44. Raymond LW. Pulmonary barotrauma and related events in divers. Chest 1995; 107:1648–1652.
45. Berquist TH, Bailey PB, Cortese DA, Miller WE. Transthoracic needle biopsy: Accuracy and complications in relation to location and type of lesion. Mayo Clin Proc 1980; 55:475–481.
46. Miller KS, Fish GB, Stanley JH, Schabel SI. Prediction of pneumothorax rate in percutaneous needle aspiration of the lung. Chest 1988; 93:742–745.
47. Gordon CA. Respiratory emphysema during labor: With two new cases and a review of 130 cases in the literature. Am J Obstet Gyn 1927; 14:663–646.
48. Faust RC. Subcutaneous emphysema during labor. Northwest Med J 1940; 39:24–26.
49. Zuckerman H, Sadovsky E, Frankel M, Brzezinski A. Subcutaneous and mediastinal emphysema during labor. Gynaecologia 1962; 153:12–18.
50. Manco JC, Terra-Filho J, Silva GA. Pneumomediastinum, pneumothorax and subcutaneous emphysema following measurement of maximal expiratory pressure in a normal subject. Chest 1990; 98:1530–1532.
51. de Swiet M. Chest diseases in pregnancy. In: Weatherall DJ, Ledingham JGG, Warrell DA. eds. The Oxford Textbook of Medicine, 3d ed. Vol 2. Oxford, England: Oxford University Press, 1996:1746–1747.
52. Eggleston PA, Ward BH, Pierson WE, Bierman CW. Radiographic abnormalities in acute asthma in children. Pediatrics 1974; 54:442–449.
53. Pellinen TJ, Karjalainen JE. Spontaneous mediastinum. Acta Med Scand 1982; 211: 139–140.
54. Maunder RJ, Pierson DJ, Hudson LD. Subcutaneous and mediastinal emphysema: Pathophysiology, diagnosis and management. Arch Intern Med 1984; 144:1447–1453.

55. Pierson DJ. Pneumomediastinum. In: Murray JS, Nadel KA, eds. Textbook of Respiratory Medicine, 2d ed. Philadelphia: Saunders, 1994:2250–2265.
56. Abolnik IZ, Lossos IS, Breuer R. Spontaneous pneumomediastinum: A report of 25 cases. Chest 1991; 100:93–95.
57. Barrett NK, McIvar J. Mediastinal emphysema simulating aortic rupture. J R Soc Med 1988; 81:670–671.
58. Panacek EA, Singer AJ, Sherman BW, et al. Spontaneous pneumomediastinum: Clinical characteristics and natural history. Ann Emerg Med 1992; 21:1222–1227.
59. Fujiwara T. Pneumomediastinum in pulmonary fibrosis. Chest 1993; 104:44–46.
60. Colebatch HJH, Smith MM, Ng CKY. Increased elastic recoil as a determinant of pulmonary barotrauma in divers. Respir Physiol 1976; 26:55–64.
61. Colebatch HJH, Ng CKY. Decreased pulmonary distensibility and pulmonary barotrauma in divers. Respir Physiol 1991; 86:293–303.
62. Brooks GJ, Pethybridge RJ, Pearson RR. Lung function reference values for FEV_1, FVC FEV_1/FVC ratio and FEF_{75-85} derived from the results of screening 3788 Royal Navy submariners and submariner candidates by spirometry. Proceedings of the XIV annual meeting of the EUBS. Aberdeen, Sept 5–9, 1988.
63. Agarwal PK, Miller SEP. Spontaneous rupture of the oesophagus: Case report of a delayed diagnosis and subsequent management. J R Soc Med 1995; 88:149–150.
64. Smith BA, Ferguson DB. Disposition of spontaneous pneumomediastinum. Ann Emerg Med 1991; 9:256–259.
65. Macnaughton PD, Morgan CJ, Denison DM, Evans TW. Measurement of carbon monoxide transfer and lung volume in ventilated subjects. Eur Respir J 1993; 6: 231–236.
66. Shekerdemian LS, Shore DF, Lincoln C, et al. Negative pressure ventilation improves the cardiac output after right heart surgery. Circulation 1995; 92 (suppl 1):1–122.
67. Adams BH, Polak IB. Traumatic lung lesions produced in dogs by simulating submarine escape. Nav Med Bull 1933; 31:18–20.
68. Kolobow T, Morettii MP, Fumigalli R, et al. Severe impairment in lung function induced by high peak airway pressure during mechanical ventilation: An experimental study. Am Rev Respir Dis 1987; 135:312–315.
69. Carlon GC, Cole R, Pierri MK, et al. High-frequency jet ventilation: Theoretical considerations and clinical observations. Chest 1982; 81:350–354.
70. Gattinoni L, Pesenti A, Avalli L, et al. Pressure-volume curve of total respiratory system in acute respiratory failure: Computed tomographic scan study. Am Rev Respir Dis 1987; 136:730–736.
71. Dreyfus D, Soler P, Basset G, Saumon G. High inflation pressure pulmonary edema: Respective effects of high airway pressure, high tidal volume and positive end-expiratory pressure. Am Rev Respir Dis 1988; 137 1159–1164.
72. Dreyfus D, Saumon G. Pulmonary microvascular injury related to mechanical ventilation. Curr Opin Anesthesiol 1991; 4:257–260.
73. Lenaghan R, Silva YJ, Walt AJ. Hemodynamic alterations associated with expansion rupture of the lung. Arch Surg 1969; 99:339–343.

74. Coelho JCU, Tonnesen AS, Allen SJ, Miner ME. Intracranial hypertension secondary to tension subcutaneous emphysema. Crit Care Med 1985; 13:512–513.
75. Morris WP, Butler BD, Tonnesen AS, Allen SJ. Continuous venous air embolism in patients receiving positive end-expiratory pressure. Am Rev Respir Dis 1993; 147:1034–1037.
76. Woodring JH. Pulmonary interstitial emphysema in the adult respiratory distress syndrome. Crit Care Med 1985; 13:786–791.
77. Haake R, Schlichtig R, Ulstad D, Henschen RO. Barotrauma: Pathophysiology, risk factors and prevention. Chest 1987; 91:608–613.
78. Marcy TW. Barotrauma: Detection, recognition and management. Chest 1993; 104: 578–584.
79. Zwillich CW, Pierson DJ, Creagh CE, et al. Complications of assisted ventilation: A prospective study of 354 consecutive episodes. Am J Med 1974; 57:161–170.
80. Gammon RB, Shin MS, Buchalter SE. Pulmonary barotrauma in mechanical ventilation. Chest 1992; 102:568–572.
81. Marini JJ, Culver BH. Systemic gas embolism complicating mechanical ventilation in the adult respiratory distress syndrome. Ann Intern Med 1989; 110:699–703.
82. Firth DC. Robert Boyle 1627–1691. In Hutchings D, ed. Late Seventeenth Century Scientists. Oxford: Pergamon Press. 1969:1–32.
83. Bert P. La pression barométrique; recherches de phyiologie expérimentale. Paris: Masson, 1878.
84. Haldane JS. Respiration. Oxford, England: Oxford University Press, 1920.
85. Heath EM. Spontaneous pneumothorax in healthy young adults: with particular reference to the aetiological role of aerial ascent. Am J Med Sci 1946; 211:138–143.
86. Hitchcock FA, Whitehorn WV, Edelman A. Tolerance of normal man to explosive decompression. J Appl Physiol 1948; 1:153–164.
87. Holstrum L. Collapse during rapid decompression. J Aviat Med 1958; 29:91–96.
88. Bryan CA, Leach WG. Physiologic effects of cabin pressure failure in high altitude passenger aircraft. Aerospace Med 1960; 31:267–275.
89. Ernsting J, Denison DM, Byford GH, Fryer DI. Hypoxia induced by rapid decompression from 8,000 ft to 40,000 ft: The influence of rate of decompression. Flying Personnel Research Committee Report 1324. London: Ministry of Defence, 1973.
90. Holness DE, Porlier JAG, Ackles KN, Wright GR. Respiratory gas exchange during positive pressure breathing and rapid decompression to simulated altitudes of 18.3 and 24.4 km. Aviat Space Environ Med 1980; 51:454–458.
91. Topliff EDL. Mechanism of lung damage in explosive decompression. Aviat Space Environ Med 1976; 47:517–522.
92. Violette F. Les effets physiologiques des décompressions explosives et leur mécanisme. La Medicine Aeronautique 1954; 9:223–271.
93. Violette F. La pression pulmonaire au cours de la décompression explosive. La Medicine Aeronautique 1955; 10:70–72.
94. Luft UC, Bancroft RW. Transthoracic pressure in man during rapid decompression. J Aviat Med 1956; 27:208–220.

95. Achiary A, Cabanon A, Andre V, Richet J. Décompressions rapides et explosives en vol: etude de 15 observations. La Medicine Aeronautique 1955; 10:73–86.
96. Brooks CJ. Loss of cabin pressure in Canadian Forces ejection seat aircraft, 1962–1982. Aviat Space Environ Med 1984; 55:1154–1163.
97. Howard P, Urquhart DRH, Wagner PR, Whittingham PDGV. A report of an escape from the English Electric Lightning T4 on October 1st 1959. RAF Institute of Aviation Medicine Report 134. London: Ministry of Defence, 1959.
98. Kolesari GL, Kindwall EP. Survival following accidental decompression to an altitude greater than 74,000 ft (22,555 m). Aviat Space Environ Med 1982; 53: 1211–1214.
99. Ernsting J. The physiological effects of failure of the pressure cabins of passenger aircraft flying at altitudes between 35,000 ft and 65,000 ft. RAF Institute of Aviation Medicine Report 313. London: Ministry of Defence, 1965.
100. Ernsting J. Some effects of raised intrapulmonary pressures. Maidenhead, Berks: Technivision, 1966:63–74.
101. Cran IR, Rumball CA. Survey of spontaneous pneumothoraces in the Royal Air Force. Thorax 1967; 22:462–465.
102. Fuchs HS. Incidence of spontaneous pneumothorax in apparently healthy aircrew. Aerospace Med 1967; 38:1286–1288.
103. Fuchs HS. Idiopathic spontaneous pneumothorax and flying. Aerospace Med 1967; 38:1283–1285.
104. Hopkirk JAC, Pullen MJ, Fraser JR. Pleurodesis: The results of treatment for spontaneous pneumothorax in the Royal Air Force. Aviat Space Environ Med 1983; 54:158–160.
105. McCormick TJ, Lyons TJ. Medical causes of in-flight incapacitation: USAF experience 1978–1987. Aviat Space Environ Med 1991; 62:884–887.
106. Lim MK, Peng CM. Spontaneous pneumothorax occurring in flight. Singapore Med J 1985; 26:93–95.
107. Everett WD. Spontaneous pneumothorax: An analysis of pleurectomy vs conservative therapy in United States Air Force fliers. Aviat Space Environ Med 1988; 59:1089–1093.
108. Neidhart P, Suter PM. Pulmonary bulla and sudden death in a young airplane passenger. Intensive Care Med 1985; 11:45–47.
109. Wallace WA, Wong T, O'Bichere A, Ellis BW. Managing in-flight emergencies. Br Med J 1995; 311:374–376.
110. Rudge FW. Altitude induced arterial gas embolism: A case report. Aviat Space Environ Med 1992; 63:203–205.
111. Murrison AW, Lacey EJ, Restler M, et al. Ten years of diving-related illness in the Royal Navy. J Soc Occup Med 1991; 41:217–219.
112. Dovenbarger J, ed. Report on Diving Accidents and Fatalities. Durham, NC: Divers Alert Network, 1994.
113. Kizer KW. Dysbaric cerebral air embolism in Hawaii. Ann Emerg Med 1987; 16: 535–541.
114. Greer HD, Massey EW. Neurological injury from undersea diving. Neurol Clin 1992; 10:1031–1045.

115. Benton PJ, Woodfine JD, Francis TJR. A review of spirometry and UK submarine escape training tank incidents (1954–1993) using objective diagnostic criteria. Alverstoke, England: Institute of Naval Medicine, Report R94011, 1994.
116. Williamson J. Arterial gas embolism from pulmonary barotrauma: What happens in the lung? SPUMS J 1988; 18:90–92.
117. Bachrach AJ, Egstrom GH. Stress and performance in diving. San Pedro, CA: Best, 1987.
118. Elliott DH, Harrison JAB, Barnard EEP. Clinical and radiological features of eighty-eight cases of decompression barotrauma. In: Shilling CW, Beckett MW, eds. Proceedings of the Sixth Symposium on Underwater Physiology. Bethesda, MD: Federation of American Societies for Experimental Biology, 1978:527–535.
119. Leitch DR, Green RD. Pulmonary barotrauma in divers and the treatment of arterial gas embolism. Aviat Space Environ Med 1986; 57:931–938.
120. Neuman TS. Pulmonary disorders in diving. In: Bore AA, Davis JC, eds. Diving Medicine, 2d ed. Philadelphia: Saunders, 1990:233–238.
121. Weiss LD, van Meter KW. The applications of hyperbaric oxygen therapy in emergency medicine. Am J Emerg Med 1992; 10:558–569.
122. Edmonds C. Asthma and diving. SPUMS J 1991; 21:70–74.
123. Martin L. The medical problems of underwater diving. N Engl J Med 1992; 326: 1497.
124. Melamed Y, Shupak A, Bitterman H, Weiler-Ravell D. The medical problems of underwater diving. N Engl J Med 1992; 326:1498.
125. Neuman TS, Bove AA, O'Connor RD, Kelsen SG. Asthma and diving. Ann Allergy 1994; 73:344–350.
126. Farrell PJS, Glanvill P. Diving practices of scuba divers with asthma. Br Med J 1990; 300:166.
127. Martindale JJ. Scuba divers with asthma. Br Med J 1990; 300:609.
128. Wall SJ, Gunnyeon WJ. Scuba divers with asthma. Br Med J 1990; 300:609.
129. Cullen R. Novice recreational scuba divers and asthma: Two small surveys reported. SPUMS J 1995; 25:8–10.
130. Smith TF. The medical problems of underwater diving. N Engl J Med 1992; 326: 1497–1498.
131. Liebow AA, Stark JE, Vogel J, Schaeffer KE. Intrapulmonary air trapping in submarine escape training casualties. U.S. Armed Forces Med J 1959; 10:265–289.
132. Calder IM. Autopsy and experimental observations on factors leading to barotrauma in man. Undersea Biomed Res 1985; 12:165–182.
133. Saywell WR. Submarine escape training, lung cysts and tension pneumothorax. Br J Radiol 1989; 62:276–278.
134. Ziser A, Väänänen A, Melamed Y. Diving and chronic spontaneous pneumothorax. Chest 1985; 87:264–265.
135. Jenkins C, Anderson SD, Wong R, Veale A. Compressed air diving and respiratory disease. Med J Aust 1993; 158:275–279.
136. Unsworth IP. Pulmonary barotrauma in a hyperbaric chamber. Anaesthesia 1973; 28:675–678.

137. Benton PJ, Woodfine JD, Westwood PR. Arterial gas embolism following a 1-metre ascent during helicopter escape training. A case report. Aviat Space Environ Med 1996; 67:63–64.
138. Burki NK. Effects of immersion in water and changes in intrathoracic blood volume on lung function in man. Clin Sci Mol Med 1976; 51:303–311.
139. Taylor NA, Morrison JB. Static and dynamic pulmonary compliance during upright immersion. Acta Physiol Scand 1993; 149:413–417.
140. Broome CR, Jarvis LJ, Clark RJ. Pulmonary barotrauma in submarine escape training. Thorax 1994; 49:186–187.
141. Dean DM, Allison RS. Effects of high-explosive blast on the lungs. Lancet 1940; 2:224–226.
142. Hadfield GH, Ross JM, Swain RHA, et al. Blast from high explosive. Lancet 1940; 2:478–481.
143. Zuckerman S. Experimental study of blast injuries to the lung. Lancet 1940; 2: 220–224.
144. Wilson JV, Tunbridge RE. Pathological findings in a series of blast injuries. Lancet 1943; 1:257–261.
145. Boerhaave H. Atrois, nec descripti prius, morbi historia: Secundum medicae artis leges conscripta. Lugdini Batavorum Boutesteniana 1724 ex: Derbes VJ, Mitchell RE (transl). Bull Med Libr 1955; 43:217–240.
146. Turnbull A. A remarkable coincidence in dental surgery. Br Med J 1900; 1:1131–1135.
147. Sandler CM, Libshitz HI, Marks G. Pneumoperitoneum, pneumomediastinum and pneumopericardium following dental extraction. Radiology 1975; 115:539–540.
148. Pedersen TH, Karlsen HM, Semb G, Hatteland K. Comparison of bubble release from various types of oxygenators: An in-vivo investigation. Scand J Thorac Cardiovasc Surg 1987; 21:73–80.
149. Pearson DT, Holden MP, Poslad SJ, et al. A clinical evaluation of the performance characteristics of one membrane and five bubble oxygenators: Gas transfer and gaseous microemboli production. Perfusion 1986; 7:15–26.
150. Pearson DT, Poslad SJ, Murray A, Clayton R. Extracorporeal circulation material evaluation: Microemboli. Life Support Systems 1987; 5:53–67.
151. Torrey RG, Grosh LS. Acute pulmonary emphysema observed during the epidemic of influenzal pneumonia at Fort Hancock, Georgia. Am J Med Sci 1919; 157:170–181.
152. Gorman DF. Arterial gas embolism as a consequence of pulmonary barotrauma. Desola J, ed. Proceedings of the IXth Congress of the European Undersea Biomedical Society. Barcelona, Sept 23–25, 1984:348–368.
153. Broome JR., Smith DJ. Pneumothorax as a complication of recompression therapy for cerebral arterial gas embolism. Undersea Biomed Res 1992; 19:447–455.
154. Harker CP, Neuman TS, Olson LK, et al. The roentgenographic findings associated with air embolism in sport scuba divers. J Emerg Med 1993; 11:443–449.
155. Balk M, Goldman LM. Alveolar hemorrhage as a manifestation of pulmonary barotrauma after scuba diving. Ann Emerg Med 1990; 19:930–934.

156. James RE. Extra-alveolar air resulting from submarine escape training: A post-training roentgenographic survey of 170 submariners. Report No. 550. Groton CT: U.S. Naval Submarine Medical Center 1968.
157. Hamman L Spontaneous mediastinal emphysema. Bull Johns Hopkins Hosp 1939; 64:1–21.
158. Hamman L. Mediastinal emphysema. JAMA 1945; 128:1–6.
159. Friehs I, Friehs GM, Friehs GB. Air embolism with bilateral pneumothorax after a five metre dive. Undersea Hyperbar Med 1993; 20:155–157.
160. Dutka AJ. A review of the pathophysiology and potential application of experimental therapies for cerebral ischemia to the treatment of cerebral gas embolism. Undersea Biomed Res 1985; 12:403–421.
161. De La Torre E, Mitchell OC, Netsky MG. The seat of respiratory and cardiovascular responses to cerebral air emboli. Neurology 1960; 12:141–147.
162. Evans DE, Kobrine A, Weathersby PK, Bradley ME. Cardiovascular effects of cerebral air embolism. Stroke 1981; 12:338–344.
163. Norris JW. Effects of cerebrovascular injuries on the heart. Neurol Clin 1983; 1: 37–55.
164. Pearson RR, Goad RF. Delayed cerebral edema complicating cerebral arterial gas embolism: Case histories. Undersea Biomed Res 1982; 9:283–296.
165. Van Genderen L, Waite CL. Evaluation and treatment of traumatic air embolism. Aerospace Med 1968; 39:709–713.
166. Pearson RR. Clinical aspects of cerebral arterial gas embolism and decompression sickness with cerebral involvement. In: Francis TJR, Smith DJ, eds. Describing Decompression Illness. Bethesda: Undersea and Hyperbaric Medical Society, 1991:55–64.
167. Elliott DH, Moon RE. Manifestations of the decompression disorders. In: Bennett PB, Elliott DH, eds. The Physiology and Medicine of Diving. London: Saunders, 1993:481–505.
168. Pearson RR. Diagnosis and treatment of gas embolism. In: Shilling CW, Carlston CB, Mathias RA, eds. The Physician's Guide to Diving Medicine. New York: Plenum Press, 1984:333–367.
169. Francis TJR, Pearson RR, Robertson AG, et al. Central nervous system decompression sickness: Latency of 1070 human cases. Undersea Biomed Res 1988; 15: 403–417.
170. Kelleher PC, Pethybridge RJ, Francis TJR. A manifestation-based mathematical model to predict outcome of neurological decompression illness based on 214 cases. Aviat Space Environ Med 1996; 67:654–658.
171. Neuman TS, Bove AA. Combined arterial gas embolism and decompression sickness following no-stop dives. Undersea Biomed Res 1990; 17:429–436.
172. Francis TJR, Smith DJ, eds. Describing Decompression Illness. Bethesda, MD: Undersea and Hyperbaric Medical Society, 1991.
173. Hallenbeck JM, Bove AA, Elliott DH. Mechanisms underlying spinal cord damage in decompression sickness. Neurology 1975; 25:308–316.
174. Gorman DF, Edmonds CW, Parsons DW, et al. Neurologic sequelae of decompression sickness: A clinical report. In: Bove AA, Bachrach AJ, Greenbaum LJ,

eds. Proceedings of the 9th Symposium on Underwater and Hyperbaric Physiology. Bethesda, MD: Undersea and Hyperbaric Medical Society, 1987:993–998.

175. Hodgson M, Beran RG, Shirtley G. The role of computed tomography in the assessment of decompression sickness. Arch Neurol 1988; 45:1033–1035.
176. Yiannikas C, Beran NR. Somatosensory evoked potentials, electroencephalography and CT scans in the assessment of the neurological sequelae of decompression sickness. Clin Exp Neurol 1988; 25:91–96.
177. Moon RE, Gorman DF. Treatment of the decompression disorders. In: Bennett PB, Elliott DH, eds. The Physiology and Medicine of Diving. London: Saunders, 1993:506–541.
178. Hodgson M, Smith DJ, MacLeod MA, et al. Case-control study of cerebral perfusion deficits in divers using ^{99m}Tc hexamethylpropylene amine oxime. Undersea Biomed Res 1991; 18:421–431.
179. Evans SA. An investigation of the potential use of Tc-HMPAO-SPECT scanning in decompression illness. PhD thesis. Aberdeen: Robert Gordon University, 1994.
180. Lowe VJ, Hoffman JM, Hanson MW, et al. Cerebral imaging of decompression injury patients with 18-F-2-fluoro-2-deoxyglucose positron emission tomography. Undersea Hyperbar Med 1994; 21:103–113.
181. Murrison AW. The contribution of neurophysiologic techniques to the investigation of diving-related illness. Undersea Hyperbar Med 1993; 20:347–373.
182. Murrison AW, Glasspool E, Pethybridge RJ, et al. Neurophysiological assessment of divers with medical histories of neurological decompression illness. Occup Environ Med 1994; 51:730–734.
183. Murrison AW, Glasspool E, Pethybridge RJ, et al. Electroencephalographic study of divers with histories of neurological decompression illness. Occup Environ Med 1995; 52:451–453.
184. Murrison AW, Glasspool E, Francis TJR, Sedgwick EM. Somatosensory evoked potentials in acute neurological decompression illness. J Neurol 1995; 242:669–676.
185. Miller AC, Harvey JE. Guidelines for the management of spontaneous pneumothorax. Br Med J 1993; 307:114–116.
186. Light RW. Management of spontaneous pneumothorax. Am Rev Respir Dis 1993; 148:245–248.
187. Northfield T. Oxygen therapy for the resolution of spontaneous pneumothorax. Br Med J 1971; 4:86–88.
188. Daugherty CG. Inherent unsaturation in the treatment of pneumothorax at depth. Undersea Biomed Res 1990; 17:171–177.
189. Broome JR, Smith DJ. Pneumothorax as a complication of recompression therapy for cerebral arterial gas embolism. Undersea Biomed Res 1992; 19:447–455.
190. Jerrard DA. Diving Medicine. Emerg Clin North Am 1992; 19:329–338.
191. Francis TJR, Gorman DF. Pathogenesis of the decompression disorders. In: Bennett PB, Elliott DH, eds. The Physiology and Medicine of Diving. London: Saunders, 1993:455–480.

192. Broome JR, Dick EJ, Dutka AJ. Multifocal CNS hemorrhage as a cause of recompression treatment failure in a pig model of neurological decompression illness (DCI). Undersea Hyperbar Med 1994; 21(suppl):69–70.
193. Hallenbeck JM, Leitch DR, Dutka AJ, Greenbaum LJ. The amount of circumscribed brain edema and the degree of postischemic neuronal recovery do not correlate well. Stroke 1982; 13:797–804.
194. Lanier WL, Stangland KJ, Scheithauer BW, et al. The effect of dextrose solution and head position on neurologic outcome after complete cerebral ischemia in primates: Examination of a model. Anesthesiology 1987; 66:39–48.
195. Drummond JC, Moore SS. The influence of dextrose administration on neurologic outcome after temporary spinal cord ischemia in the rabbit. Anesthesiology 1989; 70:64–70.
196. Robertson CS, Goodman JC, Narayan RK, et al. The effect of glucose administration on carbohydrate metabolism after head injury. J Neurosurg 1991; 74:43–50.
197. Van Allen CM, Hrdina LA, Clark J. Air embolism from the pulmonary vein—A clinical and experimental study. Arch Surg 1929; 19:567–599.
198. Atkinson JR. Experimental air embolism. Northwest Med 1963; 62:699–703.
199. Gorman DF, Browning DM, Parsons DW, Traucott FM. Distribution of arterial gas emboli in the pial circulation. SPUMS J 1987; 17:101–115.
200. Hills BA, James PB. Microbubble damage to the blood-brain barrier: Relevance to decompression sickness. Undersea Biomed Res 1991; 18:111–116.
201. Dutka AJ. Therapy for dysbaric central nervous system ischemia: Adjuncts to recompression. In: Bennett PB, Moon RE, eds. Diving Accident Management. Bethesda, MD: Undersea and Hyperbaric Medical Society, 1990:222–234.
202. Gorman DF. The redistribution of cerebral arterial gas embolism. PhD thesis. University of Sydney, 1987.
203. Gorman DF, Browning DM. Cerebral vasoreactivity and arterial gas embolism. Undersea Biomed Res 1986; 13:317–335.
204. Helps SC, Parsons DW, Reilly PL, Gorman DF. The effect of gas emboli on rabbit cerebral blood flow. Stroke 1990; 21:94–99.
205. Anderson D, Nagasawa G, Norfleet W, et al. O_2 pressures between 0.12 and 2.5 atm abs, circulatory function, and N_2 elimination. Undersea Biomed Res 1991; 18:279–292.
206. Wells CH, Bond TP, Guest MM, Barnhart CC. Rheologic impairment of the microcirculation during decompression sickness. Microvasc Res 1971; 3:163–169.
207. Obrenovitch TP, Kumaroo KK, Hallenbeck JM. Autoradiographic detection of ^{111}Indium-labelled platelets in brain tissue sections. Stroke 1984; 15:1049–1056.
208. Hallenbeck JM, Dutka AJ, Tanashima T, et al. Polymorphonuclear leucocyte accumulation in brain regions with low blood flow in the early post-ischemic period. Stroke 1986; 17:246–253.
209. Helps SC, Gorman DF. Air embolism of the brain in rabbits pre-treated with mechlorethamine. Stroke 1991; 22:351–354.

210. Hammarlund C. The physiologic effects of hyperbaric oxygen. In: Kindwall EP, ed. Hyperbaric Medicine Practice. Flagstaff AZ: Best Publishing, 1995:17–32.
211. Workman RD. Treatment of bends with oxygen at high pressure. Aerospace Med 1968; 39:1076–1083.
212. Gorman DF, Browning DM, Parsons DW. Redistribution of cerebral arterial gas emboli: A comparison of treatment regimens. In: Bove AA, Bachrach AJ, Greenbaum LJ, eds. Proceedings of the 9th Symposium on Underwater and Hyperbaric Physiology. Bethesda, MD: Undersea and Hyperbaric Medical Society, 1987: 1031–1050.
213. Leitch DR, Greenbaum LJ, Hallenbeck JM. Cerebral arterial air embolism: I. Is there benefit in beginning treatment at 6 bar? Undersea Biomed Res 1984; 11: 221–235.
214. Leitch DR, Greenbaum LJ, Hallenbeck JM. Cerebral arterial air embolism: III. Cerebral blood flow after decompression from various pressure treatments. Undersea Biomed Res 1984; 11:249–263.
215. McDermott JJ, Dutka AJ, Koller WA, et al. Comparison of two recompression profiles in treating experimental air embolism. Undersea Biomed Res 1992; 19: 171–185.
216. McDermott JJ, Dutka AJ, Koller WA, Flynn ET. Effect of an increased P_{O_2} during recompression therapy for the treatment of experimental arterial gas embolism. Undersea Biomed Res 1992; 19:403–413.
217. Hart GB. Treatment of decompression illness and air embolism with hyperbaric oxygen. Aerospace Med 1974; 45:1190–1193.
218. Bove AA, Clark JM, Simon AJ, Lambertsen CJ. Successful therapy of cerebral air embolism with hyperbaric oxygen at 2.8 ATA. Undersea Biomed Res 1982; 9:75–80.
219. U.S. Navy Diving Manual. Vol 1 (Air Diving). Publication No. 0994-LP-001-9010. Washington DC: U.S. Navy Sea Systems Command, 1993.
220. Clark JM. Oxygen toxicity. In: Kindwall EP, ed. Hyperbaric Medicine Practice. Flagstaff AZ: Best Publishing, 1995:34–42.
221. Douglas JDM, Robinson C. Heliox treatment for spinal decompression sickness following air dives. Undersea Biomed Res 1988; 15:315–319.
222. Kol S, Adir Y, Gordon CR, Melamed Y. Oxyhelium treatment for severe spinal cord decompression sickness after air diving. Undersea Hyperbar Med 1993; 20: 147–154.
223. Hyldegaard O, Madsen J. Influence of heliox, oxygen and N2O–O2 on N2 bubbles in adipose tissue. Undersea Biomed Res 1989; 15:315–319.
224. Hyldegaard O, Moller M, Madsen J. Effect of He-O_2, O_2, and N_2O-O_2 breathing on bubbles in spinal white matter tissue. Undersea Biomed Res 1991; 18:361–371.
225. Evans DE, Kobrine AI, LeGrys DC, Bradley ME. Protective effect of lidocaine in acute cerebral ischemia induced by air embolism. J Neurosurg 1984; 60:257–263.
226. Evans DE, Catron PW, McDermott JJ, et al. Effect of lidocaine after experimental cerebral ischemia induced by air embolism. J Neurosurg 1989; 70:97–102.

227. McDermott JJ, Dutka AJ, Evans DE, Flynn ET. Treatment of experimental air embolism with lidocaine and hyperbaric oxygen. Undersea Biomed Res 1990; 17: 525–534.
228. Dutka AJ, Mink R, McDermott JJ, et al. Effect of lidocaine on somatosensory evoked response and cerebral blood flow after canine cerebral air embolism. Stroke 1992; 23:1515–1520.
229. Drewry A, Gorman DF. Lidocaine as an adjunct to hyperbaric therapy in decompression illness: A case report. Undersea Biomed Res 1992; 19:187–190.
230. Dutka AJ, Mink RB, Pearson RR, Hallenbeck JM. Effects of treatment with dexamethasone on recovery from experimental cerebral arterial gas embolism. Undersea Biomed Res 1992; 19:131–141.
231. Brooks GJ, Green RD, Leitch DR. Pulmonary barotrauma in submarine escape trainees and the treatment of cerebral air embolism. Aviat Space Environ Med 1986; 57:1201–1207.
232. Denison DM. Physiological principles. In: Parkes WR, ed. Occupational Lung Disorders, 3d ed. Oxford, England: Butterworth Heinemann, 1993:18–34.
233. Giertsen JC, Sandstad E, Morield I, et al. An explosive decompression accident. Am J Forens Med Pathol 1988; 9:94–101.

9

Long-Term Pulmonary Effects of Diving

JAMES W. REED

University of Newcastle
Newcastle upon Tyne, England

EINAR THORSEN

Norwegian Underwater Technology Centre A/S
Laksevåg, Norway

I. Introduction

With diving, the lungs are exposed to several factors that have long been known to have detrimental effects on pulmonary function. The consequences of hyperoxia, venous gas microemboli, and increased respiratory mechanical loads are well established and have been reviewed in previous chapters of this book. In the light of increasing knowledge, periodic reassessment of the diving tables and the development of more sophisticated diving equipment over the last decades have resulted in revised diving procedures that have limited the risks of exposure and the likelihood of acute diving-related disease. Any deleterious effect of diving on the lung not associated with either a catastrophic event or a documented decompression incident has been largely discounted. The role of lung-function testing has therefore been seen to be confined to the assessment of medical fitness to dive. This has led to much debate and indeed some controversy over the significance of preexisting conditions such as asthma, bronchitis, and so on.

There is, however, an accumulating body of evidence to suggest that lung function is altered by diving, albeit mainly from studies undertaken in conjunction with the development of procedures for deep saturation diving. For the last

15 to 20 years, saturation diving to depths of 300 m and deeper has been considered experimental and borderline with respect to both the divers' operational capability and established technical procedures. Extensive studies have therefore been done on divers participating in such dives, both at depth and after surfacing. In contrast, studies of the routine, shallower saturation diving in the depth range of 50 to 150 m, which is the depth range of most of the operational diving on offshore oilfields, and air-bounce diving to depths of less than 50 m are very scarce.

Whether operational diving in accordance with established procedures can result in subtle functional changes, which over time accumulate to long-term effects of clinical significance, is still to be resolved.

II. Diving Exposure

The basic physical parameters characterizing a dive are pressure, time, and gas mixture; these form the basis for the calculation of oxygen exposure, decompression stress (inert gas accumulation and elimination), and respiratory mechanical load (gas density). These primary parameters are independent of the method of diving and can be used to characterize both short air-bounce dives and long, deep saturation dives. Differences between different methods of diving are, therefore, quantitative rather than qualitative.

Aside from the basic physical attributes of the dive, exposure is also characterized by the equipment used and the surrounding environment. Both the breathing apparatus and submersion will contribute additional respiratory mechanical loading. Physical activity during the dive will influence local circulation and the rate of inert gas exchange in various tissues. The temperature and humidity of the respired gas partially determine respiratory heat and water loss, which may induce a bronchoconstrictive response. In addition, the diver may be exposed to toxic contaminants in the breathing gas, particularly while inside welding habitats. Finally, the diving may take place in environments with bacteriological, chemical, or radioactive contamination.

This multifactorial nature of the diving exposure contributes to the complexity of studies into the underlying mechanisms of functional changes. In studying a single dive, most of these factors can be monitored and controlled; but in epidemiological studies based on historical exposure data, there are considerable difficulties. Ideally, cumulative diving exposure should be calculated from data in the divers' logbooks, but logbooks describing diving activity several years in the past are not easily obtained. Exact data have not been available in the cross-sectional studies published so far. Less specific exposure data—such as number of years of occupational diving, the number of dives performed, number of days in saturation, and depth range—are more easily obtained, as these data are usually transferred to successive logbooks and used by the divers as documentation of experience. These simple measures of cumulative exposure constitute all factors related to the diving.

The usefulness of more specific characterization of the diving exposure in epidemiological surveys may be questioned. As hyperoxia, venous gas microembolism, and gas density are all dependent on the same basic physical variables of pressure, time, and gas mixture, indices of cumulative exposure to each over a diving career are strongly interrelated. The problems of colinearity that such interrelationships introduce (see Sec. III) may obscure a significant effect or complicate evaluation as primary or secondary (1). Detailed knowledge of the exposures are necessary, however, when effects of single exposures are studied or when improvements in diving procedures are to be considered. In such studies, it is important to standardize exposure to all factors but that under investigation. When the simple general measures of overall diving exposure are used, the risk of missing effects related to diving is reduced, but the specificity of the analyses with respect to cause-effect relationships is also reduced.

There is no general agreement on how diving exposure can best be quantified. Only for hyperoxia is there an established method of quantifying exposure—i.e., the calculation of the unit pulmonary toxic dose (UPTD) as introduced by Clark and Lambertsen (2). The concept has recently been revised as the integrated product of time and partial pressure of oxygen in excess of 21 kPa (3). Venous gas microemboli (VGM) may be considered as an exposure factor with respect to the lung as long as most of the microemboli are filtered in the pulmonary circulation, but VGM are essentially dependent upon the rate of inert gas elimination from other tissues. Methods for the assessment of the total load of venous gas microemboli are technically difficult, with no universally accepted index; at best the methods are only semiquantitative and not practical for long-term monitoring. The pulmonary mechanical load depends on several factors related to both internal and external influences, but as far as internal airway resistance is concerned, it is essentially proportional to gas density.

III. Assessment of Lung Function and Association with Exposure

Epidemiological studies of the effects of diving on lung function are complicated by the multifactorial nature of the diving exposure, with different exposure factors having differing or even opposing effects with dissimilar time courses. Thus, a reduction in vital capacity caused by oxygen toxicity may be opposed by an increase as a result of a training effect on respiratory muscles (Fig. 1). The sensitivity and reproducibility of the methods used, time of assessment with

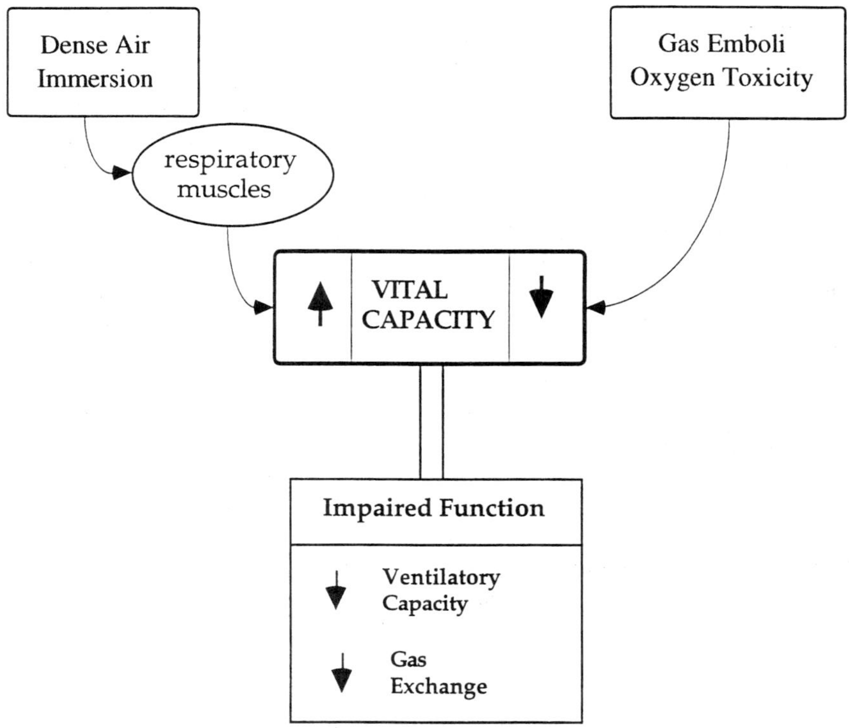

Figure 1 Conflicting influences of diving factors on vital capacity.

respect to the last dive, and quantification of diving exposure are critical. Following a single dive, the acute effects on lung function have a half-life of approximately 4 to 6 weeks (4–6).

It is not out of place to stress that the methods must be appropriate, equipment suitable and calibrated correctly, and the operator well trained in its use. A description of methodology and associated problems is too extensive to be presented in detail here; the reader is referred to publications from the American Thoracic Society (7,8) and European Respiratory Society (9). A succinct description of methodologies and the establishment of an association of impaired respiratory function with occupational exposure is given by Cotes (10,11).

In relation to diving, the demonstration of an effect on the lung depends upon:

1. Evidence for impaired lung function or, if overall lung function is within the normal range, an increased rate of deterioration with age

2. An association between lung function and diving exposure that cannot be explained by other interrelated variables

The former implies knowledge of a ''normal'' or ''reference'' value, the latter involves an adequate quantitative index of the exposure.

A. Detection of Impairment

Historically, the forced vital capacity (FVC) and forced expiratory volume (FEV_1) have been used to assess ventilatory capacity, with changes in vital capacity being used as marker of oxygen toxicity. Other indices of relevance that are currently not measured routinely on divers include indices of peripheral airway function. These are the maximal flow rates that can be developed at different lung volumes (when 25, 50, and 75% of the FVC remains to be exhaled; MEF_{25}, MEF_{50}, and MEF_{75}, which can throw light on the patency of the small airways. These are derived from the same maximal exhalation as is used to measure the FVC and FEV_1. They are difficult to interpret without a knowledge of lung volumes, and the prognostic value is in doubt.

Measurement of static lung volumes, diffusing capacity (transfer factor) for carbon monoxide, and assessment of exercise capacity are necessary for any detailed understanding of the mechanisms of change. However, the tests are time-consuming and require expensive and complicated equipment. The accuracy and reproducibility of the measurements are not as good as for FVC or FEV_1, and the specificity in detecting significant change is less. For these practical reasons, they are not generally considered to be suitable for inclusion in larger epidemiological studies.

Reference Values

The categorization of ''normal'' or ''impaired'' is dependent upon whether or not the measured value falls within acceptable limits. A measured value at one point in time can be compared with either a reference value for a healthy subject of the same age, stature, gender, and ethnic group or with a result for a control group of persons chosen to be similar to the divers in all relevant respects other than their occupation. Interpretation of longitudinal changes in lung function with time can be made in a similar manner, using local reference values.

Criteria for reference values have evolved with time. They are now more stringent with respect to the methods of measurement and include criteria for the exclusion of subjects on account of smoking and respiratory symptoms. The effects of the changes have summated with those due to improved nutrition and other factors to progressively increase the levels of reference values, and the process is continuing. Regular review and updating of reference values is-therefore essential, but can complicate interpretation, particularly when published limits of "normality" differ between North America and Europe and even within different geographical areas of Europe. Some of these difficulties can be avoided by using a control group, particularly if allowance is made for lung size, which is on average larger in divers and some other occupational groups than in the general population.

Confounding Factors

Confounding factors that can affect function and potentially influence interpretation include smoking, exposure to welding fumes, and other environmental agents not directly connected with the actual dives. The effects can be troublesome to quantify because of difficulties in assessing exposure. In the case of fumes, the noxious agent may not even have been identified. For smoking, although the number of cigarettes smoked per day can be recorded, it is now apparent that "passive" smoking may affect lung function; hence the level of exposure to tobacco fumes is essentially unquantifiable. The fumes from different sources can exert separate effects on the lungs; they can also interact both with each other and with other variables, especially age. This variable is usually correlated with indices of diving exposure. It is correlated with cigarette consumption expressed in pack-years; in many populations, it is also negatively correlated with stature. Before an effect can be attributed to diving, an allowance should have been made for possible errors due to colinearity between the relevant variables.

B. Association with Exposure

For purposes of comparison with lung function, diving exposure can be relatively elementary, as when it is classified simply as either present or absent; alternatively, the exposure can be expressed quantitatively. The former approach requires a suitable control group of nondivers and the latter a knowledge of individual exposures (Sec. II).

Comparison with Control Group

This approach is a first step to a more detailed analysis, since it groups all divers together, without taking into account differences in exposure between individuals. The study is usually cross-sectional at one point in time, but a longitudinal approach is also possible. The comparison is with healthy nondivers—who should be matched for the variables relevant to divers and not merely for age, gender, size and ethnic group, as is the case for reference values.

Successful and meaningful interpretation of the outcome depends upon any differences being due entirely to the diving exposure. In practice, the identification and recruitment of a suitable control group can be difficult to achieve. For example, professional firefighters also tend to have the larger lungs commonly found in divers and have a high level of physical activity; they would therefore seem to provide an appropriate control group. In practice, firefighting as an occupation is associated with exposure to noxious fumes, and relatively few firefighters have not been so exposed. In addition, many firefighters are overweight.

Such comparisons give limited information. The classification of diving exposure as "present" or "absent" may also lead to an erroneous conclusion, as no account can be taken of differing exposures; subtle effects may be overlooked.

Cross-sectional studies in which divers' values are compared with reference values from a general population or from an improperly selected control group can be misleading. Even if the measured values are within the predicted range, significant changes in function may have taken place—an accelerated rate of decline is as significant as a low absolute value. Comparisons with predicted values or control groups may be helpful but are not definitive in establishing or excluding occupationally related effects.

Analysis with Graded Exposure

Grades of exposure can be used to explore possible stimulus/response relationships within the data without reference to a control group. By this means the difficulties inherent in identifying a control group are avoided, but the analysis is dependent upon the existence of a suitable index of diving exposure (see Sec. II). A common approach is to take measurements at one point in time and attempt to correlate either the absolute value of the variable of interest or the degree of impairment (with reference to a standardized value), with the index of exposure. The results can give valuable information. However, this form of cross-sectional analysis is critically dependent on the accuracy of retrospective data (diving history) and is influenced by other factors. For example, the apparent effect of age includes a component due to the cohort effect (12,13). As a consequence, cross-sectional analysis cannot be used to describe longitudinal changes. The alternative is a longitudinal study, in which the subjects are followed over a period of several years. The longitudinal study has many advantages; each subject acts as his or her own control, diving exposure can be detailed, there is no interaction of diving exposure with age, no cohort effect, and differences between subjects can be both allowed for and subjected to scrutiny.

The successful completion of a longitudinal study is complicated by its duration. A relatively long study may lead to poor subject compliance (and hence loss of data) and bias due to some subjects becoming lapses as a result of nonrandom factors related to diving. In addition, there may be changes in personnel or instrumentation that affect the quality of the measurements. This can be of critical importance, since the normal annual changes are small in relation to the variability of the measurement. Accuracy is then influenced by the interval between measurements and the number of replicate observations. The optimal time interval between the initial and final measurements appears to be between 5 and 7 years (14,15), while the number of intermediary observations is less important. The only published data known to the authors that allow for an estimate of the time course for the expression of cumulative effects of diving exposure would suggest that it is likely to be not less than 5 years (16).

A major drawback is the lack of appropriate reference values; where these do exist, the interpretation of the observed changes may be materially affected by concurrent changes in smoking habit, body mass, and other variables.

Longitudinal models tend to predict lower rates of change for indices of ventilatory capacity than cross-sectional models (17,10). From Table 1 it can be seen that for this diver, the change in vital capacity over a period of 9 years might be expected to be a loss of 260 ml when using cross-sectional reference values for which the effect of age is treated as being the same at all ages, but an increase of 170 ml using the longitudinal reference value where the change is related to the mean age over the period of follow-up. Relative to the latter, the actual loss of 220 ml cannot be regarded as innocuous.

IV. Observations

A. Effects of a Single Dive on Pulmonary Function

A single dive may result in symptoms from the upper respiratory tract or lung and in functional pulmonary changes. In a study of 43 saturation divers exam-

Table 1 Lung Function Data from a Saturation Diver Obtained from Medical Examinations 9 Years Apart

	Age 25	Age 34	Predicted change		Actual change
			Cross[a]	Long[b]	
FEV_1 (L)	3.85	3.12	−0.27	−0.04	−0.73
VC (L)	6.56	6.34	−0.26	+0.17	−0.22
FEV/VC (%)	58.7	49.0	−3.3	−3.5	−9.7
PEFR ($L \cdot sec^{-1}$)	8.80	7.50	−0.27	−0.11	−1.30

[a] Predicted from cross-sectional reference values (11).
[b] Predicted from longitudinal reference values (17).

ined after deep saturation dives to 300 to 450 m, 20 divers reported retrosternal discomfort, nonproductive cough, or undue breathlessness on exertion in the first 2 weeks after the dive (18). Such symptoms are nonspecific and can be due a number of factors, including oxygen toxicity and respiratory decompression sickness (''chokes''). Physical detraining during long decompression periods could be the basis for the perception of undue breathlessness on exertion but not for the other symptoms. Clinical examination and chest x-rays do not usually reveal any abnormalities after single uncomplicated dives, but functional tests in the first weeks after deep saturation dives have consistently demonstrated at least transitory changes in lung volumes and gas-transfer function.

Effects on Static and Dynamic Lung Volumes

An increase in vital capacity of 4 to 7% has been seen after several saturation dives. It was first described by Fisher et al. (19) and later by Wright et al. (20) after a 14-day saturation dive to a pressure of 4.0 ata with an atmosphere of 5.2% oxygen (normoxia), balance nitrogen. There was also an increase in maximal voluntary ventilation. This pattern of change is commonly observed following swim training or a period of training with increased respiratory loads (21,22); the mechanism is presumably related to training of the respiratory muscles. The hyperinflation can be opposed by an effect of oxygen toxicity, which would cause a decrease in vital capacity but decreases in vital capacity after otherwise uncomplicated dives have not been reported.

An increase in vital capacity after saturation dives has not, however, been a consistent finding. It was found after the deep dives reported by Cotes et al. (4), Yamasaki et al. (23), and Smith et al. (24) but was seen in only three of eight deep dives in the Norwegian study (18) and not at all by Suzuki et al. (6). Similarly, static lung volumes (total lung capacity, residual volume) have been described as either increasing (16,18) or not changing (4). Respiratory muscle training could account for an increase in total lung capacity but not in residual volume (22). The increases in static lung volumes are transient and return to predive levels within 4 to 6 weeks after exposure.

Reduced maximal expiratory flows, particularly at low lung volumes, are consistently demonstrated in divers compared with control groups in cross-sectional studies. In contrast, no such changes are seen immediately after deep saturation dives. However, interpretation of these indices is critically dependent on concurrent lung volume; if not measured at the same absolute lung volume, any effects of a reduction in airway conductance on the flow indices might be expected to be nullified by an increase in vital capacity as a result of a dive (11).

In a study of the effects of hyperoxia associated with deep saturation dives (25), eight subjects were exposed to a partial pressure of oxygen of 40 to 50 kPa for 28 days at a pressure of 0.25 MPa. The oxygen levels were chosen to be the same as in a deep saturation dive to a pressure of 3.7 MPa in an attempt to remove the potentially confounding influence of the hyperbaria. Oxygen at these partial pressures would not be expected to result in any changes in vital capacity (2).

There were, in fact, no significant changes in static lung volumes, but there was a decrease in forced expiratory flow rates. There was also an increase in inspiratory lung compliance and a trend toward a decrease in elastic recoil pressure (26). These findings are opposite to the classical description of pulmonary oxygen toxicity but are consistent with a loss of elastic properties of the lung, via destruction of elastic tissue or changes in surfactant function. The changes in lung compliance are also consistent with the increases in total lung capacity and residual volume after saturation dives. Thus, it would appear that changes in vital capacity and other static lung volumes after saturation dives are not simply an effect of mechanical loads associated with the dives.

Effects on Pulmonary Gas-Transfer Function

A reduced transfer factor for carbon monoxide is the most consistent finding immediately after deep saturation dives (4,6,18). This reduction, approximately 10 to 15%, may persist for up to 6 weeks. In a shallow experimental dive to 0.25 MPa with hyperoxia (25), the reduction in transfer factor for carbon monoxide (Tl_{CO}) was the same as in a deep saturation dive, suggesting that exposure to hyperoxia is a significant contributing factor. This finding has recently been confirmed (6,27). One possible interpretation of this loss of gas-exchanging capacity independent of ambient pressure and in the absence of changes in vital capacity is that Tl_{CO} is a more sensitive indicator of oxygen toxicity.

There are also, however, studies showing an effect of venous gas microemboli after both deep saturation dives (3,28) and air-bounce dives (29,30). The time course for the changes caused by the different protocols may, however, be different. In the shallow air-bounce dives, the changes were normalized within 2 days, but the cumulative load of venous gas microemboli must have been very different between the two decompression procedures.

Gas transfer across the lung is related to hemoglobin levels and alveolar volume. Both can be materially affected by a dive; therefore they influence the estimation of gas-exchanging capacity. All the quoted studies have taken such effects into account.

Effects on Exercise Performance

Progressive exercise testing up to a symptom-limited maximum gives information not only of the maximal working capacity of the subject but also characterizes the ventilatory, cardiovascular, and metabolic responses to increasing physiological stress. There is less information about exercise capacity after single dives compared with other lung-function characteristics, but the studies of Smith et al. (24), Cotes et al. (4), and Thorsen et al. (28) have shown a reduction in maximal oxygen uptake of about 10 to 15% after deep saturation dives. There are certain characteristic changes in the pattern of ventilatory and gas-exchange response. Resting heart rate is significantly increased and ventilation is increased relative to oxygen uptake and carbon dioxide output, which may indicate an increase in physiological dead space. There is a decrease in anaerobic threshold as assessed from gas-exchange parameters, but the study of Ørnhagen et al. (31) did not demonstrate any changes in anaerobic threshold from measurements of lactate in venous blood samples. In this latter study there was a reduction in measured maximal oxygen uptake of 15%. Maximal oxygen uptake and changes in gas-exchange characteristics are normalized within 4 to 6 weeks after the dive, the same as for the changes in other lung-function variables.

The reduction in aerobic capacity could have been due to a detraining effect as a result of the long periods of physical inactivity during decompression, typically on the order of 2 weeks. The deterioration in performance is, however, larger than would be expected after 2 weeks' detraining of athletes, where Coyle et al. (32) found a reduction in maximal oxygen uptake of 7%. The effect on anaerobic threshold after deep dives is equivocal, and changes indicating increased physiological deadspace are not expected to be caused by detraining alone.

The changes in pulmonary function described so far are mostly from studies of deep experimental saturation dives. Very few studies have looked into effects of shallow or air-bounce dives. Catron et al. (33) did not find any changes in pulmonary mechanical function after air dives to a pressure of 0.9 MPa in which venous gas microemboli were found in all of the six subjects. Dujic et al. (29) and Thorsen et al. (30) found changes in transfer factor for carbon monoxide after dives to 45 and 39 m that were ascribed to venous gas microemboli. Thus, different forms of diving result in quantitatively different exposures to various factors that are fundamentally similar.

B. Long-Term Effects on Pulmonary Function

There is little doubt that single experimental dives of the type described above result in changes in the mechanical and gas-exchanging properties of the lung. However, the relevance of these studies to normal operational diving can legitimately be questioned. The effects of these acute studies usually have a half-life of approximately 4 to 6 weeks; the existence of any residual effect with the potential to accumulate over time to a long-term effect is effectively unknown. For this, a more structured epidemiological approach is necessary. There are still very few such studies, most coming from England and Norway reflecting the high diving activity associated with the offshore oil production in the North Sea.

Cross-Sectional Studies

The first studies from England showed that divers in general had larger vital capacities than predicted (34–37) (Table 2). There was a positive correlation between vital capacity and the maximal depth the divers had ever dived to, indicating an effect of respiratory muscle training, which is consistent with the findings seen immediately after single dives. In one of the studies, however, this effect was seen only in divers less than 30 years of age (34). The later Norwegian study (38), which used different control groups, did not find any differences in vital capacity between divers, policemen, offshore workers, and the general Scandinavian population. However, if compared with the common European standard for lung function indices at that time (39), vital capacity and the FEV_1 were larger and comparable with those of the former studies. Thus, there could be a selection of subjects with large lungs as divers or an adaptation to diving, as suggested by Bouhuys and Beck (40). This question is still not definitively answered, although there are data relating vital capacity to diving history (36,37).

These studies and a later study from the former Soviet Union (41) have in common the finding that the FEV_1 and maximal expiratory flow rates at low lung volumes are smaller than expected when compared with the vital capacity. This pattern is characteristic of airway obstruction, but it must be stressed that as the forced expired volume is still within the normal predicted range, it is more appropriately described as an indication of small airway dysfunction. Significantly, there was a negative correlation between FEV_1 and cumulative diving

Table 2 Association of Indices of Lung Function with Diving Exposure

Subjects	Study	Index	Maximum depth	Years diving
858 [a]	Cross-sectional	FVC	0.13	
		FEV/FVC	−0.15	0.16
255 [a]	Longitudinal	FVC	0.12	
81 [b]	Cross-sectional	MEF_{25} [c]		
115 [b]	Cross-sectional	FEV	0.15	
		MEF_{25}		−0.032

[a] Logbook data.
[b] Laboratory data.
[c] Value reduced when compared to a control group of firebrigadesmen.
Source: Adapted from Refs. 36 and 42.

exposure measured either as number of years of diving or number of days in saturation. The conclusions were in agreement with those of Elliott et al. (42) and have recently been confirmed by Ramaswami and Watt (43), who in addition demonstrated an additive effect of cigarette smoking. In the Norwegian study only, active North Sea divers with saturation diving experience were included; there were significant negative correlations between FEV_1 and diving exposure measured as number of days in saturation dives. The same negative relationships were seen for the forced expired flow rates at low lung volume.

There are very few published studies on other lung-function variables. In the Norwegian cross-sectional study (38), there was a reduction in transfer factor for carbon monoxide which was related to increasing diving exposure, but there was no diminution in maximal oxygen uptake (43). There was, however, an increased ventilatory equivalent for both oxygen uptake and carbon dioxide output at the highest workloads, which was consistent with the exercise response reported by Davey et al. (36) in a subgroup of the English divers.

B. Longitudinal Studies

There are no adequate longitudinal studies of populations of divers followed over time in which rates of change in lung function have been related to diving exposure. In a retrospective study of 255 divers (Table 2), where diving history was derived from logbook data and lung function extracted from records held by the Diving Registry of the University of Newcastle, U.K., analysis confirmed an association of FVC with diving exposure and a positive correlation of the rate of change of FVC with the annual progression in maximal depth (36). Those divers who progressed to deeper depths year upon year had an increase in FVC, reversing the normal downward trend, whereas those whose maximal depth was relatively static or decreased exhibited a reduction in FVC. The population included a significant proportion of nonsaturation divers.

Some information is available from follow-up studies performed on selected groups of divers. Following experimental saturation dives to depths of 300 m or more, 26 divers were followed for 3 to 4 years and their lung function was compared to that of a control group of 28 professional divers who had never taken part in deep experimental diving (45). One year after the deep dive, there was a significant reduction in FEV_1 and maximal expiratory flow rates, after which the rate of change was not different between the two groups (Fig. 2). The deep divers had resumed normal commercial operational diving approximately 3 months after the experimental dive, and the subsequent diving history was not different from that of the controls.

A reduction in maximal expiratory flow rates as a consequence of exposure to hyperoxia (25) has been shown to persist for 3 years after the dive in subjects who did not take part in any diving activities over the follow-up period (46).

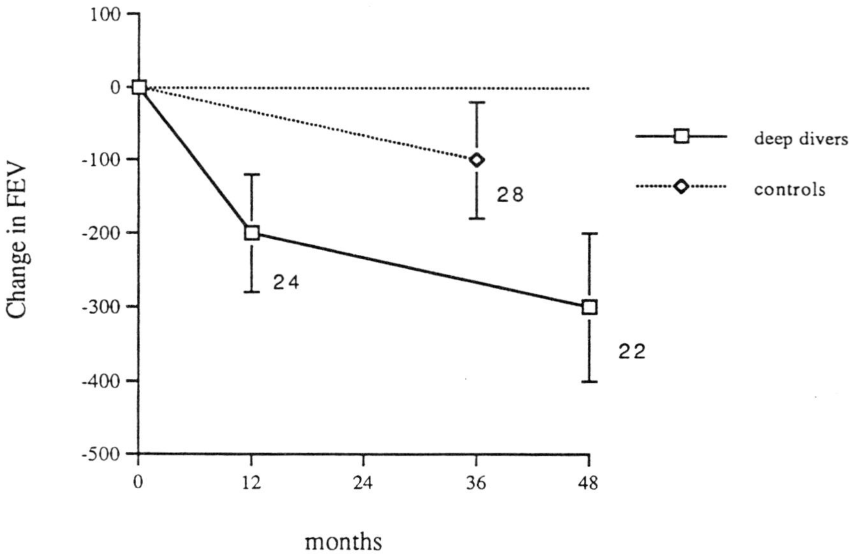

Figure 2 Reduction in FEV_1 following a deep saturation dive. Numbers 28, 24, and 22 indicate numbers of divers assessed at examination.

V. Mechanisms Underlying Observed Changes

The associations between diving exposure and changes in lung function suggest a causal relationship. It is therefore not unreasonable to assume that potential causative agents will include the major exposure factors of oxygen toxicity, decompression stress, and respiratory mechanical load. The mechanisms underlying the induced changes are reviewed in previous chapters but are essentially those relating to localized inflammatory reaction. In the case of venous gas microemboli, there will also be a mechanical effect that will disrupt the pulmonary microcirculation. This is likely to result in increased ventilation/perfusion inequality, with a secondary involvement of the small airways and alveolar ducts.

The lung has historically been considered to be a very resilient organ, resistant to abuse and with large "reserves" of functionality. Any demonstrable long-term effects have usually been accepted as positive adaptations—for example, the larger vital capacities commonly seen in divers are seen as a result of a training effect on the respiratory muscles. However, an alternative interpretation is that prolonged diving exposure causes an overdistention of the lung and therefore an increased risk of damage (34,35). In other words, an argument can be made for the situation to be viewed as the effect of work (diving exposure) on health (changes in lung function) rather than the effect of health (preexisting lung function) on work (ability to dive safely). This view was challenged (40) but recently has received some support. The suggestion has been put forward that the lung is in fact quite a fragile organ which, when stressed, operates very close to its mechanical limit (47,48). Although there is little to support this concept in man, it is consistent with the finding that lung tissue density is inversely related to lung size (49).

It might therefore be considered that diving causes a hyperinflation of the lung, which, by overstretching it, renders it more susceptible to damage from the known exposure factors. If so, it would then be logical to expect that those divers with the greatest degree of hyperinflation would exhibit the greatest loss of function. This has yet to be demonstrated.

VI. Implications for Health and Lifestyle

The clinical significance of the observed effects, which are consistent with a peripheral lung lesion affecting gas exchange, is debatable. Much depends on whether these changes are progressive or reversible and whether they continue after retirement from active diving. With the present state of knowledge, it is impossible to make a definitive statement; the information is not yet available. As with other physiological systems, the absence of reported symptoms is frequently taken to indicate that any impairment is trivial and of no clinical significance. However, symptoms will not usually be reported until there is significant loss of functionality; in the case of divers whose lung function tends to be above average, the functional loss can be material. This impairment may not lead to actual loss of ability to carry out routine tasks but may have significant implications for state of health and lifestyle in later years.

The long-term health effect of diving was the subject of an international consensus conference arranged in Norway in 1993 (50). Most of the studies referred to in this review were subjected to evaluation by a working group (which included the authors), which came to the following conclusions:

> "There are slight but definite long term effects on the lung...these would be increasingly obvious in retirement, with age."
>
> "There is evidence that changes in...the lung can be demonstrated in some divers who have not experienced a diving accident or other established environmental hazard."
>
> "The changes are in most cases minor and do not influence the diver's quality of life. However, the changes are of a nature that may influence the diver's future health."

VII. Concluding Remarks

There is little doubt that diving has acute transient physiological effects on the lung. Similarly, functional changes can be associated with indices of diving exposure in both cross-sectional and longitudinal studies in populations of divers who have not exceeded normal operational depths and which include a significant proportion of nonsaturation divers. The patterns of change are not dissimilar, which strongly suggest that the effects of single dives may be cumulative, leading to a long-term loss of pulmonary function. The association cannot, however, be considered conclusive.

Further studies of the time course and mechanisms for the acute effects are needed to establish the link between short- and long-term effects together with comprehensive longitudinal multicenter studies of both current and ex-divers to determine clinical significance.

Clarification will ultimately be dependent on the generation and maintenance of a comprehensive medical and physiological database that can be analyzed in conjunction with a detailed history of diving exposure.

References

1. Cotes JE, Steel J. Work-related lung disorders: Occupational respiratory surveys. London: Blackwell, 1987:106–121.
2. Clark JM, Lambertsen CJ. Oxygen toxicity: A review. Pharmacol Rev 1971; 23: 37–133.
3. Thorsen E, Segadal K, Kambestad BK. Mechanisms for reduced pulmonary function after a saturation dive. Eur Respir J 1994; 7:4–10.
4. Cotes JE, Davey IS, Reed JW, Rooks M. Respiratory effects of a single saturation dive to 300 m. Br J Ind Med 1987; 44:76–82.
5. Thorsen E, Segadal K, Pasche A, Gulsvik A. Pulmonary mechanical function and diffusion capacity after deep saturation dives. Br J Ind Med 1990; 47:242–247.
6. Suzuki S, Ikeda T, Hashimoto A. Decrease in the single breath diffusing capacity after saturation dives. Undersea Biomed Res 1991; 18:103–109.
7. American Thoracic Society. Lung function testing: Selection of reference values and interpretive strategies. Am Rev Respir Dis 1991; 144:1202–1218.
8. American Thoracic Society. Single breath carbon monoxide diffusing capacity (transfer factor): Recommendations for a standard technique. Am J Respir Crit Care Med 1995; 136:2185–2198.
9. Quanjer Ph, Tammeling GJ, Cotes JE, et al. Standardised lung function testing: Lung volumes and forced ventilatory flows—1993 update. Eur Respir J 1993; 6(suppl 16):4–40.
10. Cotes JE, Chinn DJ. Is respiratory function diminished? Ann NY Acad Sci 1991; 643:149–156.

11. Cotes JE. Lung Function: Assessment and Application in Medicine, 5th ed. Oxford, England: Blackwell, 1993.
12. Van Pelt W, Quanjer Ph, Borobrook G. Cohort effects in ventilatory function and chronic respiratory symptoms in a 12 year follow-up study. Eur Respir J 1989: 2(suppl 5):366s.
13. Van Pelt W, Borsboom G, Rijcken B, et al. Discrepancies between longitudinal and cross-sectional change in ventilatory function in 12 years of follow-up. Am J Respir Crit Care Med 1994; 149:1218–1226.
14. Berry G. Longitudinal observations, their usefulness and limitations with special reference to the forced expiratory volume. Bull Physiopathol Respir 1974; 10:643–655.
15. Burrows B, Lebowitz MD, Camilli AE, Knudson RJ. Longitudinal changes in forced expiratory volume in one second in adults: Methodological considerations and findings in healthy nonsmokers. Am Rev Respir Dis 1986; 133:974–980.
16. Gulyar SA, Ilyin VN. Adaptation of breathing to hyperbaria: Many years monitoring and correction. In: Hope A, Lund T, Elliott DH, et al., eds. Long-Term Heath Effects of Diving, Bergen: NUTEC 1994:343–357.
17. Chinn DJ, Cotes JE, Reed JW. Longitudinal effects of change in body mass on measurements of ventilatory capacity. Thorax 1996; 51:699–704.
18. Thorsen E, Segadal K, Myrseth E, et al. Pulmonary mechanical function and diffusion capacity after deep saturation dives. Br J Ind Med 1990; 47:242–247.
19. Fisher AB, Dubois AB, Hyde RW, et al. Effects of 2 months undersea exposure to N2-O2 at 2.2 ATA on lung function. J Appl Physiol 1970; 28:70–74.
20. Wright WB, Fisher AB, Hendricks PL, et al. Pulmonary function studies during a 14 day continuous exposure to 5.2% O_2 in N_2 at pressure equivalent to 100 fsw (4 ATA). Aerospace Med 1973; 44:837–843.
21. Leith DE, Bradley M. Ventilatory muscle strength and endurance training. J Appl Physiol 1976; 41:508–516.
22. Clanton TL, Dixon GF, Drake J, Gadek JE. Effects of swim training on lung volumes and inspiratory muscle conditioning. J Appl Physiol 1987; 62:39–46.
23. Yamasaki M, Taya Y, Fujiie K, et al. Effect of a simulated saturation dive to 31 ATA on pulmonary function Ann Physiol Anthropol 1986; 5:191–196.
24. Smith RM, Hong SK, Dressendorfer RH, et al. A 17 day dry saturation dive at 18.6 ATA: Cardiopulmonary functions. Undersea Biomed Res 1977; 4:267–281.
25. Thorsen E, Segadal K, Reed JW, et al. Contribution of hyperoxia to reduced pulmonary function after deep saturation dives. J Appl Physiol 1993; 75:657–662.
26. Reed JW, Elliott C, Thorsen E. Increased lung compliance in response to a moderate hyperoxic exposure. In: Sipinien SA, Leiniö M, eds. Proceedings of the XXIth annual meeting of the European Undersea and Biomedical Society. Helsinki, 1995: 30.
27. Suzuki S. Probable lung injury by long term exposure to oxygen close to 50 kilopascals. Undersea Hyperbar Med 1994; 21:235–243.
28. Thorsen E, Hjelle J, Segadal K, Gulsvik A. Exercise tolerance and pulmonary gas exchange after deep saturation dives. J Appl Physiol 1990; 68:1809–1814.
29. Dujic Z, Eterovic D, Denoble P, et al. Effect of a single air dive on pulmonary diffusing capacity in professional divers. J Appl Physiol 1993; 74:55–61.

30. Thorsen E, Risberg J, Segadal K, Hope A. Effects of venous gas microemboli on pulmonary gas transfer function. Undersea Hyperbar Med 1995; 22:347–353.
31. Örnhagen H. Thorsen E, Gennser M. Physical work capacity after three different saturation dives. In: Schriers LM, ed. Proceedings of the XIIth annual meeting of the European Undersea and Biomedical Society. Rotterdam, 1986:141–148.
32. Coyle EF, Martin WH, Bloomfield SA, et al. Effects of detraining on responses to submaximal exercise. J Appl Physiol 1985; 59:853–859.
33. Catron PW, Bertoncini J, Layton RP, et al. Respiratory mechanics in men following a deep air dive. J Appl Physiol 1986; 61:734–740.
34. Crosbie WA, Clarke MB, Cox RAF, et al. Physical characteristics and ventilatory function of 404 commercial divers working in the North Sea. Br J Ind Med 1977; 34:19–25.
35. Crosbie WA, Reed JW, Clarke MC. Functional characteristics of the large lungs found in commercial divers. J Appl Physiol 1979; 46:639–645.
36. Davey IS, Cotes JE, Reed JW. Relationship of ventilatory capacity to hyperbaric exposure in divers. J Appl Physiol 1984; 56:1655–1658.
37. Watt SJ. Effect of commercial diving on ventilatory function. Br J Ind Med 1985; 42:59–62.
38. Thorsen E, Segadal K, Kambestad BK, Gulsvik A. Divers' lung function: Small airways disease? Br J Ind Med 1990; 47:519–523.
39. Quanjer P. Standardized lung function testing. Bull Eur Pathophysiol Respir 1983; 19(suppl 5):7–10.
40. Bouhuys A, Beck GI. Large lungs in divers? J Appl Physiol 1979; 47:1136.
41. Dmitrouk AI, Gulyar S, Ilyin VN, Moiseenko EV. Physiological mechanisms of adaptation of divers to the condition of deep water dives in the arctic. In: Sterk W, Geeraedts L, eds. Proceedings of the XVIth annual meeting of the European Undersea and Biomedical Society. Amsterdam, 1990:311–319.
42. Elliott C, Reed JW, Cotes JE, et al. Narrowing of small lung airways in commercial divers. In: Sterk W, Geeraedts L, eds. Proceedings of the XXIth annual meeting of the European Undersea and Biomedical Society. 1990:197–202.
43. Ramaswami RA, Watt SJ. Dynamic lung function in professional divers. In: Sipinien SA, Leiniö M, eds. Proceedings of the XXIth annual meeting of the European Undersea and Biomedical Society. Helsinki, 1995:22–29.
44. Thorsen E, Segadal K, Kambestad BK. Characteristics of the response to exercise in professional saturation divers. Undersea Biomed Res 1991; 18:93–101.
45. Thorsen E, Segadal K, Kambestad B, Gulsvik A. Pulmonary function one and four years after a deep saturation dive. Scand J Work Environ Health 1993; 19:115–120.
46. Thorsen E, Kambestad BK. Persistent small-airways dysfunction after exposure to hyperoxia. J Appl Physiol 1995; 78:1421–1424.
47. Denison D. Pulmonary function—Long term effects of Diving on the Lung. In: Long-Term Health Effects of Diving. Consensus document. Bergen, Norway: John Grieg A/S, 1994:319–323.
48. Costello ML, Tsukimoto K, Prediletto R. High lung volume increases stress failure in pulmonary capillaries. J Appl Physiol 1992; 73:123–133.

49. Brudhin LH, Rhodes CG, Valind SO, et al. Regional lung density and blood volume in nonsmoking and smoking subjects measured by PET. J Appl Physiol 1987; 63: 1324–1334.
50. Hope A, Lund T, Elliott DH, et al. Long-Term Health Effects of Diving. Consensus document. Bergen, Norway: John Grieg A/S, 1994:387–391.

10

Drowning and Near-Drowning

A. JOSEPH LAYON

University of Florida and Shands Hospital
Gainesville, Florida

JEROME H. MODELL

University of Florida College of Medicine
Gainesville, Florida

I. Introduction/Epidemiology

Drowning is the third leading cause of accidental death in the United States (1); it ranks second in children aged 5 to 14 years of age and is the leading cause of accidental death among children below 2 years of age (National Centers for Health Statistics, unpublished mortality statistics, 1988). Based upon data reported for 1984 through 1987, there were approximately 80,000 near-drownings each year (2) and nearly 6000 deaths from drowning in the United States alone (1,3). In 1990, the number of deaths decreased to 3979 (4). Worldwide, approximately 150,000 deaths per year are thought to occur from drowning (3). Given the incidence of 1 death per 13 near-drownings in the United States each year, this suggests that there are approximately 2 million near-drowning events annually throughout the world. Nearly half of all persons who drown are under the age of 20 years, and 35% are accomplished swimmers (5). Factors contributing to drowning include alcohol or other drug abuse in up to 50% of cases involving adolescents or adults (6), limited swimming ability, exacerbation of existing medical problems (for example, seizure disorder or syncope), and/or attempted suicide. While most drownings and near-drownings occur in private swimming pools (50%), lakes, rivers, streams, storm drains (20%), or bathtubs

(15%) (7), there are also other unusual sites where these accidents occur. For example, the suction generated in some hot tubs has been known to be of sufficient force to trap children under water (8). Also, because of the difference between torso and lower-body size, toddlers can become trapped in a bucket or toilet when they lean over to play in the water contained in these vessels (3,7,9).

II. Definitions

There has been some confusion regarding the terminology used to describe persons who have ''drowned.'' *Dorland's Medical Dictionary* offers the following definition of drowning: ''suffocation and death resulting from filling of the lungs with water or other substance or fluid so that gas exchange becomes impossible'' (10). It is well known, however, that victims of drowning frequently aspirate only relatively small quantities of water, and the lungs are seldom ''filled with water.'' Furthermore, drowning implies death, yet many victims are resuscitated and eventually recover. Thus, the following subdefinitions delineate drowning and near-drowning events with greater accuracy. To *drown without aspiration* is to die secondary to respiratory obstruction and asphyxiate while submerged in water. To *drown with aspiration* is to die secondary to asphyxia resultant from aspiration of water while submerged. To *near-drown without aspiration* is to survive, at least initially, after an asphyxic event resultant from submersion in water. To *near-drown with aspiration* is to survive, at least initially, after submersion in and aspiration of water or other liquid material (5).

No two cases of drowning and near-drowning are identical. The type, temperature, and quantity of water aspirated may differ, and the victim's state of health prior to drowning may be important (11). One individual might have become submerged in the water secondary to complete physical exhaustion, while another may have dived into the water, hit her or his head, and suffered a concussion. A third may have severe myocardial ischemia while swimming, lose consciousness, and then aspirate water and drown. Another important factor may be the temperature of the water in which the victim was submerged; cold water, which may result in rapid hypothermia, may decrease the victim's requirement for oxygen, thereby prolonging the period of time he or she may be submerged and still completely recover (12,13). On the other hand, significant hypothermia may also lead to severe delays in myocardial conduction, arrhythmias, and cardiac arrest. Additionally, as has been shown by several groups (14–16), exposure to or immersion in cold (0 to 15°C) water increases minute ventilation and decreases maximal duration of breath holding. This may decrease the effectiveness of the dive response and increase the likelihood of drowning or near-drowning. Each of these factors must be initially evaluated when a patient is rescued from an immersion event.

III. Pathophysiology

A. Pulmonary Changes and Acid-Base Balance

The pathophysiology of drowning and near-drowning has been extensively studied (5,17–24); the central issue of most concern clinically is the effect on the pulmonary and central nervous systems. The alterations noted are primarily related to abnormal gas exchange induced by pulmonary injury and resultant cerebral hypoxia. Later, cerebral edema may follow from these processes (22–24). Interestingly, at least in endothermic animals, hypoxia results in both a lowered set point of the thermoneutral zone and vasodilation (25); the result is hypothermia without shivering and thus a decrease in oxygen consumption ($\dot{V}_{O_2}$) of about 11% per degree Celsius. Whether this phenomenon is of any significance in humans is unclear.

Drowning and Near-Drowning Without Aspiration

It has been estimated that approximately 10% of human drowning victims die without aspirating the liquid in which the event occurs (26); that is, they die from hypoxic cardiac arrest during laryngospasm or breath holding. In a canine model of asphyxia, Kristoffersen and colleges (27) separated out the effects of hypoxia, hypercarbia, and acidosis during death. This study found that hypercarbia without hypoxia was not fatal, but that when the arterial oxygen tension (Pa_{O_2}) decreased to between 10 to 15 torr, the animals inevitably died.

Craig (28,29) studied the breath-holding breaking point (the point at which a breath would be taken involuntarily) in human volunteers during simulated underwater swimming. He found that at rest, the breath-holding breaking point was 87 sec; at that time, the partial pressures of CO_2 and O_2 in alveolar air were 51 and 73 torr, respectively. After hyperventilation, breath-holding could be maintained for a full 146 sec; at this time, the partial pressure of alveolar CO_2 increased to only 46 torr, whereas alveolar oxygen tension decreased to 58 torr. When exercise followed hyperventilation, the breath-holding break point was only 85 sec. In this instance, while the alveolar partial pressure of CO_2 was only 49 torr, alveolar oxygen tension had dropped to 43 torr. Craig concluded that while exercise, such as swimming, increased metabolically produced CO_2, the Pa_{CO_2} was relatively low because stores had been depleted during hyperventilation; thus, the urge to breathe was delayed. With exercise, the Pa_{O_2} decreased to levels incompatible with maintaining consciousness prior to the time the level of Pa_{CO_2} had become unbearable. Thus, he surmised that loss of consciousness during underwater swimming was a result of cerebral hypoxia rather than hypercarbia. This work was sentinel in our understanding of the pathophysiology of near-drowning without aspiration.

From data such as these, we now know that hypoxia is the signal abnormality in death resultant from acute respiratory obstruction. While it is possible that the added effects of acidosis and hypercarbia may contribute secondarily to the terminal event, the primary phenomenon in these cases is hypoxemia. Reinstitution of adequate ventilation and oxygenation before the occurrence of circulatory arrest or irreversible nervous system damage results in complete and dramatic restoration of function. If, however, spontaneous ventilation begins while the patient is still submerged in water, aspiration will occur, resulting in a more complicated and persistent pathophysiology.

Drowning and Near-Drowning with Aspiration

Approximately 85 to 90% of human drowning and near-drowning victims aspirate aqueous media into their lungs (26,30). While multiple models have been devised to study the phenomena of near-drowning and drowning with aspiration and different methods have been used to measure oxygenation, all authors agree that hypoxia occurs immediately upon aspiration of the fluid. Although there are some differences in the degree of hypoxemia, depending on whether large or small volumes of fluid are aspirated, profound alterations in arterial oxygenation may occur when as little as 1 to 2.2 mL/kg water is aspirated into the lungs (17,19,31,32). Unlike near-drowning without aspiration, in which reinstitution of ventilation and circulation results in the immediate reversal of hypoxemia, when aspiration of water occurs, the hypoxemia is persistent. For example, Modell (18) showed that after instillation of 22 mL/kg of fresh water or normal saline solution into the tracheas of anesthetized dogs, significant arterial hypoxemia persisted even though the animals were breathing spontaneously and hyperventilating when the 60-min postaspiration blood samples were drawn. Hypoxemia also resulted when volumes as small as 2.2 mL/kg were instilled intratracheally and treatment was limited to restoring spontaneous ventilation and circulation (17). In another study, when 11 mL/kg of fresh water or seawater was instilled into the trachea, Pa_{O_2} was reduced for at least 72 hr after the aspirative event (33). As discussed by Modell and colleagues (33), the hypoxia and intrapulmonary shunting seen immediately after near-drowning with aspiration of fresh water are due in large measure to alteration of the surface-tension properties of alveolar surfactant (34). Seawater aspiration does not alter surfactant surface-tension properties; however, fluid-filled but perfused alveoli cause shunting after seawater is aspirated (34). Thus, aspiration of either type of water leads to the functional collapse of terminal gas-exchanging airways. Differences in the pathophysiology of hypoxemia seen after freshwater versus seawater near-drowning are discussed in more detail below.

In a study of 91 patients, Modell and colleagues (30) analyzed arterial blood for Pa_{O_2}, Pa_{CO_2}, and pHa at various times after an immersive event in either seawater, fresh water, or brackish water. In many of these cases, profound arterial hypoxemia was noted; the Pa_{O_2} to inspired oxygen fraction (FI_{O_2}) ratio ranged from 30 to 585 torr. Only one patient with a Pa_{O_2}:FI_{O_2}>150 torr died; this individual was judged neurologically unsalvageable and therapy was withdrawn. Two patients had Pa_{O_2} above 80 torr while breathing room air; both these individuals were thought to be victims of near-drowning without aspiration (30). While in some patients the Pa_{O_2} returns to normal within 48 hr, others show persistent hypoxia for days and even weeks following an episode of near-drowning (30,35,36).

Mechanism of the Pulmonary Effects Seen with Near-Drowning

One of the first investigators to suggest a mechanism for the events seen with drowning was Karpovich (37), who suggested that water in the alveoli and conducting airways impaired ventilation by mechanical blockage during subsequent resuscitation. Since this initial work, other investigators have demonstrated that aspiration of seawater leads to an increase in the volume of fluid within the air spaces of the lungs (19,38). Halmagyi (31) showed that the weight of rat lungs increased threefold above the weight added by instilled seawater. Other studies (19,38) have shown that if one attempts to drain the lungs of dogs by gravity or mechanical suction after aspiration of seawater, more fluid is harvested than was initially instilled into the trachea. Indeed, in a canine model of massive seawater aspiration—40 to 91 mL/kg—Redding and colleagues (38) noted that volume drained from the lungs in excess of 14 to 33 mL/kg was associated with survival only when replacement of intravascular volume was provided.

Conversely, after freshwater aspiration, the lungs of rats did not increase in weight (31). When a sublethal amount of fresh water was aspirated into anesthetized dogs (17,33,39), it was absorbed so rapidly that significant amounts of water could not be recovered from the airway by gravity drainage after only 3 min.

Since seawater is hypertonic, it is relatively easy to understand why pulmonary edema occurs in patients who have suffered a near-drowning event in seawater; it is not quite as clear why this may occur with fresh water. Studies of the effects of aspirated water on the surface-tension properties of pulmonary surfactant have partially explained this question (34). Pulmonary surfactant extracted from the lungs of animals that died while totally immersed in fresh water exhibit abnormal surface-tension properties, thus promoting alveolar instability and collapse. In contrast, during total immersion in isotonic saline or in seawater, while some surfactant is washed from the lungs, significant quantities of normal material remain, so that surfactant extracted at autopsy displays surface-tension properties compatible with normal function. Since alveoli deficient in surfactant are unstable and become permeable to fluid, it is quite likely that at least one factor contributing to the pulmonary edema occurring after freshwater aspiration is the loss of the normal surface-tension activity of surfactant. Another factor that may be involved is the transient hypervolemia that occurs with freshwater aspiration (17,21). The pulmonary edema that occurs after seawater aspiration, on the other hand, is probably due primarily to an osmotic gradient across the alveolar capillary membrane with accumulation of alveolar fluid.

Whether the near-drowning occurs in fresh water or seawater, the end result is pulmonary edema, a decrease in pulmonary compliance, and an increase in the ventilation/perfusion mismatch. Immediately after aspiration of either liquid, a large alveolar-arterial oxygen gradient is seen, whether the subject is breathing room air or 100% oxygen. This suggests that the hypoxia seen in near-drowning is due to ventilation/perfusion mismatch, which spans the spectrum from absolute intrapulmonary shunt to a simple imbalance in the ventilation/perfusion ratio. In a detailed and, for its time, rather elaborate investigation, Colebatch and Halmagyi (32) studied the effects of fluid aspiration on pulmonary mechanics in an ovine model. Animals were divided into groups of between three and seven, and either fresh water (1 or 3 mL/kg) or seawater (1 or 2.5 mL/kg) was instilled intratracheally. Compliance of the lung was noted to decrease by as much as 66% (from 29 to 100 to 16 to 31 mL/cmH_2O) within 5 min of liquid instillation; elastic work of breathing increased five- to ninefold (from 10 to 65 to 55 to 100 kg-m/min/10^{-2}); airways resistance increased two- to eightfold (from 1.5 to 1.8 to 2.1 to 9.4 cmH_2O/L/sec). The administration of atropine (intravenous) or isoproterenol (intravenous or inhaled) lessened the degree of compliance alteration noted (40).

During the recovery phase after aspiration of either fresh water or seawater, significant hypoxia may be seen during breathing of room air, even after the alveolar-arterial oxygen gradient while breathing 100% oxygen has returned to normal (33,35). This finding suggests that areas of nonuniform ventilation/perfusion or diffusion alteration cause hypoxia even after absolute intrapulmonary shunt is no longer clinically significant. A number of changes that occur following aspiration of fluid may also contribute to this delayed defect. These include organization of a proteinaceous exudate, injury to the alveolar-capillary membrane, or secondary infection of the lung.

A variety of microscopic findings have been reported after fluid aspiration. After instillation of small quantities of fresh water (0.1 mL/100 mg), rat lungs did not show changes when studied by electron microscopy. After aspiration of the same quantity of seawater, however, increases in lung weight and intra-alveolar hemorrhage were observed (31). When rat lungs were perfused with fresh water via the trachea, findings included a widening of the alveolar septa, collapse of capillaries, decrease in the number of red blood cells, enlargement of the endothelial and septal nuclei, swelling of the mitochondria, and obliteration of cell outlines. These changes can all be attributed, presumably, to the rapid absorption of large quantities of fresh water from the alveoli. When rat lungs were perfused intratracheally with seawater, the changes noted were less marked and the septal and endothelial nuclei were small and dark. Red blood cells were seen in the capillaries and, although there was irregular folding of cell walls, the overall architecture of the lung was preserved (41). Thus, the microscopic changes that may be seen are different when a large versus a small volume of fluid is aspirated; the differences widen depending upon whether fresh water or seawater is aspirated.

In humans and animals, another frequent finding on autopsy after death by submersion is hyperexpansion of the lungs, resembling acute emphysema (23,42,43). These changes were attributed by Milosavich (43) to rupture of alveoli due to wide fluctuations in airway pressure during violent ventilatory efforts against a closed glottis or due to airway obstruction from water during submersion; the precise mechanism is not clear. If the patient survives for at least 12 hr after near-drowning, only to die later, the lungs will frequently show evidence of pneumonia, abscesses, mechanical injury, and deposition of alveolar hyaline material from approximately 12 hr after the near-drowning event to the third day (23). The findings are not surprising in light of Fuller's report that, in 70% of humans autopsied after drowning, evidence of having aspirated material other than water—that is, vomitus, mud, sand, or algae—was found. In spite of severe changes in pulmonary parenchyma, Butt and colleagues (36) were unable to demonstrate any consistent pattern of abnormality in pulmonary function or arterial oxygenation of patients who were studied after recovery from near-drowning. It appears that, whatever the acute changes, clinical pulmonary abnormalities are usually completely reversible after recovery from near-drowning.

Finally, neurogenic pulmonary edema must be considered as a possible cause of hypoxia after aspiration of fresh water or seawater. Even though neurogenic pulmonary edema tends to be more interstitial in nature and does not result in as extreme a degree of free foam in the airways, it may still be difficult clinically to differentiate pulmonary edema caused by aspirating freshwater or seawater from that secondary to neurogenic causes.

No matter the cause, however, intrapulmonary shunting and Pa_{O_2} can be improved by the appropriate application of positive end-expiratory pressure (PEEP) or continuous positive airway pressure (CPAP) to the airway after near-drowning (44–47). Early studies on the utilization of newer modalities of therapy such as nitric oxide (48) and partial liquid ventilation (49) appear to be promising in the treatment of other causes of severe pulmonary edema, but randomized, prospective clinical studies have not yet been reported in the treatment of near-drowning patients.

B. Changes in Blood Volume and Serum Electrolytes

After the aspiration of hypo- or hypertonic fluid media, changes other than those affecting the pulmonary parenchyma were historically thought to be of considerable significance (20). A significant change in blood volume requires the aspiration of a large volume of fluid. If greater than 11 ml/kg of hypotonic fluid is aspirated, the blood volume will increase in direct proportion to the amount aspirated (17,44). If the patient is successfully resuscitated, this absorbed fluid is rapidly redistributed and, within 1 hr, hypovolemia may occur (21). When a significant quantity of hypertonic seawater is aspirated, significant hypovolemia may rapidly ensue (19). When the aspiration of significant amounts of either hypo- or hypertonic fluid is suspected, effective circulating blood volume must be followed by measuring the patient's central venous pressure, pulmonary artery occlusion pressure, or the right-ventricular end-diastolic volume (50) to assist in the determination of treatment. However, while some require significant fluid replacement, most near-drowning victims do not aspirate enough fluid to cause life-threatening changes in blood volume.

Similarly, serum electrolyte concentrations can change after drowning and near-drowning and are also dependent on the amount and type of fluid aspirated. Experimental work in a canine model has shown that with aspiration of $\leq$22 ml/kg of either fresh water (17) or seawater (19), significant long-term changes in serum electrolyte concentrations did not occur (17,19). Again, aspiration of volumes of water in excess of this amount is highly unlikely in *near-drowned* humans and is found in only 15% of humans who die in the water from drowning (51). This probably explains why life-threatening changes in serum electrolyte concentrations have not been reported in fresh-water and seawater near-drowning victims. Thus, each patient's initial intravenous fluid therapy should be 0.9% saline solution, or, less optimally, lactated Ringer's solution, and serum electrolyte concentrations should be evaluated before any specific corrective electrolyte therapy is started. There is rarely any need for emergent treatment secondary to electrolyte abnormalities unless very large volumes of water are aspirated or the near-drowning event occurs in an extremely concentrated liquid medium, such as the Dead Sea [Na^+, K^+, Cl^-, Ca^{2+}, and Mg^{2+} are 3 to 36 times as concentrated in this body of water as in the Mediterranean Sea (52)].

While there are no data evaluating the effects of hypertonic saline resuscitation in near-drowned victims, animal studies have suggested that these solutions help prevent elevation of intracranial pressure (ICP) postinjury (global ischemia as well as focal cryogenic injury). Some (53,54), but not all (55,56), studies attempting to evaluate the differential effect of hypertonic versus iso-/hypotonic fluid to resuscitate animals from hemorrhage (52,57,58) or the effect of hemodilution (54) without brain injury have noted that ICP was lower in the experimental subjects (rabbits, dogs, and pigs) in which hypertonic solutions were used. In one study (57) in which animals suffered a focal cryogenic brain injury, cerebral blood flow (CBF) was higher and ICP lower in animals infused with hypertonic sodium lactate (500 mOsm/L) as compared with lactated Ringer's solution (270 mOsm/L). We reiterate that it must be taken into consideration that these studies were not performed in a near-drowning model.

Two animal studies evaluating outcome in complete (58) or incomplete (59) cerebral ischemia suggest that fluid replacement with solutions containing glucose results in a significantly worse neurological outcome than does replacement with a crystalloid without glucose. Finally, Ashwal and colleagues (60) suggest that elevated blood glucose levels as well as reduced CBF measured by the stable xenon technique correlate with poor outcome. Thus, we use 0.9% saline solution for emergency resuscitation. Glucose is not utilized unless the measured blood glucose is subnormal.

C. Effects on Hemoglobin and Hematocrit

If large volumes of fresh water are aspirated, hemolysis of red blood cells can occur, causing plasma hemoglobin levels to rise. The cause of the hemolysis has been shown to be secondary not only to hypotonicity but also to profound hypoxemia (61). Indeed, when animals received intravenous infusion of distilled water (44 ml/kg, a sufficient volume to cause severe electrolyte changes), they showed an elevated plasma hemoglobin only when the water infusion was associated with a concomitant hypoxic event (due to an occluded endotracheal tube). When the same volume of water was instilled intratracheally, hypoxia and hemolysis occurred.

In a canine near-drowning model, chlorinated or unchlorinated distilled water or saline at a volume of 22 ml/kg was instilled into the animals' tracheas (18). Gross hemolysis was observed in 9 out of 10 animals that aspirated distilled water but in none of those having aspirated saline. Significant changes in hemoglobin and hematocrit values are rarely found in humans (30), which lends further support to the theory that near-drowned humans do not aspirate large amounts of fluid. When a sufficiently large volume of water is aspirated and hemolysis does occur, serious bleeding disorders such as disseminated intravascular coagulation may occur (62). Only one of 91 consecutive near-drowning patients reported by Modell and colleagues (30) demonstrated a plasma hemoglobin level of 500 mg/100 ml; this individual later died of massive lung consolidation.

D. Effects on Cardiovascular and Renal Systems

A wide range of electrocardiographic changes have been observed in experimental studies of both freshwater and seawater drowning. Rarely, however, is a specific therapy required, since these changes abate when adequate oxygenation has been reestablished. Death from ventricular fibrillation after freshwater aspiration is very rare but can occur if very large amounts of fluid are aspirated (20,44). In one canine study in which saline or distilled water, 22 ml/kg intratracheally, was instilled, bigeminy occurred in 9 out of 15 dogs, while T-wave elevation was noted in 6 out of 15 (18). Even when associated with ventricular fibrillation, death is generally thought to be essentially due to hypoxia. However, Karch (63) reported finding significant cardiac pathologic changes 29 min after either a freshwater or saltwater (6 ml/kg intratracheal instillation) drowning episode. Light microscopy revealed focal areas of disruption of the normal striation pattern and, on occasion, of the intercalated disks, as well as hypereosinophilia of myocytes. On electron microscopy, the damaged myocytes showed hypercontraction with swelling and an increased lucency of the mitochondria; also seen in the myocyte nuclei was chromatin clumping and crenation. These changes were not noted in the one control animal. While the clinical relevance of these findings is uncertain, they are of interest to the further study of cardiac abnormalities after near-drowning.

Renal function is usually unimpaired; however albuminuria (23), cylindruria (23), hemoglobinuria (23,64–68), oliguria (64), acute tubular necrosis (23), and anuria (64) have on occasion been noted. Several etiologies for this renal dysfunction have been implicated, including myoglobinuria due to muscle trauma, lactic acidosis, hypoxemia or hypoperfusion, and hemolysis with subsequent hemoglobinemia (5). Although these are not common problems, all should be considered possible threats to renal function and treated accordingly.

E. Neurological Effects

A variety of neurological abnormalities have been described after near-drowning. Most victims suffer a period of unconsciousness thought to be secondary to cerebral hypoxia (44). As one of the principal issues with regard to near-drowning is the status of the patient's central nervous system, frequent neurological assessment utilizing the Glasgow Coma Scale (GCS) should be performed. This issue has been investigated by both Conn and colleagues (69) and Modell et al. (70). In these studies, the investigators found that patients who are awake and oriented upon arrival to the emergency room survive without neurological sequelae if treatment of their pulmonary problem is successful. Ninety (70) to 100% (69) of patients who arrived in the emergency room with a blunted mental status (that is, stuporous but capable of being aroused, with purposeful movements to pain) survived without neurologic residua. Patients who presented to the emergency room in a coma, however, had much worse outcomes: while 44 (69) to 55% (70) recovered completely, 10 (70) to 23% (69) had severe persistent neurological sequelae, with the highest incidence occurring in pediatric near-drowning cases. Approximately 34% (69,70) of comatose patients died after presentation. In comatose children, survival with normal brain function approximated 44%, while 39% died and approximately 17% survived with incapacitating brain damage (69,70). The implication is that the healthy hearts of children, as opposed to those of adults, will respond to cardiopulmonary resuscitation (CPR) even after a significant period of hypoxemia results in brain damage.

Attempts to "resuscitate" the brain in pediatric near-drowning cases have been largely unsuccessful. Three small studies (71–73) involving 75 severe pediatric near-drownings found that in spite of aggressive cerebral resuscitation—which included fluid restriction, ICP monitoring, intravenous mannitol for elevated ICP, hyperventilation, neuromuscular blockade, barbiturates, and, in some of the children, steroids and induced hypothermia—only 12 (16%) survived neurologically intact; the remainder either died or remained in persistent vegetative state, or, in one case, survived with mild to moderate mental retardation. Extensive neuropsychological testing in a portion of the apparently intact survivors showed nearly average cognitive function with mild gross motor and coordination defects (73).

Conn and colleagues (69) attempted to use hypothermia, barbiturate coma, neuromuscular blockers, hyperventilation, and dehydration to enhance neurologic outcome; this treatment regimen was termed "HYPER therapy." While they initially thought that there was significant improvement in the number of normal outcomes in some subgroups of near-drowned patients, a comparable series presented by Modell et al. (70) found similar results without utilizing HYPER therapy. In a follow-up study to Conn's work, Bohn and colleagues (74) from the same institution were unable to substantiate Conn's findings.

Recent findings by other groups have suggested that the use of multimodality therapy for brain protection is of little use. For example, Allman and colleagues (75) studied 66 children between April 1979 and September 1984. Each patient required full CPR and had an initial GCS of 3 (the most severe presentation possible) in the emergency room. Each patient's GCS was reclassified according to the results of a repeat neurological examination upon arrival to the pediatric intensive care unit. The results showed 16 patients (24%) with apparently intact survival, 17 patients (26%) with vegetative survival, and 33 who died (50%). None of the patients who arrived in the intensive care unit with a GCS of 3 survived neurologically intact. Fifty-five patients were also treated with ICP monitoring and aggressive therapy directed at control of ICP. Despite adequate control of ICP and maintenance of cerebral perfusion pressure (CPP), only 8 (14%) of the monitored patients survived intact, 12 (22%) survived in a vegetative state, and between 33 and 35 patients died.* The authors

*Because of problems with data presentation, the exact number of deaths cannot be determined.

suggested that, while aggressive emergency room resuscitation of pediatric near-drowning victims was justified, cerebral resuscitation measures needed to be subjected to critical prospective evaluation.

In a retrospective study of 93 patients who suffered near-drowning events, Nichter and Everett (76) showed that none of the patients who required cardiotonic drugs to obtain a perfusing cardiac rhythm survived with intact neurological status. However, all patients who had reactive pupils on arrival to the emergency room survived neurologically intact. This study is flawed by the fact that it was retrospective and lacked statistical analysis. In another retrospective study of 55 patients, Biggart and Bohn (12) showed that, all other things being equal, prolonged in-hospital resuscitation and aggressive treatment of nonhypothermic near-drowning victims resulted in an increased number of survivors in a vegetative state. When accidental hypothermia occurred at the time of the near-drowning episode, a better outcome usually resulted. However, a recent study suggests that those children who show significant neurological improvement within hours after successful CPR usually recover; those who do not are more likely to have a poor outcome (13).

Despite these rather dismal data, in a study of 121 near-drowned children, of whom 51 were in the C_3 stage of coma [no response to pain, fixed/dilated pupils, absence of spontaneous respiration, hypotension, and poor perfusion as described by Conn and Modell and their colleagues (69,70)], Nussbaum (77) found that with aggressive resuscitation as noted above, 19 of 51 (37%) had complete recovery, 14 of 51 (27%) had significant brain damage, and 18 of 51 (35%) died. The correlates of outcome in the C_3 group were submersion time, mean ICP, and mean CPP. While the report of Nussbaum (77) is encouraging, the fact that aggressive therapy is so often unsuccessful suggests that the cerebral insult is related not to ICP per se but rather to the duration of the ischemic or to reperfusion injury; the mechanisms for this type of injury have been recently reviewed (78). Further work in this area is needed to sort out the inconsistencies.

F. Treatment

Prehospital Treatment

Since most episodes of drowning and near-drowning occur away from the hospital, the initial prehospital therapy clearly affects patient outcome. The central issues that the rescuer must be concerned with when encountering a near-drowned victim are: Is the victim breathing? Does the victim have a pulse? Has a cervical spinal injury occurred?

The main objective of out-of-hospital therapy is to restore normal ventilation and circulation and to normalize gas exchange, acid-base status, and the circulation as rapidly as possible. Thus, CPR must be initiated as soon as the rescuer encounters a near-drowned victim. If the victim is apneic, mouth-to-mouth resuscitation must be initiated. Ideally, the procedure is begun in the water if it can be done without putting the rescuer in danger. During mouth-to-mouth resuscitation, care must be taken to maximize forward movement of the jaw rather than hyperextension of the cervical spine, as cervical injury may be present. This point is especially important in near-drowning cases thought to be related to diving (44). The importance of maintaining an adequate airway cannot be overemphasized, as the near-drowning victim may have swallowed large amounts of water before losing consciousness. Thus, gastric distension from inadequate mouth-to-mouth ventilation may cause the patient to regurgitate and aspirate stomach contents, with resultant aspiration pneumonitis (79). Once the rescuer is able, the victim must be evaluated carefully for the presence of a pulse. Severe bradycardia due to hypothermia, vasoconstriction, and/or hypoxia may make the arterial pulse difficult to palpate. If there is any question about the existence of a pulse, closed chest cardiac compression must be initiated and artificial ventilation continued until further help arrives.

As soon as more extensively trained individuals are available, other therapeutic modalities should be considered. Ventilation with a bag-valve-mask device using 100% oxygen should be initiated as soon as available. In the unconscious or severely hypoxic patient or in a patient in whom the airway cannot be protected for some other reason, an endotracheal tube should be placed for airway protection and to facilitate mechanical ventilation and oxygenation. Additionally, a large-bore intravenous catheter should be placed for fluid and drug therapy. Fluid therapy, as discussed above, is initiated with 0.9% saline solution.

The subdiaphragmatic thrust (Heimlich) maneuver has been recommended for use in the near-drowned victim (80,81). Previous work has shown that water exiting the mouth after drowning comes from the stomach (82). Furthermore, studies by Werner et al. (83) did not show increased benefit from an abdominal thrust over gravity drainage on the outcome of experimental animals who aspirated seawater. A thorough review of publications and testimony by the Institute of Medicine in 1994 concluded that use of this maneuver is inappropriate unless a foreign object is obstructing the airway (84). Further, use of this technique may result in delay of effective CPR or in regurgitation and aspiration of gastric contents, with consequences as serious as aspiration pneumonitis, respiratory failure, and death (84–86).

Finally, no matter how well the patient appears, he or she must be taken to a hospital for evaluation, as the initial appearance of the near-drowned patient may be misleading. It is our opinion that transport to the hospital should be carried out with basic monitoring, including electrocardiography and pulse oximetry. Oxygen (100%) should be administered en route until oxyhemoglobin analysis by pulse oximetry or Pa_{O_2} demonstrates that it can be reduced safely.

Hospital Treatment

As mentioned earlier, artificial ventilation should be administered to the apneic near-drowned patient as quickly as possible. While initial therapy is being started, one member of the health care team should obtain as adequate a history of the incident as possible from whomever accompanied the patient. Important historical points include the time of the accident, the approximate period of immersion (although this is notoriously unreliable), the type and content of the fluid, and whether or not vomiting occurred (44). All near-drowned patients should be considered to have an injury of the cervical spine until this is ruled out radiographically.

Initial hospital care should emphasize pulmonary support, with treatment individualized to patient status. As soon as possible, arterial blood gas (ABG) values should be obtained to evaluate the acid-base status and pulmonary gas exchange (44). Supplemental oxygen administration should be continued while obtaining data from ABG measurements or a pulse oximeter to evaluate for the presence of hypoxemia. Awake, alert, and cooperative patients do not require endotracheal intubation unless their pulmonary pathology does not respond favorably to enriching inhaled gas with oxygen, a CPAP mask, or both (44). All comatose patients require endotracheal intubation; those with a blunted mental status must be evaluated individually.

Spontaneous breathing is preferred if the patient can support a sufficient degree of minute ventilation with intermittent mandatory ventilation added. If this arrangement does not provide adequate ventilation, the patient is fully supported with controlled mechanical ventilation. Pressure-support ventilation (starting at 10 cmH_2O) is used to overcome work imposed by the endotracheal tube (ETT) and breathing apparatus to spontaneous breathing in adult patients (87,88).

The CPAP/PEEP is titrated so as to maintain adequate oxygen saturation ($\geqslant$95%) while using the lowest possible $F_{I_{O_2}}$. Thus, we attempt to keep the Pa_{O_2}:$F_{I_{O_2}}$ ratio above 300* and the $F_{I_{O_2}}$ below 0.5. $F_{I_{O_2}}$ below this level is generally considered to put the patient at minimal risk for oxygen toxicity. Several controlled studies have shown the effectiveness of CPAP with either mechanical or spontaneous ventilation to treat the hypoxemia associated with near-drowning (45–47). As long as the mean airway pressure is not different, there is no difference in the ability of either CPAP or PEEP to increase functional residual capacity. However, as work of breathing with CPAP is less than with PEEP, we recommend the former for spontaneously breathing patients. Also, Bergquist et al. (47) found that adding mechanical breaths to CPAP in otherwise sponta-

---

*Pa_{O_2} = 120 torr and $F_{I_{O_2}}$ = 0.4 yields a ratio of 300. This suggests a pulmonary shunt of no more than 15 to 20%.

neously breathing animals who nearly drowned in fresh water decreased intrapulmonary shunting.

A pulmonary artery catheter is not required in most patients. However, if there is concern as to the adequacy of intravascular volume, invasive monitoring with either a pulmonary artery catheter or transesophageal echocardiography may be appropriate. While cardiac output may decrease when mechanical ventilation, PEEP, and CPAP are used, it will usually improve with fluid loading, and prolonged inotropic support is rarely required (21).

In general, steroids have been shown to be ineffective in treating the pulmonary lesion of near-drowning and may in fact worsen outcome by interfering with the normal healing process (30,79,89,90). Antibiotics are appropriate when and if the patient develops signs of infection or in special cases such as near-drowning in a grossly contaminated body of water. If the medium in which the individual suffered his or her near-drowning event was a heavily contaminated body of water, it is appropriate to utilize broad-spectrum antibiotics before obtaining positive bacterial cultures. Bronchospasm may be seen in these patients and may be treated with either an intravenous bronchodilator such as aminophylline or with a nebulized drug such as albuterol or glycopyrrolate.

Pulmonary edema, as discussed above, is a common finding after near-drowning with aspiration. The application of CPAP and PEEP will recruit collapsed alveoli and facilitate oxygenation while the underlying pulmonary injury recovers. However, breaking the ventilator circuit to suction or provide nebulized treatments (as above) after CPAP and PEEP have been optimized can lead to a rapid and rather dramatic recurrence of pulmonary edema and hypoxemia. Thus, interruption of the ventilator circuit should be minimized or avoided if possible.

Despite the controversial data regarding the treatment of ICP, it is reasonable to consider placing an ICP monitoring device in comatose near-drowning victims as soon as possible after arrival at the intensive care unit. Even without an ICP monitor, mild hyperventilation (Pa_{CO_2} approximately 30 torr) may be used empirically without significant risk. If ICP is elevated ($\geq$20 torr), hyperventilation to achieve a Pa_{CO_2} of 25 to 30 torr is carried out in an attempt to decrease cerebral blood flow and thereby the ICP while simultaneously keeping the CPP [which is defined as the mean arterial pressure (MAP) - ICP] at or above 60 torr. A mannitol bolus, 0.5 g/kg ideal body weight, may be used to decrease ICP if hyperventilation alone does not produce the desired result. However, as noted previously in this chapter, the damage to the brain in near-drowning is probably the result of anoxia at the time of the injury as opposed to late elevated ICP; elevated ICP in these patients may well be nothing more than a marker of damage already done.

The importance of prehospital care of near-drowning victims is now understood, and we are now more adept at providing it than we have ever been in the past. Patients who receive early basic cardiac life support have an increased chance for normal survival. We are able to treat the pulmonary and cardiovascular complications of near-drowning quite successfully in most cases. However, in spite of years of investigation, the issue of neurological outcome has remained a stumbling block that we have been unable to surmount. It appears that, in the absence of hypothermia, aggressive brain resuscitation using current techniques is of questionable value in terms of returning the patient to normal neurological function. While there appear to be no ''magic bullets'' on the horizon, study of free-radical scavengers, calcium channel blockers, prostacyclin/thromboxane manipulations, and blockers of excitatory neuropeptides as well as investigation of phenytoin (noted to increase survival and decrease neurological deficit after cardiac arrest) are ongoing (91,92).

The most important things we can do today to prevent near-drowning deaths and persistent vegetative state as a result of near-drowning are to implement standards that govern safe pool design; enforce rules that require adequate (at least 5 ft high with self-closing latches) perimeter fencing around pools (9,93); restrict the sale and consumption of alcoholic beverages in boating, pool, harbor, marina and beach areas (9); impose severe sanctions against boat drivers who are intoxicated; post signs in areas of dangerous underwater tow (6); and, perhaps most importantly, instruct the general population in basic cardiac life support (9).

References

1. Accident Facts. Chicago: National Safety Council, 1987.
2. Baker SP, O'Neill B, Karpf RS. The Injury Fact Book. Lexington: Lexington Books–DC Heath, 1984:155–165.
3. Orlowski JP. Drowning, near-drowning, and ice-water submersions. Pediatr Clin North Am 1987; 34:75–92.
4. Vital Statistics of the United States, Vol 2: Mortality, Part A. 1990.
5. Modell JH. The Pathophysiology and Treatment of Drowning and Near-Drowning. Springfield, IL: Charles C Thomas, 1971.
6. Gulaid JA, Sattin RW. Drownings in the United States, 1978–1984. MMWR 1988; 37(SS-1):27–33.
7. Wintemute GJ, Kraus JF, Teret SP, Wright M. Drowning in childhood and adolescence—A population based study. Am J Public Health 1987; 77:830–832.
8. Monroe B. Immersion accidents in hot tubs and whirlpool spas. Pediatrics 1982; 69:805–807.
9. Cardiner SD, Smeeton WMI, Koelmeyer TD, Cairns FJ. Accidental drownings in Auckland children. NZ Med J 1985; 98:579–582.
10. Dorland's Illustrated Medical Dictionary, 25th ed. Philadelphia: Saunders, 1974: 475.

11. Davis JH. Autopsy findings in victims of drowning. In: Modell JH, ed. The Pathophysiology and Treatment of Drowning and Near-Drowning. Springfield, IL: Charles C Thomas 1971:74–82.
12. Biggart MJ, Bohn DJ. Effect of hypothermia and cardiac arrest on outcome of near-drowning accidents in children. J Pediatr 1990; 117:179–183.
13. Kemp AM, Sibert JR. Outcome in children who nearly drown—A British Isles study. Br J Med 1991; 302:931–933.
14. Hayward JS, Hay C, Matthews BR, et al. Temperature effect on the human dive response in relation to cold water near-drowning. J Appl Physiol 1984; 56:202–206.
15. Keatinge WR, Nadel JA. Immediate respiratory response to sudden cooling of the skin. J Appl Physiol 1965; 20:65–69.
16. Cooper KE, Martin S, Riben P. Respiratory and other responses in subjects immersed in cold water. J Appl Physiol 1976; 40:903–910.
17. Modell JH, Moya F. Effects of volume of aspirated fluid during chlorinated freshwater drowning. Anesthesiology 1966; 27:662–672.
18. Modell JH, Gaub M, Moya F, et al. Physiologic effects of near-drowning with chlorinated freshwater, distilled water, and isotonic saline. Anesthesiology 1966; 27:33–41.
19. Modell JH, Moya F, Newby EJ, et al. The effects of fluid volume in seawater drowning. Ann Intern Med 1967; 67:68–80.
20. Swann HG, Brucer M. The cardiorespiratory and biochemical events during rapid anoxic death VI—Freshwater and seawater drowning. Texas Rep Biol Med 1949; 7:604–618.
21. Tabeling BB, Modell JH. Fluid administration increases oxygen delivery during continuous positive pressure ventilation after freshwater near-drowning. Crit Care Med 1983; 11:693–696.
22. Fuller RH. The clinical pathology of human near-drowning. Proc R Soc Med 1963; 56:33–38.
23. Fuller RH. The 1962 Wellcome prize essay—Drowning and the postimmersion syndrome. Mil Med 1963; 128:22–36.
24. Miles S. Drowning. Br Med J 1968; 3:597–600.
25. Wood SC. Interactions between hypoxia and hypothermia. Annu Rev Physiol 1991; 53:71–85.
26. Cot C. Les asphyxies accidentelles (submersion, electrocution, intoxication oxycarbonique). Etude clinique, therapeutique et preventive. Paris: Editions Medicales, N Maloine, 1931.
27. Kristoffersen MB, Rattenborg CC, Holaday DA. Asphyxial death—The roles of acute anoxia, hypercarbia and acidosis. Anesthesiology 1967; 28:488–497.
28. Craig AB. Causes of loss of consciousness during underwater swimming. J Appl Physiol 1961; 16:583–586.
29. Craig AB Jr. Underwater swimming and loss of consciousness. JAMA 1961; 176: 255–258.
30. Modell JH, Graves SA, Ketover A. Clinical course of 91 consecutive near-drowning victims. Chest 1976; 70:231–238.

31. Halmagyi DFJ. Lung changes and incidence of respiratory arrest in rats after aspiration of sea and freshwater. J Appl Physiol 1961; 16:41–44.
32. Colebatch HJH, Halmagyi DFJ. Lung mechanics and resuscitation after fluid aspiration. J Appl Physiol 1961; 16:684–696.
33. Modell JH, Moya F, Williams HD, Weibley TC. Changes in blood gases and A-aDO_2 during near-drowning. Anesthesiology 1968; 29:456–465.
34. Giammona ST, Modell JH. Drowning by total immersion: Effects on pulmonary surfactant of distilled water, isotonic saline and seawater. Am J Dis Child 1967; 114:612–616.
35. Modell JH, Davis JH, Giammona ST, et al. Blood gas and electrolyte changes in human near-drowning victims. JAMA 1968; 203:337–343.
36. Butt MP, Jalowayski A, Modell JH, Giammona ST. Pulmonary function after resuscitation from near-drowning. Anesthesiology 1970; 32:275–277.
37. Karpovich PV. Water in the lungs of drowned animals. Arch Pathol (Chicago) 1933; 15:828–833.
38. Redding JS, Voigt GC, Safar P. Treatment of seawater aspiration. J Appl Physiol 1960; 15:1113–1116.
39. Redding JS, Voigt GC, Safar P. Drowning treated with intermittent positive pressure breathing. J Appl Physiol 1960; 15:849–854.
40. Colebatch HJH, Halmagyi DFJ. Reflex airway reaction to fluid aspiration. J Appl Physiol 1962; 17:787–794.
41. Reidbord HE, Spitz WU. Ultrastructural alterations in rat lungs: Changes after intratracheal perfusion with freshwater and seawater. Arch Pathol 1966; 81:103–111.
42. Imburg J, Hartney TC. Drowning and the treatment of non-fatal submersion—I. drowning and non-fatal submersion laboratory studies and human data. Pediatrics 1966; 37;684–698.
43. Miloslavich EL. Pathological anatomy of death by drowning. Am J Clin Pathol 1934; 4:42–49.
44. Layon AJ, Modell JH. Drowning and near-drowning. In: Tinker J, Zapol WM, eds. Care of the Critically Ill Patient. London: Springer-Verlag, 1992:909–918.
45. Modell JH, Calderwood HW, Ruiz BC, et al. Effects of ventilatory patterns on arterial oxygenation after near-drowning in seawater. Anesthesiology 1974; 40:376–384.
46. Ruiz BC, Calderwood HW, Modell JH, Brogdon JE. Effect of ventilatory patterns on arterial oxygenation after near-drowning with freshwater—A comparative study in dogs. Anesth Analg 1973; 52:570–576.
47. Bergquist RE, Vogelhut MM, Modell JH, et al. Comparison of ventilatory patterns in the treatment of freshwater near-drowning in dogs. Anesthesiology 1980; 52:142–148.
48. Mizutani T, Layon AJ. Clinical applications of nitric oxide. Chest 1996; 110(2):506–524.
49. Leach CL, Fuhrman BP, Morin FC III, Rath MG. Perfluorocarbon-associated gas exchange (partial liquid ventilation) in respiratory distress syndrome—A prospective, randomized, controlled study. Crit Care Med 1993; 21:1270–1278.

50. Stachniak JB, Layon AJ, Gallagher TJ, et al. Optimizing cardiac status with right ejection fraction pulmonary artery catheter during hypervolemic-hypertensive-hemodilution therapy (abstr). Crit Care Med 1996; 24:A71.
51. Modell JH, Davis JH. Electrolyte changes in human drowning victims. Anesthesiology 1969; 30:414–420.
52. Yagil R, Stalnikowicz R, Michaeli J, Mogle P. Near-drowning in the Dead Sea—Electrolyte imbalances and therapeutic implications. Arch Intern Med 1985; 145: 50–53.
53. Prough DS, Johnson JC, Poole GV Jr, et al. Effects on intracranial pressure of resuscitation from hemorrhagic shock with hypertonic saline versus lactated Ringer's solution. Crit Care Med 1985; 13:407–411.
54. Todd MM, Tommasino C, Moore S. Cerebral effects of isovolemic hemodilution with a hypertonic saline solution. J Neurosurg 1985; 63:944–948.
55. Ducey JP, Lamiell JM, Gueller GE. Cerebral electrophysiologic effects of resuscitation with hypertonic saline-dextran after hemorrhage. Crit Care Med 1990; 18: 744–749.
56. Prough DS, Whitley JM, Olympio MA, et al. Hypertonic/hyperoncotic fluid resuscitation after hemorrhagic shock in dogs. Anesth Analg 1991; 73:738–744.
57. Shackford SR, Zhuang J, Schmoker J. Intravenous fluid tonicity—Effect on intracranial pressure, cerebral blood flow, and cerebral oxygen delivery in focal brain injury. J Neurosurg 1992; 76:91–98.
58. Lanier WL, Stangland KJ, Scheithauer BW, et al. The effects of dextrose infusion and head position on neurologic outcome after complete cerebral ischemia in primates—Examination of a model. Anesthesiology 1987; 66:39–48.
59. Hoffman WE, Braucher E, Pelligrino DA, et al. Brain lactate and neurologic outcome following incomplete ischemia in fasted, nonfasted, and glucose-loaded rats. Anesthesiology 1990; 72:1045–1050.
60. Ashwal S, Schneider S, Tomasi L, Thompson J. Prognostic implications of hyperglycemia and reduced cerebral blood flow in childhood near-drowning. Neurology 1990; 40:820–823.
61. Modell JH, Kuck EJ, Ruiz BC, Heinitsh H. Effect of intravenous vs aspirated distilled water on serum electrolytes and blood gas tensions. J Appl Physiol 1972; 32:579–584.
62. Culpepper RM. Bleeding diathesis in freshwater drowning. Ann Intern Med 1975; 83:675.
63. Karch SB. Pathology of the heart in drowning. Arch Pathol Lab Med 1985; 109: 176–178.
64. Kvittingen TD, Naess A. Recovery from drowning in freshwater. Br Med J 1963; 5341:1315–1317.
65. Rath CE. Drowning hemoglobinuria. Blood 1953; 8:1099–1104.
66. Munroe WD. Hemoglobinuria from near-drowning. J Pediatr 1964; 64:57–62.
67. King RB, Webster IW. A case of recovery from drowning and prolonged anoxia. Med J Aust 1964; 1:919–920.
68. Redding JS, Pearson JW. Management of drowning victims. Gen Pract 1964; 29: 100–104.

69. Conn AW, Montes JE, Barker GA, Edmonds JF. Cerebral salvage in near-drowning following neurological classification by triage. Can Anaesth Soc J 1980; 27:201–210.
70. Modell JH, Graves SA, Kuck EJ. Near-drowning—Collation of level of consciousness and survival. Can Anaesth Soc J 1980; 27:211–215.
71. Sarnaik AP, Preston G, Lieh-Lai M, Eisenbrey AB. Intracranial pressure and cerebral perfusion pressure in near-drowning. Crit Care Med 1985; 13:224–227.
72. Frewen TC, Sumabat WO, Han VK, et al. Cerebral resuscitation therapy in pediatric near-drowning. J Pediatr 1985; 106:615–617.
73. Bell TS, Ellenberg L, McComb JG. Neuropsychological outcome after severe pediatric near-drowning. Neurosurgery 1985; 17:604–608.
74. Bohn DJ, Biggar WD, Smith CR, et al. Influence of hypothermia, barbiturate therapy, and intracranial pressure monitoring on morbidity and mortality after near-drowning. Crit Care Med 1986; 14:529–534.
75. Allman FD, Nelson WB, Pacentine GA, McComb G. Outcome following cardiopulmonary resuscitation in severe pediatric near-drowning. Am J Dis Child 1986; 140:571–575.
76. Nichter MA, Everett PB. Childhood near-drowning—Is cardiopulmonary resuscitation always indicated? Crit Care Med 1989; 17:993–995.
77. Nussbaum E. Prognostic variables in nearly drowned comatose children. Am J Dis Child 1985; 139:1058–1059.
78. Stachniak J, Layon AJ, Fessler R, Black S. Closed head injury and the treatment of sequelae after a motor vehicle accident (Case Conference of the University of Florida). J Clin Anesth 1994; 6:437–449.
79. Wynne JW, Modell JH. Respiratory aspiration of stomach contents—A review. Ann Intern Med 1977; 87:466–474.
80. Heimlich HJ. Subdiaphragmatic pressure to expel water from the lungs of drowning persons. Ann Emerg Med 1981; 10:476–480.
81. Heimlich HJ, Patrick EA. Using the Heimlich maneuver to save near-drowning victims. Postgrad Med 1988; 84:62–73.
82. Ruben A, Ruben H. Artificial respiration—Flow of water from the lung and the stomach. Lancet 1962; 1:780–781.
83. Werner JZ, Safar P, Bircher NG, et al. No improvement in pulmonary status by gravity drainage or abdominal thrusts after seawater near-drowning in dogs (abstr). Anesthesiology 1982; 57:A81.
84. Rosen P, Stoto M, Harley J, eds. The use of the Heimlich Maneuver in Near-Drowning. Washington, DC: Institute of Medicine, 1994:1–27.
85. Ornato JP. Special resuscitation situations—Near-drowning, traumatic injury, electric shock, and hypothermia. Circulation 1986; 74(suppl IV):IV-23–IV-25.
86. Orlowski JP. Vomiting as a complication of the Heimlich maneuver. JAMA 1987; 258:512–513.
87. Banner MJ, Kirby RR, Blanch PB. Site of pressure measurement during spontaneous breathing with continuous positive airway pressure—Effect on calculating imposed work of breathing. Crit Care Med 1992; 20:528–533.
88. Banner MJ, Kirby RR, Blanch PB, Layon AJ. Decreasing imposed work of the

breathing apparatus to zero using pressure-support ventilation. Crit Care Med 1993; 21:1333–1338.

89. Calderwood HW, Modell JH, Ruiz BC. The ineffectiveness of steroid therapy for treatment of freshwater near-drowning. Anesthesiology 1975; 43:642–650.
90. Wynne JW, Reynolds JC, Hood CI, Auerbach D, Ondrasick J. Steroid therapy for pneumonitis induced in rabbits by aspiration of foodstuff. Anesthesiology 1979; 51:11–19.
91. Rolfsen ML, Davis WR. Cerebral function and preservation during cardiac arrest. Crit Care Med 1989; 17:283–292.
92. Rogers MC, Kirsch JR. Current concepts in brain resuscitation. JAMA 1989; 261: 3143–3147.
93. Centers for Disease Control. Position Papers from the Third National Injury Control Conference: Setting the National Agenda for Injury Control in the 1990s, Executive Summaries. MMWR 1992; 41(RR-6):11–12.

11

Liquid Breathing and Breath-Holding

JOHANNES A. KYLSTRA

Duke University Medical Center
Durham, North Carolina

The exchange of oxygen and carbon dioxide between multicellular organisms and their environment occurs by diffusion along partial pressure gradients that are maintained by ventilation and perfusion of their respiratory organs. The structure of these organs reflects evolutionary adaptations that meet the functional demands of the organisms in their natural surroundings. The gills of fish are adapted to an aquatic environment, but the lungs of an air-breathing animal are not. At the surface of the earth, a volume of air normally contains about forty times more oxygen than an equal volume of water. Hence, to supply the same amount of oxygen per minute to the circulating blood, the tidal flow of water into and out of the lungs should be at least forty times greater than that of air, but the lungs are not designed for tidal flow of a fluid that is much denser and more viscous than air. Furthermore, natural waters (fresh water or seawater) usually have a composition very different from that of blood, so that inhaled water can damage the lung tissues and cause fatal alterations in the volume and composition of body fluids. In the laboratory, however, it is possible to adjust the oxygen and the salt content of water or to have an animal breathe an inert synthetic liquid instead of water. Thus it has been possible to keep hypothermic mice, rats, and cats submerged in hyperbarically oxygenated saline solutions (1–2) or normobarically oxygenated FC-80 fluorocarbon liquid (3) alive for extended periods of time. Arterial oxygenation appeared to be adequate, but alveolar hypoventilation caused a progressively severe respiratory acidosis in these spontaneously liquid-breathing animals. Mice submerged in hyperbarically oxygenated FC-75 fluorocarbon liquid survived at least 10 min. at a normal or near normal body temperature (4). In normothermic anesthetized dogs ventilated mechanically with normobarically oxygenated FC-80 fluorocarbon liquid (5), a steady-state pulmonary gas exchange was observed at a normal arterial P_{CO_2}.

Replacing nitrogen in the airspaces of a diver by a liquid should eliminate the problems of decompression sickness and nitrogen narcosis. Indeed, one FC-80 fluorocarbon-breathing mouse survived compression to 100 atm for 30 sec followed by decompression in 3 sec, after which it resumed air breathing and was alive and well 1 month later (6). Such a rate of decompression is equivalent to surfacing from 3000 ft under water at a vertical speed of 700 mi/hr without signs of decompression sickness. This experimental result would tend to support the premise that a liquid-breathing diver would be immune to decompression sickness.

A breath-holding diver with liquid-filled lungs should be able to descend much deeper under water than with gas-filled lungs because the volume of his chest would not change to any appreciable extent during the dive. Also, since the lung volume remains constant, the partial pressure of oxygen in the alveoli would not change with depth, so that hyperventilating before a dive might safely extend the duration of a breath-holding dive with liquid-filled lungs, whereas hyperventilation before breath-hold diving with air-filled lungs may cause death by drowning. This topic is discussed in more detail later.

I. Ventilation of Liquid-Filled Lungs

Isovolume pressure-flow curves of saline-filled dogs' lungs resemble those of air-filled lungs except that the expiratory flows of saline are much smaller than those of air at comparable lung volumes. As in the air-filled lungs of dogs and humans, the expiratory flow at a given lung volume (except near total lung capacity) reaches a maximum as a result of dynamic airway compression and then becomes effort-independent—i.e., the flow no longer increases in spite of an increase in expiratory effort, as reflected by an increase in pleural pressure (Fig. 1). Once dynamic airway compression occurs, the expiratory flow is equal to the pressure generated by the recoil tendency of the lung divided by the resistance to flow in the airways upstream of the dynamically compressed ones (7). The recoil tendency of a liquid-filled lung is usually diminished as a result of a decrease in alveolar surface tension. Moreover, the resistance to flow of a liquid in the airways is much greater than that of air. These factors tend to limit the tidal flow of liquid in the lungs of terrestrial mammals to a mere fraction

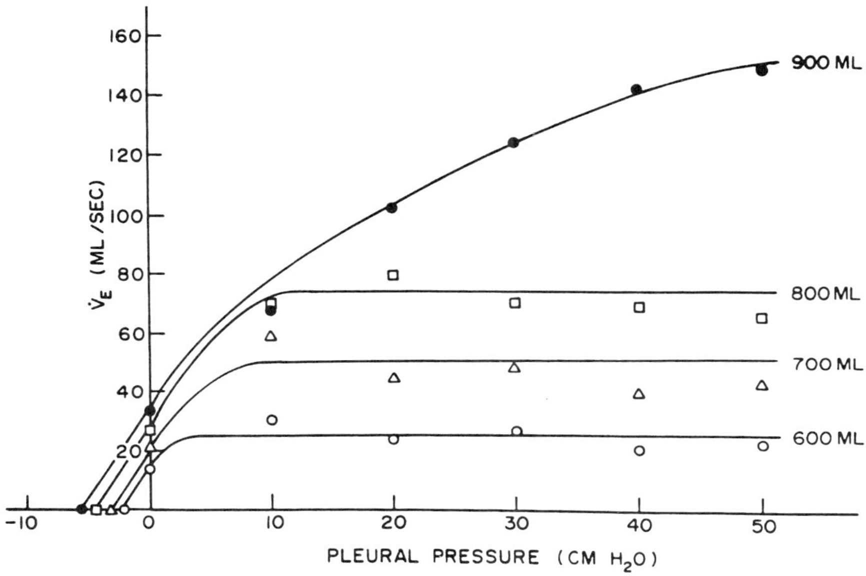

Figure 1 Relationship between pressure applied to the pleural surface of gas-free liquid-filled dogs' lungs and expiratory flow of saline at different lung volumes. (From Ref. 11.)

of the ventilation which, even at rest, is required to maintain normal partial pressures of oxygen and carbon dioxide in the arterial blood while breathing air. In excised air-filled and gas-free saline-filled lungs of dogs and rats, the static recoil pressures of saline-filled lungs were found to be less than half of those in air-filled lungs at comparable lung volumes, and maximum expiratory flows were about a hundred times less than in air-filled lungs (8,9). On the basis of these results and by extrapolation, a maximum saline ventilation of human lungs at a rate of about 3.5 L/min was predicted.

The static recoil pressure of dogs' lungs filled with a water immiscible synthetic liquid (FC-80 fluorocarbon) is greater than the static recoil pressure of saline-filled lungs (at comparable lung volumes) as a result of alveolar surface tension which, although less than in air-filled lungs, is not completely abolished, as it is in saline-filled lungs (10). Hence, at equal lung volumes, the driving force available for expiratory flow is greater in fluorocarbon-filled lungs than in saline-filled lungs. Yet the maximum expiratory flow of saline is somewhat greater than that of FC-80 fluorocarbon (11) because the fluorocarbon liquid is denser and more viscous than saline (Table 1).

Table 1 Physical Properties of Different Breathing Fluids

Property	Air	Water	FC-80
$\dot{D}_{O_2}$ (cm^2/sec)	0.178	0.0000322	0.0000133
$\dot{D}_{CO_2}$ (cm^2/sec)	0.139	0.0000255	0.0000105
α_{O_2} (cm^3/cm^3/mmHg)	0.001316	0.0000299	0.00064
α_{CO_2} (cm^3/cm^3/mmHg)	0.001316	0.000724	0.00211
η (g/sec/cm)	0.0001904	0.006947	0.0112
d (g/cm^3)	0.001117	0.99336	1.76

$\dot{D}$ = diffusion coefficient; α = solubility coefficient; d = density; η = viscosity. $\dot{D}_{O_2}$ and $\dot{D}_{CO_2}$ in air at 0° C, all other values at 37° C. $\dot{D}$ in FC-80 calculated by Scheibel's empirical equation (from Ref. 29).

During inspiration, dynamic airway compression normally does not occur, so that, theoretically, the inspiratory flow should continue to increase as the difference between the pressure in the alveoli and at the mouth increases. Interestingly, the inspiratory flow in saline-breathing dogs (breathing on their own) was about twice as great as the expiratory flow. As a result, the minute volume of ventilation was 33% greater than would have been the case had inspiration and expiration lasted equally long. Intrathoracic pressure fluctuations in these saline-breathing animals reflected the effort expended to propel the liquid through the trachea and bronchi. The pressure in the right atrium ranged from 40 mmHg below atmospheric during inspiration to 15 mmHg above atmospheric during expiration (12).

The maximum expiratory flow of saline from human lungs has been measured during therapeutic lung lavage (13,14) in a patient with alveolar proteinosis and during lavage of one lung of a healthy volunteer. These measurements were made by applying and gradually increasing suction on the outflow tube (see Fig. 2) until the rate of flow of saline ceased to increase. The minimum time required to remove 500 ml of saline from the left lung of the healthy volunteer, starting from a lung volume of 2000 ml, was 9.4 sec. The computed total lung capacity (TLC) of the left lung (0.45×TLC of both lungs measured the day before the experiment) was 2900 ml. If it is assumed that the time required for inspiration of a tidal volume is equal to the time required for expiration of that tidal volume and that there is an equal maximum expiratory flow from both lungs, then the maximum minute ventilation of this man (if he were to breathe saline) would have been 3.2 L at a tidal volume of 1 L and expiration starting at 69% of TLC. In the patient with alveolar proteinosis, 500 ml of saline could be drained from the liquid-filled left lung in 7 sec, starting at TLC. If one makes the same assumptions as before, the minute ventilation in this patient (when breathing saline) could have been 4.2 L at a tidal volume of 1 L and expiration starting at TLC.

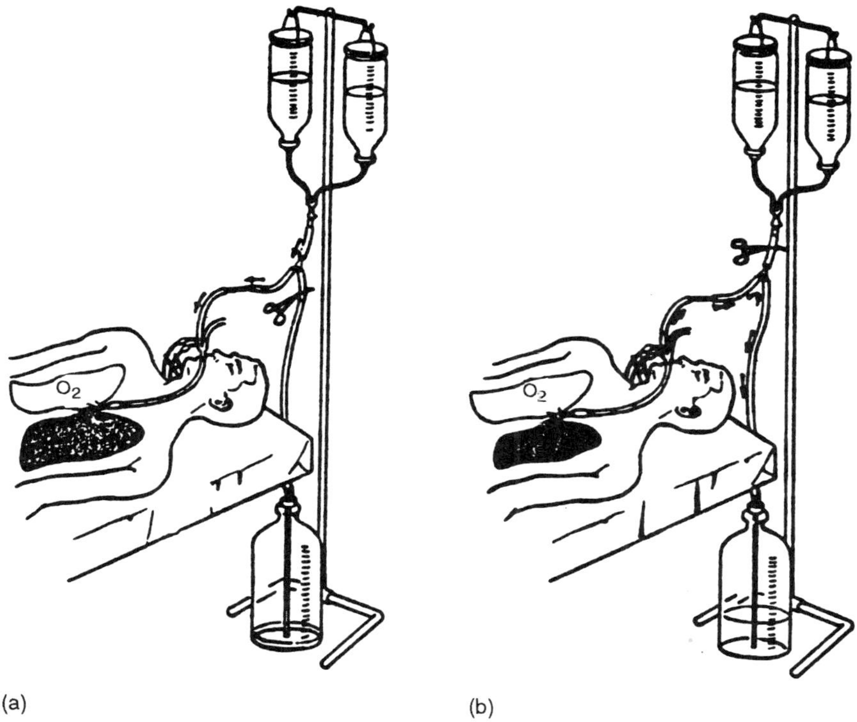

Figure 2 Volume-controlled lung lavage. (a) A tidal volume of prewarmed saline flows into the degased dependent lung. (b) Tidal volume drains from lung. The other lung is being ventilated with oxygen. (From Ref. 13.)

II. Distribution of Ventilation and Blood Flow in Liquid-Filled Lungs

The distribution of ventilation and blood flow has been studied in excised saline-filled lungs of greyhound dogs (15). The distribution of a single breath of iodinated albumin in saline was found to be uniform. At low pulmonary arterial pressures—at which regional inequality of blood flow is known to be pronounced in air-filled lungs—blood flow was evenly distributed in the saline-filled lungs, presumably because the hydrostatic pressure in the blood vessels was balanced by a corresponding pressure in the alveoli. In a lung filled with a fluorocarbon liquid that is almost twice as dense as blood, there exists a net transmural hydrostatic pressure gradient of about 1 cmH_2O/cm of vertical distance from the top to the bottom of the lung, tending to compress the blood vessels. One would therefore expect that pulmonary arterial blood flow decreases from the top to the bottom of a fluorocarbon-filled lung, which is just the opposite of what happens in air-breathing lungs (16).

III. Diffusion of Dissolved Oxygen and Carbon Dioxide in Liquid-Filled Airspaces

In dogs ventilated with a hyperbarically oxygenated isotonic salt solution, there was an unusually large difference between the end-tidal and arterial partial pressures of oxygen and carbon dioxide compatible with the existence of marked stratified inhomogeneity in the liquid-filled terminal airspaces. In dogs ventilated with normobarically oxygenated FC-80 fluorocarbon liquid at a much slower repiratory frequency, the partial pressure of carbon dioxide in end-tidal liquid and arterial blood were approximately equal, but there was a difference of 147 mmHg oxygen pressure, on the average, between end-tidal liquid and arterial blood (see Table 2). This, as we shall see, was the result of stratified inhomogeneity caused by the slow rate of diffusion of oxygen in fluorocarbon liquid.

The gas exchange in the lungs of saline-breathing dogs resembled the imaginary exchange of oxygen and carbon dioxide in a mathematical lung model consisting of identical spherical gas-exchange units. The hypothetical gas-

Table 2 Measurements Made in Anesthetized Dogs Ventilated with Hyperbarically Oxygenated Saline ($n = 7$) or Normobarically Oxygenated FC-80 Fluorocarbon Liquid ($n = 5$)[a]

	Saline	FC-80
Weight of dog (kg)	11.6 (2.0)	10.8 (1.1)
Tidal volume (ml)	300 (46)	290 (3)
Frequency (breaths/min)	10.1 (1.7)	2.8 (0.3)
FRC (liters)	0.50 (0.25)	0.479 (0.026)
PI_{O_2} (mmHg)	3434 (128)	685 (13)
$\dot{V}_{O_2}$ (ml STPD/min)	68 (15)	57 (17)
Pa_{O_2} (mmHg)	998 (747)	303 (21)
Pa_{CO_2} (mmHg)	52 (19)	44.2 (3.7)
(a-ET)P_{CO_2} (mmHg)	21.0 (8.7)	−3.6 (5.3)
(ET-a)P_{O_2} (mmHg)	1258 (338)	147 (54)

[a] Values are means and standard deviations (in parentheses) (from Refs. 4 and 18).

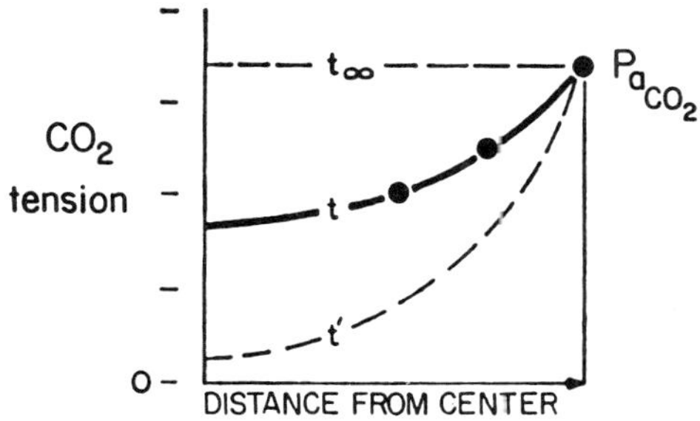

Figure 3 Partial pressure of CO_2 in a spherical gas-exchange unit as a function of distance from the center at different diffusion times t', t, t_∞. (From Ref. 19.)

exchange units fill and empty simultaneously and instantly in such a way that the liquid exhaled first is located at a greater distance from the alveolar capillaries than the liquid exhaled later. The spheres are assumed to have a uniform oxygen concentration initially, and oxygen is removed by the blood from the surface of the spheres at a constant rate. The spheres do not at first contain carbon dioxide, and the carbon dioxide concentration at the surface is assumed to remain constant. The partial pressures of oxygen and carbon dioxide inside the exchange units at any distance from the center and at any time after the beginning of inspiration can be computed from solutions to the diffusion equation (17) after some simple modifications (18,19). Figure 3 shows the partial pressures of carbon dioxide within a gas-exchange unit at different distances from the center of the unit and at different times after the beginning of a respiratory cycle. This stratified inhomogeneity tends to dissipate with time, so that, eventually, the partial pressure of carbon dioxide within the gas-exchange unit becomes homogeneous throughout and equal to the partial pressure of carbon dioxide in the alveolar capillary blood. Figure 4 shows the partial pressures of oxygen within a gas-exchange unit as a function of distance from the center at different times after the beginning of a respiratory cycle. The slope of these gradients is the same at different respiratory frequencies; it is directly proportional to the rate at which oxygen is removed by the blood at the surface of the gas exchange unit and inversely proportional to the product of the diffusion coefficient of oxygen ($\dot{D}_{O_2}$) and the solubility coefficient of oxygen (α_{O_2}) in the alveolar liquid. The difference between the oxygen tension in the inhaled liquid and the arterial blood is approximately (19) as follows:

$$\mathrm{PI}_{O_2} - \mathrm{Pa}_{O_2} = \frac{\dot{V}_{O_2}\, t}{\mathrm{V_A}\, \alpha_{O_2}} + \frac{\dot{V}_{O_2}}{20\pi\, \alpha_{O_2}\, \dot{D}_{O_2}} \frac{1}{an} \qquad (1)$$

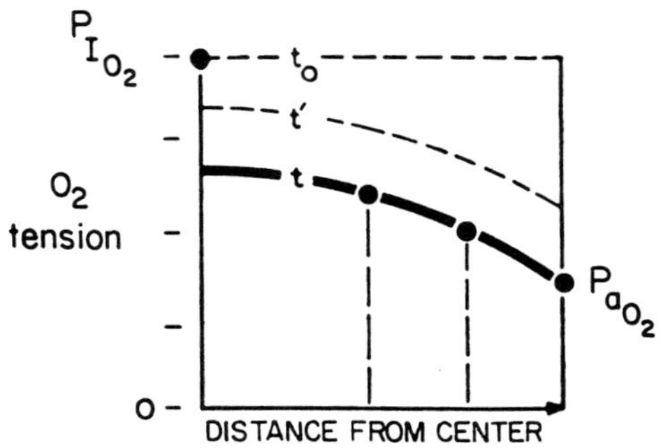

Figure 4 Partial pressure of oxygen in a spherical gas-exchange unit as a function of distance from the center at different times after the beginning of a respiratory cycle where $t_o<t'<t$. (From Ref. 19.)

where a = radius of the exchange units and n = the number of exchange units. The right-hand side of Eq. (1) is the sum of two components, of which the first increases with time while the other (the difference between the oxygen partial pressures at the center and at the periphery of the gas exchange units) remains constant as long as the oxygen transfer at the periphery of the units remains the same.

IV. Diffusion Dead Space

Persistence of diffusion gradients within individual exchange units at the end of a respiratory cycle implies differences between the mean gas tensions inside the exchange units and in the arterial blood. Such differences can be expressed in terms of respiratory dead space, which is defined as the actual or virtual volume of inhaled liquid whose gas tensions, after leaving the gas-exchange units, have failed to reach equilibrium with gas tensions in the arterial blood. The total respiratory dead space can consist of the anatomical and instrument dead spaces (where no gas exchange occurs), a distribution dead space that results fom unequal ventilation and perfusion of different gas-exchange units, and, finally, a diffusion dead space that results from persisting gradients of gas tensions within individual exchange units (see Fig. 5). Diffusion dead space for CO_2 can be minimized by decreasing the respiratory frequency when the diffusion gradient for CO_2 tends to dissipate, but the diffusion gradient for oxygen persists as long as oxygen is being removed at the same rate at the periphery of the exchange units [see Eq. (1)]. However, adequate arterial oxygenation can be maintained by increasing the partial pressure of oxygen in the inhaled liquid.

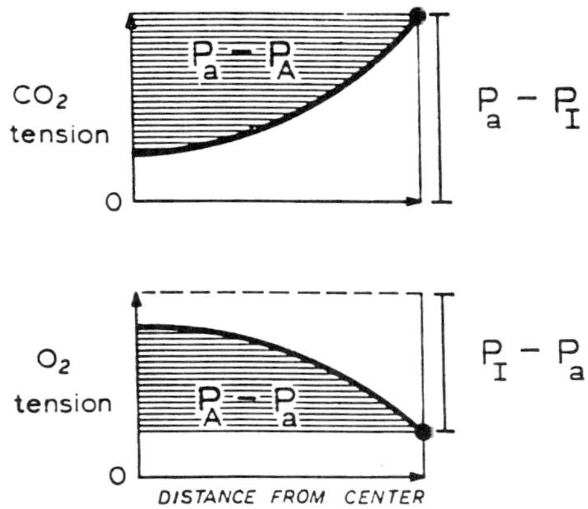

$$VD_{diff_{O_2}} = \frac{P\bar{A}_{O_2} - Pa_{O_2}}{PI_{O_2} - Pa_{O_2}} \times VA \qquad VD_{diff_{CO_2}} = \frac{Pa_{CO_2} - P\bar{A}_{CO_2}}{Pa_{CO_2} - PI_{CO_2}} \times VA$$

Figure 5 Diffusion dead space. (From Ref. 19.)

The large difference between the partial pressures of CO_2 in arterial blood and end-tidal liquid found in dogs ventilated with saline at a rate of 10 breaths per minute was not observed in dogs ventilated with FC-80 fluorocarbon liquid at a rate of 2.8 breaths per minute (see Table 2). Apparently, there was sufficient time for diffusive mixing of CO_2 in the fluorocarbon-filled terminal airspaces to be complete or very nearly so when the CO_2 diffusion dead space vanishes.

The clinical use of lung lavage (13,14) has made it possible to measure gas exchange in the saline-filled lungs of humans (20). It was found that the difference between the partial pressures of CO_2 in end-tidal liquid and arterial blood remained very nearly the same at lavage cycles lasting from 24 to 148 sec. Since differences between end-tidal and arterial CO_2 partial pressures caused by stratified inhomogeneity should decrease with an increase in the duration of the respiratory cycle, there was no evidence that stratified CO_2 inhomogeneity persisted longer than 24 sec in saline-filled human lungs.

V. Breath-Hold Diving with Liquid-Filled Lungs

Changes in lung volume during breath-hold diving with gas-filled lungs affect both the maximum duration and the maximum depth of a breath-hold dive. The duration of breath-holding depends on the diver's capacity to store metabolically produced CO_2 and his ability to resist the urge to resume breathing, which becomes irresistible at the "breaking point." The respiratory stimuli caused by a decrease in lung volume, a decrease in Pa_{O_2}, and an increase in Pa_{CO_2} interact in determining the breaking point. Breath holding following a period of sustained hyperventilation with oxygen caused an oxygen consumption–related decrease in lung volume from TLC to RV in 13 min, on the average, in men at rest at sea level (21). Inhaling hyperbarically oxygenated fluorocarbon liquid from RV to TLC following a similar period of sustained hyperventilation with oxygen might increase the maximum breath-holding time well beyond 13 min by minimizing the respiratory drive caused by a decreasing lung volume and by augmenting the CO_2 storage capacity of the lungs when the alveoli are filled with a liquid that can hold almost twice as much CO_2 as air at the same P_{CO_2} (see Table I). The depth under water to which a breath-holding diver with liquid-filled lungs can descend would not be limited by the compliance of his chest wall at and below RV and the amount of blood that can accumulate in the blood vessels of the lung without causing damage (lung squeeze). Returning to the surface when the lung volume suddenly increases would not cause a precipitous drop in $P_{A_{O_2}}$ (the so-called hypoxia of ascent), which may result in unconsciousness and death by drowning (22,23).

VI. Composite Breathing Liquids

The addition of tris (hydroxymethyl) aminomethane (THAM) to the salt solution markedly prolonged the survival of saline-breathing mice (1) and minimized respiratory acidosis in saline-breathing rats (2). One liter of an isotonic 0.3 M THAM solution titrated to pH 7.4 can hold approximately 390 ml (STPD) of CO_2 at P_{CO_2}=40 mmHg (11), whereas isotonic saline holds no more than 53 ml (STPD) of CO_2/L at P_{CO_2}=40 mmHg. The solubility of CO_2 in fluorocarbon liquids is high but not high enough to compensate for alveolar hypoventilation, so that, even at complete rest, a fluorocarbon-breathing diver would barely be able to maintain a tolerable Pa_{CO_2} while breathing at his maximum capacity. However, the advantages of a fluorocarbon liquid with a high oxygen solubility and a THAM solution with a very high carbon dioxide–carrying capacity can be combined in an emulsion. Such an emulsion can be prepared by subjecting a mixture of FC-80 fluorocarbon; a THAM solution titrated to pH 7.4; and F68 pluronic surfactant to ultrasonic energy (24). Instead of emulsions consisting of water-miscible fluorocarbon droplets suspended in water, it is also possible to prepare emulsions with a continuous fluorocarbon phase in which droplets containing NaOH are suspended. The caustic NaOH cannot enter into the water-miscible continuous phase and hence does not come into contact with the lung tissues, but CO_2 can diffuse from the blood through the fluorocarbon into the NaOH droplets when Na_2CO_3 is formed (25).

Recently, fluorocarbon emulsions prepared from perfluoro-octylbromide (PFOB) have become commercially available for medical use as oxygen and carbon dioxide carriers intended to serve as a temporary substitute for red blood cells. These emulsions are extremely stable, with a shelf life of more than 1 year at room temperature. The addition of THAM to the aqueous phase should provide an excellent breathing liquid. Oxygen and CO_2 solubilities in PFOB (0.000707 and 0.002763 cm^3/cm^3 mmHg, respectively) are greater than in FC-80 fluorocarbon liquid (see Table I). The bromine atom gives PFOB lipophilicity, which, in turn, provides for a short organ-retention time and an excellent emulsion stability (26,27). Clinical trials aimed at improving pulmonary mechanics and gas exchange in desparately ill premature infants and adults by ventilating their damaged lungs with PFOB are currently under way in several medical centers. They may open the door to liquid-breathing and breath-holding experiments in healthy divers.

References

1. Kylstra JA, Tissing MO, van der Maën A. Of mice as fish. Trans Am Soc Artif Intern Organs 1962; 8:378–383.
2. Pegg JH, Horner TL, Wahrenbrock, EA. Breathing of pressure-oxygenated liquids. Publ. no. 1181. Proceedings of the 2nd Symposium on Underwater Physiology. Washington, DC: National Academy of Sciences/National Research Council, 1963: 166–170.
3. Clark LC, Gollan F. Survival of mammals breathing organic liquids equilibrated with oxygen at atmospheric pressure. Science 1966; 152:1755–1756.
4. Lundgren CEG, Örnhagen HC. Oxygen consumption in liquid breathing mice. Aerospace Med 1972; 43:831–835.
5. Matthews WH, Balzer RH, Shelburne JD, et al. Steady-state gas exchange in normothermic anesthetized liquid-ventilated dogs. Undersea Biomed Res 1978; 5:341–354.
6. Kylstra JA, Nantz R, Crowe J, et al. Hydraulic compression of mice to 166 atmospheres. Science 1967; 158:793–794.
7. Mead JJ, Turner JM, Macklem PT, Little JB. Significance of the relationship between lung recoil and maximum expiratory flow. J Appl Physiol 1967; 22:95–108.
8. Leith DE, Mead J. Maximum expiratory flow in liquid-filled lungs (abstr). Fed Proc/Fed Am Soc Exp Biol 1966; 25:506.
9. Hamosh P, Luchsinger PC. Maximum expiratory flow in isolated liquid-filled lungs. J Appl Physiol 1968; 25:485–488.
10. Kylstra JA, Schoenfisch WH. Alveolar surface tension in fluorocarbon-filled lungs. J Appl Physiol 1972; 33:32–35.

11. Schoenfisch WH, Kylstra JA. Maximum expiratory flow and estimated CO_2 elimination in liquid-ventilated dogs' lungs. J Appl Physiol 1973; 35:117–121.
12. Kylstra JA, Tissing MO. Fluid breathing. In: Boerema I, Brummelkamp WH, Meyne NG, eds. Clinical Application of Hyperbaric Oxygen. Amsterdam: Elsevier, 1964:371–379.
13. Kylstra JA, Rausch DC, Hall KD, Spock A. Volume-controlled lung lavage in the treatment of asthma, bronchiectasis, and mucoviscidosis. Am Rev Respir Dis 1971; 103:651–665.
14. Kariman K, Kylstra JA, Spock A. Pulmonary alveolar proteinosis: Prospective clinical experience in 23 patients for 15 years. Lung 1984; 162:223–231.
15. West JB, Dollery CT, Matthews CME, Zardini P. Distribution of blood flow and ventilation in saline-filled lung. J Appl Physiol 1965; 20:1107–1117.
16. West JB. Ventilation/blood flow and gas exchange. Oxford and Edinburgh: Blackwell, 1965.
17. Crank J. The mathematics of diffusion. London and New York: Oxford University Press, 1957.
18. Kylstra JA, Paganelli CV, Lanphier EH. Pulmonary gas exchange in dogs ventilated with hyperbarically oxygenated liquid. J Appl Physiol 1966; 21:177–184.
19. Kylstra JA, Paganelli CV, Rahn H. Some implications of the dynamics of gas transfer in water-breathing dogs. In: De Reuck AVS, Porter R, eds. Development of the Lung. Boston: Little, Brown, 1967:34–58.
20. Kylstra JA, Schoenfisch WH, Herron JM, Blenkarn GD. Gas exchange in saline-filled lungs of man. J Appl Physiol. 1973; 35:136–142.
21. Klocke FJ, Rahn H. Breath-holding after breathing oxygen. J Appl Physiol 1959; 14:689–693.
22. Lanphier EH, Rahn H. Alveolar gas exchange during breath-holding with air. J Appl Physiol 1963; 18:478–482.
23. Craig AB, Jr. Causes of loss of conscienceness during underwater swimming. J Appl Physiol 1961; 16:583–586.
24. Matthews WH, Kylstra JA. A fluorocarbon emulsion with a high solubility for CO_2. Undersea Biomed Res 1976; 3:113–120.
25. Matthews WH, Kylstra JA. Investigation of a new breathing liquid. In: Shilling CW, Beckett M, eds. Underwater Physiology VI. Bethesda, MD: FASEB 1978: 179–185.
26. Weers JG. A physicochemical evaluation of perfluorochemicals for oxygen transport applications. J Fluorine Chem 1993; 64:73–93.
27. Riess JG. Highly fluorinated systems for oxygen transport, diagnosis and drug delivery: Colloids and surfaces. A: Physicochem Eng Asp 1994; 84:33–48.
28. Dittmer DS, Grebe RM, eds. Handbook of Respiration. Philadelphia: Saunders, 1958; Hodgeman CO, ed. Handbook of Chemistry and Physics. Cleveland: Chemical Rubber Publishing, 1962; 3M Company, 1976.
29. Reid RC, Sherwood TK. The Properties of Gases and Liquids. New York: McGraw-Hill, 1966:549.

12

Underwater Breathing Apparatus

JOHN R. CLARKE

Navy Experimental Diving Unit
Panama City, Florida

I. Introduction—The Free Diver's Dilemma

Consider a free diver of ordinary skill as he plunges from the surface to an easily attainable depth of 33 ft. He has made an abrupt transition from air breathing to submerged breath-holding, a transitory state that places three primary stresses on his body. The first, common to all who have swum across a pool submerged, is the unbearable urge to breathe created by an elevation of arterial CO_2. For those who defeat that physiological warning sign by hyperventilating before the dive, thereby temporarily lowering Pa_{CO_2}, the second and frequently final stress that presents itself is an acute O_2 lack. The result can be unconsciousness under water.

For those divers with the means for descending rapidly, the third barrier is pressure; a pressure imbalance between the water column outside one's chest and the air contained in the lungs at the beginning of the dive. A Boyle's law–related compression of lung volume toward residual volume can limit the depth of a free dive in ordinary individuals to depths less than 100 fsw. However, in deep-diving marine mammals and a select group of human breath-hold divers, intrathoracic blood volume increases with depth, reducing residual volume and allowing truly exceptional free dives. The current record for deep breath-hold diving in humans is greater than 400 fsw (Chap. 15).

If one is to descend under water without accumulating physical and physiological stresses, three things must be accomplished simultaneously: (1) the efficient removal of metabolically produced CO_2, (2) a constant supply of O_2 adequate to meet metabolic requirements, and (3) equalization of pressure across the thoracic boundary. These are the prime requirements for facilitating human expeditions under water using equipment called underwater breathing apparatus (UBA).

II. Primary Requirements

The UBA shares basic features in common with the dry-land breathing apparatus, the lungs, which accomplish the above primary functions. Both lungs and UBA deliver copious amounts of O_2 to the circulatory system and remove equally prodigious amounts of CO_2 from the same vasculature. To a limited extent, the thorax can respond to pressure imbalances by nature of the counterbalancing elastic properties of the lungs and chest wall. It is not, therefore, a great hyperbole to consider a UBA as an accessory respiratory organ. Its purpose is to provide O_2 and remove CO_2 when the primary organ of respiration is unable to provide that service.

The above analogy is useful because of modern medicine's twentieth-century experience with artificial organs. We know from experience that the design of an artificial organ is limited only by imagination, materials, and the laws of physics. Just as our knowledge of physiology has made possible increasingly efficacious and reliable designs for artificial organs, so it has allowed us to design increasingly improved UBA. Just as engineering skills have advanced the development of the artificial heart, so they advance the UBA.

The following sections describe how the imagination of both engineering-wise physiologists and physiology-inspired engineers have allowed UBA to solve the primary problems of sustaining life under water. We will also see that in the future, UBA will come to resemble ever more closely the organ that they mimic.

III. General Solutions to Requirements

To categorize in the broadest terms the support systems for a sojourner into a space filled with either water or a vacuum, we can describe either open systems, with a continuous flow of expendable materials, or closed systems. The closed systems can be either nonregenerative or regenerative to varying degrees. An example of a closed, nonregenerative system is one where O_2 is released from an expendable source, the sojourner converts O_2 into CO_2 through metabolic pathways, and the gaseous CO_2 is then removed from the system by chemical absorption. To date the most sophisticated diving apparatuses belong to the latter category.

A. Regenerating Systems

Before moving on to the details of actual UBAs, let us briefly dwell on ideal, conceptual life-support systems. By definition, in a regenerative closed system, the absorption of CO_2 results in the generation of O_2. One example of this type of system is photosynthesis. The earth is a grand but arguably closed system that reliably supports oxygen-dependent organisms through photosynthesis. Human efforts at reproducing this feat on a small scale have generally been less successful. The gas-exchange properties of photosynthesis have sustained mammals ranging from mice (1) to humans (2) for a number of days in sealed laboratory environments at 1 atm absolute.

Simple chemicals such as alkaline metal superoxides can be used to couple O_2 production to CO_2 uptake. Both sodium and potassium superoxide combine with CO_2 and H_2O to release O_2. Unfortunately, the enthalpies of reaction are high and in the presence of excess water can lead to near explosive results. The use of alkaline metal superoxides is therefore not well suited to the underwater environment. (These reactions are discussed in more detail in Sec. IV.E.) Even if chemical and photosynthetic systems could be made safe and efficient, they still could not used for diving without the addition of gas to the diver's lungs as he or she descends, as discussed below.

B. Pressure Imbalance

Regardless of how O_2 is supplied to a diver, there is an ever-present need to make up gas volume as pressure increases during an underwater descent. Boyle's law states that as the pressure on a deformable, gas filled system increases during descent, the system volume decreases. Assuming an ideal gas, that change in volume is described as:

$$\Delta V = -\Delta P \frac{V_f}{P_i}$$

The subscript i refers to an initial value at the start of a dive and the subscript f is the final value. ΔV and ΔP equals $V_i - V_f$ and $P_i - P_f$, respectively. To maintain normal lung volume during a descent, new gas must be added to the diver's lungs from the UBA. The moles of gas to be added is found as:

$$\Delta n = \Delta V \frac{P_f}{RT}$$

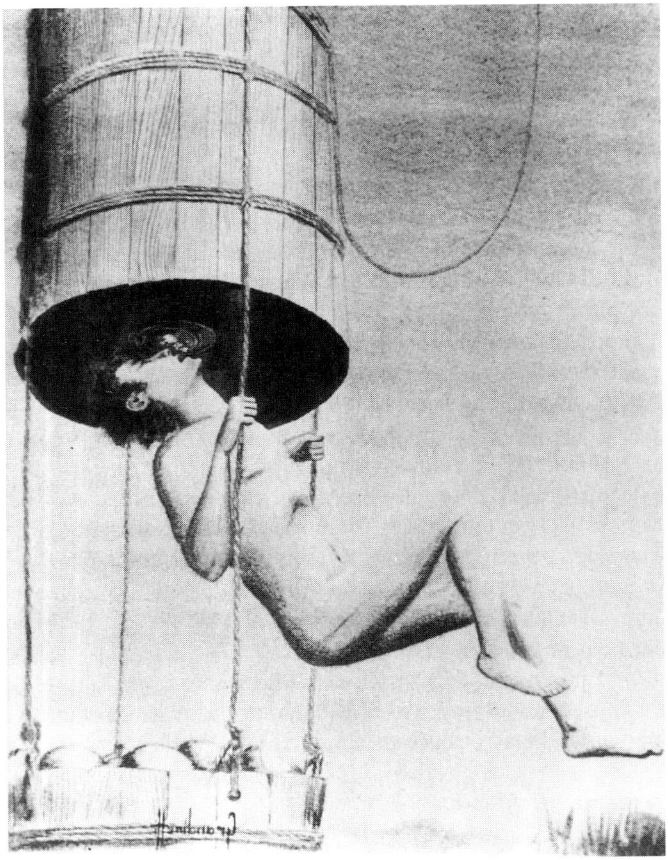

Figure 1 Free diver breathing from a barrel of air during ancient times. (From Ref. 5.)

where R is the universal gas constant and T is temperature in Kelvin. This added gas can be either O_2 or inert gas, depending on rules concerning O_2 adequacy and toxicity (Chap. 7).

Partial pressures of O_2 significantly greater than 1.6 atm abs are associated with increased risk of O_2-induced seizures. Therefore, for deep descents, gas volume must be made up with an inert gas, such as nitrogen or helium. Without the addition of gas volume, a diver would be subject to the same potentially fatal chest compression experienced by the free diver—chest compression caused by pressure gradients across the chest wall.

C. Delivery of O_2 and CO_2 Removal

Oxygen can be supplied to a diver through a variety of means. The earliest and simplest method of underwater oxygenation was the use of a bubble—a scheme invented eons ago by diving beetles (*Dysticus* and *Gyrinidae*) and spiders (*Argyronedidae*) (3,4). Humans have mimicked this prehistoric method through the use of barrels (Fig. 1), diving bells (Fig. 2), and caissons. Beetles presaged the appearance of SCUBA gear by carrying their air supply on their backs.

Spiders foresaw the appearance of underwater habitats by creating silk-enshrouded, air-filled underwater chambers (Fig. 3). Alas, insects, arachnids, and human divers share a common problem. Unless the captive air supply is refreshed, the dive must eventually be terminated due to a diminishing O_2 supply and, in some cases, an accumulation of CO_2.

The replenishment of respirable gas can be accomplished through two mechanisms. One is simple but wasteful of gas. A flow of fresh gas brings O_2 to the diver and, when dumped into the water, carries away CO_2. This is the preferred method of gas replenishment when breathing air on relatively shallow

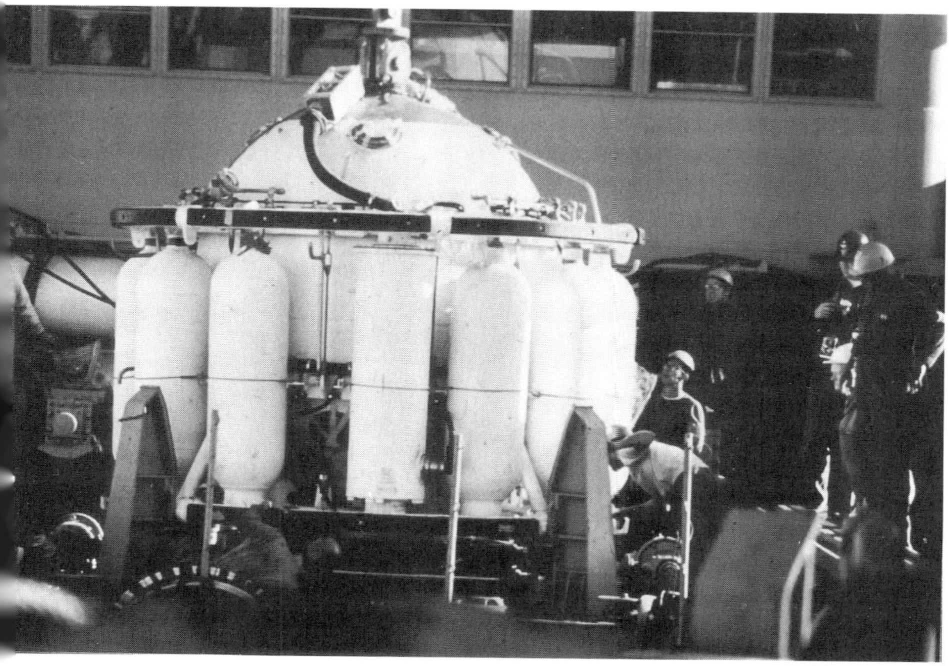

Figure 2 A diving bell or personnel transfer capsule (PTC).

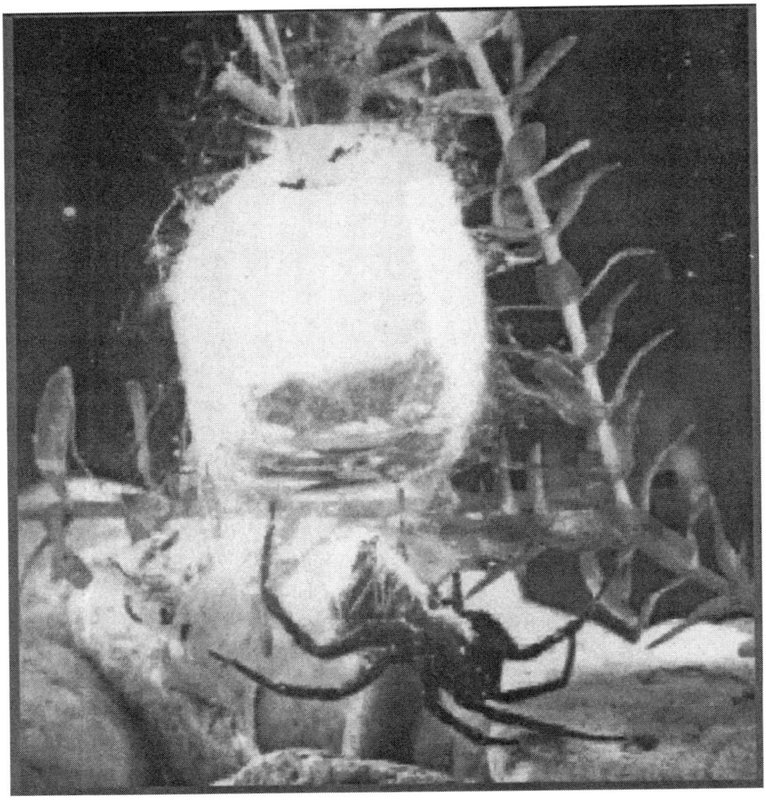

Figure 3 A water spider and air-filled nest. (*Courtesy of Microsoft, Inc., Redmond, WA.*)

dives. However, helium is frequently used as an inert gas in deep diving, and massive dumping into the water column would be extraordinarily expensive. For instance, if a diver were supplied with 170 L·min^{-1} (6 acfm, ATPD) of gas per minute at 1000 fsw [6 acfm has proven to be a good gas flow for helmet diving (5), Sec. IV.A], that would translate into approximately 5000 L·min^{-1} (~180 acfm) at 1 atm abs. A standard 3000-psi scuba cylinder contains approximately 2265 L (80 cf) at 1 atm abs. Therefore, at an open circuit flow rate of 170 L·min^{-1}, twin 207 bar (20.7 MPa or 3000 psi) bottles would be emptied in less than a minute at a depth of 1000 fsw.

A more practical approach for deep diving is to recycle the breathed gas, adding oxygen as needed and removing CO_2 through chemical absorption. The only inert gas added to the system would be that inadvertently lost through leaks or required for volume makeup during descents and small amounts dissolved in the body tissues.

IV. Specific Solutions

A. Diving Helmets

Constant Flow

Diving helmets are in principle the simplest of all UBAs. Because of their simplicity, they were also the first successful solution to our need to work under water (Fig. 4).

A helmeted diver is connected to the surface air supply by a long umbilical (Fig. 5). Just as a fetus depends on his or her umbilical blood supply to transport O_2, so must a diver trust completely in a "topside" individual to sustain his or her oxygen needs. Carbon dioxide is removed from the diver's helmet by expelling a mixture of fresh and expired gas into the water through an exhaust valve.

The principle elements of the helmet system can be described in the format of an electrical schematic (Fig. 6). The use of electrical analogs for the respiratory system is a standard tool in the field of respiratory mechanics. Some of the earliest and most complete examples of this method of describing human respiratory impedance are found in DuBois et al. (6) and Mead and Milic-Emili (7). The DuBois model of the respiratory system is referenced in essentially every modern work on respiratory impedance. We have simply extended this convention to the description of external respiratory impedances.

In the electrical analogy, the diver is represented by an alternating-current (gas-flow) generator. The diver is, in electrical terms, a constant root mean square (RMS) current source. The diver must receive the fresh gas flow required to support a given metabolic effort. He will generate whatever pressures are required to get that flow as long as he continues to work and remains conscious. Sudden loss of consciousness under water is often the first indication that a diver is not getting the gas flow required, especially during exercise in a high-P_{O_2} environment (8). [See Lanphier (9) for a full discussion of the unconscious diver.]

The circuit in Fig. 6 is divided into inspiratory and expiratory portions through the action of one-way valves (represented by diodes) on the right side of the schematic. Throughout this chapter, we use the convention of the inspiratory circuitry being at the top of the diagram and the expiratory circuitry lying below the diagrammatic diver.

The umbilical is represented schematically by a flow resistance (R_{umb}) and a shunting capacitance (C_{umb}). The shunting capacitance implies that the umbil-

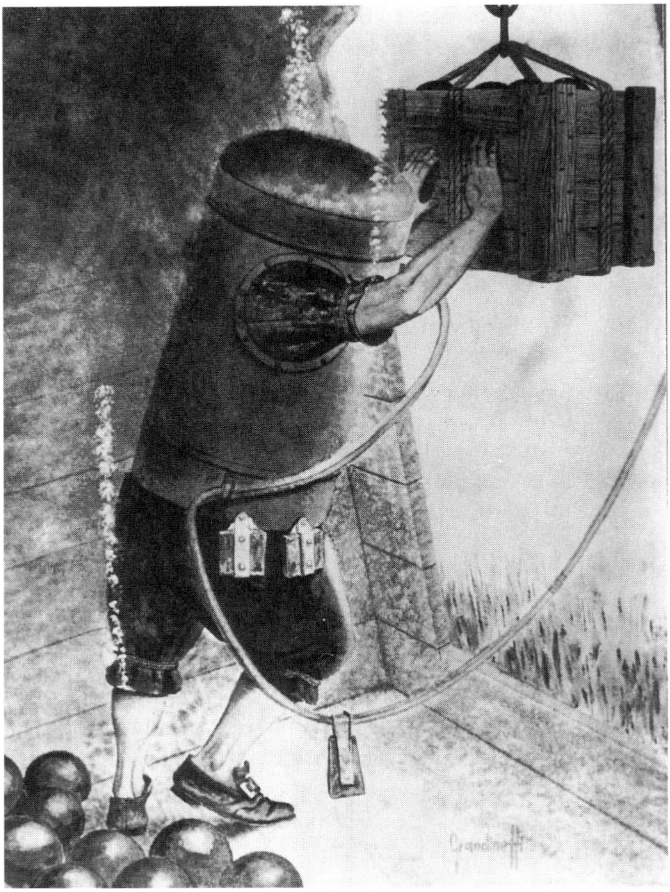

Figure 4 A 1700s salvor in a body tank for use in shallow water. (From Ref. 5.)

ical can store gas—a critical feature in certain conditions to be elaborated on in the next section. Both L_{insp} and L_{exp} are inductances [or in mechanical terms, inertances (10)] that act in the inspiratory and expiratory circuits respectively. These inductances resist sudden changes in flow and are elaborated upon in Sec. V.B.

The helmet's exhaust valve is in electrical terms a voltage-(pressure-) controlled switch and is diver-adjustable. The amount of overpressure in the helmet (relative to the surrounding water) allowed before the helmet vents is governed by the adjustment of the exhaust valve.

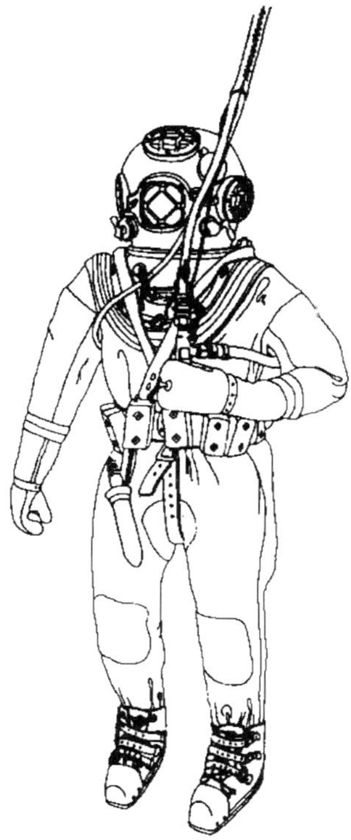

Figure 5 An MK 5 hard hat diver with umbilical. The MK 5 was used by the U.S. Navy until the mid-1980s. (From Ref. 5.)

In many diving systems, such as the U.S. Navy's MK 12 (Fig. 7), the helmet is connected to a dry suit. The suit acts as a compliant volume, represented by C_{suit} in Fig. 6. Just as the umbilical can store fresh gas, the suit can store CO_2-rich exhaled gas. The significance of this fact is addressed below. Since the flow of fresh gas through the umbilical is constant, the diver must inhale what is needed from the incoming gas flow. Gas not needed by the diver is exhausted from the helmet without passing into the diver's lungs.

An excess gas flow not only wastes gas but creates noise, which can hamper communications (the umbilical usually has an attached communication cable) and prove to be a long-term health hazard to the diver. Therefore, efforts are made to reduce gas flow whenever feasible. Herein lies a danger. While a helmet's gas flow is steady, the diver's inspiratory flow is typically sinusoidal.

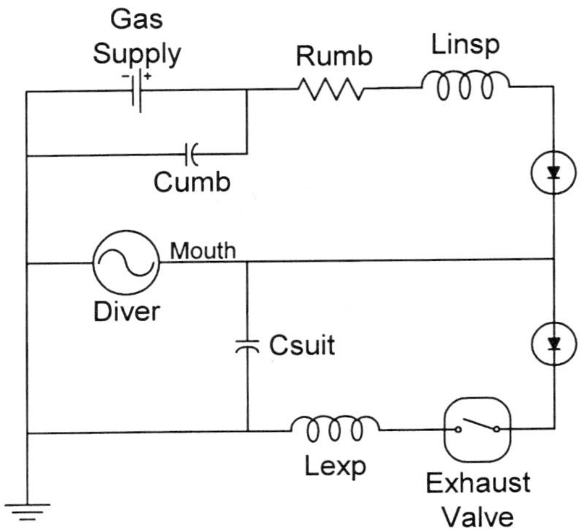

Figure 6 Electrical analog for a typical constant-flow helmet system.

Peak flow rates (in $L \cdot sec^{-1}$) for a sinusoidal breathing pattern are related to expired ventilation ($\dot{V}E$) as follows:

$$\text{Flow}_{\text{peak}} = \pi \cdot \frac{\dot{V}E}{60}$$

The continuous flow of fresh gas required by the U.S. Navy for helmeted diving is either 2.1 or 2.8 $L \cdot s^{-1}$ (4.5 or 6 acfm) (5). From the above equation, we see that the peak flow rate for sinusoidal breathing with a $\dot{V}E$ of 60 $L \cdot min^{-1}$ is about 3.1 $L \cdot s^{-1}$. Thus, there is a transient shortfall between the diver's requirements and the gas supply (11). Either the ventilation of 60 $L \cdot min^{-1}$ cannot be supported or additional gas has to come from compliant elements within the system. The most accessible alternative gas source is the suit or neck dam, which unfortunately contains CO_2 from the diver's previous exhalations.

The diver has another option: to change his or her breathing pattern. In square-wave breathing,

$$\text{Flow}_{\text{peak}} = 2 \cdot \frac{\dot{V}E}{60}$$

As shown in Fig. 8, rectangular breathing patterns allow a $\dot{V}E$ of over 60 $L \cdot min^{-1}$ to be supported by a steady flow of 2.8 $L \cdot sec^{-1}$ (6 acfm). The downside of that flow pattern is that rectangular patterns are characterized by rapid gas

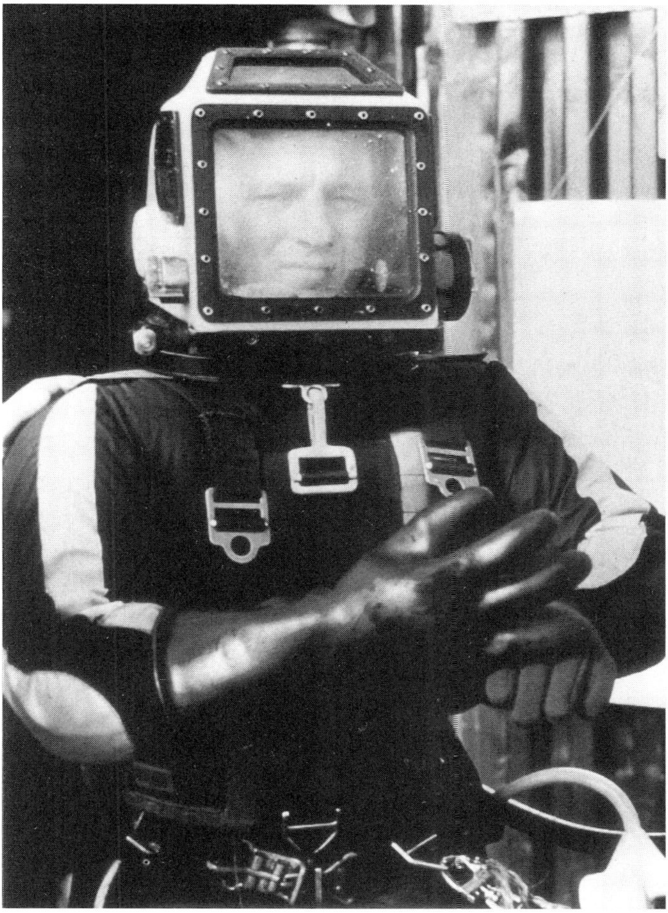

Figure 7 MK 12, umbilical-supplied hard hat diver. The MK 12 replaced the MK 5 in the U.S. Navy inventory.

acceleration, which is impeded by UBA inertance. The result can be brief but pronounced spikes of respiratory pressure.

Compared to other types of UBA, the dead space in diving helmets is large, essentially consisting of the floodable volume of the helmet minus the volume of the diver's head. [The UBA dead space is that volume where fresh gas and exhaled CO_2 mix.) The volume of a typical constant flow helmet such as the U.S. Navy's MK 12 is approximately 11 L (12).] For a nominal head

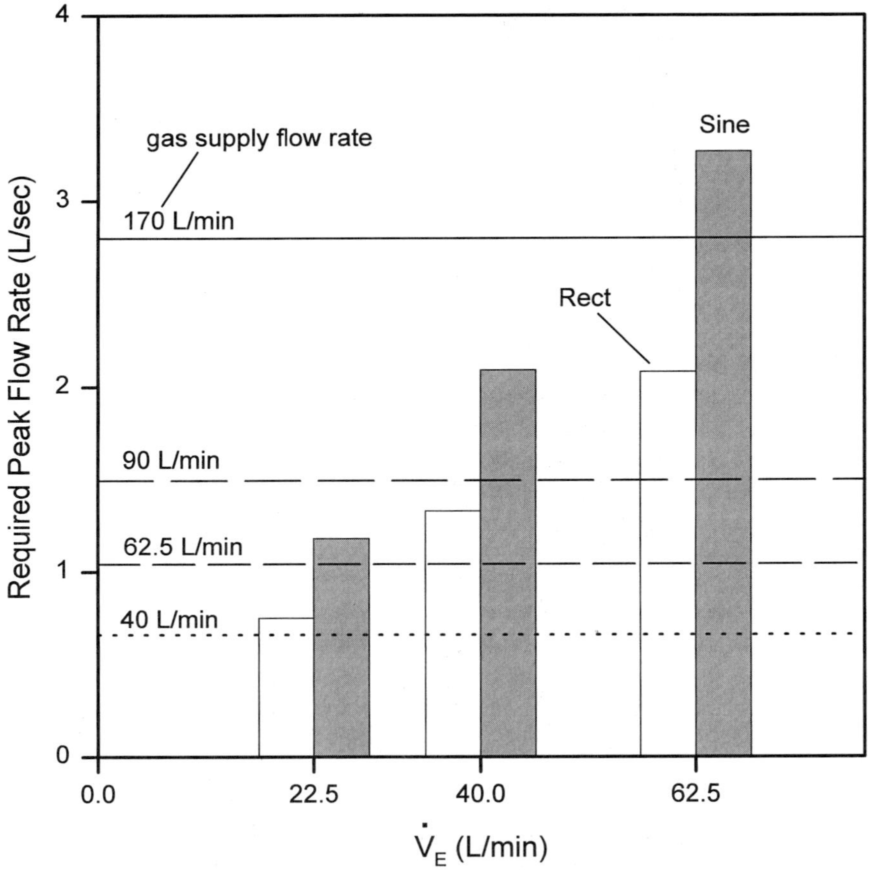

Figure 8 The diver's breathing requirements (vertical bars): peak inspiratory flow rates in L/sec required by various expired ventilations (in L/min) during sinusoidal breathing (gray bars) and rectangular breathing (white bars). Umbilical flow rates: the horizontal lines indicate the equivalent flow rates in L/sec for various constant flow rates (in L/min) delivered by the UBA gas supply. A gas supply flow rate of 170 L/min does not meet peak flow demands for a $\dot{V}_E$ of 62.5 L/min when breathing is sinusoidal. However, it will meet peak flow demands during rectangular breathing at the same $\dot{V}_E$. (Adapted from Ref. 11.)

and neck volume of about 6.5 L, helmet dead space would be about 4.5 L. Compared with a diver's anatomical dead space of roughly 150 ml, the helmet dead space is a large volume. Because of this large dead space, inspired CO_2 is usually elevated. In fact, CO_2 elevation is such a common occurrence in free-flow helmet diving that the U.S. Navy allows inspired CO_2 to rise to 15 mmHg (equivalent in partial pressure to 2% CO_2 at 1 atm abs) (5) without corrective action being taken.

The following equation, based on the law of mass balance, has been used to estimate the partial pressure of CO_2 in a helmet as a function of diver CO_2 production ($\dot{V}CO_2$) and umbilical gas flow at depth (13):

$$P_{CO_2} = 760 \cdot \left(\frac{\dot{V}_{CO_2}}{\dot{V}_{depth}} + F_{SCO_2} \cdot \frac{D + 33}{33} \right)$$

where D is depth in fsw and 33 is the approximate conversion factor from fsw to atm. F_{SCO_2} is the fraction of CO_2 in the supply gas. If there is no CO_2 in the gas supply, P_{CO_2} is governed by the ratio of diver CO_2 production to supply gas flow at depth and, not surprisingly, bears a resemblance to the alveolar ventilation equation. For a $\dot{V}_{CO_2}$ of 3 $L \cdot min^{-1}$ and an umbilical flow of 170 $L \cdot min^{-1}$ (6 acfm), the expected helmet P_{CO_2} is 13.4 mmHg, just below the allowed limit of 15 mmHg. If helmet flow were to drop to 142 $L \cdot min^{-1}$ (5 acfm), the helmet P_{CO_2} would be expected to rise to just over 16 mmHg.

For the above computation, gas in the helmet dead space is considered well mixed. In fact, helmet gas is poorly mixed, as revealed by flow visualization analysis of internal helmet flow (14). Figures 9a and 9b show results of model studies where Reynolds-number scaling was used to visualize inspiratory flow around a diver's idealized spherical head and circular mouth opening. The test medium was water instead of air, and visualization was allowed by transient injections of dye along the interior of a gas supply tube placed just below the ''diver's'' mouth. An exhaust orifice was located on the left side of the helmet from the diver's perspective (right side of the photo). The left side of the photo is the right side of the diver's head reflected in a mirror. The arrangement of helmet inlet and outlet is comparable to that in an MK 12 constant-flow helmet.

In Fig. 9a, the diver's ventilation was 40 $L \cdot min^{-1}$ and helmet gas flow was 170 $L \cdot min^{-1}$ (6 acfm). The dark area emanating from the diffuser gas inlet bar is colored water, representing CO_2 free gas. The clear liquid in the photo is well-mixed ''gas'' containing CO_2 from the diver's last expiration.

For a $\dot{V}E$ of 40 $L \cdot min^{-1}$, peak flow during sinusoidal breathing is 2.09 $L \cdot sec^{-1}$. A gas supply rate of 170 $L \cdot min^{-1}$ equals 2.83 $L \cdot sec^{-1}$. Therefore, the gas supply should more than meet peak inspiratory demands. Midway through inspiration, low-CO_2 supply gas (colored water) surrounds the mouth opening. Gas supplied to the diver is therefore relatively pure as long as the supply rate

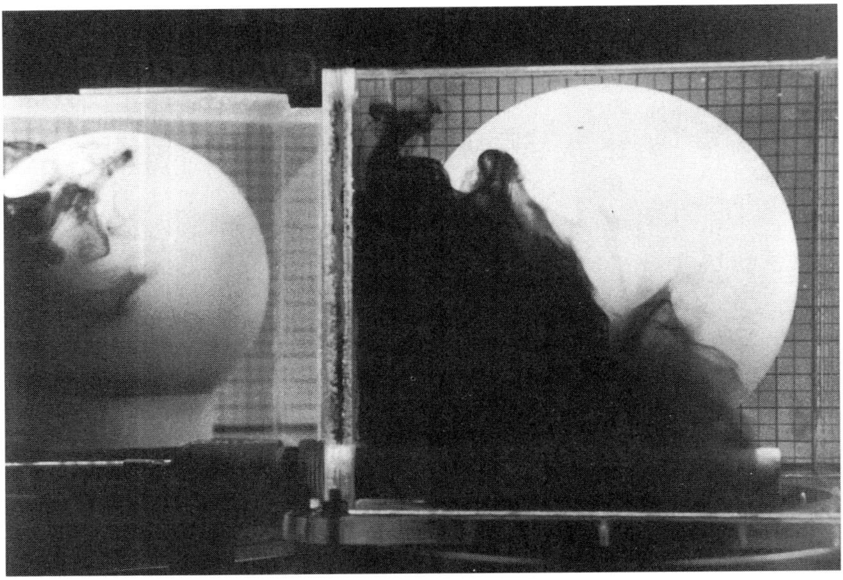

A

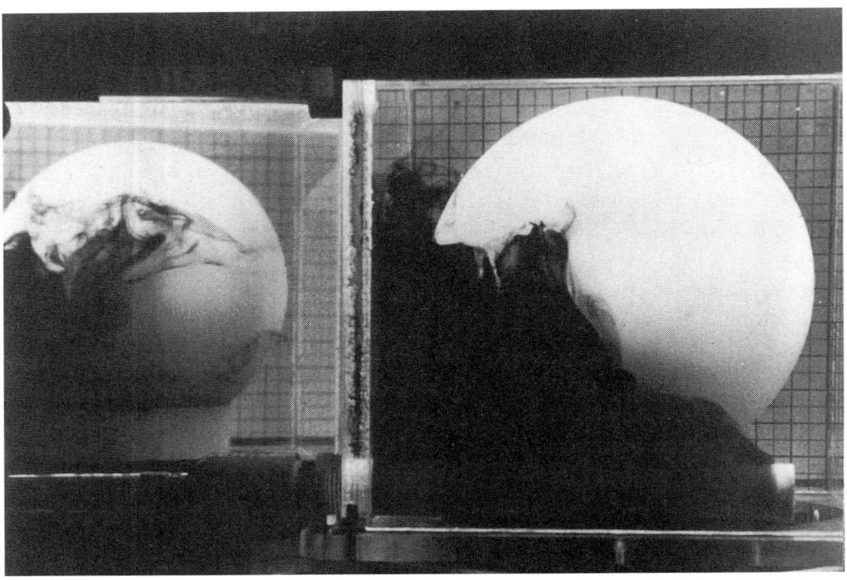

B

Figure 9 Model study with visualization of inspiratory flow in a constant flow diving helmet similar to the MK 12. (A) ''Diver'' ventilation = 40 $L \cdot min^{-1}$, helmet fresh gas supply = 165 $L \cdot min^{-1}$. (B) ''Diver'' ventilation = 40 $L \cdot min^{-1}$, helmet fresh gas supply = 125 $L \cdot min^{-1}$.

is 170 L·min^{-1}. When steady flow is reduced to 125 L·min^{-1} (or 2.08 L·sec^{-1}), peak inspiratory demand from the diver and gas supply should be matched. However, as seen in Fig. 9b, even with matched flows, CO_2-fouled gas (clear liquid) is present at the oral margin. The ''diver'' is breathing a mixture of both fresh supply gas and the previous expired breath.

Use of helmet CO_2-reducing techniques to justify reduction of steady flow for gas conservation and noise reduction has had little success to date. However, studies such as those illustrated in Fig. 9 may change this trend. Because of the points illustrated in Fig. 8, such efforts are destined to limit a diver's work capacity unless the diver has available a large compliant volume filled with low CO_2 gas.

Demand Flow

The use of steady-flow helmets such as the U.S. Navy's MK 12 (Fig. 7) has been largely supplanted by demand-flow helmets with oronasal masks fitting snugly around the mouth and nose (Figs. 10–12). These helmets minimize dead space by using the oronasal mask to limit the amount of exhaled gas exchanging with the helmet.

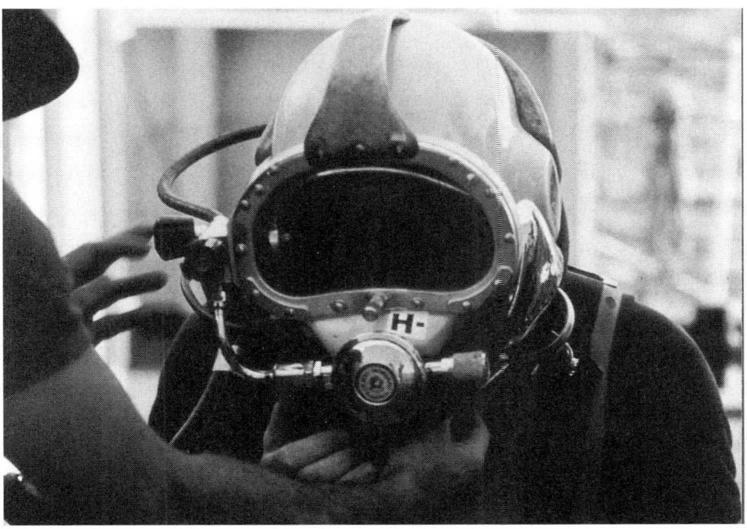

Figure 10 MK 21 demand flow, umbilical-supplied hard hat. This helmet is similar to the Superlite 17 extensively used by the commercial diving industry. In the U.S. Navy, this helmet has replaced the MK 12.

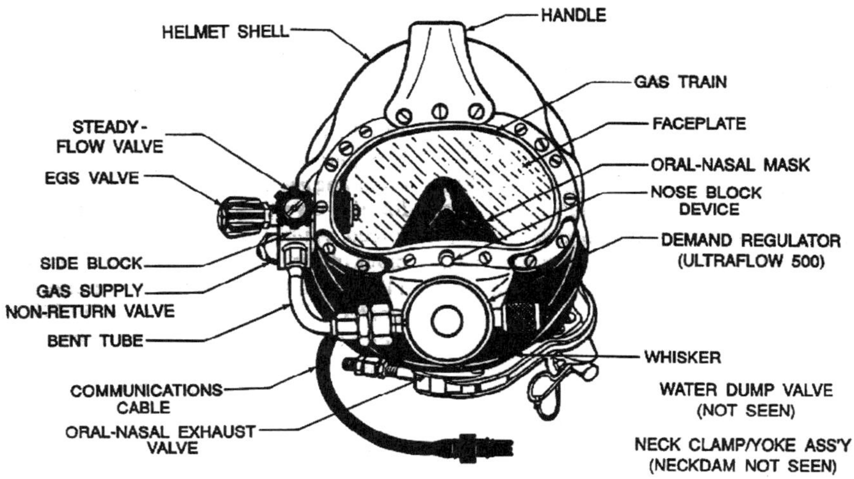

Figure 11 Diagram of the U.S. Navy's MK 21 Mod 0 helmet. (From Ref. 5.)

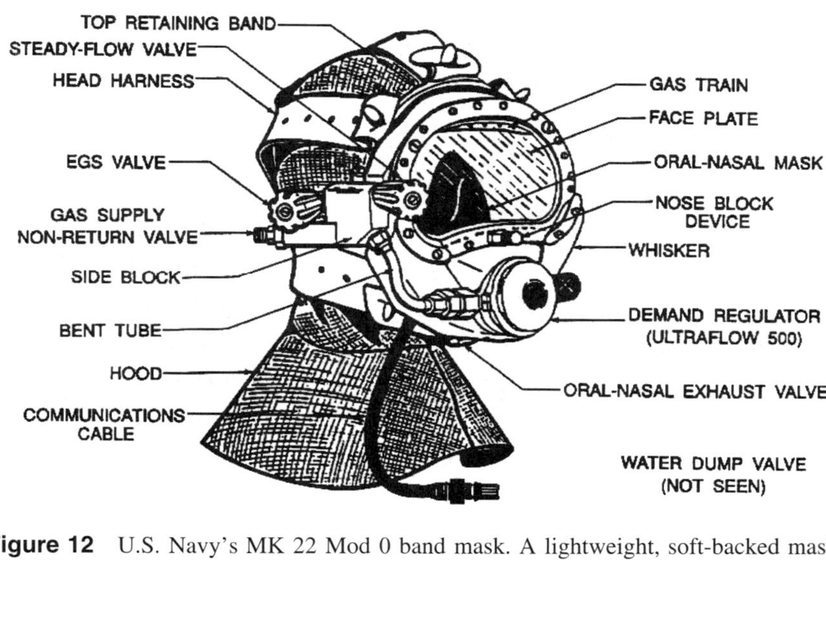

Figure 12 U.S. Navy's MK 22 Mod 0 band mask. A lightweight, soft-backed mask.

A demand regulator provides gas only when required by the diver. The demand regulator is symbolized in Fig. 13 as a voltage-controlled switch triggered by a negative pressure generated by the diver's inspiratory efforts. Since gas is supplied only on demand instead of continuously, the overall gas consumption is reduced considerably, ranging between 40 and 90 $L \cdot min^{-1}$ for typical and emergency flow requirements, respectively. In theory, the helmet dead space is reduced to only that volume within the oronasal cup and a portion of the demand-regulator body, a volume of roughly 200 mL. Therefore, inspired CO_2 concentration is minimal.

In some demand diving systems, the greatest impediment to flow occurs within the gas console itself. The console is the system of regulators, valves, and tubing immediately downstream of the gas storage flasks. The console is represented by R_{con} in the top left of Fig. 13. When the diver's demand exceeds the gas console's output, the gas stored in the umbilical becomes a useful source of additional gas (Fig. 14). If the gas stored in an umbilical 200 m long with an internal diameter of 9.5 mm (13-L floodable volume) were depressurized from 11.4 bar (165 psi) above ambient down to ambient pressure (the water pressure at depth), then approximately 35 L of gas would be made available to the diver. This additional gas can make possible the maintenance of umbilical pressure between breaths (Fig. 14b, dashed line), which, in turn, keeps the diver's mouth pressure close to zero (Fig. 14a). When the umbilical or other compliant source is lacking, umbilical pressures can drop, thereby leading to highly negative inspiratory pressures (Fig. 14, solid lines). The addition of a compliant volume to the gas supply line is known to reduce the breathing effort

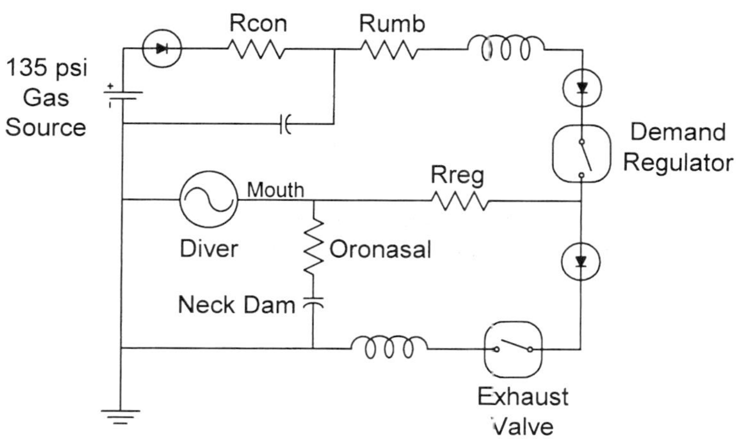

Figure 13 Electrical analog for an umbilical supplied helmet with demand regulator.

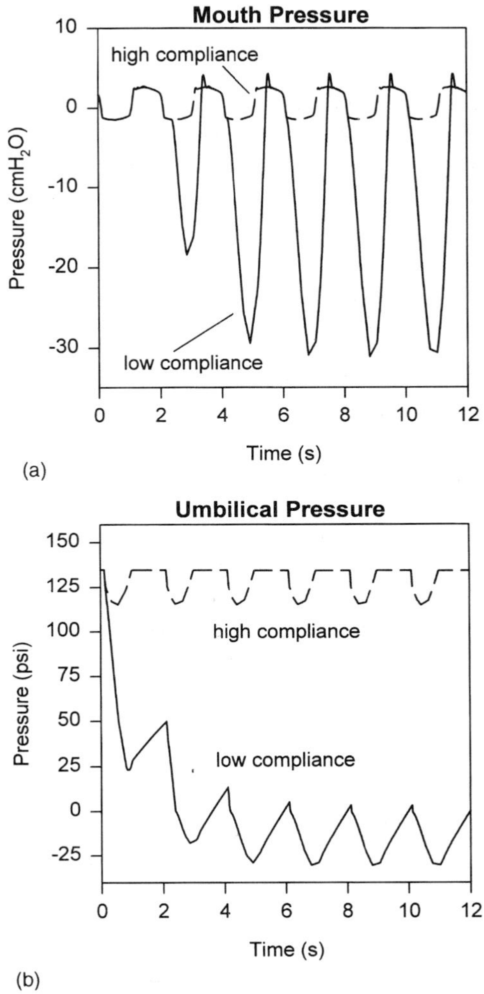

Figure 14 (a) Modeled mouth pressure and (b) umbilical pressure for low compliance (solid line) and high compliance (broken line) systems. (From Ref. 11.)

of both the MK 21 and its progenitor, the Superlite 17B, whenever gas supply is marginal (15,16).

The additional gas stored in the umbilical would be available for only a short time, of course, unless the gas-supply console were able to repressurize the umbilical during the period when the diver was making no inspiratory demands—i.e., while the diver was exhaling. Except for the highest breathing frequencies where exhalation time is very short, most diving consoles do have time to return umbilical pressure to its normal value between breaths.

Many demand helmets use a neck dam, a pliable rubber closure on the bottom of the helmet through which the diver inserts his head when putting on the helmet. The dam is intended to form a seal around the diver's neck. If the resistor in Fig. 13, identified as the oronasal resistor, is high, then little gas will communicate with the neck dam compliance. If the resistance is low—that is, if there is a poor oronasal seal—then the helmet and neck dam become a compliant gas source capable of exchanging CO_2-rich gas with the diver. Obviously, a proper oronasal seal is a critical requirement of demand helmets.

B. SCUBA

Description

By definition, the self-contained diving apparatus (SCUBA) does not rely on an umbilical to supply gas to the diver. Modern SCUBA equipment provides unparalleled freedom, exceptional reliability, and economy that is unequaled among other types of diving equipment. While the sport of SCUBA diving has expanded greatly since the 1960s, the concept of self-contained diving is quite old. Envisioned by Da Vinci in the 1500s and expounded on by Borelli in 1680, a reasonable but apparently untried design was generated as early as 1825 by the Englishman William James. The first successful compressed-air SCUBA dive (17) is believed to have been conducted in 1832. Two Frenchmen developed a demand valve in 1865, which allowed semi-self-contained diving. By 1918 the Japanese had developed an air-demand SCUBA, which was tested to 324 ft (98.8 m). Another Frenchman, Yves Le Prieur, patented a SCUBA that was a forerunner of the now famous Cousteau-Gagnan ''Aqualung'' developed in 1943. All modern-day SCUBA regulators have evolved directly from the two-hose Cousteau-Gagnan regulators of the 1940s.

The essential elements of modern SCUBAs are a high-pressure (typically 207 bar, 3000 psi) aluminum cylinder that allows a diver to carry his or her own air supply and a regulator (Fig. 15) that continuously senses and corrects pressure imbalances between the gas it delivers and the surrounding water. In modern regulators, this depressurization occurs in two stages, the first to an intermediate pressure somewhere between 8 and 14 bar (116 and 203 psi), the

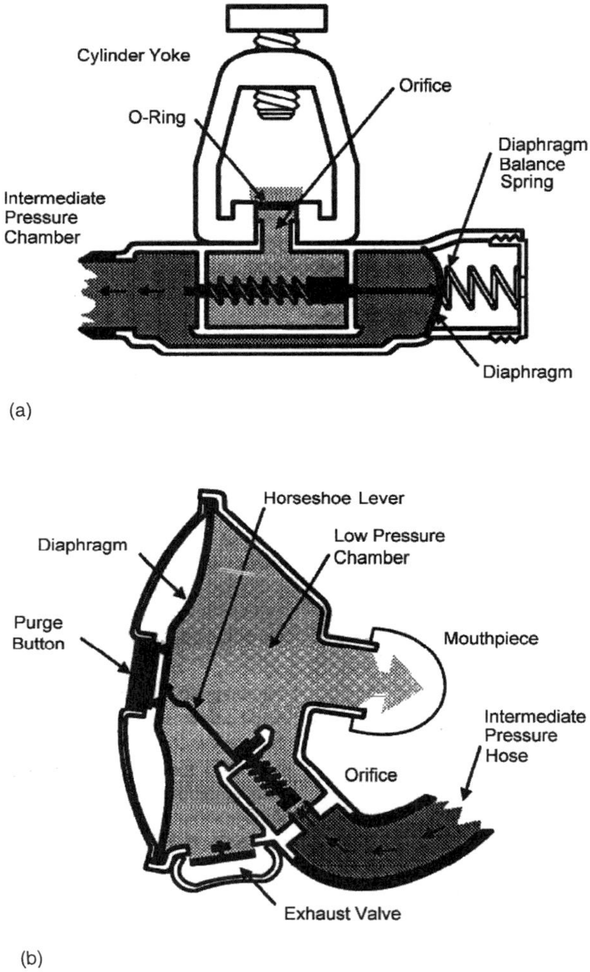

Figure 15 Internal structure of SCUBA (a) first and (b) second stage regulators. (From Ref. 5.)

second to a pressure equivalent to hydrostatic pressure at the diver's mouth (Fig. 16). The second-stage SCUBA regulator is virtually identical to the demand regulators used in demand helmets (Sec. IV.A).

The SCUBA device is characterized by an extremely low equipment dead space. Low-volume SCUBA mouthpieces and second-stage regulators keep equipment dead space to a size similar to that of anatomical dead space (150 ml) or less.

Venturi Assistance

A relatively recent advance in regulator design has been the use of flow-separation plates or other devices to generate vortices within the second-stage regulator housing during inspiration. These vortices create a low-pressure area centered on the second-stage diaphragm, thereby reducing the suction that the diver must generate to hold the inspiratory valve open. The device creating the inspiratory assist is colloquially termed a *venturi* The reduction in respiratory pressures afforded by a venturi can be significant. For example, during unmanned testing using mechanical breathing simulators (18), a U.S. Divers Conshelf XIV regulator without a flow-separation plate produced peak inspiratory pressures of -41 cmH_2O at a depth of 40 msw and a ventilation rate of 62.5

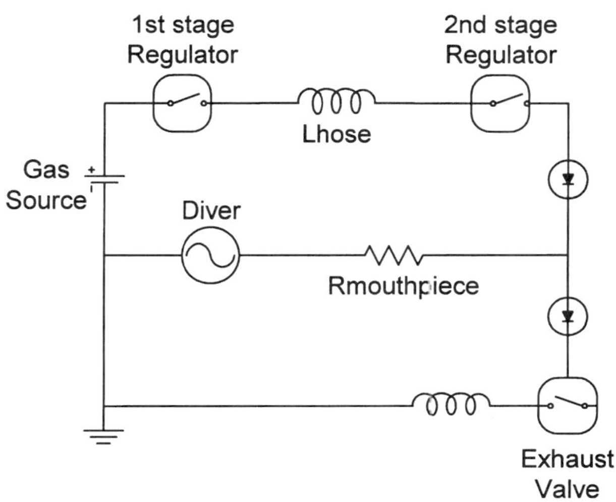

Figure 16 An electrical analog of SCUBA.

$L \cdot min^{-1}$. With the plate installed, peak inspiratory pressure was only -16 cmH_2O.

C. Rebreathers

Description

The UBAs that recycle a diver's exhaled breath are termed *rebreathers*. There are three main categories of rebreathers (19) (Fig. 17). They all remove CO_2 from the exhaled breath by passing it through a CO_2-absorbent scrubber before collecting it in a breathing bag, or, as it is sometimes termed, a counterlung (Fig. 18). The three categories of rebreathers are (1) pure O_2 rebreathers; (2) mixed gas, variable-O_2 UBAs; and (3) mixed gas, controlled-O_2 UBAs. The last of these are often referred to as electronic UBAs because of their use of electronic O_2 sensing and gas-makeup mechanisms.

Semi–Closed Circuit UBAs

Semi–closed circuit UBAs are, as the name implies, a cross between the open-circuit UBA described in Secs. IV.A and B and the closed-circuit UBAs described below. Semiclosed UBAs conserve gas without the mechanical complexity of mixed-gas, fully closed-circuit UBAs. They conserve gas by dumping into the water only a portion of each exhaled breath and feeding fresh gas into the UBA from a fixed O_2-content gas cylinder. Exhaled CO_2 is removed by chemical absorption, described in more detail in Sec. IV.E.

The first successful semiclosed UBAs used for military purposes were built essentially simultaneously by the British and an American physician and educator. The British device was termed the clearance divers breathing apparatus, or CDBA. The American UBA was given the tongue-in-cheek name FLATUS (20,21), owing presumably to its habit of intermittently releasing bubbles. The design was by Christian J. Lambertsen of the University of Pennsylvania, a researcher and practitioner of environmental medicine, pharmacologist, inventor, and humorist. The FLATUS eventually became the U.S. Navy's first semiclosed UBA, after being given the less colorful designations of MK 5 and MK 6 SCUBA (22).

Semiclosed UBAs such as the MK 6 and its modern counterparts use a critical orifice to supply gas to the diver and a high enough pressure gradient across the orifice to generate sonic flow—that is, flow with a linear velocity equal to the speed of sound. That velocity cannot be exceeded regardless of the upstream pressure (23–25). However, the mass flow through the orifice does change. When a regulator is used to maintain upstream pressure at a fixed value over ambient under sonic conditions, the mass flow through the orifice is linearly dependent upon ambient pressure or depth.

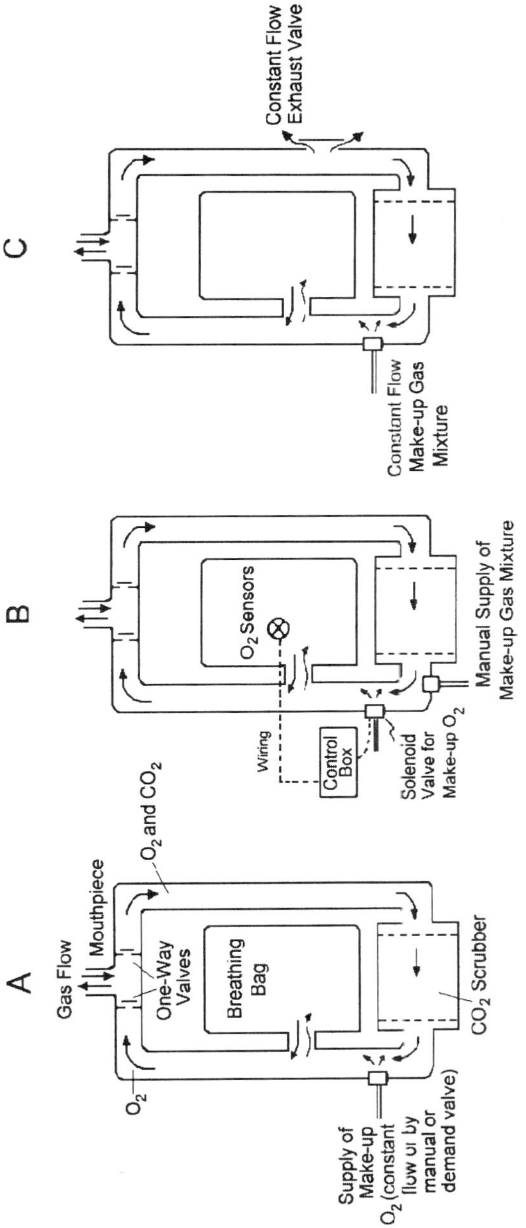

Figure 17 Three rebreathers: (A) closed-circuit oxygen UBA, (B) closed-circuit mixed gas UBA, and (C) semiclosed mixed-gas UBA. (From Ref. 19.)

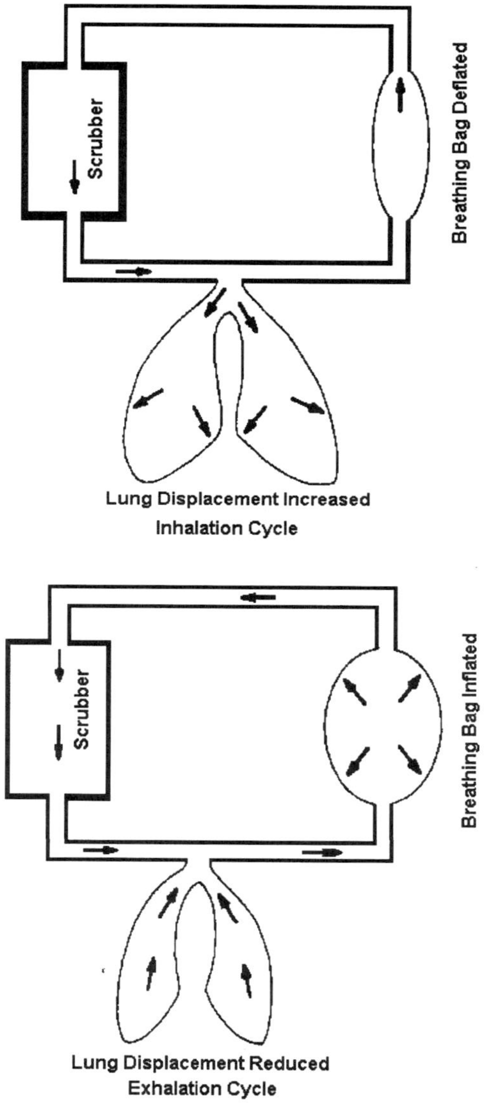

Figure 18 The breathing bag in a closed-circuit UBA is often called a counterlung, for reasons made apparent above. (From Ref. 5.)

The variation with time of the oxygen fraction within a semiclosed, constant-injection UBA is expressed as an equation with both transient and steady-state terms (26):

$$y(t) = C \cdot e^{-\frac{(\dot{V}_{inj} - \dot{V}_{O_2})}{\dot{V}_{tot}}} + \frac{(FS_{O_2} \cdot \dot{V}_{inj}) - \dot{V}_{O_2}}{\dot{V}_{inj} - \dot{V}_{O_2}}$$

where

$$C = \frac{\left[(1 - y(0)) \cdot \dot{V}_{O_2}\right] - \left[(FS_{O_2} - y(0)) \cdot \dot{V}_{inj}\right]}{\dot{V}_{inj} - \dot{V}_{O_2}}$$

and y(t) is the oxygen fraction within the UBA at any time t; y(0) is the oxygen fraction within the UBA at time zero (the beginning of a change in oxygen consumption); FSO_2 is the fraction of O_2 in the UBA gas supply; $\dot{V}_{O_2}$ and $\dot{V}_{inj}$ are the diver's oxygen consumption rate and the UBA's gas injection rate, respectively; and V_{tot} is the average gas volume in the UBA. This equation applies to STPD conditions.

Figures 19 and 20 illustrate two examples of the difficulties inherent in the use of semi–closed circuit UBAs. In Fig. 19 we assume that the diver's

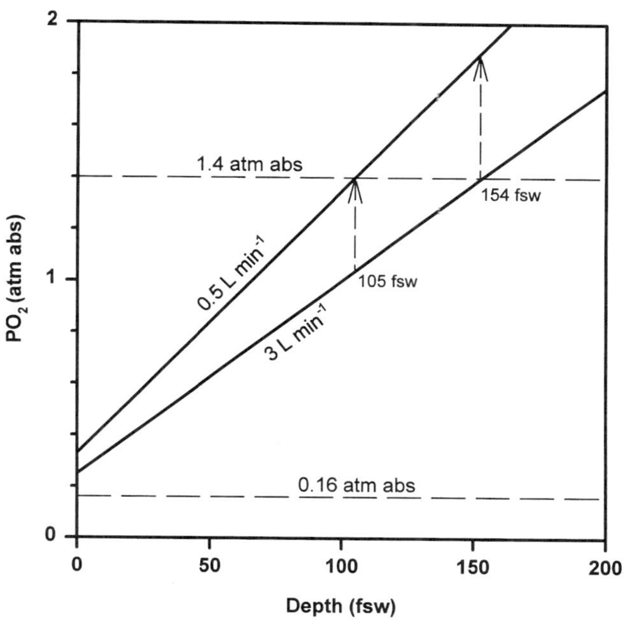

Figure 19 PO_2 versus depth for two $\dot{V}o_2$ values in a semiclosed UBA.

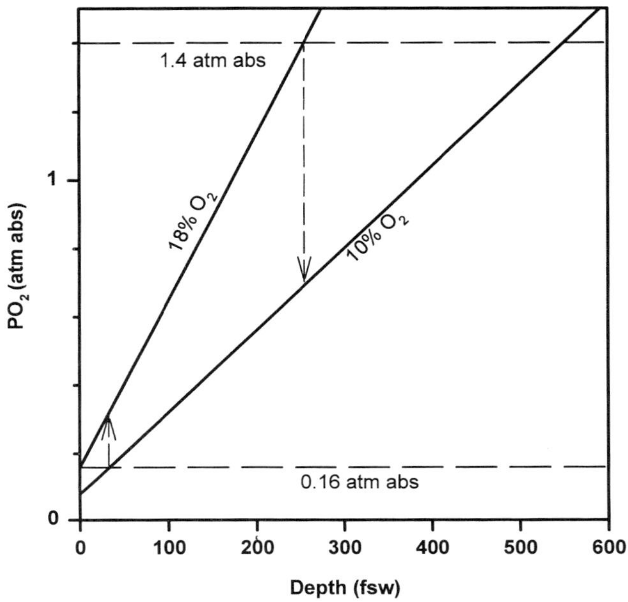

Figure 20 PO_2 versus depth for two gas mixes in a semiclosed UBA.

UBA is adjusted to provide a steady injection rate of 22 L·min^{-1} (STPD) of mixed gas containing 35% O_2. The horizontal dashed lines are high and low PO_2 limits, for this example assumed to be 1.4 and 0.16 atm absolute, respectively. The two diagonal lines represent the inspired P_{O_2} (PI_{O_2}) as a function of depth for two values of $\dot{V}O_2$, 0.5 and 3.0 L·min^{-1}, STPD. At shallow depths, PI_{O_1} is greater than the required minimum of 0.16 atm. As long as $\dot{V}_{O_2}$ remains at 3 L·min^{-1}, that gas mix can be breathed down to 154 fsw without significant risk of O_2 convulsions due to hyperoxia. However, if the diver stopped working on the bottom, reducing $\dot{V}_{O_2}$ to 0.5 L·min^{-1}, then inspired O_2 would rise to almost 2 atm abs. The maximum depth that would allow the diver to safely reduce his $\dot{V}_{O_2}$ to 0.5 L·min^{-1} STPD is 105 fsw. [This result is found by multiplying equilibrium y(t) values by ambient pressure in atm abs to yield P_{O_2}.]

Because of the high PO_2 in the gas mix, gas flow could be reduced to 10 L·min^{-1} STPD, thereby conserving gas, while still enabling wide work ranges down to at least 112 fsw. However, near the surface, if the diver encountered unexpectedly high work rates, he would quickly lapse into unconsciousness unless he raised the gas-mix flow rate to at least 15 L·min^{-1} STPD.

In Fig. 20, the diver is making a deep dive to 550 fsw with two gas mixes available, 10% and 18% O_2. Since this is to be a deep dive, the gas diluent would be helium to avoid incapacitation due to nitrogen narcosis (Chap. 1). To simplify the example, the gas injection rate is maintained at 22 L·min^{-1} STPD, as in the last example. To prevent hypoxia as the dive begins, the diver has to select an 18% O_2 mix. However, as the diver exceeds 200 fsw, that gas mix nears the hyperoxic limit. To continue deeper, the diver must switch to a 10% O_2 mix. Again on ascent, the diver will become hypoxic unless he switches back to the 18% mix before rising above 35 fsw.

A recent trend has been to reduce the weight of the semiclosed UBA by carrying smaller volumes of supply gas at relatively high O_2 fractions. Gas injection rates ($\dot{V}_{inj}$) can therefore be reduced, thus maintaining a reasonable dive duration even with a reduced gas supply. However, there is a major drawback to this strategy. With low injection rates, the P_{O_2} within the UBA becomes very sensitive to changes in the diver's O_2 consumption, as illustrated in Fig. 21. As long as the diver's O_2 requirements are moderate at a given depth, P_{O_2} stabilizes at a safe level. However, if the diver's work rate increases, the UBA's P_{O_2} would plummet within a few minutes to potentially dangerous levels. The diver can add additional gas manually to the breathing loop from the gas supply, but the UBA's oxygen level will not be known with certainty, since semiclosed UBAs are not generally equipped with oxygen sensors. The development of reliable oxygen sensors for use with low-flow, semiclosed UBAs will likely be the next advance in these types of UBAs.

In summary, the primary advantage of semi–closed circuit UBAs over closed-circuit UBAs is their simplicity, which translates into high reliability and relatively low cost. The primary disadvantage is that inspired P_{O_2} varies widely throughout the dive. This variation in O_2 tension not only increases the risk of hypoxia and hyperoxia but is not convenient for use with decompression schedules that use relatively fixed and elevated P_{O_2} to speed decompression.

Available Devices

The U.S. Navy employed the MK 6 and MK 11 semiclosed UBAs to depths of 200 and 650 fsw, respectively (27), through the 1970s and into the 1980s. However, both UBAs have now been largely replaced by UBAs with fully closed circuits. The French developed a MIXGERS semi-closed UBA that has been used to at least 80 msw (28). The Spirotechnique (U.S. Divers) DC-55 has been used successfully by French combat divers since 1955. It differs from most semiclosed UBAs in that fresh gas is injected in proportion to the divers' ventilation instead of being injected at a fixed flow rate. The fresh gas–dosing mechanism consists of an ingenious bellows within a bellows arrangement of the UBA breathing bag.

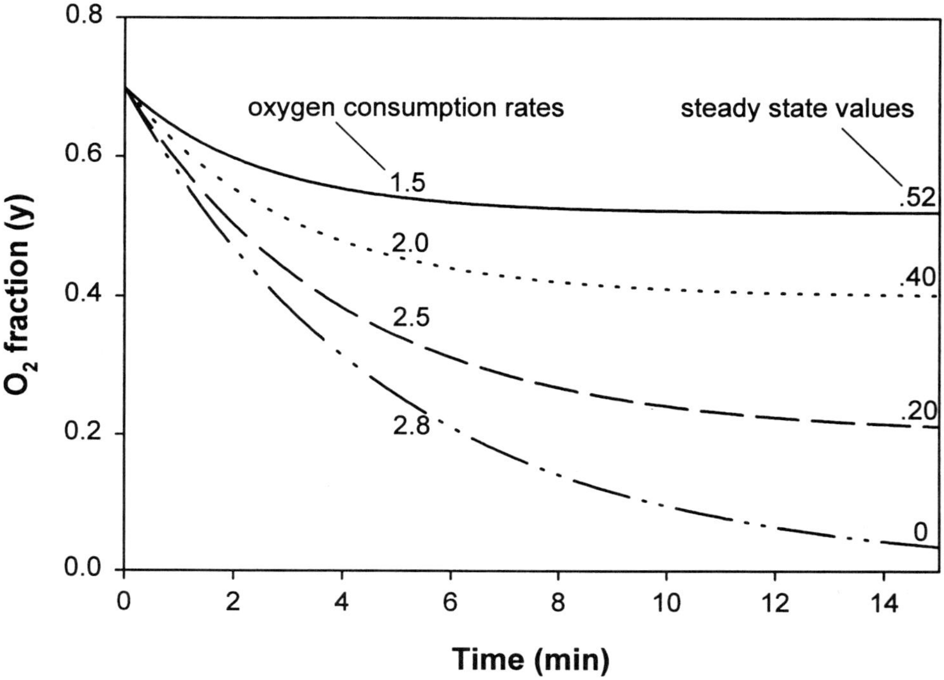

Figure 21 Dynamics of inspired O_2 fraction (y) for various diver oxygen consumptions (in $L \cdot min^{-1}$). The starting fraction is 0.7. Steady state values are those O_2 fractions obtained when the UBA has reached steady state. The time to reach steady state extends off the graph for $\dot{V}O_2$ values of 2.5 and 2.8 $L \cdot min^{-1}$. Dive depth is assumed fixed.

The Japanese recently developed a minimalist semiclosed UBA called the OBA. Since the gas supply lasts only 10 min, and because it contains 80% O_2, dives with this device are required to be both short and shallow, with a maximum depth of 5 m (29,30). Japan also markets the Fieno. United States manufacturers sell the BMR 155 (Biomarine), CCS (Oceanic), and Odyssey (RBC). InterSpiro of Sweden has produced the DCSC UBA (and its predecessor, the ACSC; Sec. IV.C), which, like the DC-55, uses a ventilation-dependent fresh gas–injection method. The DCSC is used by both the Swedish and Danish navies. The Swiss sell the RI 2000, and Canadian companies produce the SCR (BMD Tech) and the SIVA (Fullerton Sherwood). In response to interest from the civilian technical diving community, the German company Draeger is developing a promising unit called the Extreme, which is in many respects an updated but low-flow version of the original FLATUS.

Closed-Circuit UBAs

100% Oxygen UBA

The simplest closed-circuit UBA is an O_2 rebreather, so named because the gas supply contains pure O_2. The simplest of these UBAs have been pendulum rebreathers (Figs. 22 and 23a). Their simplicity amounted to an absence of valves separating inspiratory and expiratory gases (31). The obvious drawback to the pendulum rebreathers was a high dead space. In fact, the advantage of low breathing resistance accruing from the absence of valves is virtually elim-

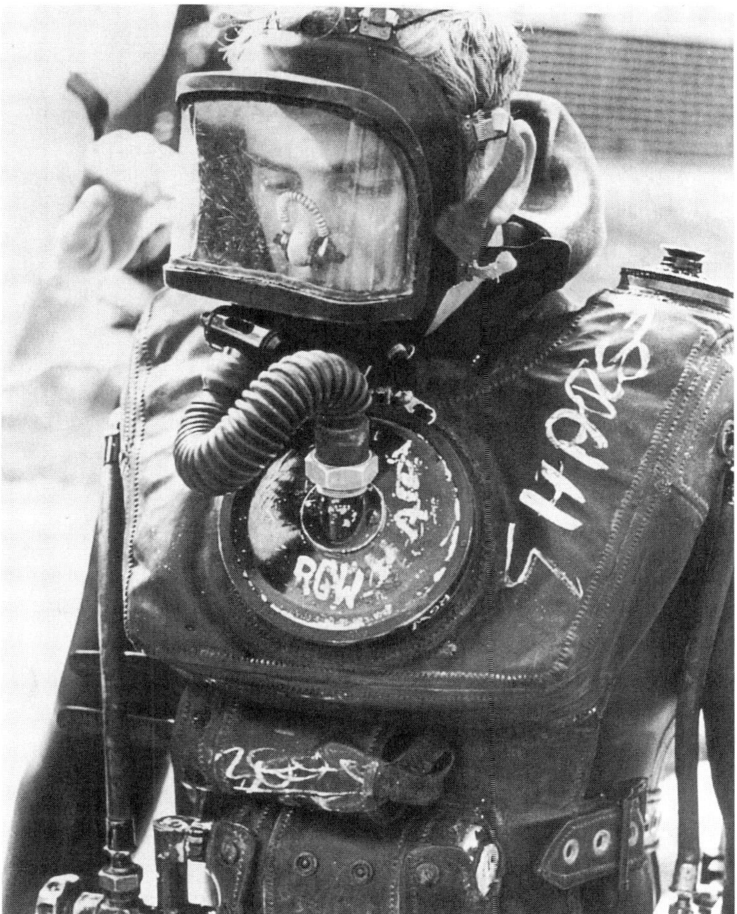

Figure 22 Pendulum breathing 100% O_2 UBA.

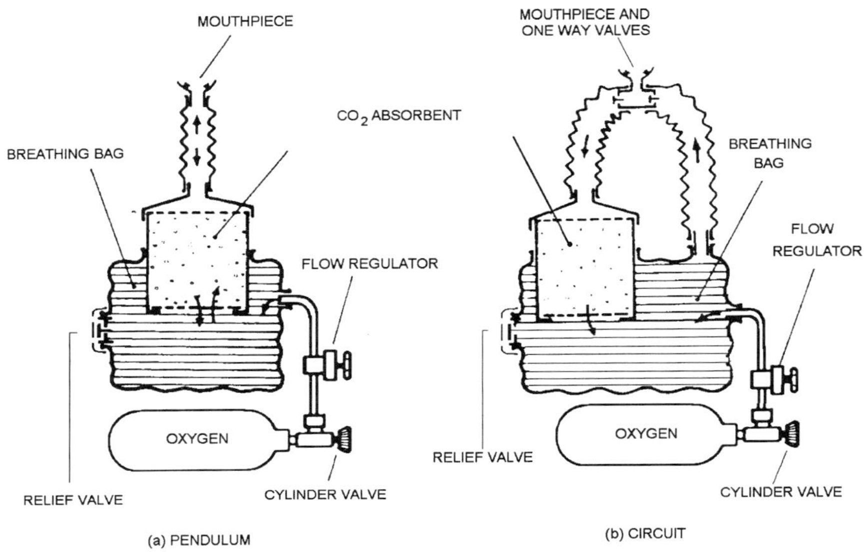

Figure 23 Pendulum and circuit 100% O_2 UBA. (From Ref. 31.)

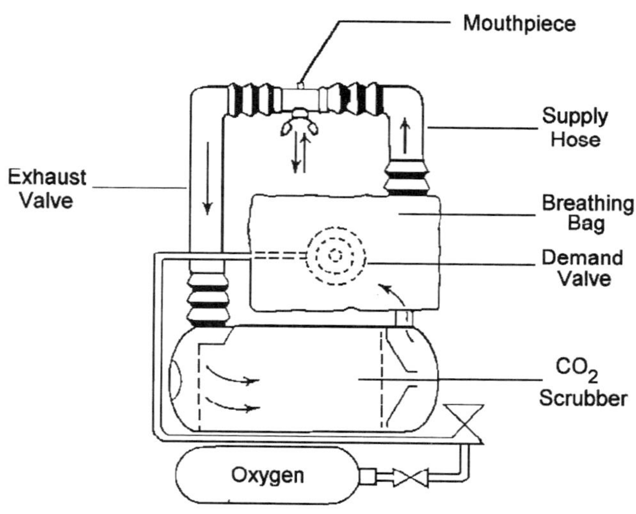

Figure 24 LAR V schematic. A pure oxygen breathing apparatus.

inated by an increase in ventilation in response to CO_2 accumulation in the UBA's dead space.

For that reason, modern 100% O_2 UBAs use a continuous-circuit gas flow path (Fig. 23b). Modern examples of O_2 UBAs are the Draeger LAR V (Figs. 24 and 25), Interspiro's Oxydive, Carleton Technology's COBRA, the Prism (Cochrane Undersea Tech), the Biomarine CCR, and the U.S. Diver's Oxy-NG.

All of the above O_2 UBAs are derived from the Lambertsen Amphibious Respiratory Unit (LARU) (22), named for the already mentioned physician-inventor of the FLATUS. The LARU was used by the U.S. Office of Strategic Services (OSS) during and after World War II.

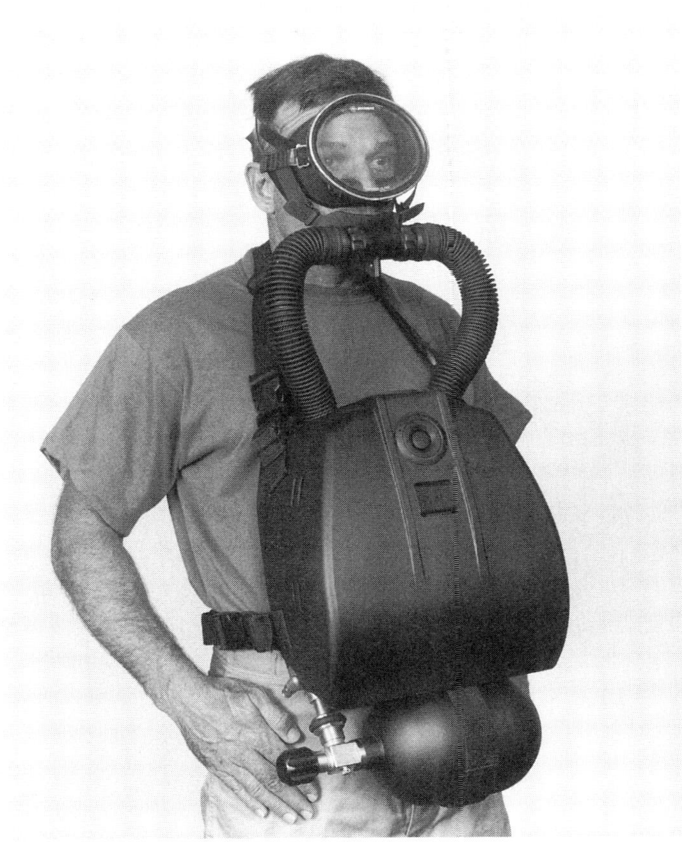

Figure 25 A LAR V UBA.

Just as in the semi–closed circuit UBA, exhaled CO_2 is removed (scrubbed) from the gas loop of an oxygen rebreather by a CO_2-absorbent canister. As a diver consumes O_2 metabolically, a breathing bag containing O_2 decreases in volume. When the bag reaches the point of collapse on inspiration, a demand valve opens, causing oxygen from a high-pressure cylinder and pressure regulator to be dumped into the breathing bag, thereby reinflating the bag. Reinflation also occurs when the breathing bag is collapsed by an increase in ambient pressure as the diver descends in the water column.

An O_2 rebreather is a relatively old idea (32,33); Henry Fleuss developed and successfully tested an O_2 rebreather in 1879. The O_2 rebreather has two primary advantages over other UBAs; it is small in size and mechanically simple. Furthermore, because there is no inert gas to be taken up by the diver's tissues, decompression sickness is extremely unlikely. On the other hand, the useful depth of the UBA is limited because of concerns for central nervous system (CNS) O_2 toxicity (Chap. 5). The risk of convulsions (and resultant drowning) from CNS toxicity can be greatly reduced by following U.S. Navy O_2 exposure limits (5): diving no deeper than 50 fsw and by limiting 50 fsw dives to durations of no more than 10 min.

B. Mixed-Gas UBA

A mixed-gas closed-circuit UBA is similar to semiclosed UBAs in that inert gas (N_2 or He) is used to make up gas volume during descents while keeping P_{O_2} within safe limits (Fig. 26). Both the mixed-gas and the 100% O_2 UBAs differ from semiclosed UBAs in that gas is released from the UBA into the water only during ascent, when gas expansion would otherwise rupture the breathing bags. The main feature distinguishing mixed-gas UBAs from all others is that P_{O_2} is electronically maintained within strict limits. Oxygen concentration in the diver's inspired gas is measured by miniature Clark electrodes. Since an electrode failure could lead to either hypoxia or hyperoxia, sensors are redundant, usually in triplicate. In the case of an electrode failure, electronic logic circuits ignore the faulty reading and maintain control with the remaining electrodes. In principle, inspired P_{O_2} (PI_{O_2}) can be accurately controlled with only one functioning sensor. PI_{O_2} is usually controlled at 0.7 ata, with high and low limits of 0.8 and 0.6 atm, respectively. New UBAs are currently being designed to maintain PI_{O_2} at 1.3 atm abs at depths deeper than 20 fsw to take advantage of reduced decompression times.

Figure 27 is an electrical schematic of the gas-flow circuitry of the MK 16 UBA. Mouthpiece resistance (Rm), canister resistance (Rcan), and inductance (L) are shown. The inhalation and exhalation sides of the breathing loop are described by ''inh'' and ''exh,'' respectively. The breathing bag is a compliant element or capacitance located in the inspiratory portion of the circuit. The diver

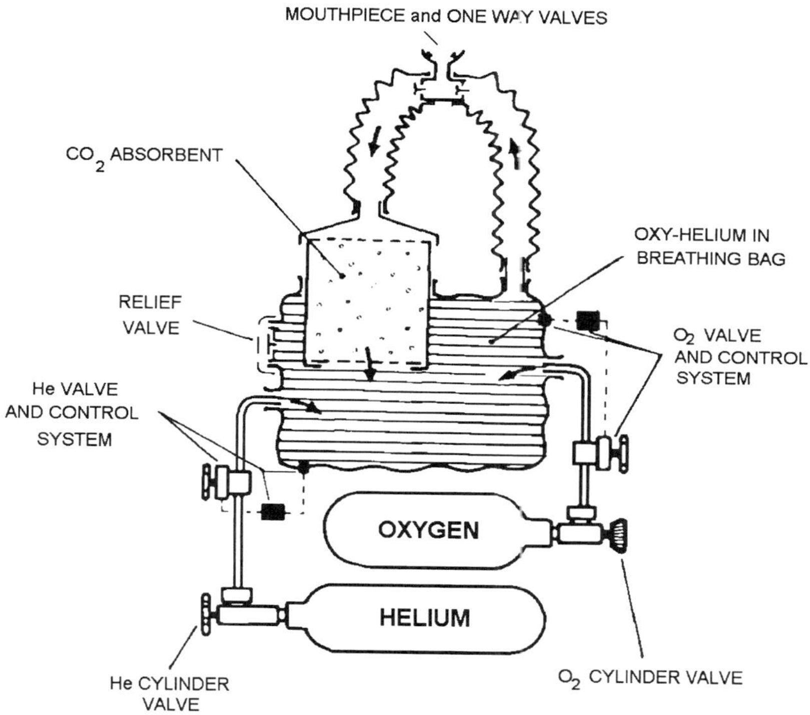

Figure 26 Closed-circuit mixed gas rebreathing UBA. (From Ref. 31.)

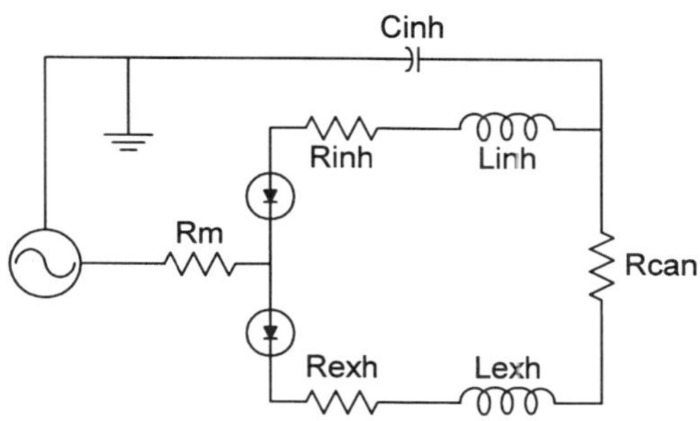

Figure 27 Electrical analog of the breathing loop of a MK 16 closed-circuit UBA.

is once again represented by the sinusoidal current source on the far left center of the figure.

As with the O_2 UBA, gas is added to the breathing circuit during descent when ambient pressure increases enough to collapse the breathing bag. But unlike the O_2 UBA, the added gas contains an inert diluent, either N_2 or He, mixed with O_2. Pure O_2 is added to the circuit only when the O_2 sensors signal a P_{O2} lower than the lower O_2 set point; typically 0.6 atm abs.

In the event of a total electronic failure in an electronically controlled closed-circuit UBA, the diver still has a way to control O_2 tensions while the dive is being aborted. Both O_2 and the breathable diluent gas can be added manually by button-controlled valves on the UBA. The diver can control his PI_{O_2} by monitoring an analog gauge connected to the Clark electrodes. Since the electrodes produce their own current, the gauge readout is independent of the UBA electronics and batteries.

As discussed in section IV.C, semi–closed circuit UBAs can provide dangerously hyperoxic gas mixtures if dived too deeply. However, even so-called fixed P_{O2} closed-circuit UBAs can create seriously high O_2 tensions if dived too rapidly (34). If a UBA is properly controlling P_{O2} at 0.7 atm abs at the surface and a diver then plummets to the bottom, diluent gas will be added to prevent the breathing bag(s) from collapsing. Since the breathable diluent may contain as much as 21% O_2, the O_2 pressure will rise during the descent. The only way that O_2 pressure can be returned to normal is through metabolic consumption. If the dive is deep and rapid enough, then PI_{O_2} can exceed 2 atm abs by the time the diver reaches the bottom. At this partial pressure, an O_2-sensitive individual could experience a convulsion due to CNS O_2 toxicity. Once on the bottom, the O_2 tension should fall fairly rapidly, but it could take as long as 20 min to return to control levels (0.7 ata) (28).

Because of the complexity and expense of fully closed mixed-gas UBAs, few are available commercially. Aside from the Carleton MK 16 used by the U.S. Navy, Cochrane Undersea markets the Prism in a mixed-gas mode and Cis-Lunar offers the MK-5P.

C. Cryogenic Closed-Circuit UBAs

A cryogenic closed-circuit, mixed-gas UBA, the S-1000, was built in the late 1960s by the Sub-Marine Systems Corporation (35). It had a nominal duration of 4 to 6 hr at a depth of 200 msw. Oxygen partial pressures were adjustable between 0.2 and 2.0 atm but contained no electronic controls. An equilibrium between the O_2 liquid and vapor phase was regulated by the rate of boil-off of liquid helium or nitrogen. A CO_2 scrubber was optional, since CO_2 was frozen out of the recirculated gas mixture as it passed the heat exchanger. As much as 0.23 kg of CO_2 could be frozen out of the gas mixture each hour, leaving a recirculating gas mixture with only 25 ppm of CO_2—more than an order of magnitude lower than the desired maximum inspired CO_2 level in closed-circuit UBAs. The rate of CO_2 removal of 0.23 kg $CO_2 \cdot hr^{-1}$ would support a $\dot{V}_{O_2}$ of about 2 $L \cdot min^{-1}$.

Closed/Semiclosed Hybrid

One self-contained closed-circuit UBA design, an alternating closed and semiclosed (ACSC) mixed-gas UBA (36), is a true hybrid that has been in use by the Swedish Navy for the past 20 years. It is also used by the Danish and Finnish navies. Like the FLATUS, it was designed by a physician-inventor; in this case, Claes Lundgren, presently of the University of New York at Buffalo. Instead of constantly injecting a metered amount of fresh gas into the UBA, this device injects fresh gas only when triggered by a certain amount of ventilation—ventilation inferred from the movements of the semirigid breathing bag (Fig. 28). Since there is a qualitatively predictable relationship between a diver's ventilatory requirements and oxygen consumption, the $\dot{V}_E/\dot{V}_{O_2}$ ratio, ventilation can be used to trigger addition of fresh gas when the O_2 in the UBA should, by calculation, require replenishment. As fresh gas is added, an equal portion of stale gas is exhausted. The rest of the time, the circuit is fully closed. Carbon dioxide is constantly absorbed, but fresh gas is not readmitted until signaled by a predetermined amount of ventilation.

Rather than expend fresh gas at a rate adequate for a presumed worst-case work load, as in the semiclosed UBA, the ACSC injects gas only as required by the actual work rate. This device therefore shares the gas-on-demand features of SCUBA without the high gas wastage typical of UBA with a fully open circuit. To emphasize that fact, the UBA has recently been renamed the DCSC, for demand-controlled semiclosed UBA. In effect, it uses the diver's ventilation—and therefore his internal chemoreceptors—to control CO_2 and O_2 without the complex electronic circuitry of UBAs with fully closed circuits.

D. Gas Recovery Systems

For diving at depths of 100 to 450 msw, umbilical-supplied helmet systems are preferred over self-contained mixed-gas UBAs because of their lower breathing resistance and other safety considerations. However, the dumping of helium into the water column during exhalation, as happens with umbilical-supplied open systems, would be prohibitively expensive. For that reason, gas-recovery systems have been developed for deep umbilical-supplied diving. In such systems, exhaled gas is collected in an exhaust umbilical that returns the gas to "topside" for processing—i.e., removal of CO_2 and addition of O_2 before being returned to the diver.

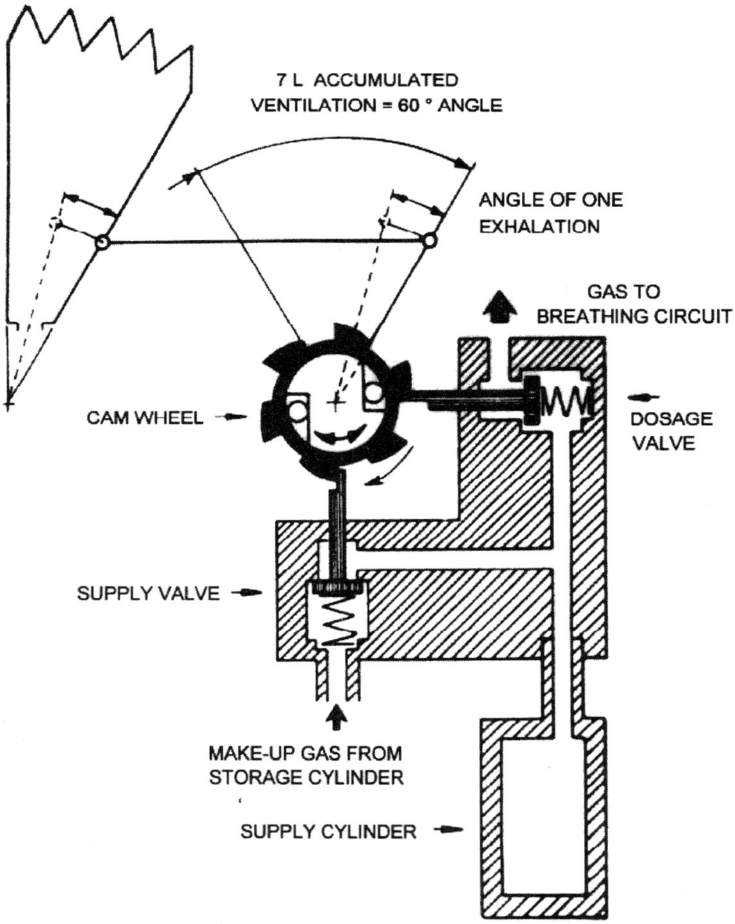

Figure 28 The Swedish ACSC alternating closed/semiclosed UBA. (From Ref. 36.)

Pressure-Gradient Systems

Fortunately, the diver does not have to force exhaled gas through the quarter mile or so of exhaust umbilical. The pressure required to supply gas to a diver at a depth of 300 msw is roughly 3 MPa (444 psi). The pressure gradient from the diver's end of the umbilical to the surface is more than enough to return exhaled gas to the surface. In fact, it is enough to return virtually anything to the surface, such as lungs or intestines. For that reason, the diver must be protected through fail-safe mechanisms such that the pressure inside the diver's helmet never becomes significantly lower than the surrounding water pressure. Likewise, if the gas inflow exceeds the gas withdrawal by an appreciable amount, excessively high pressures will be generated, which could overexpand the diver's lungs or even lift the helmet off a diver's head. The problem of maintaining steady-state gas flow in such a helmet is similar to the physiological challenges experienced by the heart. The heart has a compensatory mechanism described by Starling's law, which ensures that all the blood supplied to the right ventricle is expelled back to the body by the left ventricle, even in the face of widely varying cardiac demands. Even a slight inequality in cardiac input and output could quickly lead to death. A diver with a gas inflow and outflow mismatch in his helmet would similarly be at great risk.

In deep diving, the flow of gas back to the surface typically occurs in two stages (37). The first is to a diving bell (personnel transfer capsule or PTC; Fig. 2) located relatively close to the diver. The second stage of return flow is from the PTC to the surface. As long as the diver is deeper than the PTC, there is a single gradient of pressure driving gas from the diver to the surface. However, should the diver move above the PTC, the diver's regulator would provide gas at a lower pressure than that within the PTC. The diver's expired gas then could not flow down to the PTC without assistance. The Gassaver (Gas Services Offshore Limited) and Comex Gas Reclaim Systems (Comex Industries) are examples of closed-circuit recovery systems without upward excursion capability in closed-circuit mode. Such systems can tolerate upward excursions above the PTC only by having the diver go on open-circuit and dumping exhaled gas into the water column.

Some pressure-gradient gas recovery systems provide exhalation assistance and thus allow excursions above the PTC. Those systems use a so-called back-pressure regulator (BPR) within the PTC to maintain exhaust umbilical pressure at the PTC more negative than the ambient pressure at the diver. Therefore, the diver's exhaled gas follows a continuous pressure gradient down to the PTC and then up to the surface. The Gas Services Gasmizer is a BPR-controlled pressure-gradient system with upward excursion capability.

Push-Pull Systems

A so-called push-pull gas-recovery system pumps fresh gas to the diver and pulls exhaled gas away. The pumps may be mounted either on the PTC or topside on the dive support vessel. Back-pressure regulators for push-pull systems are often located directly on the diver or his helmet. Depending on the manufacturer, helmets may be free-flow only or either demand or free-flow. Push-pull systems have been built by Divex (Arawak), Normalair-Garrett, and Submarine Products Limited.

E. Carbon Dioxide Absorbents

Carbon dioxide is removed from a closed or semiclosed breathing system or apparatus by chemical absorption. The first recorded CO_2 absorbent canister or ''scrubber'' was used by Henry Fleuss in 1879 to absorb CO_2 in his O_2 rebreather (38). The scrubbing material consisted of rope yarn soaked in a solution of caustic potash (KOH).

Superoxides

Potassium superoxide, KO_2, formed by the spontaneous oxidation of potassium, would at first glance seem to be an ideal CO_2 absorbent; it reacts with CO_2 and water to yield bicarbonate and oxygen, as follows (38):

$$4\ KO_2 + 4\ CO_2 + 2\ H_2O \rightarrow 4\ KHCO_3 + 3\ O_2$$

or

$$4\ KO_2 + 2\ CO_2 \rightarrow 2\ K_2CO_3 + 3\ O_2$$

Another alkaline metal superoxide (39) reacts thus:

$$4\ NaO_2 + 2\ CO_2 + 2\ H_2O \rightarrow 4NaHCO_3 + O_2$$

or

$$4\ NaO_2 + 2\ CO_2 \rightarrow 2\ Na_2CO_3 + 3\ O_2$$

In the process of absorbing CO_2 and moisture, both superoxides release O_2. On a molar basis, however, sodium superoxide is not as efficient at removing CO_2 and producing O_2 as the potassium superoxide. Unfortunately, the amount of O_2 released depends on the extent to which water participates in the reaction. The anhydrous reactions tend to produce a surplus of O_2 relative to the CO_2 absorbed, whereas the hydration reactions do not.

The major drawback to both of these reactions is that they are very exothermic, capable of producing dangerously high inspired gas temperatures. An excess of water can yield a violent reaction, releasing noxious fumes. For that reason, the superoxides are typically used only in dry-land applications; for example, in mine safety equipment or some firefighters' breathing apparatus.

Sodium Hydroxide

The first widely used CO_2 absorbents for commercial and military diving consisted of pellets of sodium hydroxide (NaOH), commercially termed *Shell Natron*. Carbon dioxide is taken up by NaOH with the release of water and heat. Unfortunately, under certain unusual circumstances, the caustic mixture of NaOH and water can be accidently aspirated, with catastrophic consequences.

For that reason, modern absorbents for diving applications use various less caustic hydroxide mixtures to improve safety.

Sodalimes

One of the first such mixtures was *Baralyme*, which eliminated NaOH altogether. Baralyme consists primarily of hydrated lime (calcium hydroxide), with potassium hydroxide (KOH) added as a chemical activator. Baralyme contains 74% $Ca(OH)_2$, 11% $Ba(OH)_2 \cdot 8H_2O$, 5% KOH, and 10% H_2O. More recently, its absorbent efficiency was improved (40) by replacing $Ba(OH)_2$ with a small amount of NaOH in sodalimes such as *Sodasorb* and *Sofnolime*. These sodalimes typically contain 80% $Ca(OH)_2$, about 5% NaOH, and 1% KOH. The product typically contains 14 to 19% of water before use.

Several steps are involved in the chemical reaction of CO_2 with sodalime (41). Below is the net result:

$$CO_2 + Ca(OH)_2 \rightarrow CaCO_3 + H_2O$$

One mole of $Ca(OH)_2$ ideally reacts with one mole of CO_2 to form calcium carbonate, water, and heat. Figures 29a to c are scanning electron micrographs showing the tortuous surface of a sodalime granule. The rough surface features increase the gas-exchanging surface area far beyond what it would be if the granule's surface were smooth.

Anhydrous lithium hydroxide (LiOH) is a very effective CO_2 absorbent used in submarine and space applications. However, because of its high toxicity, it has been used only in experimental diving applications where gas-permeable but water-repellent cloth (Versapel) can keep the absorbent dry. Unlike sodalime, LiOH maintains absorption efficiency at temperatures near 0°C. For additional information, see Nuckols et al. (25), chap. 5.

Usage

Carbon dioxide absorbent is packed into canisters placed in line with a diver's exhaled gas flow circuit (Figs. 23 to 26). On exhalation, a diver must generate a respiratory pressure sufficient to force the expired breath through the absorbent canister. The flow resistance of the canister depends on the length of the flow path through the canister and the porosity of the granule bed (41,42).

Canister efficiency is affected by the size of the absorbent granules. Small granules expose a greater surface area per volume to the exhaled CO_2 molecules than do large granules and therefore extract a greater amount of CO_2 for a given path length. Furthermore, reaction products, especially water, build up within the outermost layer of each granule, creating a diffusion barrier that prevents CO_2 from penetrating more than 1 mm or so into each granule. If a granule is only 2 mm in diameter, essentially the entire granule is available for reaction.

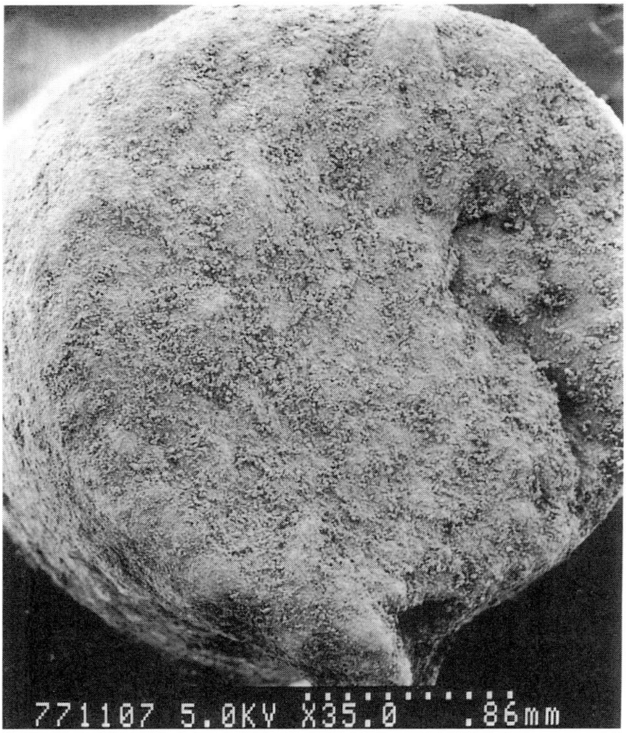

A

Figure 29 Scanning electron micrographs of Sofnolime CO_2 absorbent granules. Magnification is (A) 35x, (B) 200x, and (C) 1000x. (*Courtesy of Molecular Products Ltd., Thaxted, England.*)

With a granule 5 mm in diameter, on the other hand, most of the granule will remain unreacted.

For the above reasons, small absorbent granules would appear preferable to larger granules, However, small granules pack more tightly than larger granules, thereby decreasing void volume and canister porosity (39). As a result, the flow resistance of the canister increases appreciably, increasing the diver's work of breathing. Typically, granules in the size range of 2.4 to 4.8 mm result in a compromise between canister efficiency and resistance. They are therefore used for the majority of diving applications, at least in the United States. Where greater canister endurance is required for long diving missions and the attendant

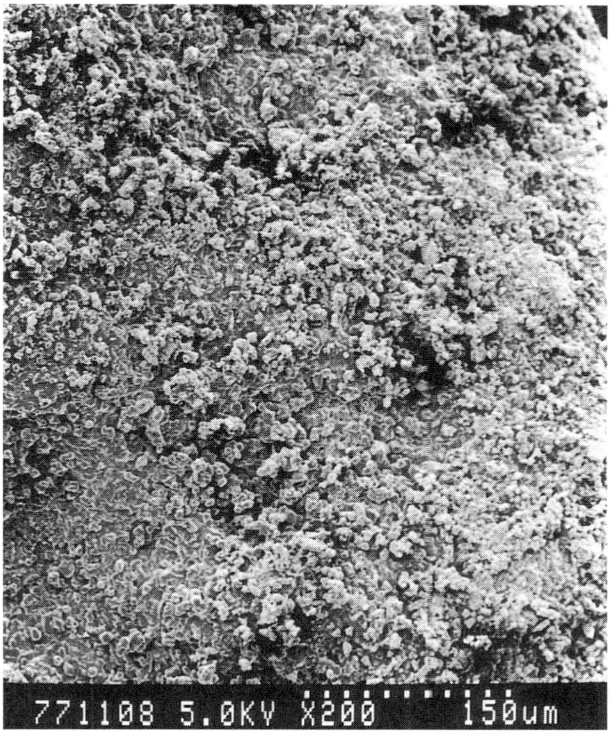

B

Figure 29 Continued

higher breathing resistance can be tolerated, granules in the diameter range of 1.4 to 2.0 mm are used.

Lung and Scrubber Similarities

As far as CO_2 concentrations are concerned, a UBA's CO_2 scrubber serves functionally the same purpose as the lungs. A fluid enters fouled with CO_2, and leaves cleansed.

Venous blood (CO_2 high) → lung → arterial blood (CO_2 low)
Exhaled gas (CO_2 high) → scrubber → inspired gas (CO_2 low)

Interestingly, the similarities between lungs and scrubbers extend beyond the obvious. The effectiveness of gas exchange across the walls of pulmonary al-

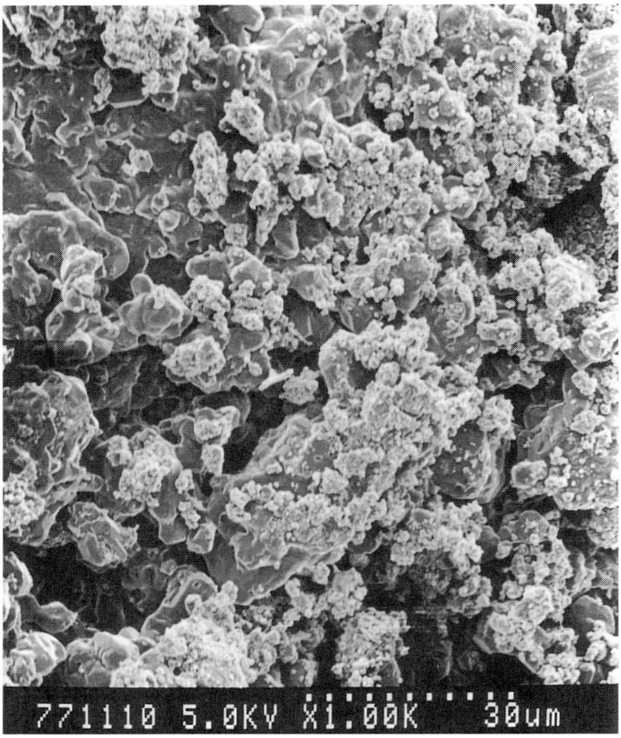

C

Figure 29 Continued

veoli is often measured by diffusing capacity. Anything that impairs diffusion, like a pathological thickening of the alveolar wall, will impair the transport of gas. A loss of alveolar surface area, as from emphysema, can also hinder gas exchange, as can a marked decrease in residence time for red blood cells in the pulmonary capillaries (43–45).

Analogous events hinder CO_2 clearance by a UBA scrubber canister. The diffusion rate of CO_2 through a dense gas can impair scrubber effectiveness (46–48), and a layer of water surrounding absorbent granules can eventually become an overwhelming diffusion barrier. Large absorbent granules have a smaller surface area per volume than smaller granules and thus are capable of absorbing less CO_2 than absorbents of smaller grain size. A large granule is therefore analogous to the large alveoli resulting from destruction of alveolar septa in emphysema. To complete the analogy, the ''contact time'' of the CO_2-rich gas stream has a significant influence on scrubber CO_2 clearance.

Residence time is affected by UBA design. Figure 30 compares the gas flow rates over time through two modeled closed-circuit UBAs (Sec. VII.B), one with two small breathing bags and one with one large bag. Gas flows through the scrubber of the one-bag UBA only during exhalation, and then at a high rate, reducing CO_2 residence time within the scrubber. The modeled two-bag UBA maintains a more even flow, with lower average flow rates and therefore longer residence times. The increased residence times associated with a two-bag UBA can be especially important to scrubber efficiency as diffusion barriers increase in dense gas environments (48) or with increases in absorbent water content.

The main difference between a CO_2 scrubber and a lung is that CO_2 leaving the venous blood via the lungs enters a virtually infinite sink—the atmosphere. On the other hand, use of a UBA scrubber is similar to pouring garbage into a trash receptacle. At some point the receptacle will overflow. When this happens to a CO_2 scrubber, the diver experiences a potentially cataclysmic rise in inspired CO_2.

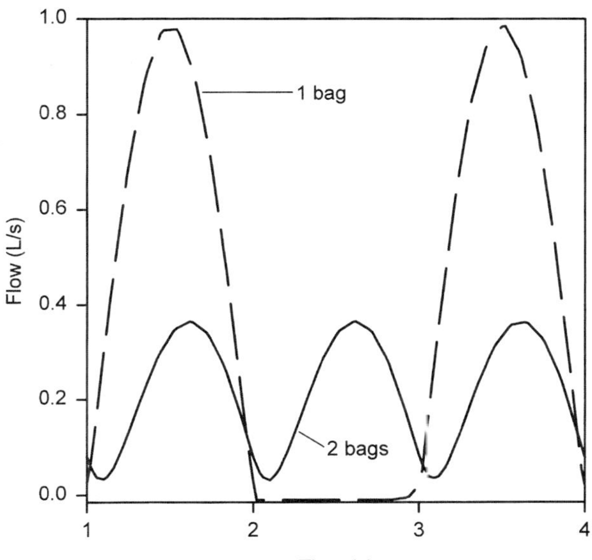

Figure 30 Computed gas flows through a CO_2 absorbent canister in a single breathing bag (dashed line) and dual breathing bag (solid line) closed-circuit UBA model.

V. The Problems with Solutions

Each solution to the primary requirements for work under water is attended by its own peculiar difficulty. To reiterate, those requirements are the efficient removal of metabolically produced CO_2, a constant supply of O_2 adequate to meet metabolic requirements, and equalization of pressure across the thoracic boundary. Some elements of these requirements that have not already been discussed are described below.

A. Cold-Water Freeze-ups

A diver venturing beneath Arctic or Antarctic ice (Fig. 31) has to be concerned with the effects of very low water temperature (about $-2°C$) on both the body and the diving equipment. By insulating the body (Chap. 6), a diver can tolerate relatively prolonged exposures to frigid water. However, the breathing equipment is not insulated and can quickly freeze both externally and internally.

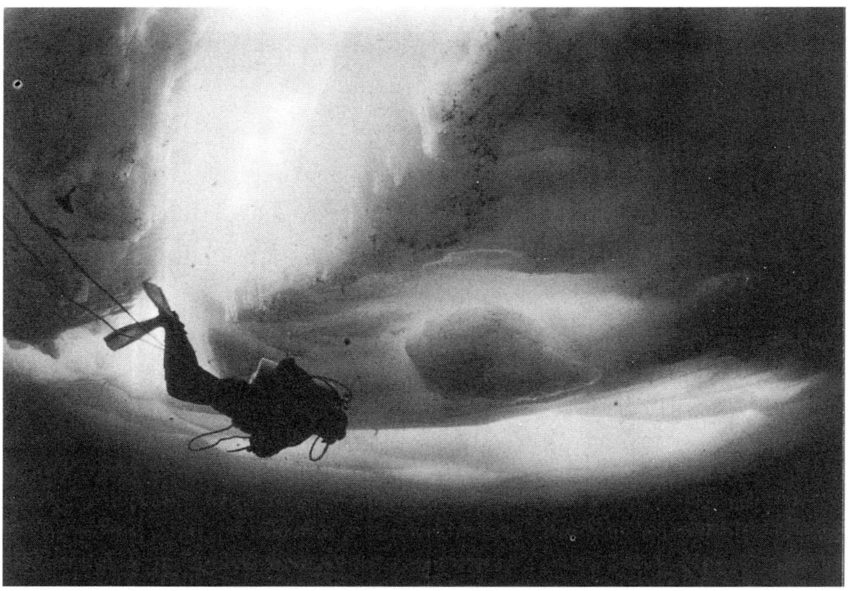

Figure 31 A SCUBA diver underneath the Arctic ice. (*Courtesy of A. Kirkbride.*)

Breathing gas experiences a large pressure drop across first and second stage SCUBA regulators. The pressure drop across the first-stage regulator may be almost 200 bar (20 MPa, 2900 psi). The resulting rapid and therefore adiabatic gas expansion causes a correspondingly large drop in temperature within the regulators. If the water surrounding the regulator is within a few degrees of freezing, the adiabatic cooling of the regulator body will cause the water to freeze. In turn, this freezing can interfere with the action of the first-stage diaphragm spring (Fig. 15). The result can be either a complete blockage of gas flow or an unrestrained free flow. For that reason, divers are advised to protect their first stages from freezing in cold water by applying an oil, grease, or dry air-filled cap, thus isolating sensitive mechanisms from the water. In spite of the use of so-called cold-water kits, if water vapor is present within the regulator, ice can form inside the regulator, disrupting gas flow and leading to a potentially catastrophic freeze-up event.

Freeze-up of SCUBA cylinder regulators is governed by the rules of probability. It is dependent upon the probability of water gaining entry to the inside of a regulator's second stage (P_{we}), and the probability of low temperatures in the second stage (P_{1T}). P_{1T} is, in turn, governed by a balance between adiabatic processes producing regions of low temperature and heat flux toward those cold regions. In general mathematical terms:

$$P_f = P_{we} \cdot P_{1T}$$

where P_f is the probability of regulator failure due to freezing. The probability of water entry into the second stage (P_{we}) is a function of exhaust-valve design (controlling the ease of exhaust-valve leakage) and the magnitude of respiratory pressures. High respiratory pressures are, in turn, generated by high ventilatory rates and high gas densities related to depth when a diver works against inspiratory resistance (another feature of regulator design). Therefore, $P_{we}=f(\dot{V}_E, D,$ and $M_{1...n})$ where $\dot{V}_E$ is expired ventilation, D is depth, and M is a number of manufacturer-determined parameters (e.g., M_1 = exhaust-valve leakage pressure, M_2 = inhalation resistance, etc.).

The temperature (T_f) of gas expanding adiabatically across orifices and valves is given by

$$T_f = T_i \cdot \left(\frac{V_i}{V_f}\right)^{\gamma - 1}$$

where T_i is the preexpansion temperature in Kelvin. V_i and V_f are the respective gas volumes, and γ is the ratio of specific heats for constant pressure and constant volume (γ = 1.4 for air). However, the balance between adiabatic cooling and the countering heat flow is controlled by $\dot{V}_E$ and also by certain design features.

Based on the foregoing, we can hypothesize an instantaneous risk or hazard function for any particular regulator model:

$$r\ (t) = (a \cdot D) \cdot (b \cdot \dot{V}\text{E}) \cdot \left(\prod_{i=1}^{N} c_i \cdot M_i \right)$$

where a, b, and c are various proportionality constants.

The influence of depth and $\dot{V}$E can be combined into an expression of mass flow. Mass flow is defined as:

$$\dot{M} = \rho \cdot \dot{V}\text{E} \cdot \frac{P_{amb}}{P_0}$$

where ρ is gas density at 1 atm abs and 0°C, $\dot{V}$E is expired ventilation in $L{\cdot}min^{-1}$, and P_{amb} is ambient pressure in absolute units. P_0 is the absolute pressure at 1 atm. Mass flow rate reflects the mass of gas flowing through the regulator each minute, with units of $g{\cdot}min^{-1}$.

The total probability of cold induced failure is based on the survivor function (49):

$$P_f = 1 - e^{-\int_0^T r(t)dt}$$

The use of survival functions in defining other diving-related probabilistic events has been described by Weathersby et al. (50) and Harabin et al. (51).

Figure 32 shows experimentally determined incidences of cold-induced high respiratory pressures in one model of SCUBA regulator (52). The probability of encountering high respiratory pressures increased monotonically with mass flow and time of exposure to cold water. (A mass flow of about 400 g/min is obtained with an expired ventilation of 75 $L{\cdot}min^{-1}$ of air at a depth of 99 fsw, or 62.5 $L{\cdot}min^{-1}$ at a depth of 132 fsw.) The least risky dives are those occurring for short periods of time, at shallow depths, and with low respiratory flow rates.

B. Ventilatory Loading—General Concepts

The use of any lung, be it anatomical or engineered, requires the user to overcome respiratory impedance—i.e., respiratory resistance, elastance, and inertance. In certain pulmonary diseases, airway resistance and tissue elastance can be elevated enough to impair breathing. External respiratory apparatus, especially underwater breathing apparatus, can likewise hamper breathing through the action of analogous impedances.

A UBA represents a complex impedance (Z) that opposes flow, changes in volume, and acceleration. Figure 33 shows a diver using a closed-circuit UBA with breathing bags. The diver is exposed to flow resistance, breathing-bag elas-

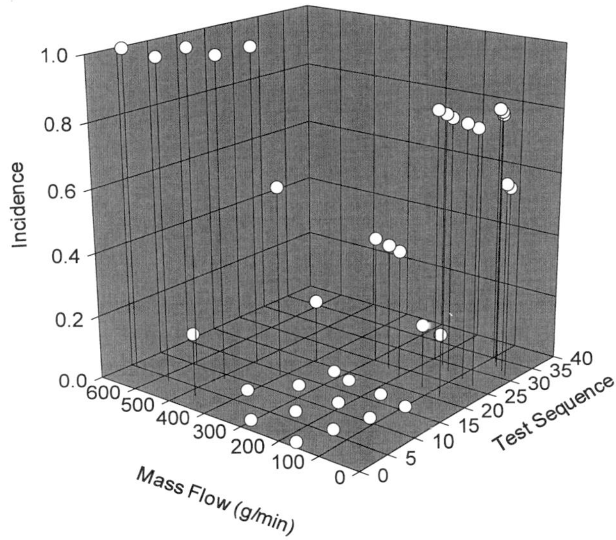

Figure 32 Incidence of high respiratory pressures in a SCUBA regulator designed for use in cold water. (From Ref. 52.)

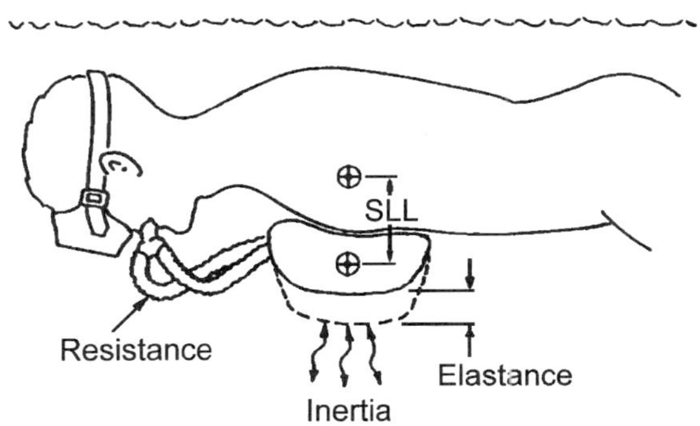

Figure 33 The mechanical respiratory loads encountered by a diver using a UBA with breathing bags. SLL is static lung loading. (From Ref. 53.)

tance (due to the change of gas volumes in a water environment), static lung loading (SLL), and inertial loads (53).

A simple electrical analog for a so-called lumped-parameter description of the above UBA is found in Fig. 34. With impedance elements arranged in series, Z is defined as:

$$Z = \sqrt{R^2 + \left(\frac{E}{\omega} - I\omega\right)^2}$$

where R is resistance, E is elastance, I is inertance (also termed L for inductance in electrical schematics), and ω is the breathing frequency in radians per second.

In the following sections, we discuss separately the components of impedance, R, E, and I and discuss their relevance to UBAs. The influence of all three types of impedance on a diver's ventilation has been examined from a theoretical standpoint by Clarke et al. (54) as well as Van Liew (55,56). (In electrical analogies such as those of Figs. 6, 13, 16, and 27, inertance is usually indicated by L in place of I so as to avoid confusion with the electrical symbol for current.)

Resistive Impedance

Flow resistance is the predominant impedance found in all UBAs except constant-flow diving helmets (Sec. IV.A). The majority of the procedures for characterizing the respiratory impact of breathing devices are based upon measures in one form or another of resistive impedance (57). Gas flow resistance (*R*) in humans occurs primarily from the friction of gas moving through respiratory airways. The characteristics of this flow through the internal respiratory system are described in detail by Pedley, Schroter, and Sudlow in Vol. 3 of this series (58) and Chap. 1 of this volume. Clarke et al. (59) described the elevated respiratory resistance of divers at pressures up to 46 atm abs and suggested that

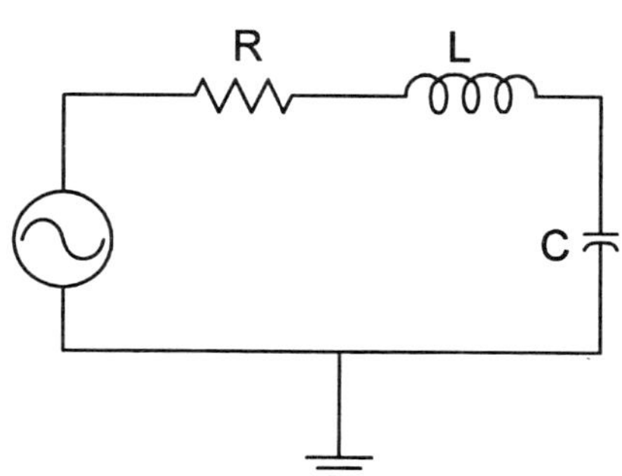

Figure 34 Series equivalent circuit for a closed-circuit UBA.

small differences in airway resistance at the surface could lead to substantial differences at great depth.

Pedley et al. (58) proposed an equation [Eq. (35), page 248 of their reference] relating pressure drop in an airway to geometry, gas flow rate, and gas density. To emphasize changes in viscous resistance (ΔR) as a function of airway geometry, their equation can be rearranged to yield:

$$\Delta R = \Delta K \cdot (\mu\rho\dot{V})^{1/2}$$

where K is a geometrical factor; for example, the reciprocal of airway or hose diameter, volumetric flow rate is $\dot{V}$, and ρ is gas density. This equation describes, at least qualitatively, how changes in airway geometry can affect flow resistance in high-density environments (59).

Flow resistance is also contributed by the airways within the UBA; notably hoses, orifices, valves, and CO_2-absorbent canisters. As noted above for internal resistance (59), small differences in UBA resistance may result in large differences at depth—a trend noticeable in tests of different makes of SCUBA regulators (60). Darcy's formula for static pressure losses in pipes (found in any text on fluids engineering) can be arranged to yield a result qualitatively similar to that predicted from the above equation.

From a UBA designer's perspective, the above paragraphs teach us that a reduction in UBA resistance at the surface should yield increased benefits for the diver at depth. Recognition of the importance of resistance reduction has led to the design of new low-resistance mouthpieces for closed-circuit UBAs (61) and even to valveless breathing circuits for use in deep diving (62).

Elastic Impedance

Elastance (E) is a measure of the pressure-volume characteristics of an enclosed system. It is the reciprocal of compliance, with units of pressure divided by volume (e.g., $kPa \cdot L^{-1}$). When a diver breathes against an elastic load he must elevate respiratory pressures, contributing to discomfort (63), fatigue (64), and even unconsciousness (65).

As in the case of resistance, sources of elastance may be internal or external to the diver. Internally, it exists in the form of lung and chest wall elasticity (66,67). Externally, it is in diving helmets with neck dams, wet suits, and buoyancy compensators (68) as well as in the hoses, CO_2 canisters, and breathing bags of UBAs (69).

Inertial Impedance

Inertial impedance, or inertance, is that property of a system which resists acceleration of masses within the system. It is related linguistically and mechanistically to inertia and shares a kinship with other impedances in that it is the proportionality between one component of pressure and a derivative of displacement. For example, elastic pressure (P_E) is the component of the total pressure at any given moment attributable to system elastance. Therefore, in linear systems $P_E = E \cdot V$, where V is UBA volume. Likewise, resistive pressure (P_R) equals $R \cdot \dot{V}$, and inertial pressure (P_I) equals $I \cdot \ddot{V}$.

The inertance (I) of a fluid in a cylindrical tube such as the trachea or a UBA breathing hose is defined as:

$$I = \frac{m}{A^2}$$

where m is the mass of the fluid in motion, and A is the cross-sectional area of the tube (70). An alternative expression is:

$$I = \frac{\rho \cdot L}{A}$$

where ρ is gas density and L is the length of the tube. The masses that have to be accelerated by a diver are inspired gas, the chest wall, moving UBA components such as breathing bags, and the water displaced by moving equipment parts.

Both gas and tissue components of respiratory inertance in nonimmersed, normal individuals are negligibly small at 1 atm abs (10,71). In morbidly obese individuals, however, chest wall inertance may be more than double the normal value (72,73).

In diving, since the mass of inhaled gas is related to gas density, which increases with depth, a deep dive with a dense gas will involve more inertance than a shallow, low-density dive—a fact confirmed by a number of authors (10,74). A reasonable approximation for respiratory inertance in humans at 1 atm (55) is 0.01 $cmH_2O \cdot L \cdot sec^{-2}$. However, at depths of 46 atm (1500 fsw) or more, inertance can theoretically rise as high as 0.1 to 0.2 $cmH_2O \cdot L \cdot sec^{-2}$ due to elevations of gas density.

Such inertances may indeed have some impact upon a diver. High inertance within pulmonary airways can in theory influence the distribution of ventilation within a diver's lungs (75). Even a diver's choice of respiratory waveform (76) may be influenced by high inertance within the UBA.

Unlike resistance and elastance, inertance is not always bad. One benefit of high inertance is that it can partly offset the elastic impedance associated with wet suits or UBA breathing bags, thereby reducing the total effective flow impedance. That effect is described by the impedance equation for a series arrangement of R, I, and E elements (Sec. V.B) where $I\omega$ is subtracted from E/ω. That equation also shows that inertial impedance is most significant at higher respiratory frequencies, while elastic impedance predominates at low frequencies. At the resonant frequency of the system, the two reactive impedances cancel, leaving only resistive impedance (77) (Fig. 35). The remaining pure resistance is the minimum impedance that can be presented to the diver. It is conceptually possible to build a UBA that maintains resonance (78,79) at the diver's respiratory frequency, thereby minimizing UBA impedance (Sec. VIII.F).

Mixed Impedance

Resistive and elastic impedances are equally detrimental to a diver's ventilatory effort (80–82). For that reason, design goals for UBAs limit resistance and elastance when applied separately (Secs. VI.B and D). When both loads exist simultaneously, it makes sense to reduce the design tolerance on each to keep the total input impedance of the UBA at a comfortable level.

Hydrostatic Loading

During immersion, a pressure gradient is applied to the chest wall due to the depth-dependent variation of hydrostatic pressure in a column of water (Fig. 36). Gas in a diver's lungs, on the other hand, is at a pressure determined by

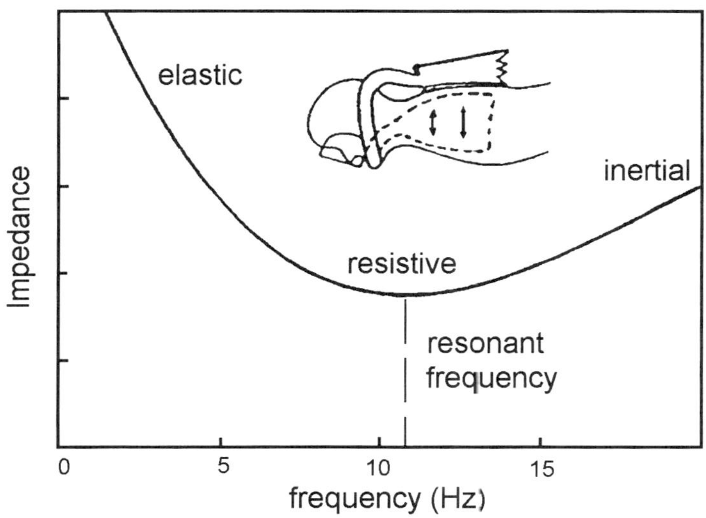

Figure 35 A typical impedance magnitude spectrum of the idealized circuit in Fig. 34. Elastic impedance predominates below the resonant frequency; inertial impedance predominates above.

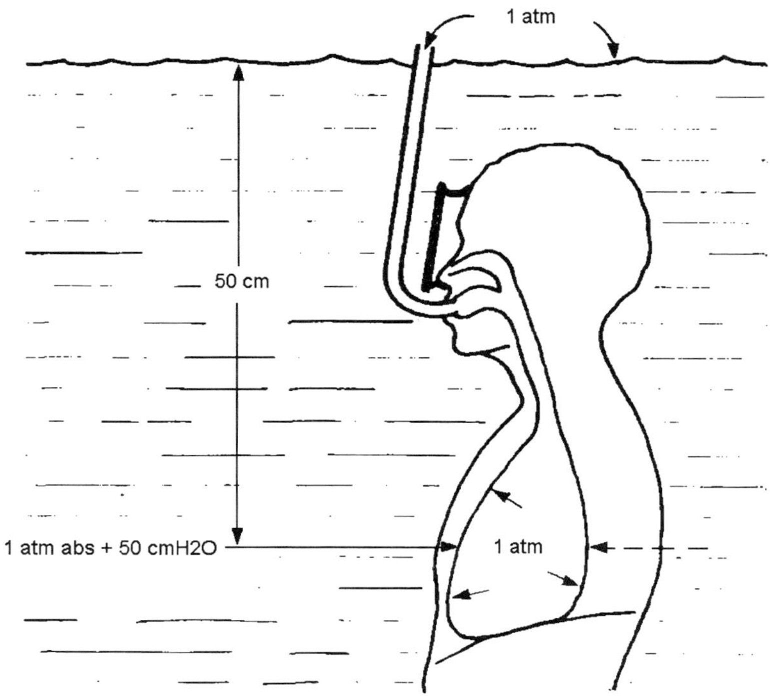

Figure 36 Pressure gradients across a submerged chest during use of a snorkel. (From Ref. 31.)

the breathing apparatus and may not match the mean pressure external to the chest wall. Under certain conditions, the resulting pressure imbalance, referred to as *hydrostatic loading*, can lead to diver discomfort or impair ventilatory ability. This topic is discussed further in Sec. VI.E.

VI. Minimizing Problems—UBA Design Standards

Measurements of the physiological response of divers to respiratory loads have led to the establishment of various UBA design standards (60,83–89), which have historically addressed (1) peak pressures, a reflection of the overall respiratory impedance; (2) flow resistance; and (3) a variation on the work of breathing.

A. Pressure Limits

According to Bradley et al. (90), up to 1970 the criteria used by the U.S. Navy Experimental Diving Unit for determining the acceptability of breathing resistance in SCUBA was based upon the observations of Lanphier (91): ''At moderate work rates, the average diver is reasonably comfortable for considerable periods if the inspiratory and expiratory pressures do not exceed 10–15 cmH_2O at peak flow. Subjects usually report definite discomfort when the pressures rise above 20 cmH_2O.'' That statement is probably the basis for the original military specification for SCUBA regulators, which allowed as much as 20 cmH_2O inspiratory and expiratory pressure at a depth of 200 ft (92).

This pressure limit gained further credence when Bentley et al. (87) determined the effect of inspiratory resistance on 158 mine rescue workers at 1 atm abs. In their subjects, respiratory comfort correlated inversely with peak mouth pressures. Bentley et al. suggested that during unmanned tests of respiratory protective equipment, the inspiratory pressure drop should not exceed 20 cmH_2O.

B. Resistance Limits

Fifty years ago, Silverman (84) specified that breathing apparatus used at high ventilatory rates should have an inspiratory resistance no greater than 4.5 $cmH_2O \cdot L^{-1} \cdot sec$ (0.44 $kPa \cdot L^{-1} \cdot sec$) and an expiratory resistance no higher than 2.9 $cmH_2O \cdot L^{-1} \cdot sec$ at a flow rate of 1.42 $L \cdot sec^{-1}$. (Most UBA resistances are that inspiratory resistance is, in general, nonlinear with flow, therefore the flow rate at which the resistance was measured must be stated.) Cain and Otis (93) drew similar conclusions from their related work. Both laboratories demonstrated that inspiratory resistance is, in general, better tolerated than expiratory resistance. However, experienced divers improve their tolerance to respiratory loading over that of naive subjects by altering their breathing pattern to counteract the asymmetrical resistances (inspiratory>expiratory) commonly encountered in diving (94).

Addressing breathing resistance at increased ambient pressures, Mead (85) stated that total breathing resistance, internal plus external (intrathoracic and UBA), should be no greater than 12 $cmH_2O \cdot L^{-1} \cdot sec$ (1.18 $kPa \cdot L^{-1} \cdot sec$). He suggested that during air breathing, internal resistance alone would reach this value at 70.8 msw (231 fsw). Silverman later observed that subjects tolerated higher resistances during moderate work rates than during heavy work (95). Therefore, both Silverman and Mead noted that increases in internal resistance due to increased flow rate or high gas density lead to reductions in tolerated external resistance. The implications of these observations are addressed in Sec. VI.C.

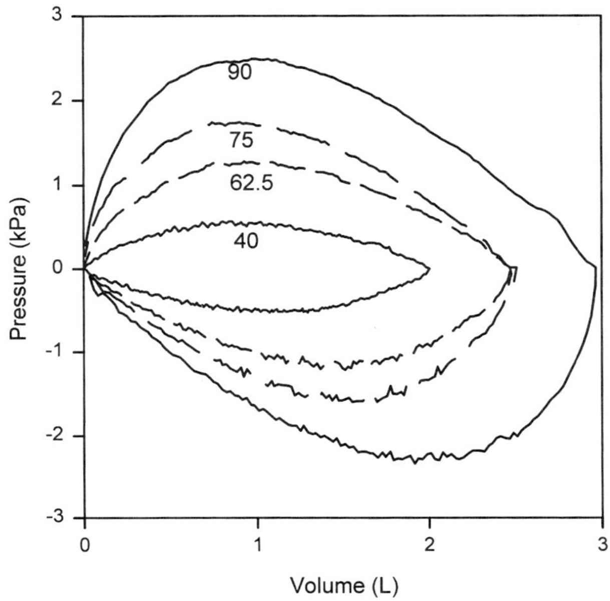

Figure 37 Pressure-volume loops for an orifice resistor at several $\dot{V}_E$. (From Ref. 97.)

C. Work of Breathing

Description

Mechanical work (W) is defined as the product of force multiplied by displacement, or, for fluid systems, the change in system pressure (ΔP) multiplied by the change in system volume (ΔV). Expressed as an integral,

$$W = \oint P dV$$

with units of kgf·m or joules (J).

The work involved in breathing is normally a small fraction of the total energy expended by exercising humans. However, in the underwater hyperbaric environment, dense gas and UBA impedance can raise the work of breathing to overwhelming levels. For that reason, ventilatory work and its variants have long been of interest to UBA designers and evaluators.

Computation of the work of breathing for respiratory equipment begins with the measurement of the area inside a plot of mouth pressure versus UBA volume when a UBA is ventilated on a breathing machine (Fig. 37), or:

$$W = \int_0^{V_T} P_{ex} \cdot dV - \int_0^{V_T} P_{inh} \cdot dV$$

where W is the classically defined resistive work of breathing with units of joules, P_{ex} is pressure during exhalation, and P_{inh} is inhalation pressure.

Fig. 37 is a series of breathing loops generated by ventilating an orifice resistor over a range of $\dot{V}_E$ from 40 to 90 L·min^{-1}. The areas within the loops, and therefore the work of breathing, was 1.5, 4.2, 5.7, and 9.9 kPa·L (or joules) for the 40, 62.5, 75, and 90 L·min^{-1} loops, respectively.

The loops in Figs. 38 and 39 are the 62.5 L·min^{-1} loop of Fig. 37, displaced upward so that all pressures are positive. Figure 38 shows the expiratory work against the orifice resistance, while Fig. 39 shows inspiratory work, represented by vertical lines. The difference between inspiratory and expiratory work is the dotted area inside the loop, representing the resistive work of breathing.

In Fig. 37, tidal volumes (V_T) increase from 2 to 3 L as $\dot{V}_E$ increases. To account for differences in V_T, it has been customary in the diving literature to

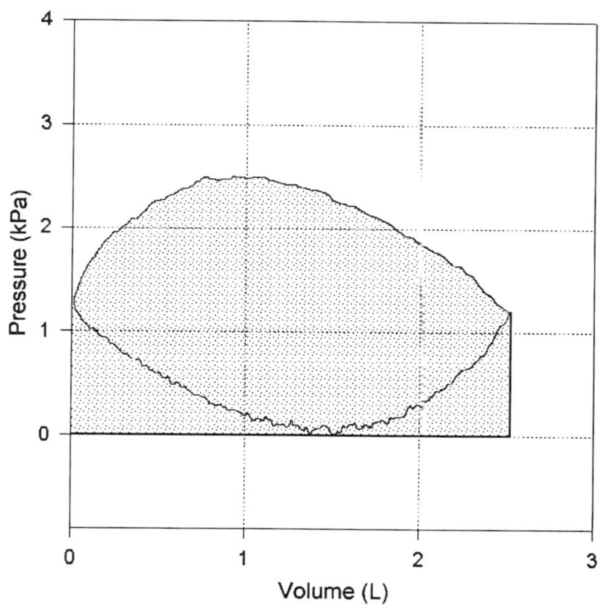

Figure 38 Expiratory work of breathing. (From Ref. 97.)

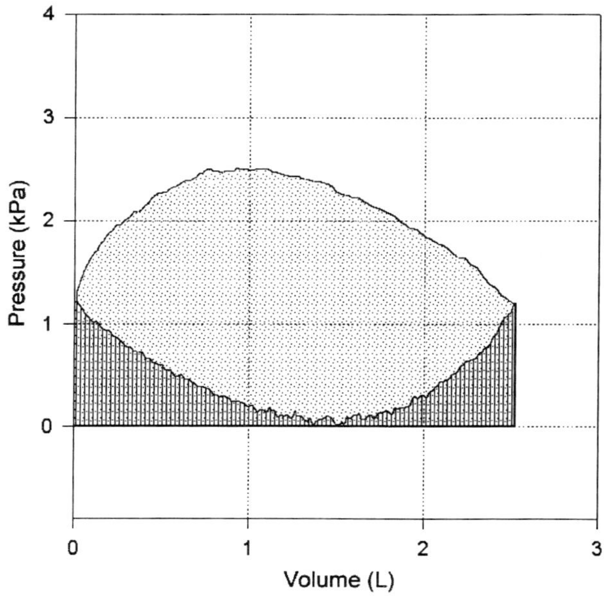

Figure 39 Calculation of work. The area under the inspiratory curve (vertical lines) is subtracted from the area under the expiratory curve (dotted area). (From Ref. 97.)

divide W by V_T. The result is a volume-averaged pressure, or, as described by Warkander et al. (89), volume-weighted mean pressure ($\overline{P}_V$):

$$\overline{P}_V = \frac{W}{V_T} = \frac{1}{V_T} \oint P \cdot dV$$

$\overline{P}_V$ is pressure averaged over the tidal breath, with units of kPa or J/L. The volume-averaged pressures for the four loops in Fig. 37 are 0.8, 1.7, 2.3, and 3.3 kPa, or $J \cdot L^{-1}$. With a little imagination, it can be seen that the 1.7-kPa value for the loops of 62.5 $L \cdot min^{-1}$ $\dot{V}_E$ in Figs. 38 and 39 corresponds to the average difference between expiratory pressure and inspiratory pressure across the tidal volume (Fig. 40).

$\overline{P}_V$ can be transformed into an estimate of breathing resistance (89,90). Since $\overline{P}_V$ is an average pressure, dividing by average ventilation yields an average resistance (R), an average over the entire tidal breath (96,97):

$$\overline{R} = \frac{120 \cdot \overline{P}_V}{\pi^2 \cdot \dot{V}_E}$$

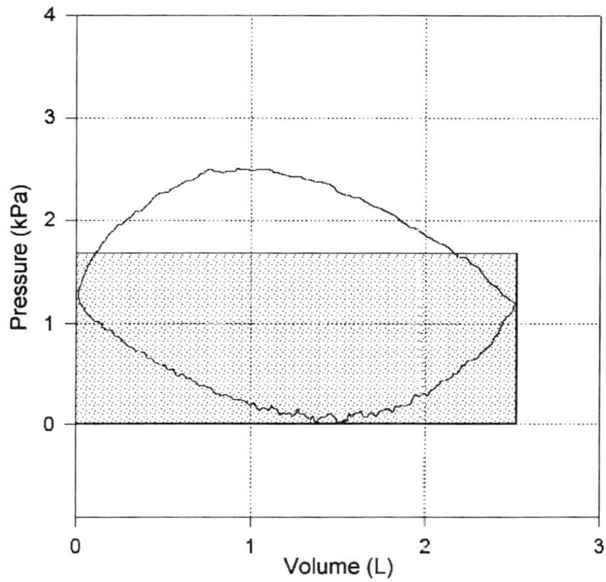

Figure 40 The work of breathing for the loop is identical to that of a rectangle with a height equal to the volume-averaged pressure for the loop and a length equal to the tidal volume. (From Ref. 97.)

where $\dot{V}_E$ is the expired ventilation in effect during the measurement of $\bar{P}_V$.

Figure 41a shows a plot of $\bar{P}_V$ for the orifice resistor of Fig. 37 at 5 $\dot{V}_E$. Figure 41b is the plot of the computed average resistance for that same orifice using the above equation.

The last two figures show various waveforms for a MK 16 closed-circuit UBA. Figure 42 was derived from a mathematical model of the MK 16, while Fig. 43 shows data from an actual UBA. The lower left panels (c) of both figures are P-V loops for the UBA. $\bar{R}$ was the average resistance computed from $\bar{P}_V$ and $\dot{V}_E$. On the lower right of the figure (d) is a pressure-flow loop with a linear regression line drawn through it. The slope of that line, the classical definition of resistance, was equal to the average resistance computed above. Thus, UBA resistance could be computed by either transforming the $\bar{P}_V$ data, or by regressing the pressure-flow data.

During testing of UBA at the Navy Experimental Diving Unit, the U.S. Navy's UBA evaluation laboratory, flow is not recorded; only pressure and volume (98). In Fig. 43 are waveforms from a modified MK 16 at 33 fsw being

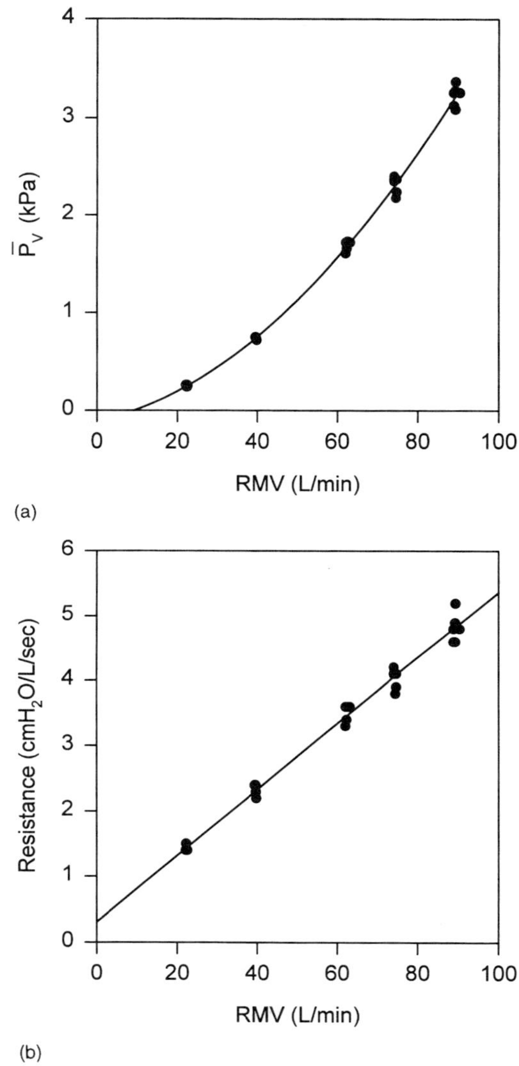

Figure 41 (a) Volume-averaged pressure ($\bar{P}_V$) and (b) average resistance for an orifice resistor at $\dot{V}_E$ of 22.5–90 $L \cdot min^{-1}$. (From Ref. 97.)

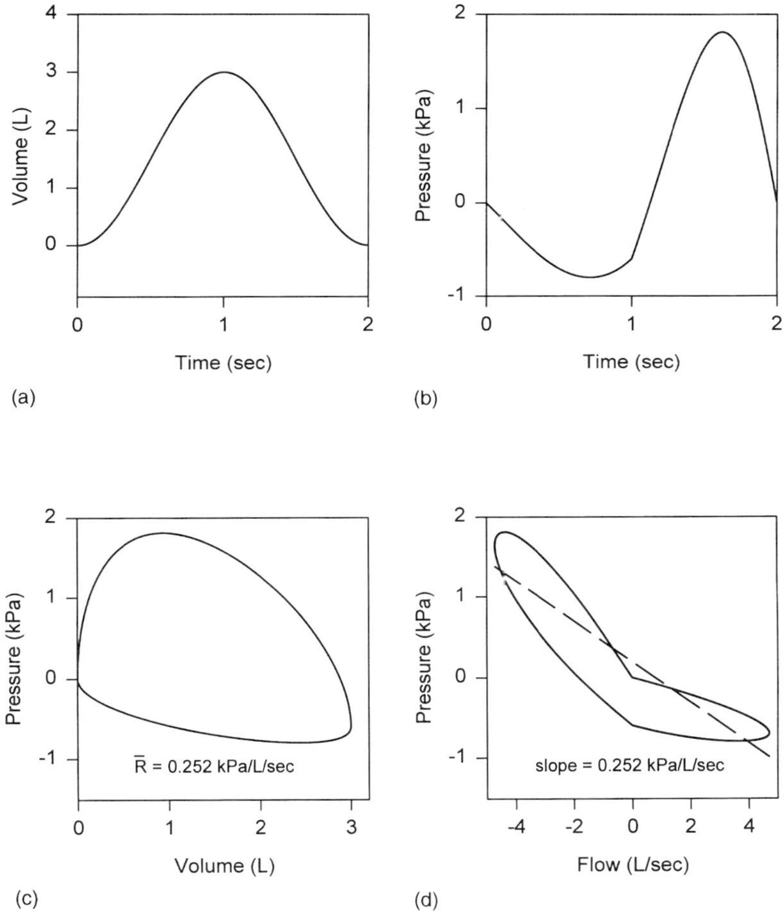

Figure 42 Model MK 16 UBA. $\bar{R}$ is the average resistance computed from $\bar{P}_V$ and $\dot{V}_E$. The slope of the regression of pressure against flow is the conventional measure of resistance. (From Ref. 97.)

ventilated at a $\dot{V}_E$ of 62.5 $L \cdot min^{-1}$. The majority of those waveforms are very similar to the mathematically modeled result in Fig. 42 (the flow data in the lower right quadrant are noisy due to the differentiation procedure used to extract it from the volume data). Nevertheless, the general shape of the pressure-flow curve is discernible, and the linear regression can be computed. These illustra-

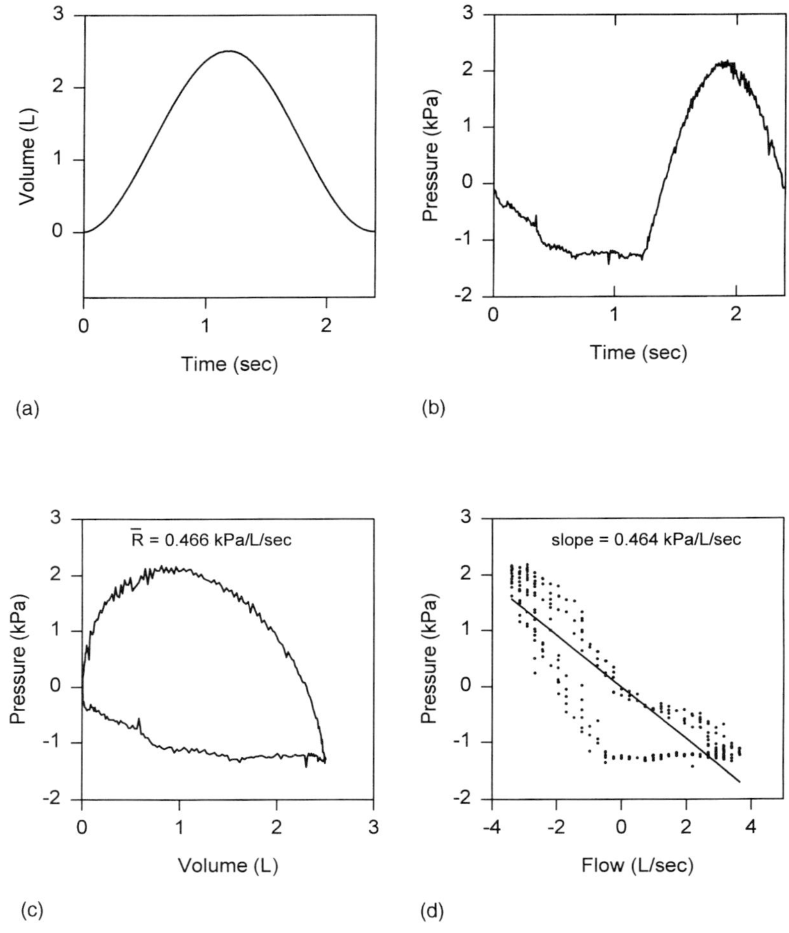

Figure 43 Actual MK 16 UBA. $\overline{R}$ and slope mean the same as in Fig. 42. (From Ref. 97.)

tions show that the resistance obtained from the above equation or from linear regression represents an average for the entire breath.

Work-of-Breathing Limits

Cooper

The attention to work as a physical descriptor of UBA, as opposed to pressure or resistance, seems to have sprung from various interpretations of Cooper's

1960 paper (57) on methods for testing respiratory protective equipment. Cooper emphasized work rate ($\dot{W}$), the product of inspiratory work per breath and respiratory frequency, with units of kgf·m·min^{-1}.

Work rate is equivalent to power, with 1 W of power equaling 6.13 kgf·m·min^{-1} or 60 J·min^{-1}. Cooper proposed that when respiratory protective equipment is tested with a breathing machine, the measured work rate should increase linearly with ventilation. Furthermore, for the comfort of the user, the slope relating work rate to ventilation should not exceed a critical limit.

In Fig. 44a are both the desired and maximum work rates (power) recommended by Cooper as a function of expired ventilation ($\dot{V}_E$). Cooper expressed the maximum tolerated external work rate as being proportional to one-quarter of the $\dot{V}_E$. The slope of that limit line is constant at 0.25 kgf·m·L^{-1} (Cooper's units). Since kgf·m is a unit of work, the slope defining the design limit is expressed as a constant work per liter, equivalent in modern units to 2.45 J·L^{-1}.

Since 1 J·L^{-1} is equal to 1 kPa, a unit of pressure, in the simplest terms, Cooper's limits translate to constant pressure limits of 25 cmH_2O (maximum) and approximately 12.5 cmH_2O (desired) (Fig. 44b). His expression of a standard in terms of work rate and flow rate obscured a much simpler observation.

Bentley et al.

Bentley et al. (87) were the first to describe acceptable resistive loads in probabilistic terms. They studied the effects of graded inspiratory resistances on 158 men exercising on a treadmill. An acceptable resistance was one where no more than 10% of the test population experienced discomfort. The maximum acceptable load was "0.17 kg-m per liter of air breathed," or a $\bar{P}v$ of 17 cmH_2O (1.67 kPa, Fig. 45). When $\bar{P}v$ was raised to 0.26 kgf·m·L^{-1} or 26 cmH_2O, with peak inspiratory pressures of 33 cmH_2O, the probability (p) of discomfort rose to about .50, with 95% confidence limits ranging from 0.4 to 0.7.

The limit of $p \leq .1$ of Bentley et al. was close to the average of Cooper's two limits. Bentley's standard of 0.17 kgf·m·L^{-1} for surface respiratory equipment was promulgated by Reimers in 1974 in proposed standards for underwater breathing apparatus (99).

Middleton and Thalmann

In 1980, Middleton proposed design goals (60) for SCUBA, which were extended in 1981 by Middleton and Thalmann to include performance goals for all U.S. Navy UBA (88). There were various "work-of-breathing (WOB)" limits; 0.14 kgf·m·L^{-1} (14.0 cmH_2O) for SCUBA, 0.17 kgf·m·L^{-1} (17 cmH_2O) for umbilical-supplied demand helmets. For other types of UBA, the goals varied directly with $\dot{V}_E$; at a $\dot{V}_E$ of 62.5 L·min^{-1}, the goal for WOB or $\bar{P}v$ ranged

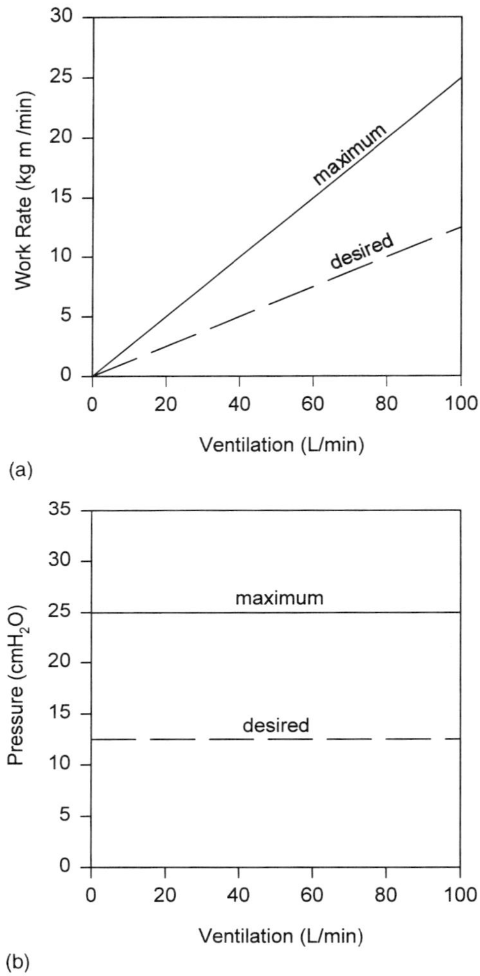

Figure 44 (a) Cooper's limits for work rate as a function of ventilation. (b) Cooper's limits replotted as average pressure.

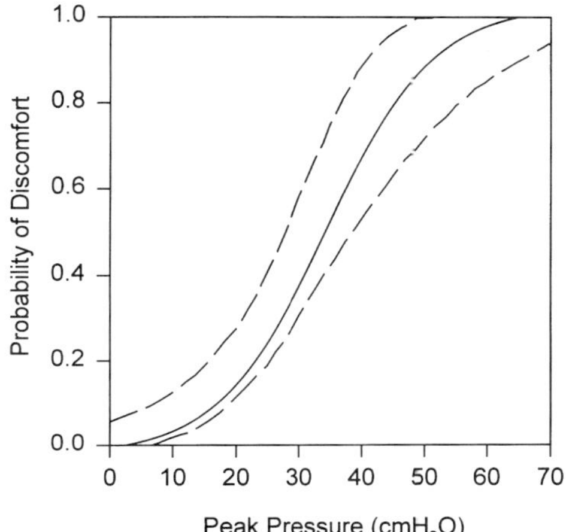

(a)

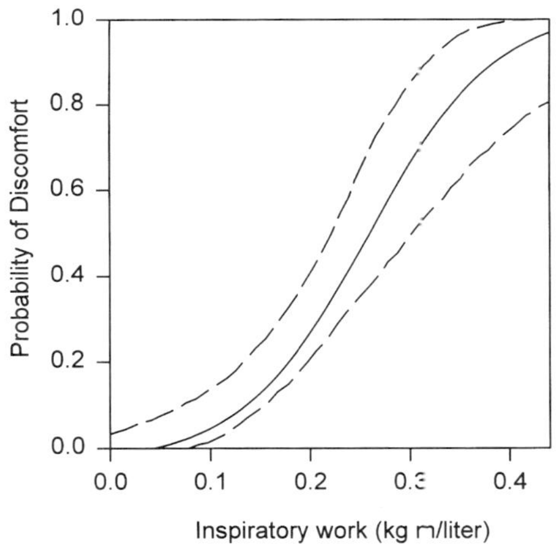

(b)

Figure 45 Probability of subject discomfort as a function of (a) peak inspiratory pressure and (b) inspiratory work. Dashed lines are 95% confidence limits. (From Ref. 87.)

from 0.12 kgf·m·L^{-1} to 0.157 kgf·m·L^{-1} (12 to 16 cmH_2O) for closed and semi–closed circuit UBA in air and helium environments, respectively.

Morrison and Reimers

Morrison and Reimers (60) proposed UBA design goals that also allowed $\bar{P}v$ to rise with mean ventilation,

$$\bar{P}v = 0.5 + 0.04\ \dot{V}E\ J/L$$

where $\dot{V}E$ has units of L/min. The above equation delineated a region of work tolerance, not diver comfort. The authors proposed a separate limit that would assure the diver's comfort.

$$\bar{P}v = 0.5 + 0.02\ \dot{V}E\ J/L$$

Warkander et al.

In what is arguably the most complete study of hyperbaric breathing limits to date, Warkander et al. (89) proposed limits in 1992 for breathing resistance in diver's breathing gear based on their studies of resistance tolerance at 3 and 57 msw. Six divers performed immersed exercise on a prone bicycle at a workload corresponding to 60% of each subject's maximum oxygen consumption determined under nonimmersed conditions. The subjects breathed through orifices that provided low, moderate, and high resistances. The highest resistance was chosen for each diver as one that was tolerated for 25 min but not 30 min. That resistance typically ranged from 8 to 12 $cmH_2O{\cdot}L^{-1}{\cdot}sec$ at flow rates of 2 to 3 $L{\cdot}sec^{-1}$, in the range of Mead's suggested limit (85) for total resistance (12 $cmH_2O{\cdot}L^{-1}{\cdot}sec$). Peak-to-peak pressure excursions averaged 46 cmH_2O at 1 atm abs and 43 cmH_2O at 6.8 atm abs. The other resistors were sized to yield about 85 and 65% of the highest resistance.

These authors observed that a bad dive outcome may result from either CO_2 retention, with the possibility of loss of consciousness, or dyspnea. The two results are often mutually exclusive. While dyspnea is by definition a respiratory discomfort, divers affected by high CO_2 levels due to hypoventilation are sometimes comfortable up to the moment of collapse.

Warkander et al proposed a volume-weighted mean pressure ($\bar{P}v$) limitation at 190 fsw during air breathing of between 1.5 and 2.0 J/L (~15 to 20 cmH_2O) over the $\dot{V}E$ range from 30 to 75 $L{\cdot}min^{-1}$. From the last equation in Sec. VI.C, this translates to an average resistance of as little as 2.5 $cmH_2O{\cdot}L^{-1}{\cdot}sec$. These authors' minimum limits lie just above those of Middleton and Thalmann for use with SCUBA.

Clarke et al.

Clarke et al. (65,100,101) supplemented the probabilistic approach initiated by Bentley (87) and combined it with the premise of Mead (85) that the total flow resistance or ventilatory load to which a diver is exposed should be limited (Sec. VI.B). Total resistance is composed of the summation of internal and external sources of resistance—human airways and UBA, respectively. As a diver descends, gas density increases; consequently internal resistance also increases. Since, according to Mead's premise, the total resistance should be fixed, the tolerated external resistance must decrease with depth. In probabilistic terms, as gas density increases in response to dive depth and mouth pressure increases in response to UBA resistance, the probability of a diver successfully completing a period of heavy exercise diminishes.

Whereas several design limits have used ventilatory rate as an independent variable, the probabilistic approach assumes ventilation is reasonably well fixed at that required for heavy work, with $\dot{V}_E$ roughly between 60 and 75 $L \cdot min^{-1}$. Instead, the independent variable is gas density (ρ). The total impedance (Z) to which a diver is exposed can be estimated by the following empirical equation:

$$Z = k \cdot \Delta P + a \cdot \rho + b$$

where Z has units of resistance ($cmH_2O \cdot L^{-1} \cdot sec$) and ΔP is peak-to-peak pressure measured at the diver's mouth. ΔP is an index of external resistance if $\dot{V}_E$ is constrained. The parameter k was assumed to be of unity magnitude with units of $sec \cdot L^{-1}$. The probability that a particular respiratory load would cause a diver difficulty, prove to be eventful, can be described by the Hill equation,

$$P = \frac{Z^n}{(Z^n + Z_{50}{}^n)}$$

where P is the probability of some untoward event and Z_{50} is the impedance that results in a 50% probability of that event. The event can be either respiratory distress or impending CO_2 narcosis due to hypoventilation (Fig. 46).

The above equations were fitted to a database of 237 well-documented human dives involving a variety of diving equipment under a wide range of conditions using a fixed exercise protocol. The dive outcomes were rated in a binary fashion as either eventful or uneventful, and the parameters a, b, n, and Z_{50} were found by maximum likelihood estimation techniques.

Figure 47 is a plot of event probabilities vs. mouth ΔP for various gas densities. It differs in two respects from Bentley's probability estimates (Fig. 45). First, pressure is peak-to-peak instead of just peak inspiratory. Secondly, the probability estimates cross the abscissa far from 0, due to a modeled threshold in diver tolerance.

Isoprobability lines (Fig. 48) were determined from a rearrangement of the above two equations.

$$\Delta P = \frac{Z_{50}}{\left(\frac{1}{P} - 1\right)^{1/n}} - a \cdot \rho + b$$

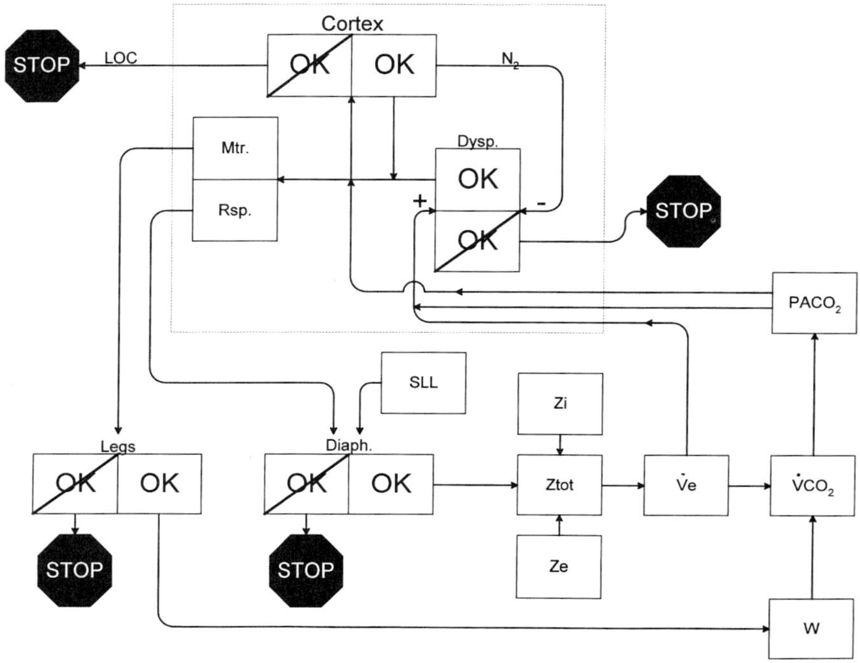

Figure 46 Sources of dive events (work stoppages). The fatigue of limb skeletal muscles was not considered an event due to respiratory loading. The rectangular dashed line consolidates CNS centers. SLL = static lung loading, Zi = internal impedance, Ze = external impedance, Ztot = total impedance, W = work, Mtr. = motor centers, Rsp. = respiratory centers, LOC = loss of consciousness, N_2 = nitrogen [postulated to have a salutary (−) effect on dyspnea]. In this drawing, high PA_{CO_2} and ventilation ($\dot{V}E$) were assumed to have a stimulatory (+) effect on dyspnea. In some individuals, however, high PA_{CO_2} may not be stimulatory.

When the event probability (P) approaches 0, the above reduces to:

$$\Delta P = b - a \cdot \rho$$

This line marks a demarcation below which the probability of an event is essentially zero. The probability of an event occurring rises as pressures increase above this line. Isoprobability lines ranging from event probabilities of 0.01 up to 0.9 are shown in Fig. 48.

For the same gas density, the event probability in a nitrogen atmosphere was approximately 60% of the probability in a heliox atmosphere (Fig. 48). This means that either high-pressure helium atmospheres exacerbate diver discomfort

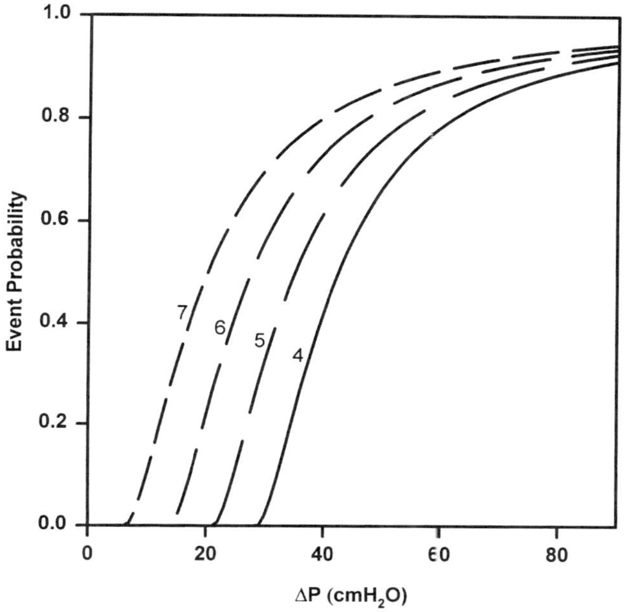

Figure 47 Event probability in a non-narcotic environment as a function of peak-to-peak pressure for various gas densities (4 to 7 g/L).

or that potentially narcotic nitrogen atmospheres tend to ameliorate the diver's perceptions of effort. In the work of Fothergill and Carlson, there is evidence of narcotic-induced reductions in perceived respiratory effort both at 1 atm (102) and at depth (103). When divers were exposed to isodensity narcotic and non-narcotic nitrogen mixtures at depth, the narcotic mixtures resulted in lower $\dot{V}_E$, esophageal pressures, and perceived respiratory effort than did the nonnarcotic mixes.

D. Elastic Loading

Description

Elastance is relatively unchanged by depth, unlike resistance, W, and $\overline{P}v$. It is governed by the depth-independent properties of material and by the displacements of gas within a water column (104). In mechanical systems, elastic elements are usually assumed not to dissipate energy. Energy put into an elastance is fully recovered. However, in physiological systems, elastic loads increase the O_2 cost of breathing almost as much as matched resistive loads (105).

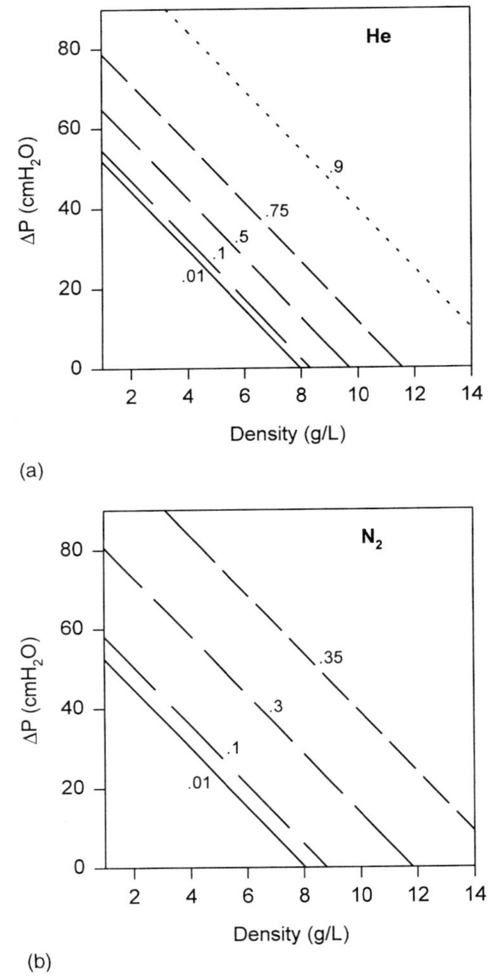

Figure 48 Isoprobability lines for eventful, hard working (high flow rate) dives. (a) Helium-oxygen dives; (b) air or nitrox dives.

Normal respiratory system elastance is between 5 and 10 $cmH_2O{\cdot}L^{-1}$. The range between barely detectable and barely tolerated external elastic loads (106–108) lies between 1 and 150 $cmH_2O{\cdot}L^{-1}$. As in resistive loading, the perceived magnitude of external elastic loads is highly correlated with the peak mouth pressure generated against the load (109).

Rohrer (110) suggested in 1925 that when respiratory loads are increased, respiratory rate and frequency might vary to minimize the total work of breathing. This idea was explored on theoretical grounds by Otis et al. (111) in 1950. Five years later, McIlroy et al. (112) studied the ventilatory response of human subjects to a purely elastic load (an air-filled 200-L tank). Due to the compressibility of gas at 1 atm abs, this noncollapsible volume provided an elastic load of 5.6 $cmH_2O \cdot L^{-1}$. As predicted, subjects increased respiratory rate and reduced tidal volume in response to this load—a strategy that reduced respiratory work. The tachypnea associated with elastic loads of approximately 6 $cmH_2O \cdot L^{-1}$ is apparently a reflex response (113).

DiMarco et al. (114) reported on the increase in elastic loading afforded by strapping of the rib cage and abdomen. (Strapping studies give some insight into the potential effects of restrictive diving garments such as wet suits.) A doubling of respiratory system elastance caused an approximately 30% reduction in vital capacity and FRC. In animal studies, a doubling of inspiratory elastance limits ventilation, causing hypoxemia and hypercapnia. The alveolar-arterial oxygen gradient (A-a$\dot{D}_{O_2}$) may increase during electrically stimulated exercise of anesthetized animals exposed to elastic loads, leading some to suggest that large negative intrapleural pressures combined with increased cardiac output may cause transient interstitial edema during elastic loading (115).

Elastic Load Limit

Warkander and Lundgren (80,81) exposed immersed divers to a range of elastic loads during prone underwater exercise at 60% of their maximum $\dot{V}_{O_2}$. Elastic loads greater than 7 $cmH_2O \cdot L^{-1}$ resulted in either excessive end-tidal CO_2 (>65 mmHg) or excessive dyspnea. They therefore proposed that for diving applications, UBA elastance should not exceed 7 $cmH_2O \cdot L^{-1}$ during normal operation. This would allow an approximate doubling of the elastic load to which a diver is normally subjected on dry land and is 50% of the elastic load which reduces tolerance to near maximal workloads at 1 atm abs (116).

The limit proposed by Warkander and Lundgren is met by the majority of UBAs tested by the U.S. Navy. When oriented vertically in the water column, the MK 16 closed-circuit mixed-gas UBA, and the Gasmizer gas recovery UBA in backpack mode have elastances of approximately 4 and 6 $cmH_2O \cdot L^{-1}$, respectively. When a UBA with small breathing bags is overventilated, however, bag collapse or over extension can lead to disturbingly high respiratory pressures. It is not too unusual to find elastances of 15 $cmH_2O \cdot L^{-1}$ in over extended LAR V UBA.

The use of breathing apparatus is usually associated with combinations of various respiratory loads and their interactions. Hydrostatic loading, discussed in the next section, is a good example. An imbalance between airway pressure

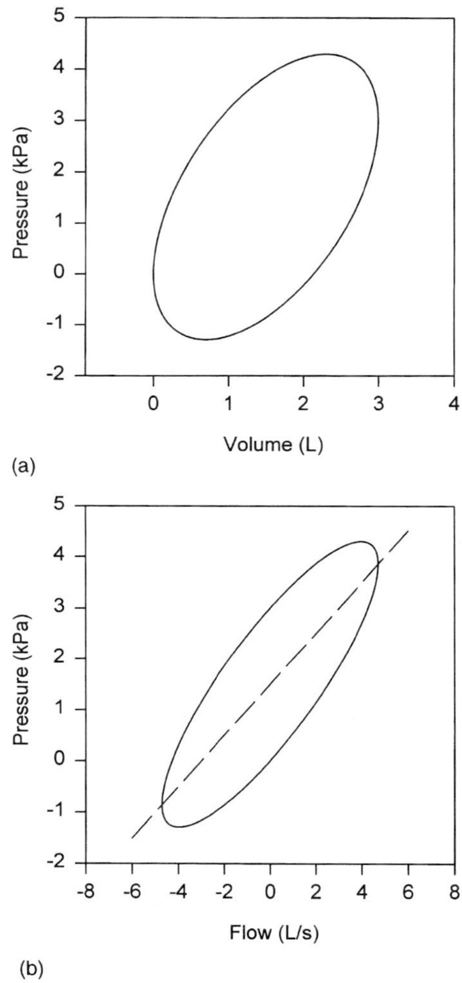

Figure 49 (a) UBA resistance yields an open P-V loop, while (b) elastance causes the P-V loop to slope upwards from horizontal. The slope of the linear regression of P vs. $\dot{V}$ (dashed line in part b) is a measure of R, and the openness of the P vs. $\dot{V}$ loop is due to elastance.

and mean hydrostatic pressure exerted upon the chest alters lung volumes and thus perturbs intrinsic respiratory elastance. When lung volumes are too low by reason of inadequate intrapulmonary pressure (negative-pressure breathing), then respiratory elastance is increased, presumably reducing a subject's tolerance to added elastic loads.

Figure 49 shows theoretical pressure-volume (a) and pressure-flow loops (b) for a UBA with combined resistance and elastance. The area of the loop in (a) is an index of UBA resistance. The slope of the loop is an indicator of elastance. In (b), just the opposite applies. The slope of the loop is a measure of resistance, and the area of the loop is an index of elastance.

Resistance, elastance, and hydrostatic loading can also act independently. On the basis of their results, Warkander and Lundgren have proposed that respiratory loads are additive (82,83). That is, if a barely acceptable elastance is combined with a barely acceptable resistance or hydrostatic load, the combined result will be unacceptable. Therefore, any given limit on a respiratory load should be reduced when combined with other types of loading.

E. Hydrostatic Loading and Imbalance

Description

Although both hydrostatic and elastic loads may be experienced underwater, the two respiratory loads are in at least one sense independent. In Fig. 50, a diver in a horizontal position is shown with a counterlung (breathing bag) on his back (a) or chest (c). Mouth pressure oscillates as the diver breathes. The vertical displacement of the pressure waveform is governed by the position of the counterlungs relative to the diver's lungs. This vertical displacement is termed *hydrostatic loading*.

The pressure of the water acting on a diver's rib cage can make it difficult to breathe unless that inward force is counterbalanced by the outward force of gas filling the diver's lungs. If breathing bags are placed high on the chest or back of an upright diver, a pressure imbalance will exist with the inspired gas being at a lower pressure than the mean hydrostatic pressure surrounding the lungs. Relative to the external pressure, the inspired pressure is negative in sign, and therefore a negative pressure balance is said to exist.

Negative-pressure breathing also occurs when a diver is snorkeling while prone or using a mouth-held demand regulator while upright. There is a net force acting to compress the diver's lungs and rib cage. To inflate his lungs against this force, the diver has to create an unusually high negative intrapleural pressure. Negative-pressure breathing increases the inspiratory work of breathing (117) and decreases maximum voluntary ventilation (MVV) and physical work capacity (118,119). These changes are accompanied by a reduction in functional

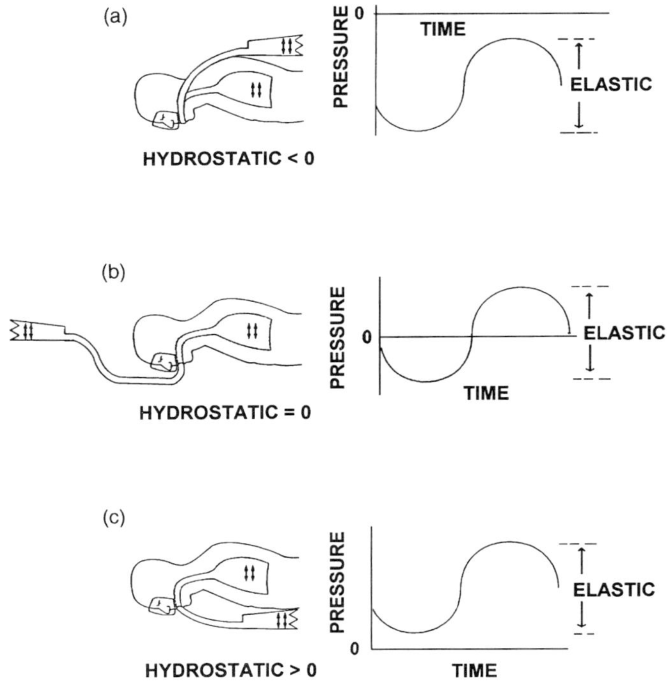

Figure 50 Hydrostatic loading. (From Ref. 104.)

residual capacity (FRC) and a resultant increase in airway resistance and elastic work (120,121).

Breathing bags placed low on a diver (Fig. 50c) means the gas supply is at a higher, more positive pressure than the hydrostatic pressure surrounding the diver's chest. Therefore, gas flows down a pressure gradient into the diver's lungs, easing inspiration. Unfortunately, to exhale, the respiratory muscles must contract forcefully to expel gas back to the breathing bags. Both forceful inhalation from negative-pressure breathing or forceful exhalation from positive-pressure breathing can result in diver fatigue.

The transrespiratory pressures likely to be found in various UBA range from -25 to $+40$ cmH_2O with respect to the hydrostatic pressure at the seventh cervical vertebra or to -32 to $+33$ cmH_2O with respect to the suprasternal notch (Fig. 51). The hydrostatic load depends on the diver's orientation in the water and the location of breathing bags and regulator demand valves (118). Under usual conditions, the effects of these pressures only rarely affect the acceptability of a diving rig. Nevertheless, when both human and machine are

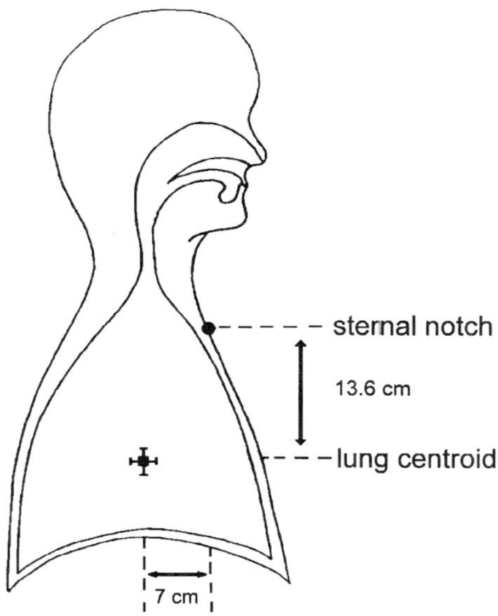

Figure 51 Lung centroid relative to the suprasternal notch. (From Ref. 123.)

stressed by high work levels, commonly found hydrostatic loads can exert a profound influence on comfort and work tolerance (119).

The effects of hydrostatic imbalances on diver comfort and performance, recently reviewed by Lanphier and Camporesi (122), has been one of the most extensively researched topics in diving physiology during the last decade. The central question has been the following: What respiratory pressures are optimal for counterbalancing the inward force of the water column?

Hydrostatic Limits

The selection of an optimum airway pressure as a criterion for UBA design is complicated by the naturally occurring balance between physiological and sensory cues. In attempting to correct an imbalance created by an unusual environment, an apparent physiological improvement may come at considerable sensory expense. Most authors contend that lung centroid pressure (P_{LC}) appears to be the optimal pressure for diver comfort during immersion (123). In an upright immersed person, P_{LC} is 13.6 cm below the sternal notch and 7 cm above the plane of the sternal notch in the supine (horizontal, face down) position (Fig. 51).

Higher pressures are not well tolerated in nonhelmeted divers because high transpharyngeal pressures cause uncomfortable inflation of the cheeks and oropharynx (124,125). By using diving helmets to eliminate transpharyngeal pressure gradients, pressures equal to P_{LC}+13.6 cmH_2O (pressure respect to the extracorporeal pressure at the level of the sternal notch) are readily tolerated, resulting in an improvement in exercise ventilation (126). However, an airway pressure of approximately P_{LC}+20 cmH_2O is required to return maximum voluntary ventilations and functional residual capacity during immersed spontaneous breathing to its normal value in the dry (117). Carlson (125) observed that when faced with strenuous ventilatory requirements, pressures of P_{LC}+20 cmH_2O or more have proven beneficial to the ventilatory endurance of severely stressed immersed divers.

There has been some concern that under more moderate conditions high airway pressures might decrease respiratory endurance by increasing the work of the expiratory muscles (126). Interestingly, Derion et al. (127) found that divers may not always sense the body position and static loading that is best from a physiological standpoint. Their work added to the literature that positive static lung loads are preferable from a respiratory mechanical standpoint over negative static lung loads. These authors also found that the prone body position is preferred over the upright position. This combination of postures and static lung loads is found in the swimming of only one type of closed-circuit UBA, 100% O_2 UBA, such as the LAR V (Fig. 24).

Hazardous Hydrostatic Loads

Freedman and Campbell (107) reported that the maximum sustained static inspiratory load that could be tolerated was 75 cmH_2O. Even short exposure to loads of 100 cmH_2O, as in snorkeling at 1-m depths, resulted in ventricular extrasystoles in three of five subjects (128). With immersion to 1 m while snorkeling, the right ventricle is exposed to 1 atm pressure, but the left ventricle must pump against the sum of arterial resistance and the 100-cm pressure head. In a 1911 study, an athletic individual attempted to breath through a tube while submerged 2 m below the surface. Due to the 200-cmH_2O pressure gradient across his chest wall, his respiratory efforts were ineffectual. The unfortunate subject apparently suffered ''delirium cordis'' and acute cardiac dilatation as a result (128). A temporary increase in heart size during submersion and negative-pressure breathing has been more recently observed by Risch (129,130).

F. Hydrostatic and Elastic Loads

In the descriptions of UBAs found earlier in this chapter, they were described as various combinations of resistance, elastance, and inertance (inductance).

What then is hydrostatic loading (SLL of Fig. 33), and where does it fit in this description? Hydrostatic loading is not a mechanical load in the same sense as resistance and elastance. It is rather a description of the potential of the system—of the pressure bias. In electrical terms, it determines the operating point of the circuit; it is a measure of the degree to which capacitors are charged at the beginning of current flow (breathing). Hydrostatic loading determines the value of elastance around which the diver's pulmonary system oscillates. When hydrostatic loading is optimal, the respiratory system is operating in the linear, low-elastance portion of the chest wall and lung compliance curve (Chap. 3).

G. Synthesis

Theory

Fifty years of design standards for UBA were summarized in Secs. C, D, and E. Some were engineering-based standards, while others were physiologically based. We will attempt to unify these diverse treatments into a scheme that is physiologically based but which maintains much of the character of the engineering based limits.

We first assert that the key element determining a diver's comfort and safety under water is respiratory impedance. The impedance due to external sources may come from UBA resistance, elastance, inertance, or various combinations. As yet we have no reason to believe that one impedance acting alone is any more debilitating than the others (80–83).

When each impedance is applied separately, respiratory pressures increase during breathing. From this, we obtain an obvious but cardinal rule for UBA standards development: *Respiratory pressures should be kept as low as possible.*

Even the lowest-impedance UBA will produce respiratory pressures that increase monotonically with density and flow. Therefore, design goals that allow respiratory pressures to rise somewhat with increasing flow or gas density, such as those of Middleton and Thalmann (60) or Morrison and Reimers (66) are necessary from an engineering standpoint and reasonable from a psychophysical standpoint. The psychophysical power laws of Stevens (131,132) and Borg (133) as well as their antecedent, the Weber-Fechner law [described in Geldard (134)], are all rationales for reducing respiratory pressures at low flow rates, and allowing it to rise at higher flow rates.

The second cardinal rule is the following: *The sum of UBA and internal respiratory impedance has a maximum value that will allow useful work.*

This is a restatement of the claims of Mead (85). Expressed mathematically,

$$Z_{allowed} = Z_{max} - Z_{aw}$$

where $Z_{allowed}$ is the allowed UBA impedance, Z_{max} is Mead's proposed impedance (resistance) limit (12 $cmH_2O \cdot L^{-1} \cdot s$), and Z_{aw} is the flow impedance of the diver's airways. Since

$$Z_{allowed} = \frac{\Delta P_{allowed}}{\dot{V}}$$

then

$$\Delta P_{allowed} = Z_{max} \cdot \dot{V} - \Delta P_{aw}$$

For ΔP_{aw}, we use the equation of Pedley et al (58):

$$\Delta P_{aw} = a \cdot (\rho^{0.5} \cdot \dot{V}^{1.5}) + b \cdot (\rho \cdot \dot{V}^{2})$$

where the first term describes flow in lower airways (primarily laminar), and the second term represents a combined kinetic energy term and a term for flow in the upper airways, which is largely transitional or turbulent.

$\Delta P_{allowed}$ Surface

When $\Delta P_{allowed}$ is plotted against gas density and flow, we obtain a curved surface as in Figs. 52 and 53. Figure 52a is a three-dimensional mesh plot of the allowed pressure surface, while Fig. 52b is a contour plot of the same surface. In Fig. 52, coefficients a and b were equal to 0.2 and 0.35 respectively. (*The waviness of the zero flow intercept with the density axis is an artifact of the mesh generation process.*) In Fig. 53, the mesh plot of Fig. 52 has been rotated to show the ΔP - density presentation of the three-dimensional surface. This view shows that for a given flow rate, $\Delta P_{allowed}$ varies inversely and linearly with gas density.

Figure 53b illustrates this point with a plot of $\Delta P_{allowed}$ for flow rates of 2.0 and 3.9 $L \cdot sec^{-1}$. The higher flow rate, resulting in a more steeply sloped line, is the peak flow rate associated with an expired ventilation ($\dot{V}_E$) of 75 $L \cdot min^{-1}$ during sinusoidal breathing. The coefficients a and b were selected such that the above line approximates the 0.01 isoprobability lines in Fig. 48, described in Section VI.C.

The resulting surface represents a UBA design goal that follows the guidance of Mead and that allows UBA pressure to increase with flow in keeping with both psychophysical laws and existing engineering based design standards (60,66), at least at moderate gas densities. This surface also explains the results of Clarke et al. (100,101), who found that at high workloads and high $\dot{V}_E$'s, the peak mouth pressures tolerated by Navy divers dropped linearly as gas density increased (Fig. 48). In effect, the surface described by the $\Delta P_{allowed}$ equation unifies existing design goals.

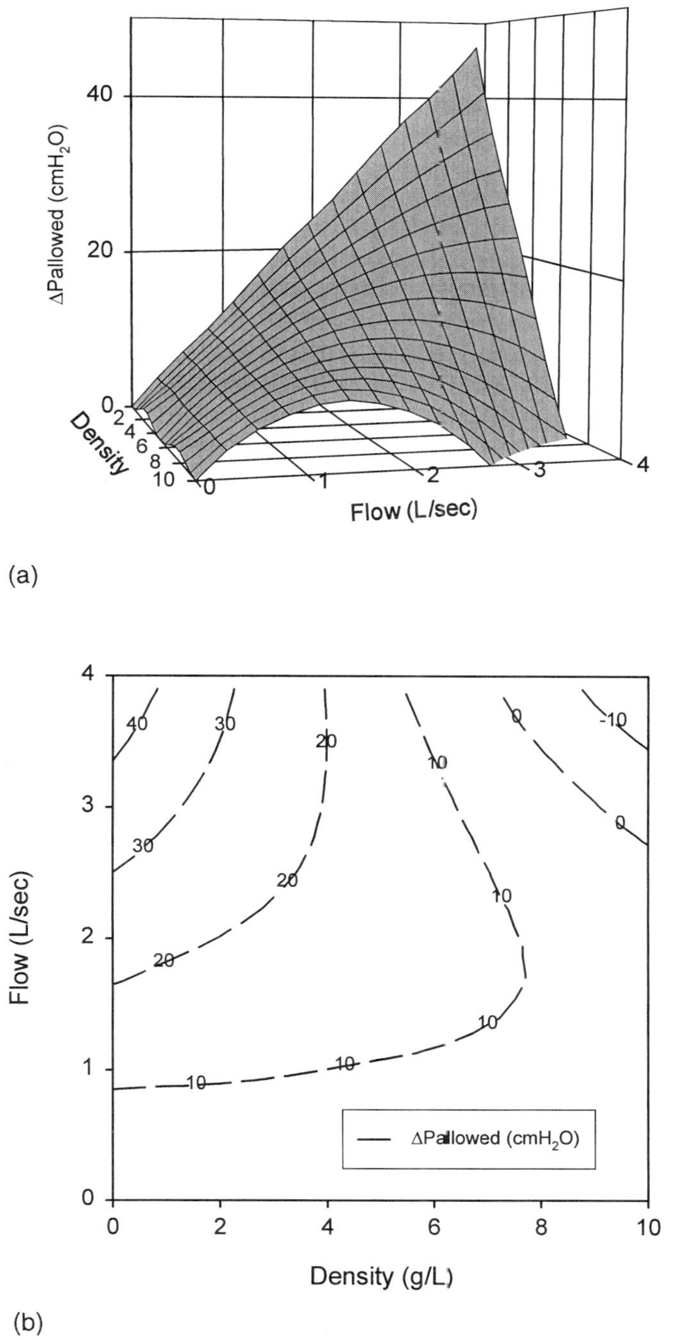

Figure 52 (a) $\Delta P_{allowed}$, $\dot{V}$, ρ surface for coefficients of a=.2, b=.35; (b) a contour graph of the above surface. Curving dashed lines are iso-pressure lines with $\Delta P_{allowed}$ ranging from 10 to 40 cmH_2O.

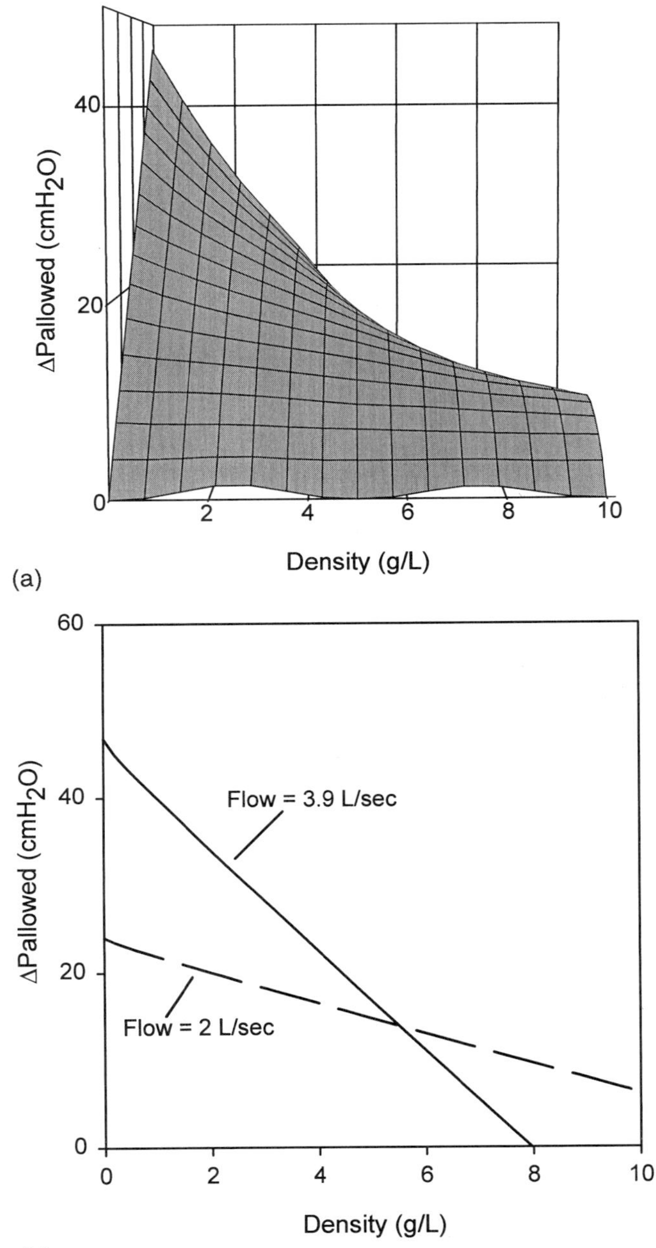

Figure 53 (a) Density and pressure projection of the $\Delta P_{allowed}$, $\dot{V}$, ρ surface; (b) gas density versus $\Delta P_{allowed}$ for two peak flow rates (in $L \cdot sec^{-1}$), showing the approximately linear relationship.

By keeping UBA pressures on the allowed ΔP, $\dot{V}$, ρ surface, the probability of experiencing a troublesome dive should be low. To the extent that actual UBA pressures rise above the $\Delta P_{allowed}$, $\dot{V}$, ρ surface, the probability of a diver encountering an untoward event would rise. This point is illustrated by Figs. 54 and 55, which show the surface from two angles. Figure 54 also contains a scatter plot of the ΔPs measured during breathing machine tests of a state of the art SCUBA regulator at depths down to 30 msw with $\dot{V}_E$'s up to 90 $L \cdot min^{-1}$ (peak flow to 4.7 $L \cdot sec^{-1}$). A few of the data points from that regulator are seen just emerging from the surface in Fig. 54a. Figure 54b shows that the majority of the regulator data points lie well below that surface.

Data from a poorly performing regulator is shown in Fig. 55. Most of the data points lie considerably above the $\Delta P_{allowed}$, $\dot{V}$, ρ surface. Even at low gas densities, the data points lie very close to the surface. This particular regulator was involved in a diving fatality, so the height of the data points above the surface is of more than academic interest.

Respiratory pressures must eventually extend far above the $P_{allowed}$ surface as gas density and flow rate continues to rise, at least in passive mechanical devices. The region of declining UBA tolerance on the front right corner of Fig. 52 therefore describes an area where a UBA appreciably limits the diver's ventilation. It also suggests a region of flow and density where active ventilatory assistance might be of most benefit.

VII. Modeling

A. Mathematical

In principle, the most accurate way to model UBAs is to describe the system of equations pertaining to the system of state of the UBA defined over a period of time. As long as the system has few degrees of freedom, the mathematical description may be straightforward. As an example, Clarke et al. (135) derived the single differential equation controlling the oxygen content in a semiclosed UBA at STPD conditions. The solution to that equation is plotted in Fig. 21 (Sec. IV.C).

Unfortunately under more complex conditions, complete mathematical models require information on a multitude of physical parameters, some of which are likely to be known with little precision. As a result, the mathematical parameters for these models are often altered empirically to provide realistic results (18). Undoubtedly, when the operation of a UBA is required to be understood in great detail, the mathematical treatment so required is by necessity complicated (136). In fact, a complete description of a seemingly simple UBA breathing bag can entail a considerable modeling effort (137). Some of the most

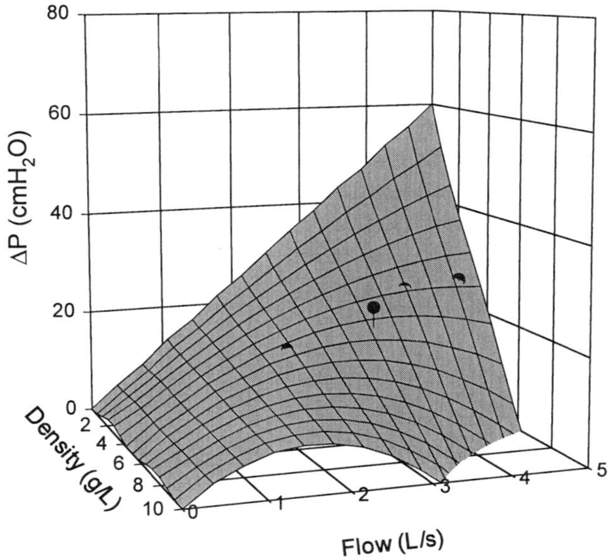

(a)

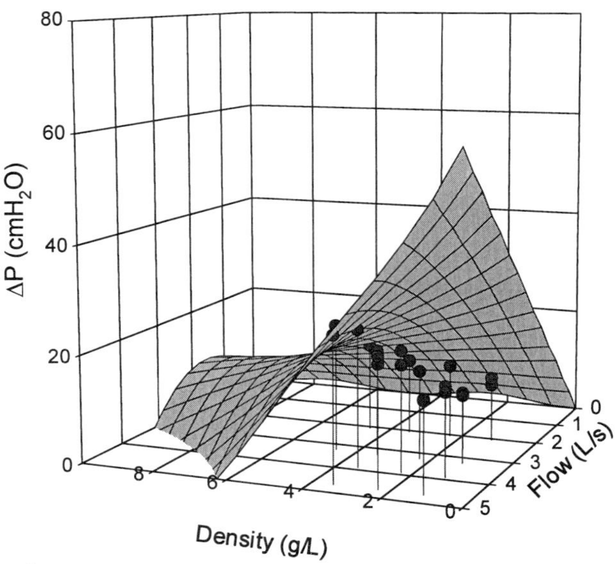

(b)

Figure 54 (a) Scatterplot of breathing machine data for a state-of-the art SCUBA regulator superimposed on the $\Delta P_{\text{allowed}}$, $\dot{V}$, ρ surface. (b) The same plot from a different angle. Regulator data lies mostly within or below the $\Delta P_{\text{allowed}}$, $\dot{V}$, ρ surface.

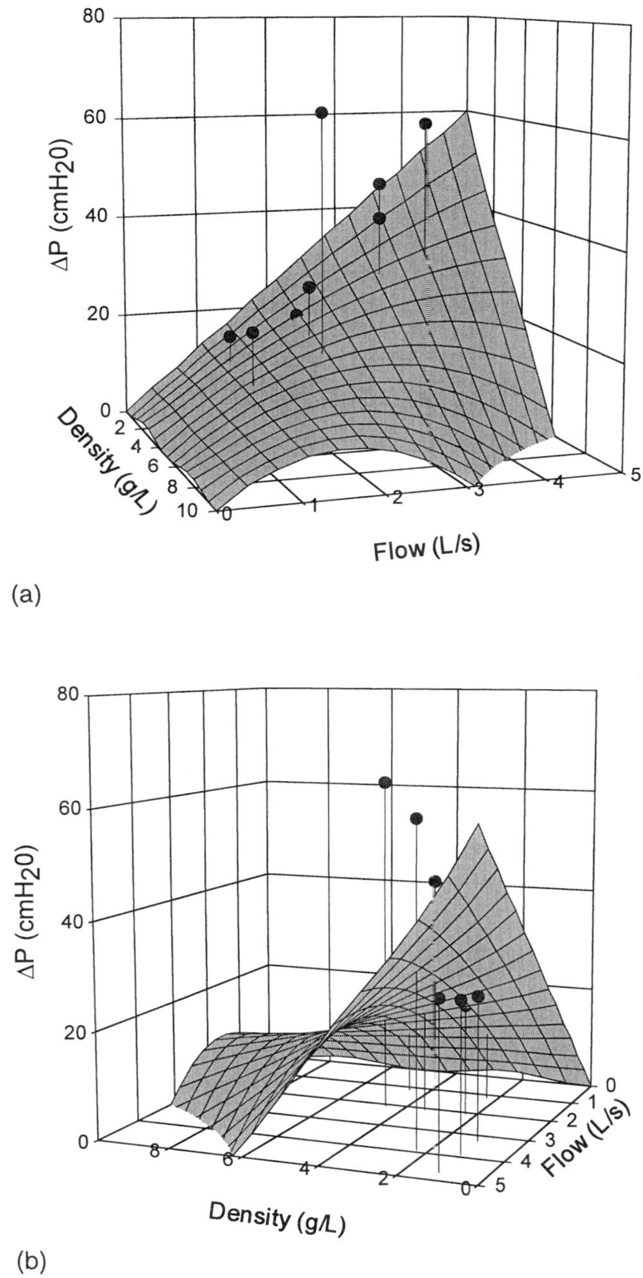

Figure 55 (a) Scatterplot of breathing machine data for a poorly performing SCUBA regulator superimposed on the $\Delta P_{allowed}$, $\dot{V}$, ρ surface. (b) The same plot from a different angle. Many of the regulator data points lie far above the $\Delta P_{allowed}$, $\dot{V}$, ρ surface.

didactic discussions of this topic are found in the writings of Sexton and Nuckols (138), Antoon et al. (139), and Mittleman (140).

B. Electrical

Description

This chapter uses circuit diagrams throughout to illustrate the key UBA components involved in gas flow, just as Mead and Milic-Emili (7) and Van Liew (55) used circuit diagrams to illustrate the mechanical structure of the human respiratory system at normal and elevated gas densities, respectively. Circuit diagrams serve more than a didactic function, however. They are a graphical representation of computer code that can be used to explore the properties of UBA under a wide range of conditions. Simulations can be performed that would be difficult or impossible to conduct in real laboratories.

The early electrical circuit models of the respiratory system (6) defined systems of linear differential equations which were solved by analog computers. With the ascendancy of digital computers, the Department of Electrical Engineering and Computer Sciences at the University of California at Berkeley developed algorithms that allowed faithful simulation of analog electronic circuitry. The Berkeley SPICE (Simulation Program with Integrated Circuit Emphasis) algorithms have become the de facto world standard for analog circuit simulation (141,142). Below are some examples of the simulation output that can be obtained by applying SPICE algorithms to various UBA schematics.

Analogs of Open-Circuit UBAs

Figure 56 is an analog of the U.S. Navy MK 21 demand helmet UBA (Fig. 10), similar to the commercially produced SuperLite 17. The schematic is a simplified version of Fig. 13. This is an open-circuit device in that gas is supplied from a compressed source and is exhausted to the water column. A regulator drops the gas supply to a pressure usable by the diver, who is seen as a sinusoidal current source. The gas flow path is determined by two diodes (valves) and an exhaust valve. The neck dam is a flexible rubber seal around the diver's neck, attached to the bottom of the helmet opening. The neck dam presents a shunting, compliant gas-flow path whose availability is dependent upon the resistor preceding it. That resistor represents the seal on an oronasal cup, and can vary from being very high (tight seal) to nonexistent (ineffective seal). The coiled elements in the inspiratory and expiratory circuits represent inductances (inertance).

Figure 57 is a pressure-volume loop of an actual open-circuit demand UBA such as the MK 21. Figure 58 is a model prediction for the same P-V loop. (No attempt was made to model the high frequency regulator chatter seen

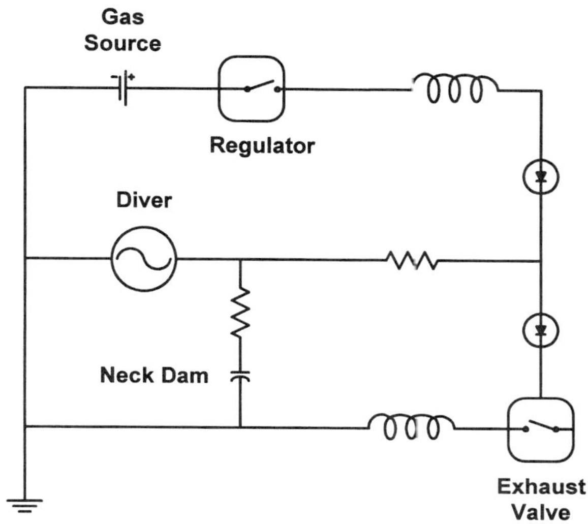

Figure 56 Electrical analog of the MK 21 demand helmet UBA.

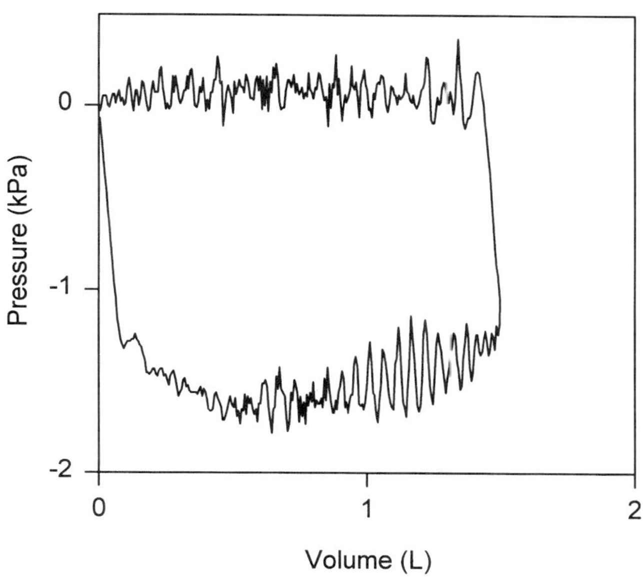

Figure 57 P-V loop from an actual demand, open-circuit UBA.

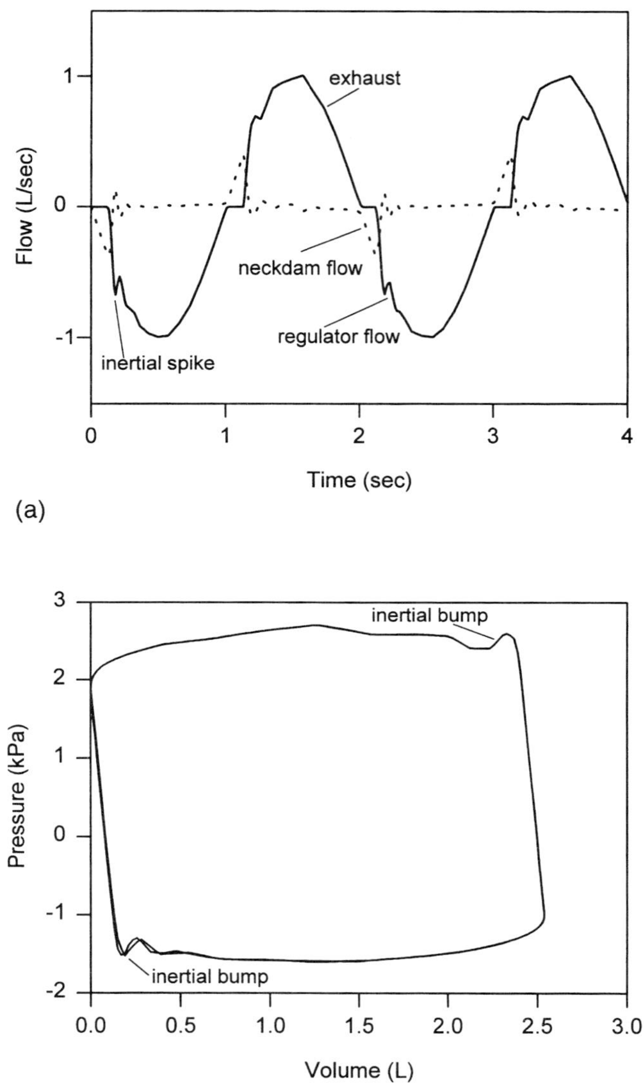

Figure 58 PSpice simulation results. (a) Variation with time of various flows, including flow to and from the neck dam (dotted line). The solid line is flow from the regulator (negative flow) and through the exhaust valve (positive flow). (b) The P-V diagram. The spikes in (a) and the bumps in (b) as flow reverses direction are due to the inertances in the inhalation and exhalation limbs of the circuit of Fig. 56.

in Fig. 57.) The overall loop characteristics are identifiable in the modeled output from the circuit of Fig. 56.

One of the benefits of an electrical analog model is that the shunted flow through the oronasal resistor can be calculated. The shunted gas accumulates within the neck dam compliance; since that gas is CO_2-rich, it can significantly raise the diver's inspired CO_2 level when reinhaled. Therefore, the oronasal shunting resistance should be as high as possible (i.e., a tight seal maintained) to minimize to-and-fro gas flow within the neck dam region of the helmet.

A highly sloping P-V loop is a telltale sign of a poor oronasal seal and a compliant neck dam (Fig. 59). In Fig. 59a, we see that with a poor seal a considerable portion of the diver's gas comes from the neck dam area (dotted line) rather than the demand regulator. The result is CO_2 rebreathing and, in effect, a large dead space.

Analogs of Closed-Circuit UBAs

Figure 60 is a schematic of the breathing loop of a UBA with dual breathing bags, one for inspiration, and one for expiration. The force of the diver's exhalation forces CO_2-rich gas into the exhalation bag (C_{exh}) and then through the CO_2 scrubber canister represented by a relatively large resistance (R_{can}). Once through the canister, the scrubbed gas collects in an inspiratory breathing bag or compliance (C_{inh}). The pathway from the inspiratory bag to the diver is relatively effortless since both R_{inh} and L_{inh} have low values.

Figure 61 is the result of the simulation based on the circuit of Fig. 60, and Fig. 62 is an actual pressure-volume loop from a prototype two-bag UBA. The similarities in loop shape are obvious.

VIII. The Future

A. Retrospective

In a symposium held 25 years ago, UBA designers and engineers discussed the technologies that were being explored for use in UBA. Among those technologies were electronic monitoring of CO_2 partial pressures within UBAs (143), and novel CO_2 removal methods, such as molecular sieves and electrolytic decomposition in a solid electrolyte (39). Cryogenic systems had been devised that both removed CO_2 and added O_2 to the breathing circuit (Sec. IV.F).

Unfortunately, the intervening 25 years have seen relatively little progress in underwater life support engineering. Cryogenic systems are no longer being seriously considered. In spite of an ever-increasing desire for electronic monitoring of P_{CO_2} in UBA, that goal has yet to be realized. Infrared techniques, the mainstay of commercial CO_2 monitors, are sensitive to water in both the liquid

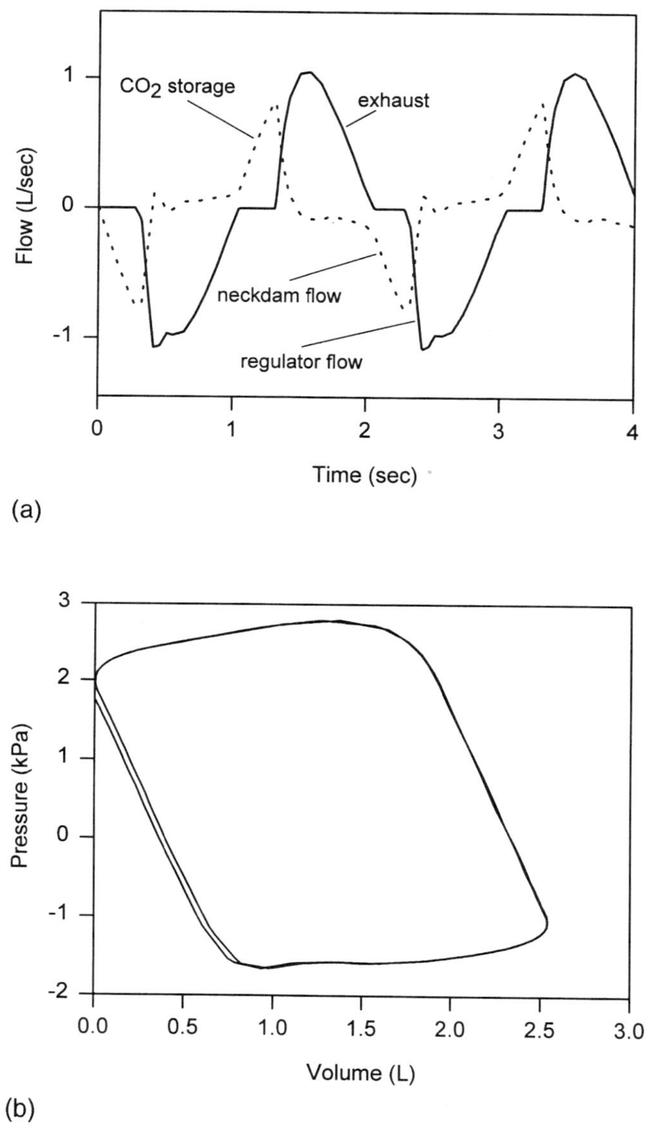

Figure 59 PSpice simulation results. Same as Fig. 58 but showing the results of poor oronasal seal and high neck dam compliance. (a) The volume of gas exchanging non-productively with the neck dam storage area is found as the area under one phase of the flow. A considerable portion of the total gas flow to and from the diver is rebreathed within the helmet. (b) The P-V diagram.

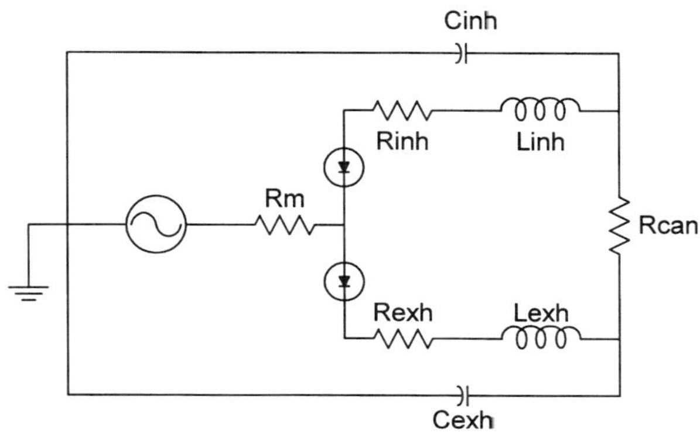

Figure 60 Electrical analog of a two breathing bag closed-circuit UBA showing the resistances (R) and inductances (L) in the inhalation (inh) and exhalation (exh) side of the circuit. Rcan is the flow resistance of the scrubber canister. One-way valves are represented by diodes, circles with arrows showing the direction of flow. The two breathing bags are identified as Cinh and Cexh. Mouthpiece resistance is identified as Rm.

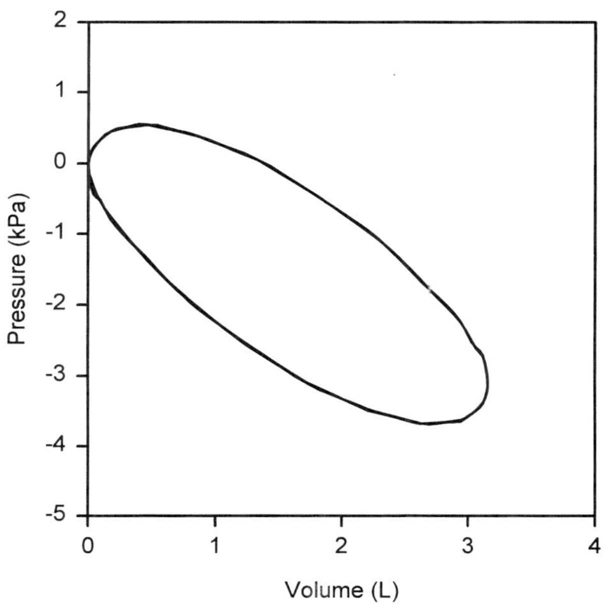

Figure 61 PSpice model results for a two breathing bag closed-circuit UBA.

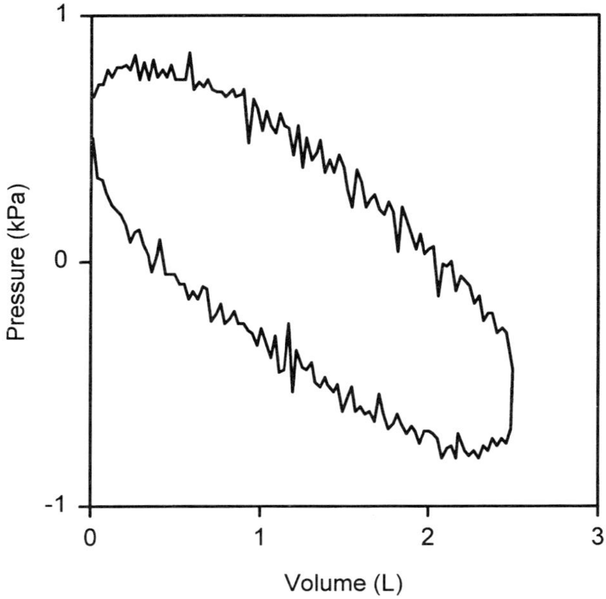

Figure 62 Actual breathing loop for a two breathing bag closed-circuit UBA. Data was collected at a lower tidal volume than in the simulation.

and vapor phase. Since water is ever-present in UBA, infrared CO_2 sensors have not been successfully applied to UBA.

B. Future Carbon Dioxide Sensing

The newest trend in gas monitoring is based on solid-state sensors that can monitor both O_2 and CO_2. These sensors are described as thick-film electrocatalytic multigas cermet microsensors. The sensing signal is based on cyclic voltametry (144) and is capable of using trained neural networks to differentiate among various gases (145). Related work from the Argonne National Laboratories is being published as this chapter goes to press (146).

C. Membrane-Based Gas Exchange

Since the first description of a semipermeable membrane oxygenator (147) in 1963, extra-corporeal membrane oxygenation (ECMO) and extracorporeal carbon dioxide removal ($ECCO_2R$) have found steady clinical application. These devices provide temporary support during pulmonary failure due to disease, injury, or lack of development in premature infants. The latest development has been the appearance of an intravenous membrane oxygenator based upon a bundle of hollow fiber membranes (148).

Polymer membranes made of cellulose acetate are used industrially to separate CO_2 from natural gas. A variety of other polymer membranes are being studied for their ability to improve gas separation processes (149). There is reason to believe that some of these polymers may be well suited to separating CO_2 from the breathing gas in UBA (150). This raises the possibility of developing a UBA with a $ECCO_2R$ device in the place of a CO_2-absorbent canister.

D. Artificial Gills

The advent of membrane gas-exchange devices, either intracorporeal or extracorporeal, could ultimately result in UBAs that provide measured doses of O_2 from compressed or liquified gas supplies while simultaneously removing CO_2. In addition, if a diver's lungs were filled with an incompressible fluid such as one of the many perfluorocarbons, then an inert gas supply would not be needed to counterbalance the compressing effects of depth. Divers could both descend and ascend as rapidly as they wished without risk of decompression sickness or arterial gas embolism. Of course, such a form of diving requires a considerable personal commitment from the diver. The topic of liquid breathing and artificial gills is addressed in detail in Chap. 11.

E. High-Frequency Ventilation

Hypoventilation and CO_2 retention is a physiological response to the high respiratory impedances encountered while breathing dense gas (Chaps. 2 and 4). High frequency ventilation (HFV) is a form of assisted ventilation that applies small volume oscillations to either the chest wall or airway opening at frequencies between 2 and 45 Hz. Even though the delivered oscillatory tidal volumes may be smaller than anatomical dead space, the resulting convection augments gaseous diffusion many fold over what it would have been in the absence of HFV. A detailed discussion of HFV's role in clinical applications is found in Vol. 26 of this series.

At 1 atm, a large percentage of the energy transmitted to human airways via the mouth by a high frequency oscillator is shunted by upper-airway gas compression. Due perhaps to these inefficiencies, HFV finds its greatest use in neonates where ventilation requirements are low, and both convection and diffusion distances are short. Lunkenheimer et al. (151) found that prolonged HFV can be effective in animals the size of adult humans, but only with high bias flow rates, adequate mean airway pressures, and powerful ventilators. It is not known if high-frequency percussive ventilation, of use in patients with inhalation injury (152), will be more adaptable to the diving environment. However, that possibility is worth exploring.

In theory, the efficiency of HFV should increase when upper-airway shunting is reduced by pressure induced decreases in gas compressibility. The effect of reduced gas compressibility on gas exchange within the intrathoracic airways is not known. However, there is some evidence that elevations in gas density alone do not impede the efficiency of HFV once changes in airway impedance are taken into account (153–155).

Of course the ultimate in incompressible fluids is a liquid. One might speculate that the superposition of high-frequency pressure oscillations to a perfluorocarbon-filled lung might enhance CO_2 transport during liquid breathing. Therefore, the use of high-frequency ventilators as a component of future UBA, with either gas- or liquid-filled lungs, remains an intriguing possibility.

F. Reactive Impedance Reduction

In the past 25 years, the manufacturers of diving equipment have reduced the resistive work of breathing of diving equipment. Those improvements have come primarily by increasing the sizes of hoses and restrictions through which a diver must breathe. In SCUBA, venturi assistance has reduced the effort required for inhalation. However, while breathing resistance has been reduced, elastic impedances remain.

Future closed-circuit UBA may incorporate on-board computers not only to control gas concentrations within the UBA but also to continuously tune the device to present a minimal mechanical impedance to the diver. One mechanism for doing this is to continuously compute and adjust the inertance that would be required to cancel UBA elastance (78). The result would be a purely resistive, and therefore minimal, UBA impedance (Sec. V.B). Such a device would be ''reactive'' not only because it would eliminate so-called reactive or frequency dependent impedance but also because it would continuously react to the diver's breathing pattern. The technological challenge will be to accomplish this in a manner that does not coincidentally increase resistance and in a mechanism that can survive the abuses of diving.

References

1. Eley JH Jr, Myers J. Study of a photosynthetic gas exchanger, a quantitative repetition of the Priestly experiment. Texas J Sci 1964; 16:296–333.
2. Bovee HH, Pilgrim AJ, Sun LS, et al. Large algal systems. In: Prince AE, Kitzes G, eds. Biologistics for Space Systems Symposium. Report AMRL-TDR-62-116. Aerospace Medical Division, Wright-Patterson Air Force Base, Dayton, Ohio, 1962.

3. Arnett RH Jr. American Insects, A Handbook of the Insects of America North of Mexico. Gainesville, FL: Sandhill Crane Press, 1993.
4. Mafan R, Mafan K. Spiders of the World. New York: Facts on File Publications, 1984.
5. U.S. Navy Diving Manual, Vol. 1. Washington, DC: U.S. Navy, 1979.
6. DuBois AB, Brody AW, Lewis DH, Burgess BF Jr. Oscillation mechanics of lungs and chest in man. J Appl Physiol 1956; 8:587–594.
7. Mead J, Milic-Emili J. Theory and methodology in respiratory mechanics with glossary of symbols. In: Fenn WO, Rahn H, eds. Handbook of Physiology: Respiration I. Washington, DC: American Physiological Society, 1964:363–376.
8. Barlow HB, MacIntosh FC. Shallow water blackout. Royal Navy Physiological Laboratory Report RNP 44/125 UPS 48(a), 1944.
9. Lanphier EH, ed. The Unconscious Diver: Respiratory Control and Other Contributing Factors. Bethesda, MD: Undersea Medical Society, 1982.
10. Mead J. Measurement of inertia of the lungs at increased ambient pressure. J Appl Physiol 1956; 9:208–212.
11. Baiss D, Southerland DG, Clarke JR. MK 3 Mod 0 Lightweight Dive System (LWDS) Air Flow Capacity. Navy Experimental Diving Unit Technical Report 12-95, 1995.
12. Thalmann ED. Determination of the adequacy of helmet ventilation in a prototype Navy MK-12 and the MK-5 hard hat diving apparatus. Navy Experimental Diving Unit Technical Report 16-74, 1974.
13. Flynn ET, Catron PW, Bayne CG. Diving Medical Officer Student Guide, 2d ed. Course A-6A-0010. Washington, DC: U.S. Naval School Diving and Salvage, 1981: 6–2.
14. Camperman J. Investigation of Carbon Dioxide Transport in Life Support Helmets. Ph.D. dissertation. Boca Raton, FL: Florida Atlantic University, 1995.
15. Andersson L, Bengtstrom C, Dahlback GO, et al. Unmanned Testing of the Bailout system in a Deep Diving Helmet. Report R11:0983. Goteborg, Sweden: Division of Underwater Technology, Chalmers University of Technology, 1983.
16. Ross CM. Evaluation of the Gates 33 HB ⅜ inch ID Divers Umbilical for Use with the MK 20 and MK 21 Mod 1 UBA. NEDU Technical Memorandum 91-10, 1991.
17. Larson HE. A History of Self-Contained Diving and Underwater Swimming. NAS/NRC Publication 469. Washington, DC: National Academy of Sciences, 1959.
18. James AT. Mathematical modeling of Conshelf XIV demand regulator (U.S. Divers Co.). Document TP2152, Somerset, U.K.: Normalair-Garett Limited, 1982.
19. Lundgren C. A physiologist's approach to breathing gear design. In: Proceedings of First Annual Canadian Ocean Technology Congress. Toronto: March 11–12, 1982; 216–243.
20. Dwyer JV. FLATUS mixed-gas SCUBA. Navy Experimental Diving Unit Formal Report 13-54, 1954.
21. Hollingsworth WC. FLATUS II semi-closed circuit mixed gas SCUBA. Navy Experimental Diving Unit Report 6-56, 1956.
22. Searle WF. A history of man's deep submergence. United States Naval Institute Proceedings 1966; 92:80–92.

23. Harter JV. Orifice selection in semi-closed circuit mixed gas underwater breathing apparatus. Navy Experimental Diving Unit Research Report 1-67, 1967.
24. Riegel PS, Harter JV. Design of breathing apparatus for diving to great depths. ASME Paper 69-De-22. New York: American Society of Mechanical Engineers, 1969.
25. Nuckols ML, Tucker WC, Sarich AJ. Life Support Systems Design—Diving and Hyperbaric Applications. Needham Heights, MA: Simon & Schuster, 1996.
26. Clarke JR, Knafelc ME, Junker DL, Allain SC. Evaluation of the Fullerton Sherwood S-24 (SIVA) semi-closed underwater breathing apparatus. Navy Experimental Diving Unit Technical Report 9-96, 1996.
27. U.S. Navy Diving Manual: Vol. 2. Mixed-Gas Diving. Change 1 to Revision 1, Navy Department, Washington, 1982.
28. Giry P, Galland FM, Meliet SL. Measurement of FIO_2 and $FetO_2$ during dives of ten minutes at 80 meters, using MIXGERS UBA equipped with a new injector. Centre d'Etudes et de Recherches Biophysiologigues Appliquees a la Marine, Toulon FR. 1988; CERB Report 88-12.
29. Oshima S, Takahashi M, Shirane Y, Hatsumoto K. Development of a semi-closed underwater breathing apparatus, the "OBA." Ann Physiol Anthropol (Jpn) 1990; 9:299–304.
30. Kakitsuba N, Nakayama H. Evaluation of a semi-closed underwater breathing apparatus, the "OBA." Ann Physiol Anthropol (Jpn) 1990; 9:305–310.
31. Edmonds C, Lowry C, Pennefather J. Diving and Subaquatic Medicine, 3d ed. Oxford, England: Butterworth-Heinemann, 1992.
32. Foregger R. Development of mine rescue and underwater breathing apparatus: Appliances of Henry Fleuss. J Hist Med Allied Sci 1974; 29:317–330.
33. Bauer JA, Bauer SE. The hard-hat diving helmet. In: Bachrach AJ, Desiderati BM, Matzen MM, eds. A Pictorial History of Diving. San Pedro, CA: Best Publishing, 1988:16–37.
34. Nuckols ML. Oxygen levels in closed-circuit UBAs during descent. Life Supp Biosphere Sci 1996; 2:117–124.
35. Fischel H. Closed-circuit cryogenic SCUBA. In: Mitchell EB, ed. Equipment for the Working Diver: 1970 Symposium. Washington, DC: Marine Technology Society, 1970:229–244.
36. Lundgren CEG. Applying physiology in the design of breathing gear for divers. In: Lin Y-C, Niu AKC, eds. Hyperbaric Physiology and Medicine. San Pedro, CA: Best Publishing, 1988:155–170.
37. Sisman D, ed. The Professional Diver's Handbook, 2d ed. Houston: Gulf Publishing, 1985.
38. Kotz JC, Purcell KF. Chemistry and Chemical Reactivity, 2d ed. Philadelphia: Saunders, 1990.
39. Lower BR. Removal of CO_2 from closed-circuit breathing apparatus. In: Mitchell EB, ed. Equipment for the Working Diver: 1970 Symposium. Washington, DC: Marine Technology Society, 1970:261–282.
40. Middleton JR. A comparison of the relative merits of Baralyme and Sodasorb. Navy Experimental Diving Unit Technical Report 12-78, 1978.
41. Nuckols ML, Purer A, Deason GA. Design Guidelines for Carbon Dioxide Scrub-

bers. NCSC TechMan 4110-1-83A. Panama City, FL: Naval Coastal Systems Center, 1985.

42. Purer A, Deason GA, Hammonds BH, Nuckols ML. The effects of pressure and particle size on CO_2 absorption characteristics of high performance Sodasorb. NCSC Technical Memorandum TM 349-82. Panama City, FL: Naval Coastal Systems Center, 1982.
43. Riley RL, Shepard RH, Cohn JE, et al: Maximal diffusing capacity of the lungs. J Appl Physiol 1954; 6:573–587.
44. Wagner PD, West JB. Effects of diffusion impairment on O_2 and CO_2 time courses in pulmonary capillaries. J Appl Physiol 1972; 33:62–71.
45. Piiper J. Alveolar-capillary gas transfer in lungs: Development of concepts and current state. Adv Exp Med Biol 1994; 345:7–14.
46. MacGregor CD, Fraser MG. The effect of pressure on the efficiency of carbon dioxide absorbents. In: Nuckols ML, Smith KA, eds. The Characterization of Carbon Dioxide Absorbing Agents for Life Support Equipment. New York: American Society of Mechanical Engineers, 1982:75–82.
47. Radic SB, Gosovic NM. Effect of ambient pressure and diluent gas on CO_2 chemisorbtion by soda lime. In: Schmutz J, Wendling J, eds. Proceedings of the joint meeting of the 3rd Swiss Symposium on Hyperbaric Medicine and XVIII European Union of the Undersea Biomedical Society (EUBS). Basel: Foundation for Hyperbaric Medicine, 1992.
48. Lin MJ, Jaeger MJ. CO_2 binding by Baralyme in three different carrier gases. Undersea Hyperbar Med 1994; 21:329–340.
49. Elandt-Johnson RG, Johnson NL. Survival Models and Data Analysis. New York: Wiley, 1980.
50. Weathersby PK, Survanshi SS, Homer LD, et al. Predicting the time of occurrence of decompression sickness. J Appl Physiol 1992; 72:1541–1548.
51. Harabin AL, Survanshi SS, Homer LD. A model for predicting central nervous system oxygen toxicity from hyperbaric oxygen exposures in humans. Toxicol Appl Pharmacol 1995; 132:19–26.
52. Clarke JR, Rainone M. Evaluation of Sherwood SCUBA regulators for use in cold water. Navy Experimental Diving Unit Technical Report 9-95, 1995.
53. Warkander DE. Ergonomics of Breathing Apparatus, with Special Reference to Work of Breathing, Dead Space and Breathing Resistance. Ph.D. dissertation. Göteborg, Sweden: Chalmers University of Technology, 1994.
54. Clarke JR, Fisher MA, Jaeger MJ. Inertance as a factor in uneven ventilation in diving. In: Bachrach AJ, Matzen MM, eds. Underwater Physiology. VII: Proceedings of the Seventh Symposium on Underwater Physiology. Bethesda, MD: Undersea Medical Society, 1981:225–233.
55. Van Liew HD. The electrical-respiratory analogy when gas density is high. Undersea Biomed Res 1987; 14:149–160.
56. Van Liew HD. Components of the pressure required to breathe dense gas. Undersea Biomed Res 1987; 14:263–276.
57. Cooper EA. Suggested methods of testing and standards of resistance for respiratory protective devices. J Appl Physiol 1960; 15:1053–1061.
58. Pedley TJ, Schroter RC, Sudlow MF. Gas flow and mixing in the airways. In: West

JB, ed. Bioengineering Aspects of the Lung. New York: Marcel Dekker, 1977:163–265.
59. Clarke JR, Jaeger MJ, Zumrick JL, et al. Respiratory resistance from 1 to 46 ATA measured with the interrupter technique. J Appl Physiol 1982; 52:549–555.
60. Middleton JR. Evaluation of commercially available open circuit SCUBA regulators. Navy Experimental Diving Unit Technical Report 2-80, 1980.
61. Giedraitis RB, Crepeau LJ. Evaluation of Carleton Technology Incorporated mouthpiece utilized in LAR V UBA with two grades of Sofnolime CO_2 absorbent. Navy Experimental Diving Unit Technical Report 2-92, 1992.
62. Zwingelberg KM, Jaeger MJ. Application of a valveless anesthesia circuit for deep diving. Undersea Hyperbar Med 1994; 21:443–458.
63. Pope H, Holloway R, Campbell EJM. The effects of elastic and resistive loading of inspiration on the breathing of conscious man. Respir Physiol 1968; 4:363–372.
64. D'Urzo AD, Chapman KR, Rebuck AS. Effect of elastic loading on ventilatory pattern during progressive exercise. J Appl Physiol 1985; 59:34–38.
65. Clarke JR, Vila D, Cabeca A, et al. The testing of physiological design criteria for underwater breathing apparatus (UBA). In: Diving and Hyperbaric Medicine, Proc 15th European Undersea Biomedical Society (E.U.B.S.), Israeli Navy Publications 1989:171–176.
66. Morrison JB, Reimers SD. Design principles of underwater breathing apparatus. In: Bennett PB, Elliott DH, eds. The Physiology and Medicine of Diving, 3d ed. London: Bailliére Tindall, 1982.
67. Fishman AP, ed. Handbook of Physiology: Sec 3. The Respiratory System. Bethesda, MD: American Physiological Society, 1986.
68. Lanphier EH, Camporesi EM. Respiration and exercise. In: Bennett PB Elliott DH, eds. The Physiology and Medicine of Diving. San Pedro, CA: Best Publishing, 1982:99–156.
69. Morrison JB, Reimers SD. Design principles of underwater breathing apparatus. In: Bennett PB, Elliott DH, eds. The Physiology and Medicine of Diving. San Pedro, CA: Best Publishing, 1982:55–98.
70. Peslin R, Fredberg JJ. Oscillation mechanics in the respiratory system. In: Fishman AP, ed. Handbook of Physiology: Sec 3. The Respiratory System. Bethesda, MD: American Physiological Society, 1984:145–177.
71. Michaelson ED, Grassman ED, Peters WR. Pulmonary mechanics by spectral analysis of forced random noise. J Clin Invest 1975; 56:1210–1230.
72. Sharp JT, Henry JP, Sweany SK, et al. Total respiratory inertance and its gas and tissue components in normal and obese men. J Clin Invest 1964; 43:503–509.
73. Brown LK, Schwartz J, Miller A, et al. Respiratory drive and pattern during inertially-loaded CO_2 rebreathing: Implications for models of respiratory mechanics in obesity. Respir Physiol 1990; 80:231–243.
74. Peterson RE, Wright WB. Pulmonary mechanical functions in man breathing dense gas mixtures at high ambient pressures—Predictive Studies II. In: Lambertsen CJ, ed. Underwater Physiology. V: Proceedings of the Fifth Symposium on Underwater Physiology. Bethesda, MD: Federation of American Societies for Experimental Biology, 1976:67–77.
75. Clarke JR, Fisher MA, Jaeger MJ. Inertance as a factor in uneven ventilation in

diving. In: Bachrach AJ, Matzen MM, eds. Proceedings of the Seventh Symposium of Underwater Physiology. Bethesda: Undersea Medical Society, 1981:225–233.

76. Clarke JR, Survanshi S, Flynn ET. Respiratory waveform efficiency during the use of underwater breathing apparatus (UBA) (abstr) Undersea Biom Res 1990; 17(suppl):31.
77. Clarke JR. Impedance and power measurements in the testing of closed-circuit UBA. In: Flook V, Brubakk AO, eds. Lung Physiology and Diver's Breathing Apparatus. Aberdeen: BPCC-AUP, 1992:85–99.
78. Clarke JR, Joye DD, Carlson NA, Wechgelaer P. Reactive, Closed-Circuit Underwater Breathing Apparatus. U.S. Patent No. 5,315,988. Washington DC: U.S. Patent Office, 1994.
79. Joye DD, Mints WH, Clarke JR, Wechgelaer P. Manually Tunable, Closed-Circuit Underwater Breathing Apparatus. U.S. Patent No. 5,485,834. Washington DC: U.S. Patent Office, 1996.
80. Warkander DE, Lundgren CEG. Respiratory performance in divers during exposure to combinations of ventilatory impediments (abstr). Undersea Hyperbar Med 1993; 20(suppl):36–37.
81. Warkander DE, Lundgren CEG. Effects of graded combinations resistance and elastance on divers' respiratory performance (abstr). Undersea Hyperbar Med 1994; 21(suppl):96–97.
82. Warkander DE, Lundgren CEG. Effects of combinations of resistance and elastance on divers' respiratory performance during exposure to a negative static load (abstr). Undersea Hyperbar Med 1995; 22(suppl):71.
83. Warkander DE, Lundgren CEG. Effects of graded combinations of resistance and elastance on divers' respiratory performance during exposure to a positive static load (abstr). Undersea Hyperbar Med 1996; 23(suppl):17.
84. Silverman L, Lee G, Yancey AR, et al. Fundamental Factors in the Design of Respiratory Equipment: A Study and an Evaluation of Inspiratory and Expiratory Resistances for Protective Respiratory Equipment. Bulletin 5339. Washington DC: Office of Scientific Research and Development, 1945.
85. Mead J. Resistance to breathing at increased ambient pressures. In: Goff LG, ed. Proceedings of the Symposium on Underwater Physiology. Washington, DC: National Academy of Sciences/National Research Council 1955:112–120.
86. Senneck CR. Breathing apparatus for use in mines. In: Davies CN, ed. Design and Use of Respirators. Oxford: Pergamon Press, 1962:143–159.
87. Bentley RA, Griffin OG, Love RG, et al. Acceptable levels for breathing resistance of respiratory apparatus, Arch Environ Health 1973, 27:273–280.
88. Middleton JR, Thalmann ED. Standardized NEDU unmanned test procedures and performance goals. Navy Experimental Diving Unit Technical Report 3-81, 1981.
89. Warkander DE, Norfleet WT, Nagasawa GK, Lundgren CEG. Physiologically and subjectively acceptable breathing resistance in divers' breathing gear. Undersea Biomed Res 1992; 19(6):427–445.
90. Bradley ME. The interaction of stresses in diving and adaptation to these stresses. In: Human Performance and SCUBA Diving. Proceedings of the Symposium on Underwater Physiology, La Jolla, CA, April 10–11, 1970. Chicago: The Athletic Institute, 1970:63–69.

91. Lanphier EH. Physiological considerations in design of breathing apparatus. In: Submarine Medical Practice, NAVMED P-5054. Washington: US Govt. Printing Office, 1956:185–210.
92. Department of the Navy Military Specification MIL-R-24169A.
93. Cain CC, Otis AB. Some physiological effects resulting from added resistance to respiration. J Aviat Med 1949; 20:149–160.
94. Robinet C, Calas P, Giry P. Tolérance aux résistances ventilatoires asymétriques. CERB Report 91-14. Toulon, France: Centre D'Études et de Recherches Biophysiologigues Appliquées a La Marine, 1991.
95. Silverman L, Lee G, Plotkin T, et al. Air flow measurements on human subjects with and without respiratory resistance at several work rates. Arch Indust Hyg Occup Med 1951; 3:461–478.
96. Clarke J. The transformation of work of breathing measurements to estimates of flow resistance (abstr). Undersea Hyperbar Med 1995; 22(suppl):26.
97. Clarke JR. Measurement of average resistance in underwater breathing apparatus. American Society of Mechanical Engineers. In: Conference Papers of Energy Week '96, Book 3, Vol. 2, 1996:227–230.
98. U.S. Navy Unmanned Test Methods and Performance Goals for Underwater Breathing Apparatus. Navy Experimental Diving Unit Technical Manual 1-94, 1994.
99. Reimers SD. Proposed standards for the evaluation of breathing resistance of underwater breathing apparatus. Navy Experimental Diving Unit Report 19-73, 1973.
100. Clarke JR, Survanshi S, Thalmann ED, Flynn ET. Limits for mouth pressure in underwater breathing apparatus (UBA). In: Lundgren CEG, Warkander DE, eds. Physiological and Human Engineering Aspects of Underwater Breathing Apparatus. Bethesda, MD: Undersea and Hyperbaric Medical Society, 1989:21–32.
101. Clarke JR. Diver tolerance to respiratory loading during wet and dry dives from 0 to 450 m. In: Flook V, Brubakk AO, eds. Lung Physiology and Diver's Breathing Apparatus. Aberdeen: BPCC-AUP, 1992:33–44.
102. Fothergill DM, Carlson NA. Effects of N_2O narcosis on breathing and effort sensations during exercise and inspiratory resistive loading. J Appl Physiol 1996; 81: 1562–1571.
103. Fothergill DM, Carlson NA. The roles of gas density, high pressure, and inert gas narcosis on exercise tolerance and psychophysical perceptions of exertion (abstr). Undersea Hyperbar Med 1995; 22(suppl):70.
104. Joye DD, Clarke JR, Carlson NA, Thalmann ED. Characterization and measurement of elastance with application to underwater breathing apparatus. Undersea Hyperbar Med 1994; 21:53–65.
105. Cala SJ, Wilcox P, Edyvean J, et al. Oxygen cost of inspiratory loading: Resistive vs. elastic. J Appl Physiol 1991; 70:1983–1990.
106. Campbell EJM, Dickenson CJ, Howell JBL. The immediate effects of elastic loads on the breathing of man. J Physiol (Lond) 1961; 156:260–273.
107. Freedman S, Campbell FJM. The ability of normal subjects to tolerate added inspiratory loads. Respir Physiol 1970; 10:213–235.
108. Daubenspeck JA. Influence of small mechanical loads on variability of breathing pattern. J Appl Physiol 1981; 50:99–106.

109. Killian KJ, Bucens DD, Campbell EJM. Effect of breathing patterns on the perceived magnitude of added loads to breathing. J Appl Physiol 1982; 52:578–584.
110. Rohrer F. Physiologie der Atembewegung. In: Bethe ATJ et al., eds. Handbuch der normalen und pathologische Physiologie. Berlin: Springer, 1925:70–127.
111. Otis AB, Fenn WO, Rahn H. The mechanics of breathing in man. J Appl Physiol 1950; 2:592–607.
112. McIlroy MB, Eldridge FL, Thomas JP, Christie RV. The effect of added elastic and non-elastic resistance on the pattern of breathing in normal subjects. Clin Sci 1955; 14:18–25.
113. Puddy A, Younes M. Effect of slowly increasing elastic load on breathing in conscious humans. J Appl Physiol 1991; 70:1277–1283.
114. DiMarco AF, Kelsen SG, Cherniak NS, et al. Effects on breathing of selective restriction of movement of the rib cage and abdomen. J Appl Physiol 1981; 50: 412–420.
115. Chonan T, Hida W, Kikuchi Y, et al. Effects of elastic loading and exercise on pulmonary gas exchange in dogs. Tohoku J Exp Med 1991; 164:157–167.
116. D'Urzo AD, Chapman KR, Rebuck AS. Effect of elastic loading on ventilatory pattern during progressive exercise. J Appl Physiol 1985; 59:34–38.
117. Flynn ET, Camporesi EM, Nunneley SA. Cardiopulmonary responses to pressure breathing during immersion in water. In: Lanphier EH, Rahn H, eds. Man, Water, Pressure, II. Dept of Physiology, School of Medicine, State University of New York at Buffalo, Buffalo, NY 1975:78–94.
118. Morrison JB, Butt WS. Effect of underwater breathing apparatus and absolute air pressure on diver's ventilatory capacity. Aerospace Med 1972; 43:881–886.
119. Thalmann ED, Sponholtz DK, Lundgren CEG. Effects of immersion and static lung loading on submerged exercise at depth. Undersea Biomed Res 1979; 6:259–290.
120. Agostoni EG, Gurtner G, Torri G, Rahn H. Respiratory mechanics during submersion and negative-pressure breathing. J Appl Physiol 1966; 21:251–258.
121. Hong SK, Cerretelli P, Cruz JC, Rahn H. Mechanics of respiration during submersion in water. J Appl Physiol 1969; 27:535–538.
122. Lanphier EH, Camporesi EM. Respiration and exertion In: Bennett PB, Elliott DH, eds. The Physiology and Medicine of Diving, 4th ed. London: Saunders, 1993:77–120.
123. Taylor NAS, Morrison JB. Lung centroid pressure in immersed man. Undersea Biomed Res 1989; 16:3–19.
124. Thompson LJ, McCally M. Role of transpharyngeal pressure gradients in determining intrapulmonary pressure during immersion. Aerospace Med 1967, 38:931–935.
125. Carlson NA. Effect of Static Lung Loading during Immersion on Breathing Pattern and Dyspnea. Ph.D. dissertation. Madison, WI: University of Wisconsin, 1987.
126. Taylor NAS. Effect of Breathing Gas Pressure on Respiratory Mechanics on Immersed Man. Ph.D. dissertation. Burnaby, BC: Simon Fraser University, 1987.
127. Derion T, Reddan WG, Lanphier EH. Static lung load and posture effects on pulmonary mechanics and comfort in underwater exercise. Undersea Biomed Res 1992; 19:85–96.

128. Stigler R. Die Kraft unserer Inspirationmuskulatur. Pflugers Arch 1911; 139:234–254.
129. Risch WD, Koubenec HJ, Beckman U, et al. The effect of graded immersion on heart volume, central venous pressure, pulmonary blood distribution, and heart rate in man. Pflugers Arch 1978; 374:115–118.
130. Risch WD, Koubenec HJ, Gauer OH, Lange S. Time course of cardiac distension with rapid immersion in a thermo-neutral bath. Pflugers Arch 1978; 374:119–120.
131. Stevens SS. The surprising simplicity of sensory metrics. Am Psychol 1962; 17: 29–39.
132. Stevens SS. Intensity functions in sensory systems. Int J Neurol 1967; 6:202–209.
133. Borg GAV. Physical performance and perceived exerction. Stud Psychol Paedog 1962; 11:1–64.
134. Geldard FA. The Human Senses, 2d ed. New York: Wiley, 1972.
135. Clarke JR, Knafelc ME, Junker DL, Allain SC. Evaluation of the Draeger Extreme semi-closed underwater breathing apparatus. Navy Experimental Diving Unit Technical Report 7-96, 1996.
136. Tilley DG, Livesey J, Tomlinson SP, Himmens IA. An approach to the modeling of underwater breathing apparatus. In: Lundgren CEG, Warkander DE, eds. Physiological and Human Engineering Aspects of Underwater Breathing Apparatus. Bethesda, MD: Undersea and Hyperbaric Medical Society, 1989:125–137.
137. Tomlinson SP, Livesey J, Tilley DG, Himmens IA. Computer simulation of counterlungs. Undersea Hyperbar Med 1993; 20:63–73.
138. Sexton PG, Nuckols ML. Computer simulation of breathing systems for divers. Trans ASME 1983; 105:54–59.
139. Antoon TA, Middleton JR, Nuckols ML. Breathing dynamics of a surface-supplied diving system with demand flow. In: McGuinness T, Shih HH, eds. Current Practices and New Technology in Ocean Engineering. New York: The American Society of Mechanical Engineers, 1986:307–313.
140. Mittleman J. Computer modeling of underwater breathing systems. In: Lundgren CEG, Warkander DE, eds. Physiological and Human Engineering Aspects of Underwater Breathing Apparatus. Bethesda, MD: Undersea and Hyperbaric Medical Society, 1989:225–270.
141. Tuinenga PW. SPICE, A Guide to Circuit Simulation & Analysis Using PSpice. Englewood Cliffs, NJ: Prentice-Hall, 1988.
142. Kielkowski R. Inside SPICE. New York: McGraw-Hill, 1994.
143. Gafford RD, Greene MW. Monitoring carbon dioxide partial pressures in semiclosed underwater breathing systems. In: Mitchell EB, ed. Equipment for the Working Diver: 1970 Symposium. Washington, DC: Marine Technology Society, 1970:283–297.
144. Vayenas CG, Ioannides A, Bebelis S. Solid electrolyte cyclic voltammetry for *in situ* investigation of catalyst surfaces. J Catal 1991; 129:67–87.
145. Vogt MC, Shoemaker EL, MacShane DA, Turner T. An intelligent gas microsensor employing neural network technology. Sensors 1996; 13(9):54–62.
146. Vogt MC, Shoemaker EL, Dudek PJ. Cyclic voltammetry applied to an oxygen-ion-conducting solid electrolyte as an active electrocatalytic gas sensor. In: Solid State Ionics 1996; 92:285–292.

147. Kolobow T, Bowman RL. Construction and evaluation of an alveolar membrane artificial lung machine. Trans Am Soc Artif Intern Organs 1963; 9:238–243.
148. Hattler BG, Reeder GD, Sawzik PJ, et al. Development of an intravenous membrane oxygenator: enhanced intravenous gas exchange through convective mixing of blood around hollow fiber membranes. Artif Organs 1994; 18:806–812.
149. Stern SA. New developments in membrane processes for gas separations. In: Chenoweth MB, ed. Synthetic Membranes. New York: Harwood Academic, 1986: 1–37.
150. Stern SA, Lokhandwala KA. Development of membrane process for carbon dioxide separation from diving atmosphere. NCSC Contractor Report CR-20C-1-90. 1990.
151. Lunkenheimer PP, Redmann K, Stroh N, et al. High-frequency oscillation in an adult porcine model. Crit Care Med 1994; 22:S37–S48.
152. Cioffi WG Jr, Rue LW III, Graves TA, et al. Prophylactic use of high-frequency percussive ventilation in patients with inhalation injury. Ann Surg 1991; 213:575–580.
153. McCarthy EJ. The Effect of Gas Density on Gas Transport During High Frequency Ventilation. Ph.D. dissertation. Bethesda, MD: Uniformed Services University of the Health Sciences, 1985.
154. Clarke JR, Homer LD, Flynn ET, Bradley ME. Tracheal pressure and impedance as determinants of gas exchange during high frequency ventilation. Respir Physiol 1987; 68:121–136.
155. Jaeger MJ. High-frequency ventilation in dogs with three gases of different densities. J Appl Physiol 1991; 70:2188–2192.

13

Human Breath-Hold Diving

MASSIMO FERRIGNO

Brigham and Women's Hospital
and Harvard Medical School
Boston, Massachusetts

CLAES E. G. LUNDGREN

State University of New York
at Buffalo
Buffalo, New York

I. Introduction

A. Historical Background

The history of breath-hold diving is probably as old as the history of our species. Men and women have been diving for thousands of years to gather a variety of products, including food, sponges, and mother-of-pearl; to conduct salvage and military operations; and to explore. According to the Greek historian Herodotus, a diver named Scyllis was hired by the Persian King Xerxes to recover sunken treasures in the fifth century B.C. A few centuries later, halfway around the world, along the coasts of Japan and Korea, male and female divers (Ama) began to harvest food, collecting seaweed and shellfish (1). Thousands of mostly female Japanese and Korean breath-hold divers are still using techniques developed over 2000 years, diving down to a maximum of about 20 m, typically for no more than a minute at a time, with an excellent safety record. Professional breath-hold divers are also active in other parts of the world—e.g., in Indonesia (2) and, at least until recently, in the South Pacific, where pearl divers have been known to operate down to 40 m of depth, but not without accidents (3). The history of breath-hold diving lists dives to amazingly great depths. In 1913 Georghios Kaggí, a Greek sponge diver, made several dives down to 80 m of depth (more than 260 ft) to recover the lost anchor of the Italian battleship *Regina Margherita* (4). However, it was not until after World War II that breath-hold diving to great depths became an international sport, with new records established almost every year (Fig. 1) (5). Recently, several divers, including a woman, have dived down to more than 100 m (330 ft). The current record is 133 m (440 ft), set in November 1996 by Francisco ''Pipin'' Ferreras. Typically, these deep dives last around 3 to 3.5 min.

This chapter focuses on the respiratory mechanisms involved in human adaptation and on the limitations to breath-hold diving. In considering the ex-

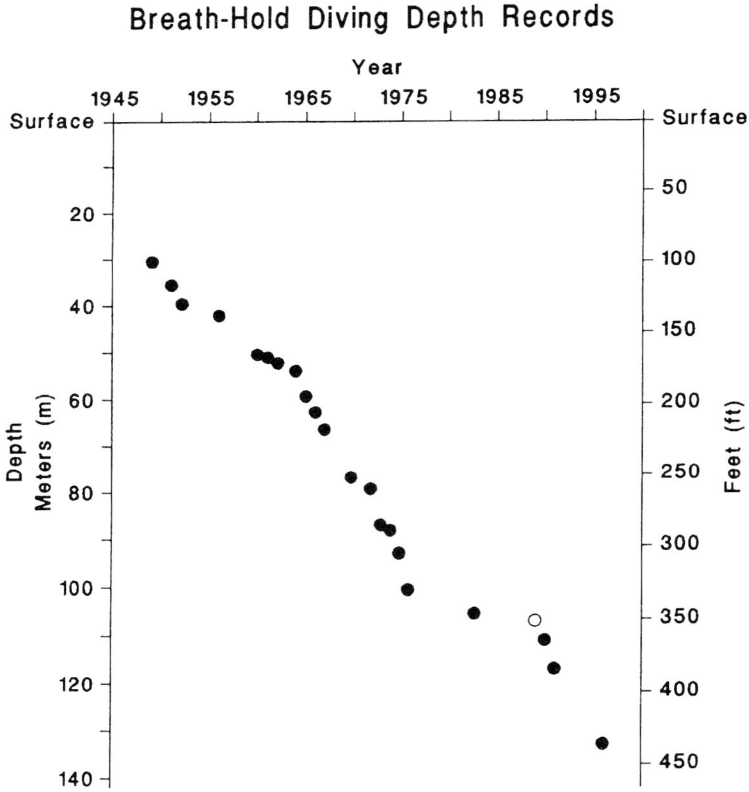

Figure 1 Depths reached in breath-hold dives over roughly a 50-year period. The record in 1989, represented by a circle, was set by a female diver. The data for this graph were derived from a multitude of mostly nonscientific sources and are not necessarily complete, although the deepest dive, to 133 m, performed in 1996, was current as of early 1998.

perimental evidence on which our understanding of the physiology of breath-hold diving is based, one should be aware of the potential problems inherent in applying data obtained in laboratory experiments to the real in-the-sea situation. The former setting is typically designed so as to isolate a particular stimulus and the responses to it, while actual diving exposes the diver to multiple and often conflicting influences. So, for instance, has the diving response in many studies been investigated during breath-holding and immersion of only the face in cold water, while in actual diving the whole body may be exposed to cold water, with potentially very different effects on respiratory drive and the circulation. Moreover, gas exchange in the lung during breath-holding at one atmosphere is quite different than during the drastic changes in ambient pressure encountered in a deep dive.

B. The Environment

As a diver descends underwater, the hydrostatic pressure acting on the body increases by 14.7 psi (1 atm) for every 33 ft of depth. For example, at 99 ft the ambient pressure will be the sum of the atmospheric pressure (1 atm) plus the hydrostatic pressure (3 atm), that is, 4 atm. Applying Boyle's law, the gas volume in a breath-hold diver's lungs will be compressed to one-fourth of the volume it had at the surface and, as a consequence, the pressure of alveolar gases will be increased four times. Also related to the changes in hydrostatic pressure during diving is the need to equilibrate pressure across the eardrums (''ear clearing'') and in the paranasal sinuses. This often involves repeated Valsalva maneuvers during descent to depth. Because the relative rate of change in pressure (and consequently in volume) is greater at shallow depths and decreases exponentially with increasing depth, ear-clearing maneuvers are required more frequently in the early phases of descent.

Commonly, immersion in water entails a cold stress for the diver, who may become hypothermic if unprotected. Water temperature in the sea varies not only with geographical location and season but also with increasing depth. For example, at the beginning of summer, a diver in the Mediterranean Sea may be exposed to a water temperature of 22°C at the surface, while at 40 m it may be about 15°C. Immersion, submersion, and depth-related pressure changes have important effects on the blood circulation. These hemodynamic changes may profoundly influence respiratory function of the breath-hold diver. During head-out immersion (discussed in Chap. 3), the hydrostatic pressure counteracts the pooling of blood in the dependent regions of the body (present in air due to the gravity force), thus causing a redistribution of blood into the chest. This redistribution, which also may occur during breath-hold diving, is crucial in achieving great depths, as discussed in Sec. II. A: ''The Challenge: Depth.'' The role of changes in water pressure is also presented in Sec. II. A: as well as in Sec. II.

B: ''Oxygen'' and ''Carbon Dioxide Stores.'' The use of these stores is influenced by submersion as described under ''The Diving Response,'' also in Sec. II. B.

II. The Challenge

Whether breath-hold diving is performed as a profession or a sport, productivity or success depends on two intimately coupled aspects, namely the diver's tolerance to the stresses of depth (high ambient pressure) and on his/her breath-holding endurance.

A. Depth

The Total Lung Capacity/Residual Volume Ratio

During a breath-hold dive, the gas-containing cavities of the body may be exposed to large and rapid changes in ambient pressure. Initially, predictions of the maximal depths that a diver could reach were based on the application of Boyle's law to lung volumes. According to the concept of ''thoracic squeeze,'' the diver could descend safely only to the depth at which his or her lungs had been compressed to residual volume (RV). That means that, if a diver started breath-hold at total lung capacity (TLC), the maximal depth could be predicted by the diver's TLC/RV ratio. However, as pointed out by Rahn (6), in predicting maximal depth, Boyle's law should also be applied to the rigid volumes of the upper airways and face mask. Agostoni (7) in his calculations of the TLC/RV of the Japanese Ama included the decrease in lung volume due to gas exchange (that is, the transfer of O_2, CO_2, and N_2 between the alveoli and the capillary blood), the effects of immersion on lung volumes and respiratory mechanics, as well as the corrections of Boyle's law for water vapor. Based on Agostoni's calculations, the maximal safe depth for an average Ama was about 16 m, which was also the typical maximum working depth for the more experienced Japanese Ama. A similar prediction for the current depth record holder, F. Ferreras, who has a total lung capacity of 9.6 L and a residual volume of 2.2 L (8), would set his safe limit of compression at about 4.4 atm (absolute pressure), corresponding to a depth of 34 m (112 ft). As mentioned earlier, he has actually reached 133 m (14.3 atm, 440 ft). This implies that if he started the dive at TLC and disregarding volume changes due to gas exchange with the blood, his RV would have been reduced to 0.67 L in order to maintain pressure equilibrium between lung air and surrounding water. This is apparently accomplished by redistribution of blood from the periphery into the blood-containing structures of the chest, as discussed further below (also see Chap. 3). It is also possible that diving may compress the chest and elevate the diaphragm to a greater extent than an RV maneuver (forced exhalation) performed at the surface (see ''Note in Proof'').

Intrathoracic Blood Pooling

Craig (9) appears to have been the first to suggest that redistribution of blood from the periphery into the chest would help to compress the gas in the lungs and contribute to the maintenance of pressure equilibrium across the chest wall. This principle is illustrated in Figs. 2A and B. Using thoracic impedance recordings on the U.S. Navy diver Robert Croft during dives to 90 and 130 fsw, Schaefer et al. (10) estimated that between 850 and 1047 ml of blood had been redistributed from the periphery into the diver's chest. More recently, Warkander

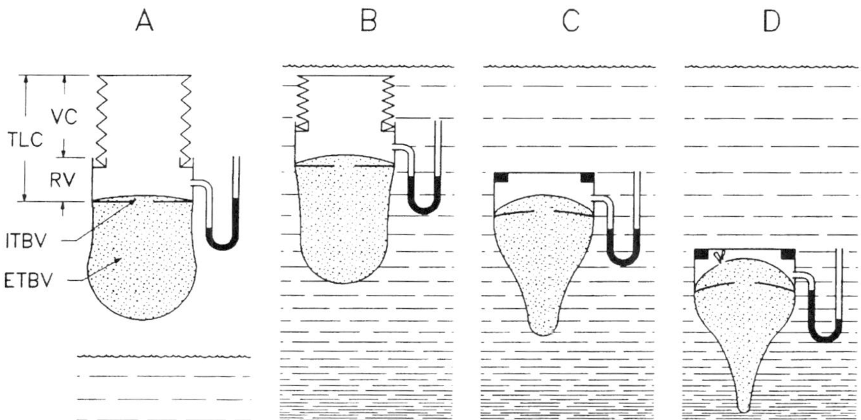

Figure 2 Schematic illustration of how pressure equilibrium between the chest cavity (lung air) and surrounding water is achieved in a deep breath-hold dive. (A) The dive starts by inhalation to total lung capacity (TLC) before entering water; vital capacity (VC) represents the portion of TLC that can be used for pressure equilibration. The manometer indicates overpressure in lung air relative to ambient atmosphere due to inward recoil of chest and lungs; the residual volume (RV) represents the "noncollapsible" fraction of TLC; the normal intrathoracic blood volume (ITBV) (in the vascular bed and heart) is modest in size; the extrathoracic blood volume is labeled ETBV. (B) Beginning of descent with pressure equilibrium relative to ambient water maintained, as indicated by manometer, by compression of chest wall and some translocation of blood from ETBV to ITBV. (C) At greater depth the limits of mechanical compression of chest wall and stretching of diaphragm have been reached but further compression of the lung air and maintenance of pressure equilibrium are achieved by redistribution of large volume of blood from ETBV to ITBV, owing to the ambient water pressure acting on the vascular bed containing the ETBV. (D) With further descent, the distensibility limit of the blood-containing structures in the chest may be reached, an underpressure develops in the lung air relative to the ambient water and therefore to the blood in the chest, with possible vascular rupture (bleeding).

et al. (11) have recorded both esophageal pressure and changes in the thoraco-abdominal volume (by inductive plethysmography) during dives to 45 to 55 m performed by three elite divers in a wet hyperbaric chamber. During these dives, the esophageal pressure recordings did not show the very low intrathoracic pressure that one would expect from the simple relationship between predive lung volume and RV; instead—except for one dive to 55 m, in which the esophageal pressure dropped to-30 cmH_2O, they typically showed pressures around zero. This relatively low pressure could be ascribed to an unusually low predive lung volume in that particular dive. The authors suggested that redistribution of blood into the diver's chest had prevented compression of the chest below RV during these deep dives. They also estimated the amount of this intrathoracic blood pooling from the difference between the changes in chest volume actually recorded during the dives and the changes in lung gas volume calculated according to Boyle's law (without taking into account the small volume loss due to gas exchange). The estimates of intrathoracic blood pooling during these dives were between 1.4 and 1.7 L. It is important to note that in these dives the normal procedure was for the subjects to stand in water to the waist level and inhale maximally before submersing themselves. Thus, they probably benefited from an optimal blood redistribution and TLC/RV ratio in terms of intrathoracic pressure equilibration. By contrast, in a separate series of measurements in the same laboratory, six subjects who made submersed chamber dives to 20 m exhibited esophageal pressures as low as about-18 cmH_2O (12). This may be explained by the fact that the dives were initiated from the immersed condition; i.e., considerable blood redistribution had occurred before the dive (13) and the subjects predive inhalations were limited to 85% of their immersed vital capacities. The importance of the transthoracic pressure equilibration is further borne out by the observation that, while the esophageal pressure drop was, on the average, 20.9 cmH_2O in these dives, it was significantly higher (i.e., 29.1 cmH_2O) when the subjects performed non-immersed dives to the same simulated depth. The mechanics behind the difference in intrathoracic pressure drop between dry and submersed dives is illustrated in Fig. 3. It depicts the pressure-volume curves for the chest wall (responsible for intrathoracic pressure) during relaxation in the dry condition (continuous line) and in head-out immersion (dotted line). Applying the mean lung volumes from the experiments of Ferrigno et al. (12) as the initial lung volumes, compression to 20 m in the dry condition would have resulted in a drop in intrathoracic pressure (ΔP_{es} in the figure) of 28 cmH_2O. For the submersed dives, the initial position on the relaxation curve was moved (to a larger lung volume) on the assumption that 0.7 L of blood (ΔV_b in Fig. 3) had been redistributed from the periphery into the chest due to submersion. Corrections for vital capacity and residual volume during head-out immersion (see Refs. 14 and 15) were also applied. According to the calculations used for this figure, compression to 20 m in the submersed condition would

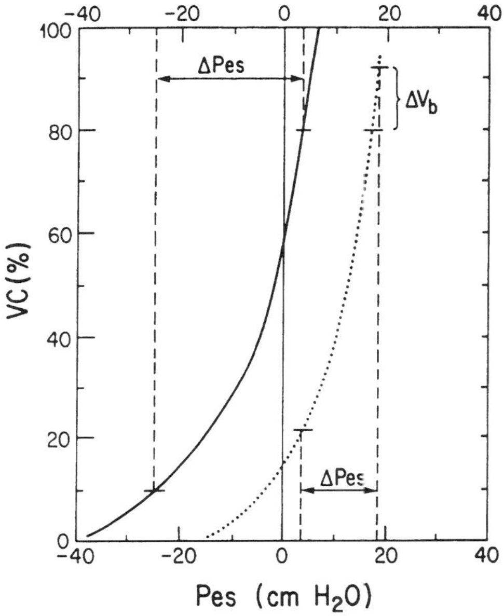

Figure 3 Pressure-volume diagram illustrating the theoretical changes in lung volume [percent of vital capacity (VC)] and intrathoracic pressure [esophageal pressure (P_{es})] during breath-hold dive to 20 m initiated after inhaling an air volume corresponding to 80% of VC. The continuous curve line represents a dry dive and the dotted curve line a submersed dive. It is assumed that submersion causes 0.7 1 of blood (ΔV_B) to be redistributed into the chest (13), thus making the actual chest volume at beginning of dive equivalent to 92% of VC. As a consequence, lung volume after compression (at about 20% VC) is larger during immersion than during nonimmersion (about 10% VC), and hence P_{es} (about 4 cm H_2O) at 20 m indicates better pressure equilibration than after a nonimmersed dive (about 24 cm H_2O). (Adapted from Ref. 16.)

have caused a drop in intrathoracic pressure of about 15 cmH_2O. The difference of 13 cmH_2O in pressure drop between dry and submersed dives, based on this theoretical analysis, should be compared with the difference of 8.2 cmH_2O calculated from the experimental dives (12). That the latter was smaller than the theoretical value could be due to the fact that the reference pressure on the chest wall, used for the calculation of the esophageal pressure during submersed dives, was not adjusted for chest compression (see Ref. 16).

Another factor that might contribute to a larger fall in intrathoracic pressure in the dry than in submersed dives is juxtathoracic venous collapse during compression in the dry situation. This phenomenon consists of the collapse of the veins entering the thorax once the intrathoracic pressure falls below zero (17). Because of this, a further decrease in intrathoracic pressure will not cause an increase in venous return. Therefore, with less blood pooling in the thorax to make up for the reduction in alveolar gas volume during the dive, the chest will be compressed to a smaller volume with a higher risk of injury. On the other hand, juxtathoracic venous collapse is not likely during the submersed dives, as the veins entering the thorax are kept open by the centralization of blood volume due to water pressure. Additional evidence that more blood moves into the chest during submersed dives than during nonimmersed compressions is the observation by Schaefer et al. (18) that thoracic electrical impedance gradually decreased during the submersed dives but not during dry compressions.

The observations reported above are in agreement with those of Craig (9), who used a different experimental approach. His subjects expired to RV and then descended as deep as 4.75 m in a lake without showing any significant changes in transthoracic pressure. The author estimated that at least 600 ml of blood entered the chest and helped to maintain intrathoracic pressure. Redistribution of such a volume of blood is entirely feasible. Indeed, mere head-out immersion in a thermoneutral bath has been shown to cause intrathoracic blood pooling of about 700 ml (13). Furthermore, measurements of reductions in vital capacity during immersion in cool water (20°C) indicate redistribution of a volume of blood twice as large (14).

It appears that, in order to maximize diving depth, the diver should start with the largest possible volume of air in the lungs. Furthermore, redistribution of as much blood as possible into the chest during the dive is desirable. It follows that the inspiration preceding the dive should be made with a minimum amount of blood competing with air for space in the chest; i.e., the predive inspiration should be made immediately before entering the water. Interestingly, the female divers of both Korea and Japan, who remain in the water between dives, whistle during exhalations prior to diving. It has been suggested (19) that the whistling serves to increase intrathoracic pressure and expel blood, so as to allow inspiration of a larger air volume before the dive. The Tuamotuan pearl divers, renowned for diving very deep, generate a "whoooeee" sound during exhalation, which may serve a similar purpose as the whistling (3). In addition, these divers raise themselves out of the water to the waist to take the final deep inspiration before descent.

B. Duration

The diving technique will determine the degree of physical effort during a dive. In assisted diving, often used in attempts to set records, the diver is pulled down (Fig. 4) by a weight during descent and pulled up by a flotation device during

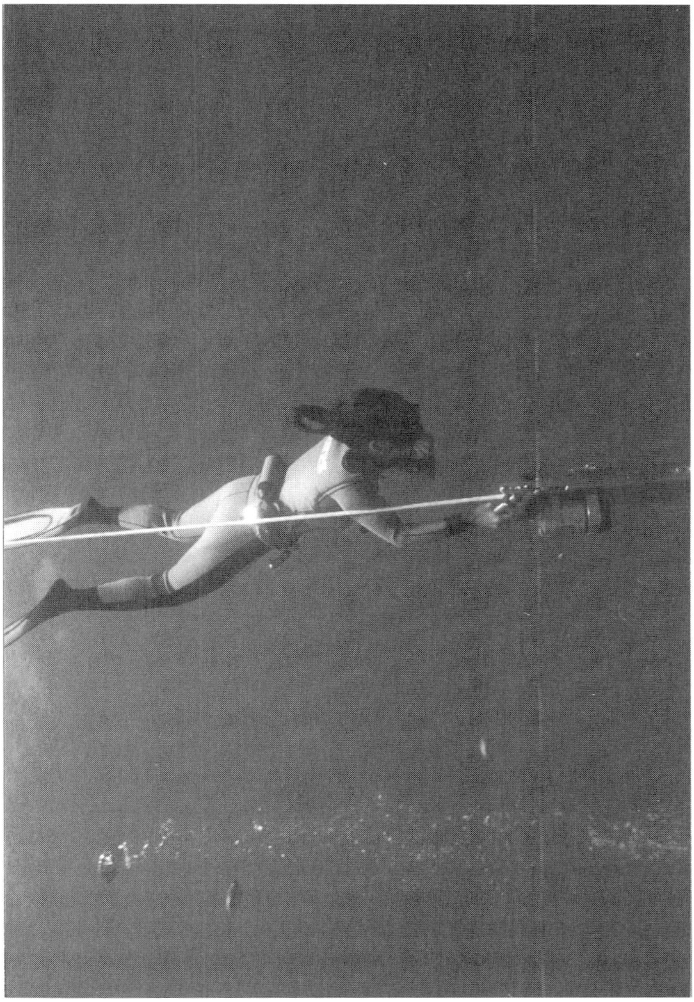

Figure 4 Diver descending for depth record attempt. Descent is aided by a weighted ‘‘sled’’ (assisted dive), which pulls the diver down along a tight rope. When the diver lets go of the handle on the sled, it locks to the rope, thus marking maximum depth reached. (*Photo courtesy Tommaso Nobili.*)

ascent (Fig. 5). Using these techniques, greater depths can be reached in a shorter time, because velocities of descent and ascent well in excess of 1 m/sec can be achieved. In addition, as compared with active swimming, this technique will decrease the rate of oxygen consumption and carbon dioxide production during a dive, allowing a longer-lasting breath-hold.

Breaking Points

When a voluntary breath-hold is sustained, two phases become apparent (20). The first one is an ''easy-going'' phase, during which the glottis is closed and the intrathoracic pressure remains stable. This phase ends with the onset of involuntary rhythmic contractions of the inspiratory muscles while the glottis remains closed, as illustrated in Fig. 6. This event is termed the *physiological breaking point*, because it is nonsubjective and is determined by the arterial P_{CO_2} and by lung volume, a large volume delaying the onset (21). Typically, in a nonimmersed breath-hold at 1 atm, the alveolar P_{CO_2} at the physiological breaking point is around 46 mmHg; during breath-holding after the lungs have been filled with oxygen, which dampens the hypercapnic respiratory drive, it is around 49 mmHg as reviewed by Lin (22). During the second, so-called ''struggle'' phase, involuntary inspiratory muscle contractions begin and increase in frequency and intensity until the airway is opened and the breath-hold is terminated. This event is termed the *conventional breaking point*. The duration of the second phase is highly variable and dependent on both physiological and psychological factors (23). Still, the alveolar CO_2 tension at the conventional breaking point is quite stable in the individual breath-holder. As shown in Fig. 7A and B, when the duration of maximal breath-hold was modified more than threefold by submersion and changes in water temperature, the breaking point P_{ACO_2} nonetheless remained unchanged in five subjects studied (24). Similarly, the end-tidal CO_2 fraction at the breaking point was unchanged in subjects whose maximal breath-hold duration varied depending on the lung volume during the breath-hold (25). Yet the asphyxia tolerance, measured as P_{ACO_2} and P_{AO_2} at breaking point, can be modified. If, at the end of a maximal breath-hold, a subject rebreathes for a few breaths into a bag without access to fresh air, a second breath-hold can be carried out to even higher alveolar CO_2 and lower O_2 levels (26). In this situation, changes in mechanoreceptor activity apparently cause a temporary reduction in respiratory drive (27). This mechanism may explain why divers approaching the limit of the breath-hold sometimes let out air, apparently getting relief from the urge to breathe. Similarly, the expansion of the chest wall during ascent may contribute to a sensation of relief (see Ref. 28), although this may also be caused by the fall in gas pressure in the lungs, which causes a reduction in alveolar P_{CO_2} (29). Other expedients to delay the conventional breaking point include swallowing, performing the Valsalva or

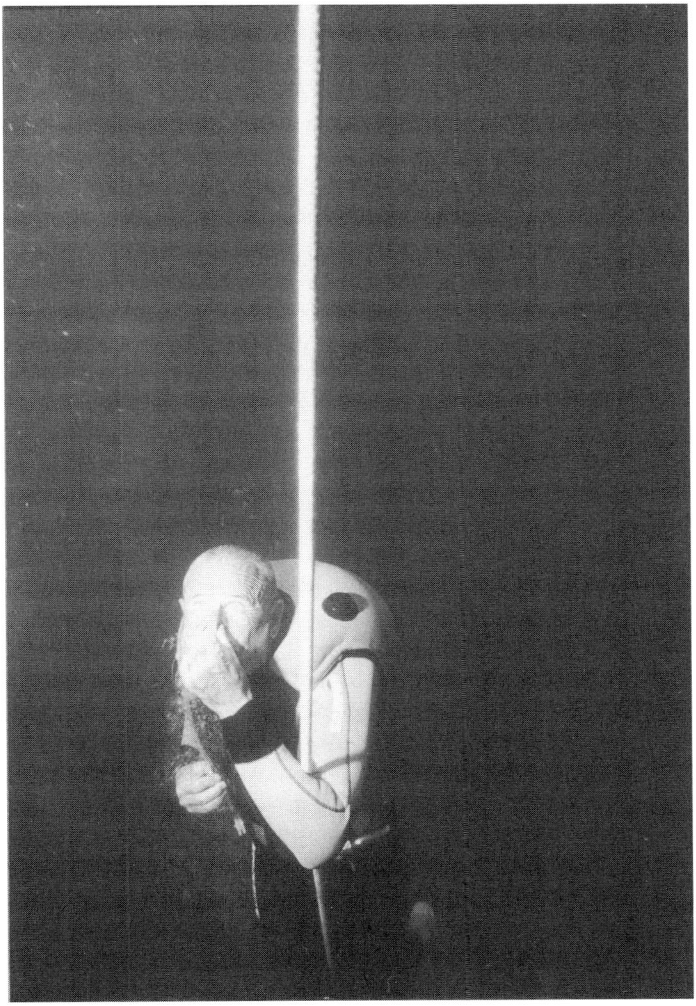

Figure 5 Ascent from deep dive using assisted technique. The diver is pulled to the surface by a bladder inflated from a small gas bottle. In this case the bladder is an integral part of the suit jacket. Note that the diver is not wearing a face mask, thus probably enhancing the diving response and keeping the incompressible gas space in his airways smaller than if a face mask covering the nose had been worn. (*Photo courtesy Tommaso Nobili.*)

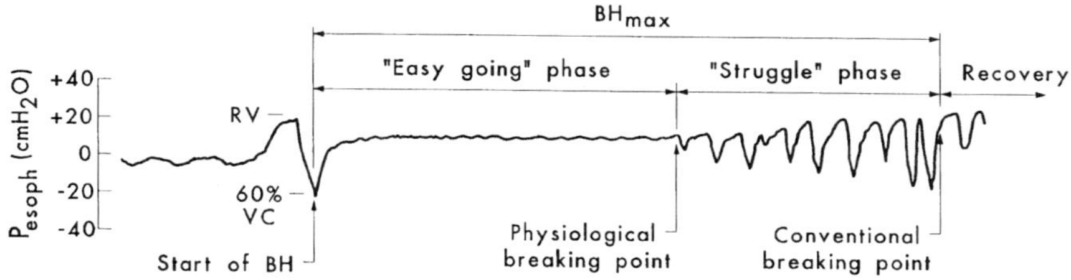

Figure 6 Recording of esophageal pressure versus time, reflecting respiratory muscle activity during a maximal breath-hold of about 120 sec duration. After expiration to residual volume (RV) and inspiration to 60% of vital capacity (VC), the breath-hold starts; during the first ''easy going'' phase, there is no respiratory muscle activity. The first involuntary inspiratory muscle activity (downward deflection) signals the physiological breaking point. The breath-hold continues while respiratory muscle activity gradually increases through the struggle phase, until breathing is resumed at the ''conventional'' breaking point. (Modified from Ref. 146.)

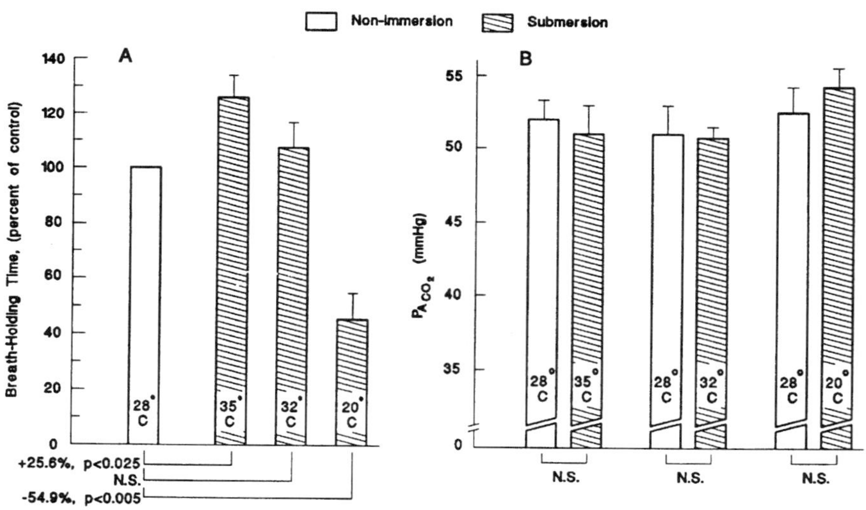

Figure 7 (A) Maximal breath-holding times during submersion in water at different temperatures expressed as percent (means $\pm$ SE) of breath-holding time during nonimmersion in five subjects. (From Ref. 24.) (B) Carbon dioxide pressures in breaking-point end-tidal air of maximal breath-holds during the same conditions as in panel A. Note the stability of breaking point P_{CO_2} despite considerable variations in breath-holding times (panel A). (From Ref. 24.)

Muller maneuver, and even squeezing a rubber ball (30) or doing mental arithmetic (31). However, the fundamental factors that determine the conventional breaking point are still the arterial P_{CO_2} and P_{O_2}—i.e., the asphyxia level at which the respiratory drive is strong enough to enforce breathing despite the breath-holder's efforts to continue breath-holding. The time it takes to reach this state of asphyxia—i.e., the duration of the breath-hold—depends on three factors: (1) the diver's tolerance to CO_2 and hypoxia, (2) metabolic rate, and (3) CO_2 and O_2 storage capacity. Typical mean alveolar gas tensions at the conventional breaking point of non-immersed breath-holds in resting untrained subjects are 43.3 to 53.5 mmHg for CO_2 and 45.6 to 80.2 mmHg for O_2; the duration of such maximal breath-holds has been between 93 and 150 sec (20,24,32–36).

Ferretti et al. (36) looked at the individual tolerance to asphyxic stimuli in trained and untrained subjects. Their three highly proficient divers, who had hyperventilated for 60 sec, were able to breath-hold for 240 to 300 sec under resting conditions. The breaking point P_{ACO_2} levels of the three divers were 53.3, 46.6, and 45.6 mmHg and the P_{AO_2} levels were 29.3, 28.0, and 40.6 mmHg, respectively (Fig. 8). The corresponding endurance for nine age-and sex-matched controls was considerably shorter at 90 to 150 sec. In the two controls who held their breaths for 150 sec, the average P_{ACO_2} could be calculated at 48.1 and 52.3 mmHg and the P_{AO_2} at 53.8 and 37.4 mmHg, respectively (36). As can be seen in Fig. 8, the alveolar P_{O_2} and P_{CO_2} values of the controls and one of the divers (PM) at the end of their maximal breath-holds fell on the breaking-point curve. On the other hand, two of the divers (EM and RM, in Fig. 8) were able to hold their breath past the limits indicated by this curve, to the boundaries of the ''anoxic collapse'' region of the O_2 to CO_2 diagram. The alveolar P_{O_2} and P_{CO_2} values of these two divers would have caused, in normal subjects, a very intense respiratory stimulation (see Ref. 36). However, trained divers exhibit an enhanced tolerance to hypercapnia and hypoxia when tested with conventional methods, as discussed further in Sec. III, ''Training and Adaptation.''

The divers who performed the nonimmersed maximal breath-holds were also studied during a total of nine deep breath-hold dives in the ocean. The end-tidal P_{O_2} values upon emersion from these dives appeared to be linearly related to the corresponding P_{O_2} values, down to a P_{O_2} of about 45 mmHg, as shown by the emersion curve in Fig. 8. This curve then turns toward the breaking-point curve, with P_{O_2} leveling off at values about 30 mmHg and P_{CO_2} values being as high as 47 mmHg (Fig. 8). Both the P_{O_2} and P_{CO_2} values appeared to be independent of dive depth (range, 40 to 70 m) and duration (80 to 150 sec). However, as noted by the authors, these values were less asphyxic than those recorded during the maximal nonimmersed breath-holds, although the estimated overall energy demand was greater during the dives. The same authors con-

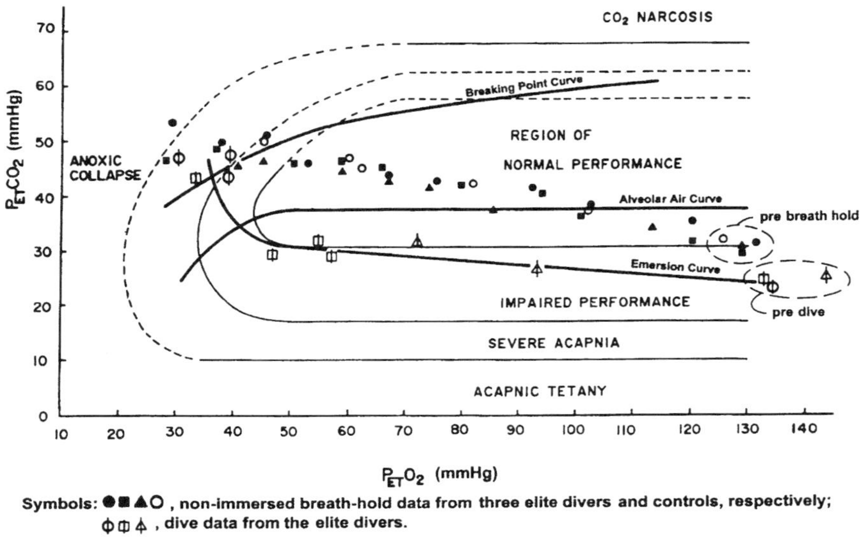

Figure 8 End-tidal P_{O_2} and P_{CO_2} of three elite divers and nine nondiving matched controls before and at termination of nonimmersed holds (BH) of increasing standardized durations (up to maximum) and deep breath-hold dives in the ocean (divers only) plotted on an O_2–CO_2 diagram (147). In addition, the following is shown: (1) the normal alveolar air curve illustrating how, during spontaneous breathing, PA_{CO_2} changes with PA_{O_2}; (2) a breath-hold breaking point curve (148); (3) lines defining the regions of normal and impaired visual contrast discrimination (149,150). (Slightly modified from Ref. 36.)

cluded that a 70-m dive does not require a maximal breath-hold and further noted that, although the end-of-dive values for P_{O_2} and P_{CO_2} appear to be marginally safe (Fig. 8), all three subjects had, on other occasions, made considerably deeper and longer-lasting dives. It seems that depletion of the oxygen stores in the deep dives is quite slow. This may be due to the blood and lung stores being primarily called on to supply the heart and brain. This would be possible, since the muscles are subject to vasoconstriction as part of the diving response (see ''The Diving Response'' in this chapter) as indicated by lactate accumulation during these dives. The data of Ferretti et al. (36) indicate that, on the average, lactate-based energy amounted to 36% of the estimated total energy expenditure during the dives. Lactate accumulation during even less demanding dives has also been noted in other studies. Thus, in relatively untrained subjects performing dives in the ocean, the blood lactate concentration increased after the first dive in a series of dives to 5 and 10 m respectively and lasting 30 to 45 sec. (37). Lactate tended to go back to normal with repetitive easy dives; but it remained elevated in the more demanding diving pattern.

To be expected, breath-hold duration is shorter during exercise than during rest. Indeed, there is an inverse relationship between breath-hold duration and oxygen consumption measured just before the breath-hold (20,24,38,39). In a study (20) that included one rebreathing breath at the physiological breaking point, the five subjects were able to breath-hold for 162 sec at rest but only for 66 sec when they were performing steady-state exercise at 167 kg m/min. At the conventional breaking point, the PA_{CO_2} was about 54 and 56 mmHg, respectively, while the PA_{O_2} was 62 and 58 mmHg. The slightly more ''asphyxic'' gas tensions in the exercise experiments probably reflect more rapid gas-exchange dynamics, secondary to an increased cardiac output, rather than changes in respiratory control sensitivity to chemical stimuli. Subjects performing breath-hold dives to different depths in studies by Craig and Medd (37) used relatively less oxygen in 10-m dives than would be predicted from the oxygen uptake in 5-m dives. The explanation offered for this was that, with increasing depth and chest compression, less work (swimming) would need to be done to overcome buoyancy. Similarly, less oxygen was used when the divers used swim fins or performed ''assisted'' dives, in which they were mechanically pulled down to depth and back to the surface (37).

The effect of the metabolic rate on breath-holding endurance was also evident in another study in which subjects were submersed in cool (20°C) water (24). In this situation, O_2 uptake, measured immediately before breath-holding, was 256% higher than during control measurements in thermoneutral (28°C) air. Underwater, the breath-holding time was about 55% shorter than in the non-immersed situation. Yet, as mentioned above, the breaking-point alveolar CO_2 tensions were the same. This lends support to the authors' explanation that the higher metabolic rate in the cool water shortened the time it took to reach alveolar gas concentrations that forced the subject to breathe. Additional respiratory drive may have been caused by cold stimulation of the skin (40,41). Such a mechanism was thought to explain why, when volunteers were suddenly dropped into water at 0 to 15°C, the breath-hold duration was 25 to 50% shorter than during presubmersion (42).

Maximal breath-hold duration increases when the breath is held on air at increasing pressures (between 1.0 and 4.0 atm) (43,44), and this is not an effect of nitrogen narcosis (44). However, it is well known that the level of alveolar ventilation resulting from a certain Pa_{CO_2} is modulated by the Pa_{O_2}, and vice versa. This also applies to respiratory drive (at the conventional breaking point), which determines the duration of a breath-hold. The relationship between alveolar P_{CO_2} and P_{O_2} at the breaking point (in the P_{O_2} range of 30 to 120 mmHg) is shown by the breaking-point curve in Fig. 8. In the study by Lin et al (20) mentioned earlier, breath-hold duration after oxygen breathing averaged 275 versus 162 sec on air when the subjects were resting and 102 versus 66 sec during exercise. Similarly, Klocke and Rahn (45) recorded breath-hold durations ranging from 3.1 to 8.5 min after oxygen breathing, with breaking-point alveolar CO_2 tensions from 51 to 91 mmHg. In air-breathing subjects exposed to high ambient pressures, the conventional breaking-point P_{CO_2} has a linear relationship to $\log_{10}$ P_{AO_2} (43,44) at P_{O_2} ranges between 60 and 300 mmHg. At oxygen pressures above 300 mmHg, however, the increase in breaking-point P_{CO_2} was less marked (44). A similar relationship between alveolar carbon dioxide and oxygen pressures has also been demonstrated for the physiological breaking point (46). The studies just referred to were made in resting subjects (43,44,46). It is noteworthy that there are observations suggesting that dangerously high CO_2 tensions may develop during conditions of hyperoxia, especially during exercise. Thus, Hill and Flack (48) reported that runners who had filled their lungs with oxygen and then attempted a fast sprint while breath-holding became incapacitated and lost consciousness, presumably from hypercapnia. Likewise, attempts at enhancing breath-holding performance in ten subjects by hyperventilation followed by inhalation of one breath of oxygen resulted in altered consciousness in one subject who held his breath for 183 sec with a breaking-point Pa_{CO_2} of 102 mmHg (49).

Oxygen Stores

The ability of the body to store O_2 and CO_2 is fundamentally important for the duration of maximal breath-holds. Moreover, at least in well-trained divers performing deep breath-hold dives, the energy balance appears to be significantly dependent on anaerobic metabolism, as discussed later. The accessibility and mode of usage of the oxygen and carbon dioxide stores are affected by various factors besides the already mentioned obvious effect of the metabolic rate. So, for instance, will the depth of the dive influence the utilization of the oxygen store in the lungs, and the presence of the physiological events known as the diving response will affect how the O_2 store in the blood is going to be used. The size of the oxygen stores of a 70-kg man with lungs at functional residual capacity is given in Table 1.

Of the total store amounting to 1546 ml, 1250 ml is contained in the blood and lungs when the latter are at functional residual capacity. Clearly, increasing the pre-breath-hold lung volume increases the O_2 stores (and the CO_2–storing capacity), thus lengthening the breath-hold time (20,39) After inspiration to total lung capacity, which usually precedes a deep breath-hold dive (assuming TLC = 5.5L and P_{AO_2} = 120 mmHg), the lung store would amount to about 820 ml for a combined lung-blood store of 1700 ml (STPD) and a total store of 1996 ml (STPD) of O_2. Several factors determine for how long this amount of O_2 can sustain metabolism. In particular, the rates of aerobic and anaerobic metabolism are important, as is the depth of the breath-hold dive. The extent to

Table 1 O_2 Stores of a 70-kg Man

Form	Site	ml STPD
Hemoglobin	Venous blood	600
	Arterial blood	280
Myoglobin	Muscles	240
Physical solution	Tissues	56
Gas	Lung	370
		Total 1546

Source: Ref. 50.

which the oxygen in the lungs can be used depends on the PA_{O_2}, which, in its turn, is influenced by the water pressure acting on the chest, as discussed further below. In the hypothetical case that the entire store of 1996 ml of O_2 could be used and given an oxygen consumption of 300 ml/min, the stores would be exhausted in about 6.5 min. Not far from this prediction, breath-hold durations of up to 5 min have been recorded in non-immersed trained divers at rest (36).

It appears that, if reaching the breaking-point PA_{CO_2} is sufficiently delayed by vigorous hyperventilation prior to breath-holding, the pulmonary O_2 store becomes the limiting factor for breath-hold duration. Three of the seven subjects who had hyperventilated for 10 min and filled their lungs with O_2 were able to use an O_2 volume roughly equivalent to their respective vital capacities and scored breath-hold times of between 12.2 and 14 min (45). In this type of experiment, the O_2 uptake causes the alveolar carbon dioxide concentration to increase. Therefore, there is no CO_2 exchange between the blood and the lungs (45,51). Hence, the theoretical breath hold duration (BHD) is

$$\text{BHD (min)} = \frac{\text{VC (L, STPD)}}{\dot{V}_{O_2}\text{(L, STPD/min)}} \tag{1}$$

and therefore

$$\dot{V}_{O_2}\text{(L, STPD/min)} = \frac{\text{VC (L, STPD)}}{\text{BHD (min)}} \tag{2}$$

Applying the breath-hold durations of 12 and 14 min and the vital capacities of the two subjects of Klocke and Rahn (45) of 4.12 L (STPD) and 4.20 L (STPD), respectively, to Eq. (2), the $\dot{V}_{O_2}$ during the breath-hold can be calculated at 0.30 L (STPD) $\cdot$ min^{-1} and 0.337 L (STPD)$\cdot\text{min}^{-1}$, respectively. These are quite reasonable values for $\dot{V}_{O_2}$ of persons who are not trained breath-hold divers, as discussed below.

The fact that the maximal breath-hold duration in the three trained divers mentioned above is close to the theoretical limit appears to be due to a component of anaerobic metabolism. That this response is particularly well developed in the divers is evident from comparisons with nondiver control subjects (36). As can be seen in Fig. 9, the O_2 uptake in the divers during nonimmersed surface breath-holds was considerably lower than in the controls. Indeed, it was lower than the normal eupneic oxygen uptake would predict. At the end of the breath-holds, this cumulative difference amounted to between 485 and 535 ml in the three divers. Since there was no accumulation of lactic acid in these experiments, the authors concluded that the missing energy derived from high-energy phosphates and/or tissue O_2 stores. The deficit corresponded to about 40% of normal O_2 stores (36). Notably, the same three divers exhibited a substantial lactic acid accumulation when performing actual breath-hold dives in the ocean. As pointed out by the authors, this is remarkable because the metabolic power output during the dives was estimated at about 20 to 30% of the subjects' maximal O_2 consumption, a level not associated with lactic acid accumulation during eupnea. The dive response was considered the likely explanation for the lactic acid accumulation in the dives, since it would cause

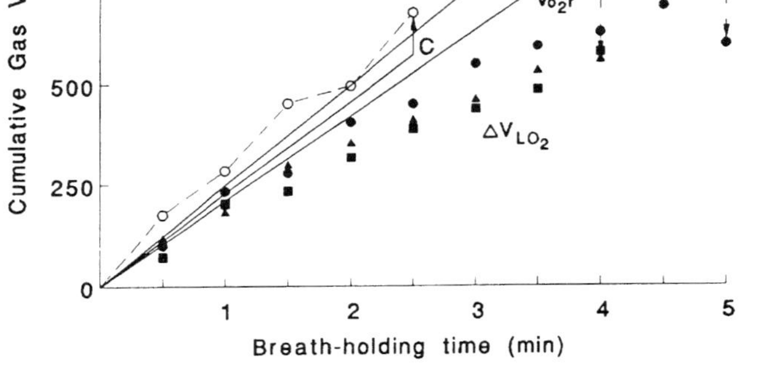

Figure 9 Cumulative volume of oxygen taken up from lungs during nonimmersed maximal breath-holds performed by three highly trained divers (EM, RM, and PM) and nine age-and sex-matched control subjects. Solid lines show hypothetical individual cumulative oxygen uptake based on measurements during eupnea. Arrows and ΔSo_2 are changes in oxygen stores. (From Ref. 36.)

peripheral vasoconstriction. It is noteworthy that the dive response, as discussed in more detail later, is more pronounced in breath-hold divers than in nondivers (see, for example, Ref.52).

The accessibility of the pulmonary oxygen stores changes with water depth during a dive because the water pressure acting on the chest determines the total alveolar gas pressure and hence the PA_{O_2}. A theoretical example will illustrate the importance of this mechanism. If a diver starts a descent with 18% O_2 in the alveoli, which yields a PA_{O_2} of 128 mmHg (P_B = 760 mmHg) and reaches a depth of 20 m (3 atm) his or her total alveolar gas pressure will be 2280 mmHg. Disregarding O_2 uptake during descent, the diver will arrive at the bottom with a PA_{O_2} of 402 mmHg. Clearly, this allows more O_2 to be used; i.e., the breath-holding time can be longer than at the surface before a dangerously low PA_{O_2} is reached. Assume that he or she lingers at the bottom until the PA_{O_2} has decreased to 60 mmHg, which is a level still compatible with unperturbed consciousness. This P_{O_2} at 3 atm represents an alveolar O_2 concentration of 2.7 %. Again disregarding O_2 uptake, ascending toward the surface with this O_2 concentration in the alveoli means that a PA_{O_2} of 30 mmHg, which is marginally compatible with consciousness (refer to Fig. 8), will be reached at a depth of 5.2 m (P_B = 1155 mmHg). The remaining ascent will occur under conditions of ever-worsening hypoxia. This phenomenon is known as the hypoxia of ascent. The situation may be further aggravated during the ascent, since the urge to breathe, which would compel the diver to return rapidly to the surface, is diminished for two reasons related to the reduction in hydrostatic pressure: (1) the fall in PA_{CO_2} as the lung gas pressure is reduced and (2) the lung and chest expansion (29). It has been shown that any given hypoxia-hypercapnia combination exerts less respiratory stimulation the larger the lung volume is (53). Not surprisingly, the hypoxia of ascent has been known to cause unconsciousness under water in divers ascending from deep dives (5,54).

In 1931, Teruoka recorded alveolar O_2 and CO_2 concentrations in the first exhalation of Japanese Ama returning to the surface from dives as deep as 25 m and lasting as long as 118 sec (55). Both the O_2 and CO_2 values were much lower (i.e., O_2 concentrations as low as 3.3% and CO_2 concentrations seldom above 5%) than the ones which would result from breath-holds of a comparable duration at the surface. It took about 30 years for researchers to understand the results reported by Teruoka. The remarkable differences in alveolar gas exchange between breath-holding at the surface and breath-hold diving were reproduced in a pressure chamber by Lanphier and Rahn (29, 56), who attributed these differences to the effects of the changing ambient pressure on the alveolar gas tensions. Linér et al. (57) examined alveolar gas exchange during surface breath-holds and simulated dives to 20 m in light of the changes in cardiac output related to increases and decreases in ambient pressure. Their results, while qualitatively similar to the pioneering observations of Lanphier and Rahn (29,

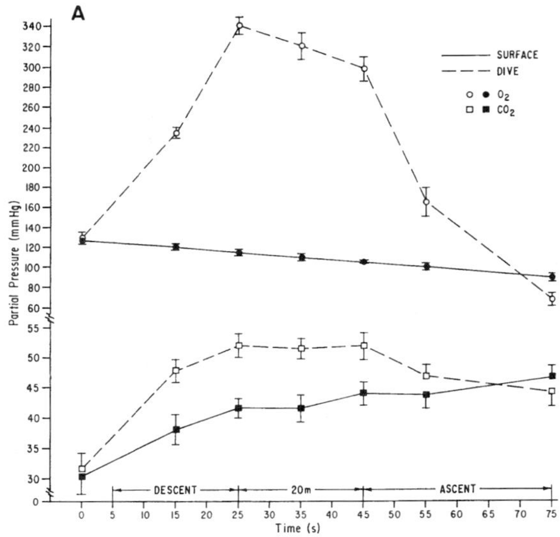

Figure 10 (A) Partial pressures and (B) volumes of oxygen and carbon dioxide in the lungs versus time during submersed breath-holds at the surface and during simulated dives to 20 m in a pressure chamber. Data points are means $\pm$ SE from three measurements in each of five subjects. Note that more oxygen was taken up from the lungs and less carbon dioxide delivered to them during the dives than during the breath-holds. (From Ref. 57.) (C) Top Panel: Exchange of oxygen from (positive values) or to the lungs (negative values) versus time during submersed breath-holds at the surface and during dives to a simulated depth of 20 m. Bottom panel: Carbon dioxide exchange under the same conditions as in top panel (From Ref. 57.) Bars show cardiac indices obtained under identical conditions in other studies in the same laboratory (12,58).

56), were derived from breath-holds of successively longer duration that were performed during submersion. By contrast, the subjects of Lanphier and Rahn were not immersed and delivered alveolar gas samples by rebreathing, which probably influenced cardiac output. Recordings of PAo_2 and $PAco_2$ (to be discussed later) during the surface breath-holds and breath-hold dives to 20 m of Linér et al. (57) are shown in Fig. 10A. The calculated O_2 and CO_2 volumes in the lungs during the two types of experiments are shown in Fig. 10B. The compression effect increasing PAo_2 during the descent is clearly evident. At 20 m, the PAo_2 fell four times faster than during the corresponding breath-hold period at the surface. Partly responsible for this rapid fall in oxygen pressure is the fact that removal of an identical number of O_2 molecules from the alveoli at depth causes a larger drop in $PAco_2$ than at the surface (29). Also evident in

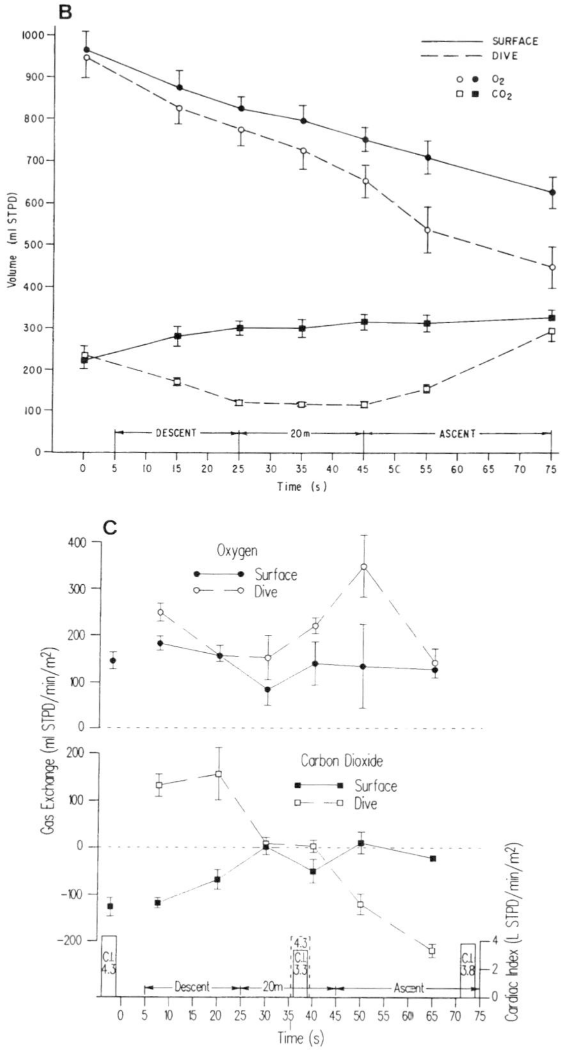
B
SURFACE
DIVE
O_2
CO_2
Volume (ml STPD)
DESCENT
20m
ASCENT
Time (s)
C
Oxygen
Surface
Dive
Carbon Dioxide
Surface
Dive
Gas Exchange (ml STPD/min/m²)
C.I. 4.3
C.I. 3.3
4.3
C.I. 3.8
Descent
20m
Ascent
Cardiac Index (L STPD/min/m²)
Time (s)

Fig. 10A is the dramatic fall in PA_{O_2}, from about 297 mmHg at the beginning of the ascent to 67 mmHg upon surfacing. This value is 22 mmHg lower than the 89 mmHg at the end of the surface breath-holds. This difference reflects the higher oxygen uptake due to both the generally higher PA_{O_2} during most of the dive and the hemodynamic changes, as discussed below. This higher oxygen uptake is shown in Fig. 10B as a gradually smaller O_2 volume in the lungs during the dive. The rates of O_2 and CO_2 exchange in this study are shown in Fig. 10C, which also depicts changes in cardiac index. Oxygen uptake was the parameter that differed the most from previous studies. After reaching the maximal depth, oxygen uptake started to increase, reaching a maximum of 346 ml (STPD)$\cdot$ $min^{-1}\cdot m^2$ (body surface area) at 50 sec, i.e., in the early part of ascent. This value exceeded the corresponding 50-sec surface breath-hold value by 214 ml (STPD)$\cdot min^{-1}\cdot m^2$ (body surface area). Later in the ascent, O_2 uptake decreased toward the corresponding surface value. As a result of the time course of $\dot{V}O_2$, the total O_2 uptake during the dives was 161 ml larger than during breath-holds at the surface. The authors argued that an increased PA_{O_2} at depth played a small role in increasing the $\dot{V}O_2$ above that recorded in the breath-holds. In fact, they estimated the extra O_2 load due to the increased PA_{O_2} to about 0.35 ml$\cdot$100 ml^{-1} of blood, which would have accounted for a total additional uptake of only about 25 ml over the duration of the dives. They explained the difference in total O_2 uptake and in the time course of $\dot{V}O_2$ between the dives and the breath-holds with hemodynamic changes related to the intrathoracic pressure, as described by Ferrigno et al. (12,58). The increased cardiac output during the simulated dives, as compared with the surface breath-holds, resulted in an enhanced pulmonary blood flow, which probably contributed to the accelerated $\dot{V}O_2$ at the bottom and early during ascent. It was calculated that over the duration of a dive, the pulmonary blood flow probably was about 1 L greater than during a surface breath-hold, and that this could account for an extra O_2 uptake of 50 ml if mixed venous O_2 concentration had remained normal. However, the authors (57) argued that venous O_2 concentration probably was lower than normal. Specifically, early in the dive, high intrathoracic pressure would have led to a reduction in cardiac output and in peripheral blood flow, with a resulting increase in O_2 extraction from the blood; they suggested that, with the fall in intrathoracic pressure during descent, about 1 L of venous blood with low O_2 content would probably have been redistributed into the chest, contributing to an increase in O_2 uptake from the lung. The delay in the rise of $\dot{V}O_2$ at the bottom was attributed to the Valsalva maneuvers used for ear clearing during compression (transiently hindering venous return by causing brief increases in intrathoracic pressure) and to the time required for the venous blood to reach and pass through the lungs. Finally, the fall in $\dot{V}O_2$ later in the ascent was ascribed not only to the rapidly decreasing PA_{O_2} but also to the rising intrathoracic pressure and the concomitant decrease in cardiac output and pulmonary blood flow. The increase in $\dot{V}O_2$ early in the ascent had not been reported earlier with the exception of a study by Schaefer and Carey (59), in which the subjects exercised during ascent. Linér et al. (57) suggested that this discrepancy may have been due to less frequent sampling in previous studies or to lack of significant transient changes in cardiac output because the dives were shallower, or to the fact that exercise and rebreathing were performed (29,60, 61).

The PO_2 changes described above for simulated nonimmersed dives also apply to the real-life diving situation, as is demonstrated by the measurement of alveolar gas tensions of two Korean female divers performing a total of six dives to 9.7 to 12.5 m of depth (60). These divers had PAO_2 levels averaging 41 mmHg (range, 28 to 53 mmHg) upon surfacing. Measurements of arterial blood gas tensions during diving to 4 to 5 m were performed by Qvist et al. (62), also in Korean female divers ($n = 5$). Their results showed a physiologically somewhat less significant hypoxemia. At depth, the PaO_2 was hyperoxic at 141 $\pm$ 24 (SD) mmHg, and at the end of the dive it had fallen to an average of 62.6 $\pm$ 13.5 mmHg (range, 32.8 to 84.0 mmHg). The apparent difference in oxygenation levels between the divers of the two studies might have been due to differences in dive depths and physical activity. The safety of the relatively shallow and brief dives is borne out by continuous recording by pulse oximetry showing arterial oxygen saturation values that never went below 96 $\pm$ 3% during routine diving (63). Interestingly, divers in this category exhibit a mechanism that may boost the O_2-carrying capacity of the blood during dives (64). Thus, the hematocrit increased by 9.5 $\pm$ 5.9% (SD) after 115 dives to 6 m over a 2.5-hr period. The authors suggest that this might have been due to immersion- and cold-induced diuresis, leading to a reduction in plasma volume as well as to a splenic contraction that reduced splenic volume in the divers by 19.5 $\pm$ 8.7% (SD) on average. The observation of cyclical increases by 8.9% in hematocrit with each of a series of breath-holds performed by Korean Amas speaks for the latter mechanism. (62). In the same study, the concentration of 2,3-diphosphoglycerate was slightly increased, causing a minor decrease in hemoglobin oxygen affinity.

An analysis of the dynamics of the O_2 and CO_2 stores during submersed breath holding at 1 atm and during diving to 20 m in a hyperbaric chamber has been performed by Linér and Linnarsson (65). As water temperature in this study was thermoneutral, it cannot be expected to have evoked a full-fledged diving response (see below). Hence, the changes in circulatory function and consequently in gas stores were due to immersion, breath-holding, and intrathoracic pressure changes (caused by descent to depth and ascent) and possibly secondary reflex mechanisms. Breath-holding at the surface, due to increased intrathoracic pressure, impedes venous return and hence cardiac output (58). A drop in cardiac index (to 73% of eupneic level) was observed by Linér and Linnarsson (65) during surface breath-holds and given as an explanation for at least part of the reduction in O_2 uptake from the lung during those conditions. The authors proposed that the reduced cardiac output would widen the arteriovenous O_2 difference, thus reducing the O_2 stores in the blood and the tissues. Furthermore, they noted that the time constant of the decrease in O_2 stores during breath-holding was about seven times slower than the time constant of the restoration of the stores after breath-holds. According to Linér and Linnarsson (65), this would be consistent with relatively slow changes in O_2 content in venous blood pooled in poorly perfused peripheral tissues during the breath-hold. The rapid restoration of blood O_2 stores after cessation of breath-holding might be explained by a sudden increase in venous return as the high intrathoracic pressure is relieved. During submersed chamber dives to 20 m, performed by the same group of subjects, the oxygen uptake from the lung was maintained roughly at eupneic levels (65). This was ascribed to the partial restoration of cardiac output at depth, as previously described by Linér et al. (57), and to reduced peripheral vasoconstriction (65).

The effects of compression and decompression on O_2 exchange in the alveoli become particularly intriguing in extremely deep dives such as those performed by a small group of divers in recent years. The literature does not offer information about blood gas tensions during such dives, but Olszowka and Rahn (66) made computer simulations of a 100-m dive lasting 220 sec. Their analysis suggests that during the last part of the ascent, when hypoxia threatens, there is a reversal of the O_2 flow, so that oxygen moves from the venous blood into the alveoli. Such a reversal of O_2 transfer was actually observed during the ascents from nonimmersed dives to 10 m in a pressure chamber (29). This mechanism slows the drop in PA_{O_2}, and consequently in Pa_{O_2}, thus offering a measure of protection against hypoxia. Based on computer simulation, this phenomenon is illustrated in Fig. 11. Notwithstanding a possible protective effect of the O_2 flow reversal, deep dives pose the risk of severe hypoxia. Thus, in two dives to 70 m in the ocean, the P_{O_2} in end-expiratory gas samples taken as the diver broke the surface were 30.6 and 39.4 mmHg, respectively (36). However, the duration of those two dives were 151 and 144 sec, respectively. Thus, it took almost three times longer for the diver to arrive at an alveolar oxygen pressure comparable to Pa_{O_2} values recorded in arterial blood in the Korean Amas after dives to 5 m lasting less than 55 sec (62) or in alveolar gas samples showing a lowest value of 28 mmHg in Amas performing 45-sec dives to 11 m (60). It appears that there is no reason to expect significant differences between alveolar and arterial gas tensions during the Amas' dives, according to Qvist et al. (62). They argued that, based on comparisons between their results and those of Hong et al. (60), there are no significant ventilation-perfusion inequalities in this type of diving. A more even distribution of alveolar gas volume relative to perfusion during breath-hold diving is also indicated by more direct

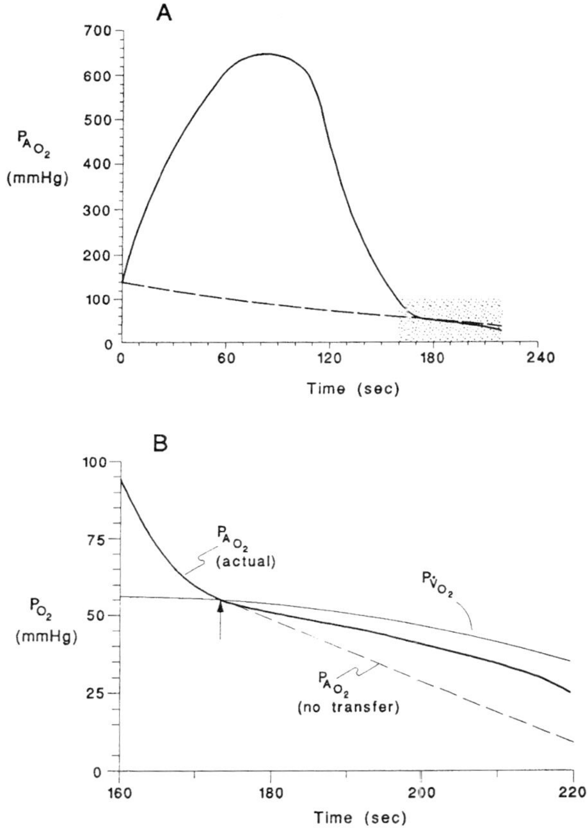

Figure 11 (A) Broken line represents computer simulation of the alveolar Po_2 versus time during breath-holding at the surface. Solid line represents breath-hold diving by the same imaginary subject descending at a rate of 0.91 m/sec, reaching a depth of 100 m at 110 sec and returning to the surface at 220 sec. Shaded area is enlarged in panel B. (Slightly modified from Ref. 66.) (B) Enlargement of shaded area in panel A showing last 60 sec of breath-hold dive to 100 m with alveolar Po_2 (heavy solid line) and the mixed venous Po_2 (light solid line). Arrow indicates the crossover point, after which venous Po_2 exceeds alveolar Po_2 and reversal of O_2 flow would occur, thus making the fall in alveolar and thus arterial Po_2 less rapid. If this retrograde O_2 flow did not occur, alveolar Po_2 would follow the interrupted line. (From Ref. 66.)

experimental evidence, as will be discussed later on. The slower development of alveolar hypoxia in the deep dives than in the briefer, shallow dives in the Amas could depend on several factors. The Amas' dives were unassisted; i.e., they swam down and up while the deep dives were assisted, the diver being pulled down by a weight and up by a flotation device. Moreover, the longer duration of the deep dives would allow more time for a full-fledged diving response (see below) to develop.

Carbon Dioxide Stores

The CO_2 stores, at about 123 L, include the bone store (67), and they are constituted mostly by tissues other than the blood, with slower gas exchange. The ''total labile CO_2 store,'' excluding bone, has been calculated by Farhi and Rahn (68) to be 16.6 L, with the muscle component being 9.6 L. Both the magnitude of the CO_2 stores and the CO_2 storage capacity are important for breath-hold endurance. The storage capacity can be thought of as the elastance of the CO_2 stores. As for the first aspect, it is obvious that if a breath-hold is started with smaller-than-normal CO_2 stores, the amount of CO_2 that can be accumulated before reaching the breaking point P_{CO_2} is larger. Pre-breath-hold hyperventilation makes use of this principle to prolong the breath-hold. For instance, a resting subject who hyperventilated by taking 20 deep breaths in the course of 1 min eliminated about 1.4 L of CO_2 (69). This exceeds the eupneic CO_2 elimination by about 1.1 L, an amount that would be equivalent to slightly less than 4 min of CO_2 production under resting conditions. However, hyperventilation does little to increase the oxygen stores. For instance, increasing the alveolar O_2 fraction from eupneic level at, say, 0.15 to 0.18 would only raise the O_2 content in the lung, at a TLC of 5 L STPD, by 0.15 L, corresponding to ½ min of eupneic O_2 usage. Since the blood is already saturated with O_2 during normal breathing, its O_2 content will not increase appreciably. Unfortunately, forceful hyperventilation prior to a dive can delay the diver's hypercapnic respiratory drive long enough for profound hypoxia to develop during the breath-hold; consequently, loss of consciousness may occur (33,70). This may cause the diver to drown, as suggested by Craig's review of 58 cases of loss of consciousness during underwater swimming (71). Similar observations in South African spearfishermen have been reported by Landsberg (54). By contrast, Korean and Japanese female divers do not hyperventilate to any great extent before diving, and loss of consciousness does not occur frequently enough to be recognized as a professional hazard by these divers (60). Hyperventilation per se, without the resulting hypocapnia (eucapnic hyperventilation), is not effective in prolonging breath-hold time (72).

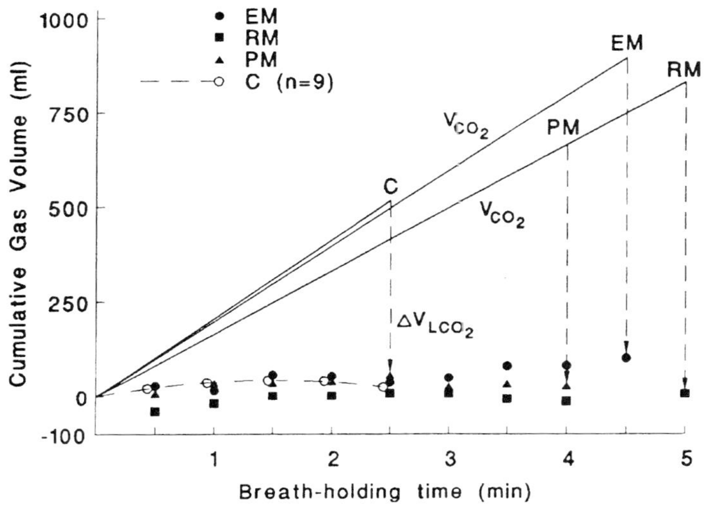

Figure 12 Cumulative volume of carbon dioxide delivered to the lung during nonimmersed maximal breath-holds performed by three highly trained divers (EM, RM, and PM) and nine age- and sex-matched control subjects. Solid lines show hypothetical individual cumulative carbon-dioxide delivery to the lungs based on measurements during eupnea. Arrows and ΔV_{LCO_2} are changes in carbon dioxide stores in the lungs (From Ref. 36.)

An important aspect of how the body handles the accumulating CO_2 load during a breath-hold relates to the CO_2 storage capacity. This dictates how much P_{CO_2} will increase from the retention of a given amount of CO_2. Other than the lungs, the tissue primarily involved in storing CO_2, in the time course of a breath-hold is the blood. As the breath-hold surpasses 1 min, the skeletal muscles and viscera come into play (73). With an unsteady state of CO_2 exchange lasting 1 to 8 min, the storage capacity for CO_2 has been given at between 0.40 and 0.50 ml of CO_2/kg of body weight and change in P_{CO_2} (in millimeters of mercury) as reviewed by Farhi (73). It is noteworthy that, in contrast to the differences in oxygen usage (Fig. 9) between untrained controls and three highly trained breath-hold divers, CO_2 exchange was quite similar in the two groups during maximal nonimmersed breath-holds (Fig. 12). In both, there was very little CO_2 delivery to the lung and eventually even some reversal of CO_2 flow. However, it took longer for the divers to reach breaking-point P_{CO_2} and P_{O_2} as recorded in the air expired after the breath-hold. The amount of CO_2 stored in the tissues by the divers was roughly twice as large as in the controls. Yet, the increase in end-expired P_{CO_2} post-breath-hold was very nearly the same in the two groups. Consequently, Ferretti et al. (36) calculated the whole-body storage capacity for the three divers to be 0.48, 0.76, and 0.66 ml·kg^{-1}·mmHg, respectively, which was considerably more than that of the controls (0.34 ml·kg^{-1}·mmHg). It is noteworthy that, in the deep dives performed by these divers, roughly the same post-apnea P_{CO_2} levels were reached as in the nonimmersed breath-holds, although the dives typically lasted only half as long.

Submersion in thermoneutral water has been shown to increase breath-holding time by 20 to 25% (24,35). Three mechanisms that could explain this prolongation of the breath-hold duration were investigated by Chang and Lundgren (35): (1) a decrease in metabolic rate, (2) a decrease in CO_2 chemosensitivity, and (3) an increase in CO_2 storage capacity. They found no change in metabolic rate or in CO_2 sensitivity during immersed breath-holds. However, in the course of a 4-min CO_2-rebreathing maneuver, the rate of rise of end-tidal P_{CO_2} was 31 % slower in head-out immersion than during nonimmersion (Fig. 13). This was considered consistent with an increase in the acute CO_2 storage capacity. The CO_2 storage capacity was estimated at 0.52 ml·kg^{-1}·mmHg for the dry control condition, and it increased to 0.66 ml·kg^{-1}·mmHg^{-1} during immersion. This increase in the acute CO_2 storage capacity (but not in steady-state CO_2 storage capacity) was ascribed by the authors to the possibility that immersion may accelerate CO_2 redistribution in the body by increasing blood

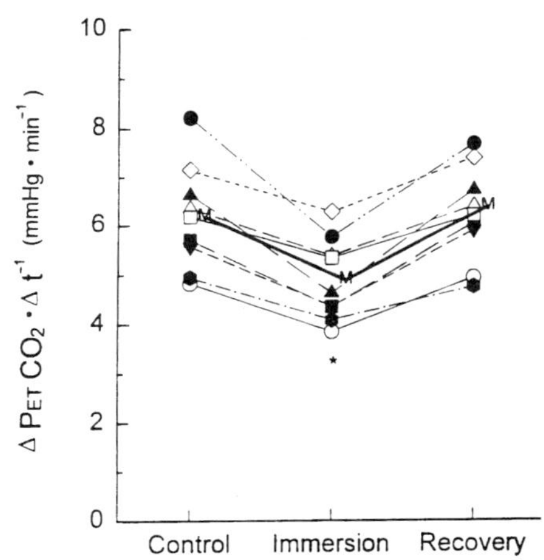

Figure 13 Rate of rise of end-tidal partial pressure of CO_2 while rebreathing into 6-L bag during nonimmersion (control), immersion, and recovery from immersion (in nine subjects; M is the mean). The end-tidal P_{CO_2} buildup rate was significantly slower during immersion, indicating a larger CO_2 storage capacity than during nonimmersion. (Slightly modified from Ref. 35.)

flow to normally low-perfused, low-metabolism, and high-capacity tissues (e.g., resting skeletal muscles).

The CO_2 dynamics as described by Linér et al. (57) during surface breath-holding and breath-hold dives to 20 m are shown in Fig. 10A, B, and C. The P_{ACO_2} increased first rapidly and then more slowly, while oxygen uptake from the lung diminished markedly in the course of breath-holds. The reduction in O_2 uptake was attributed to the limited reservoir of O_2 in the lungs. The rate of CO_2 transfer from the blood into the alveoli (Fig. 10C) showed a pattern similar to that described earlier by Mithoefer (51) and by Lanphier and Rahn (56): it decreased, becoming negligible by 30 sec and remaining so for the rest of the breath-hold. No appreciable reversal of CO_2 flow was noted during the surface breath-holds. By contrast, during the 20-sec descent phase of the dives, P_{ACO_2} increased markedly (again, due to lung compression), rising above the normal mixed venous level; CO_2 transfer was reversed and CO_2 was taken up by the blood at a rate of about 140 ml · min^{-1} · m^2 (body surface area). When the bottom was reached, P_{ACO_2} was 52 mmHg and there was no net CO_2 transfer. During ascent, the falling ambient pressure reduced alveolar P_{ACO_2}, reestablishing a normal direction for CO_2 transfer. The CO_2 volume transferred to the lungs during ascent was not enough to compensate for all the CO_2 accumulated in the blood and tissues during the dive. Therefore, the final CO_2 content in the lungs was 45 ml less than at the end of breath-holding at the surface. This drop in P_{ACO_2} could contribute, together with lung expansion, to a sense of relief experienced by the diver on ascent. Lanphier and Rahn (29) suggested that this sense of relief could reduce the divers' incentive to surface rapidly, thus further increasing the risk of hypoxia on ascent, as mentioned earlier. Linér et al. (57) suggested that, early in the descent, an increase in cardiac output would enhance the rate of rise in P_{ACO_2}. Then, once the P_{ACO_2} exceeds $P_{\bar{V}CO_2}$ the increase in pulmonary blood flow would slow the rise in P_{ACO_2}. The fact that, at the bottom, there was no CO_2 exchange indicates that the CO_2 pressure in the alveolar gas was the same as that in the venous blood. Then, early in the ascent, the CO_2 exchange would be enhanced by the improved venous return and cardiac output.

A notable feature of the comparisons of the breath-hold dives and the nonimmersed breath-holds shown in Fig. 8 is that for any given P_{O_2} level, there was a lower P_{CO_2} in lung air after the dives than after the surface breath-holds. One factor contributing to this difference in these particular experiments is that the dives were preceded by more hyperventilation. However, it is quite likely that two other factors of more general significance contributed as well. The pressure-induced reversal of CO_2 flow from the lung to the blood during descent to depth, together with the enhanced pulmonary blood flow, serves to increase the tissue CO_2 stores (65), as does the increased CO_2-storage capacity induced by immersion (37). That is to say, the CO_2 is stored at a relatively low P_{CO_2} in the tissues during the dives and cannot be delivered rapidly enough to the alveoli to keep pace with the rapid fall in alveolar Pco_2 caused by the reduction in alveolar gas pressure during ascent, a concept earlier described by Lanphier and Rahn (29). During breath-holding at the surface, on the other hand, the increase in alveolar CO_2 is driven by venous PCO_2 and the CO_2-concentrating effect of oxygen uptake. The total CO_2 retention over 75 sec in simulated breath-hold dives to 20 m studied by Linér and Linnarsson (65) was 73 $ml \cdot m^{-2}$ of body surface area. Those dives were performed 15 min apart, allowing ample time for normalization of the CO_2 stores. By contrast, in experiments by Paulev and Neraa (74), the dives, which were performed to 18.5 m in a submarine escape training tank and lasted between 36 and 124 sec were spaced only 1 to 2 min apart. An excess elimination of as much as 3.5 L of CO_2 was recorded during 16 min of sampling following a series of seven dives. The authors stated that such a large CO_2 retention may cause CO_2 narcosis. Linér and Linnarsson (65) suggested that a surface interval of about 3 min, equal to four times the time constant for CO_2 exchange (in such short-lasting events), would be adequate to avoid CO_2 retention between dives. Furthermore, they argued that redistribution of blood flow from peripheral to central vascular beds during breath-holding would increase blood flow in tissues with relatively rapid CO_2 turnover and that the similarity in the rates of O_2 and CO_2 exchange following breath-holds indicates that the largest part of the increase in tissue CO_2 stores during breath-holds occurs in blood and other rapidly equilibrating tissues.

The intrapulmonary distribution of gas exchange is altered by breath-holding, submersion, and compression to 20 m of depth (75). In particular, the alveolar plateau (phase III) of the expired CO_2 trace was flatter after a submersed breath-hold, presumably due to a more homogeneous intrapulmonary perfusion than during nonsubmersed breath-holds. However, after submersed dives, a relatively pronounced slope of the plateau was observed; it was attributed to enhanced CO_2 flow into the alveoli during expiration. Furthermore, cardiogenic oscillations in the alveolar plateau were largest after non-submersed breath-holds and smallest after submersed dives. This was considered consistent with the more even distribution of pulmonary perfusion during submersion (see Ref. 76) and compression. Finally, changes in phase IV of CO_2 and O_2 tracings in expired gas were thought to indicate less even interregional CO_2 distribution and more even O_2 distribution in the lungs after submersed breath-hold dives as compared with submersed breath-holds. These findings were supposedly linked to changes in cardiac output and in distribution of lung perfusion during different phases of the dive (75).

It is important to note that many of the experimental studies referred to above, which employed breath-holds or simulated dives, were performed under thermoneutral non-immersed conditions. By contrast, under field conditions, exposure of at least the face to cool water is likely. This typically triggers the diving response (see below), which might result in circulatory changes different from the ones observed in the thermoneutral setting.

The Diving Response

By definition, apneic submersion is synonymous with diving, and when the face is exposed to water, a number of reflexly initiated physiological events may occur that are collectively known as the diving response. These events are summarized in Table 2.

The following presentation will be limited to those circulatory aspects of the diving response that may be of consequence for respiratory function in the broadest sense and those respiratory factors that in turn, may impact on the diving response. The main manifestation of the diving response in terms of its

Table 2 Characteristics of the Diving Response

Stimuli and pathways	Responses and effects
Voluntary apnea; pathway unknown	Reinforcement of hemodynamic responses below
Cold stimulation of facial nerve	
Inhibition of somatic innervation to diaphragm and other respiratory muscles	Spontaneous apnea; reinforcement of hemodynamic responses below
Excitation of vagal nerves to heart, suppression of SA pacemaker, bronchoconstriction (78)	Bradycardia Junctional rhythm Reduced contractile force and stroke volume Reduced forced expiratory flow
Inhibition of β-adrenergic nerves to heart	Reinforcement of above
Excitation of α-adrenergic nerves to visceral, cutaneous, and muscle arteries	Peripheral vasoconstriction Reduction or interruption of peripheral blood flow; elevation of diastolic pressure; (preservation of cerebral and cardiac muscle blood flow) Economization with oxygen stored in lungs and blood
O_2 sparing through anaerobic metabolism	Temporary accumulation of lactate, CO_2, and potassium; lowering of blood pH

Source: Modified from Ref. 77.

purported biological significance is a reduction of blood flow to muscles, skin, and viscera while perfusion of the heart muscle and brain is maintained. Prominent features of this response are a slowing of the heart rate (diving bradycardia), a reduction in cardiac output, and changes in blood pressure. These changes are exemplified in Fig. 14 and 15. The diving response may be potentiated by a number of factors such as exercise (for a review, see Ref. 79), immersion of the face in cold water (e.g., Refs. 80 and 81), physical training (for a review see Ref. 82), and diving experience (e.g., Refs. 52 and 83). Factors related to respiratory function that may influence the diving response include lung volume, intrathoracic pressure, and level of asphyxia during the breath-hold. There are, however, a number of conflicting observations regarding these factors, and the reasons for these discrepancies are not clear.

Heart rate during breath-holding has been found to be directly related to the lung volume at which the breath is held. Thus, Elsner et al. (84) found that during breath-holding combined with face immersion, both bradycardia and reduction in peripheral blood flow were most pronounced in expiratory position. Similarly, according to Andersson and Schagatay (25), apneic face immersion caused lower heart rate and cutaneous blood flow when the breath was held at 60% of vital capacity than at 85% or 100% of vital capacity. Another indication that low lung volume may enhance diving bradycardia is the observation that bradycardia developed more rapidly in exercising subjects when apnea with face immersion began after a tidal-breath expiration than after an inspiration (85). By contrast, Kawakami et al. (80) saw no difference in bradycardia during apneic face immersion in cold water when they compared breath-holding at FRC

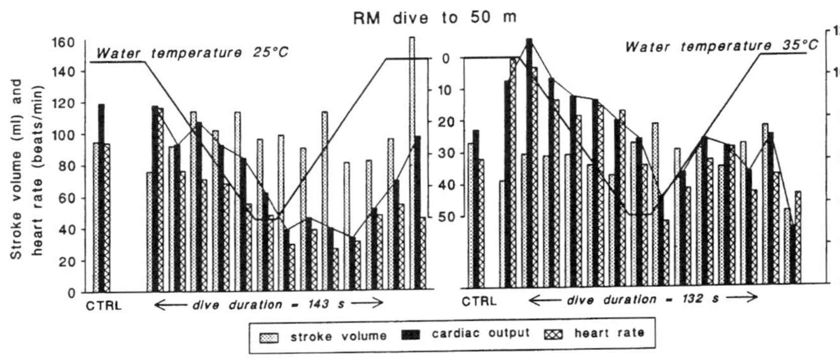

Figure 14 Cardiovascular parameters during submersed simulated dives to 50 m performed by a highly trained diver in water at 25°C and 35°C in pressure chamber. Thick line on top shows depth-versus-time profile. Thin line connects data on cardiac output, showing a greater fall of cardiac output in the cooler water. (From Ref. 125.)

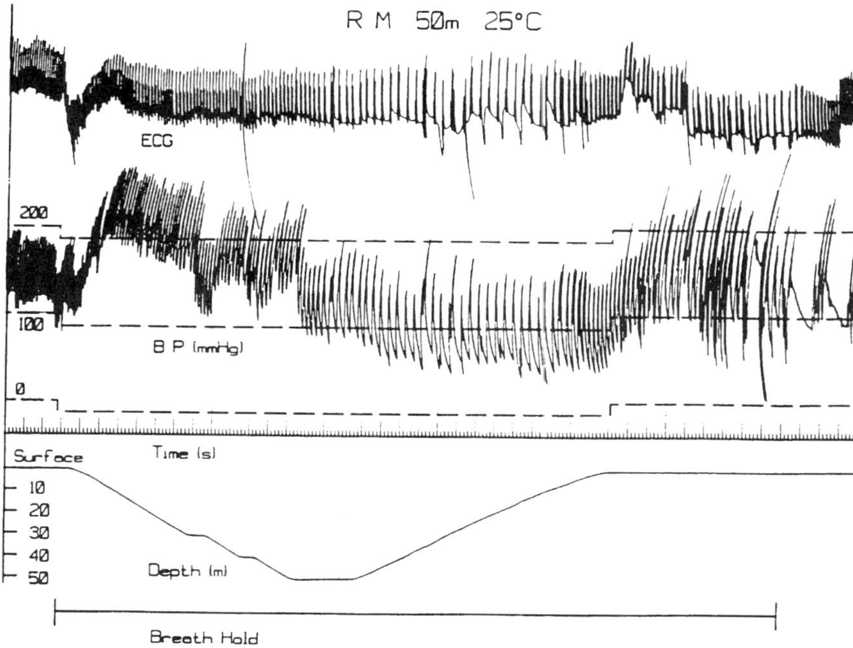

Figure 15 ECG and arterial blood pressure (measured invasively) versus time during a submersed simulated dive, performed by a highly trained diver, to 50 m in cool water (25°C). Breath-hold duration was 190 sec and dive duration 160 sec. (From Ref. 125.)

and TLC. However, their breath-hold durations were generally much shorter (30 sec or less), than in most other studies. Nonimmersed breath-holding has been reported to result in an inverse relationship between heart rate and lung volume (80,86,87). The effects of apneic lung volume in experiments by Asmussen and Kristiansson (88) are somewhat inconclusive, probably because the subjects, who were exercising, held their breaths for only 10 to 15 sec. Moreover, the subject pool was small and quite varied in terms of training.

The effects of different intrathoracic pressures on the diving response is of interest since, when the respiratory muscles are relaxed, breath-holding at volumes larger than FRC will raise the pressure. This is due to the recoil of the lungs, to which, at volumes larger than the resting volume of the thorax, is added the inward recoil of the chest wall. Thus, at TLC the intrathoracic pressure may be at least 20 $cmH_2.O$, and this pressure will counteract venous return into the chest, impair diastolic filling, and tend to decrease cardiac output. A similar effect is exerted by the Valsalva maneuver, which is often performed by the diver for the purpose of "ear-clearing" during descents. Pressor-receptor unloading during this maneuver occurs because of both a tendency of the arterial pressure to fall and because of the raised intrathoracic pressure, thus causing a tachycardia, which is often apparent at the beginning of a breath-hold dive (Figs. 14 and 15). Craig (89) has shown that when peripheral blood pooling, caused by high intrathoracic pressure, is counteracted by head-out immersion, the initial tachycardia is reduced and bradycardia develops more readily during the breath-hold than is the case during nonimmersed breath-holding. As the diver submerges the face, diving bradycardia ensues, and an additional negative chronotropic effect develops as the diver descends from the surface. This is because the increasing water pressure reduces the volume of the chest and lungs, thus lowering their recoil pressure and hence the relative overpressure in the chest.

The interruption of alveolar ventilation during breath-holding leads to hypoxia and hypercapnia. The effects of this condition of increasing asphyxia on diving bradycardia were studied by Lin et al. (90), who separated the individual effects of hypoxia and hypercapnia in subjects performing breath-holding with immersion of the face in cool water. The authors concluded that, in breath-holds lasting 90 sec, the apnea per se was responsible for an 18% reduction in heart rate and that concomitant hypoxia caused an additional 18% reduction, while hypercapnia accounted for a 6% cardioacceleration, yielding a net reduction of the heart rate of 31% during breath-holds with face immersion. A similar potentiating effect on the diving bradycardia by hypoxia was reported by Moore et al. (91), while asphyxia alone is probably not a major trigger of bradycardia (80). Measuring arterial blood gases during apneic face immersion, air breathing, oxygen breathing, and hyperventilation with oxygen, Elsner et al. (92) also found the bradycardia and the peripheral blood-flow reduction of the diving response to be basically independent of asphyxic blood gas changes.

Traditionally, the diving response is considered an important O_2 conserving mechanism in natural divers such as seals, whales, and ducks (for a review, see Ref. 93). It now appears that the preponderance of experimental observations supports the notion that the diving response can serve the same function in humans, although this may be evident only in trained breath-hold divers. The reduction in forearm blood flow, which is an element of the diving response in humans, was found to be inversely related to the fall in arterial oxygen tension during face-immersion apnea subsequent to hyperventilation with oxygen (92). This was considered as an indication that the diving response may serve an oxygen-conserving function in humans. During apneic face immersion in volunteers, Wolf et al. (94) noted that arterial O_2 saturations fell very little when the subjects exhibited a marked "oxygen-conserving reflex," whereas it fell markedly when, under identical conditions, the bradycardia and peripheral vasoconstriction were absent. While the authors just mentioned do not offer a lot of data in support of the notion of O_2 conservation, additional evidence has recently been provided by the observations of Andersson and Schagatay (95). They recorded reductions in heart rate and skin blood flow in subjects who performed apneas of equal duration in air and during face immersion in cold water. The bradycardia and reduction of peripheral blood flow were more accentuated during apneic face immersion than during nonimmersed apnea, while the reduction in arterial O_2 saturation was twice as rapid in the dry breath-holds as during apneic face immersion (Fig. 16A and B). Additional indications of an oxygen O_2-conserving effect by the diving response were obtained by the same authors (52) when they correlated maximal breath-holding time (at rest) to the intensity of the aforementioned circulatory responses triggered by apneic face immersion. They found that in subjects with actual dive training (but not in nondivers) the apneic time was significantly correlated to the reductions in heart rate and skin capillary blood flow. These observations are in agreement with those of Mukhtar and Patrick (96), who found that face immersion in cold water was connected with longer-lasting (14%) maximal breath-holds and with higher alveolar P_{CO_2} at the breaking point than apneas with face immersion in warm water. Moreover, when their subjects breathed either air or 5% CO_2 during cold-water face immersion, they exhibited transient hypoventilations of 13 to 10%, respectively. The authors concluded that apnea with face immersion in cold water modestly reduces ventilatory drive in humans and that this appears to be a component of the diving response (96). The same authors also found increases in maximal breath-holding time of 15% during apneic cold-water face immersion as compared with breath-holds without face immersion (97).

An immersion effect on CO_2 exchange has been described by Craig and Medd (37). They compared alveolar P_{CO_2} at the end of breath-holds lasting 30 sec in subjects swimming horizontally just under the surface of the sea and when they performed nonimmersed exercise on a bicycle ergometer. The oxygen uptake in the two situations was nearly identical. Yet, the $P_{A_{CO_2}}$ at the end of the breath-holds was distinctly lower (by about 10 mmHg) during swimming than during nonimmersed exercise. The authors entertained the possibility that, in the diving situation, peripheral vasoconstriction, as part of the diving response, would retard the flow of CO_2 from the tissues to the lungs, although they also discussed the possibility that body cooling in the water (27°C) may have caused a general vasoconstriction with the same effect.

In contrast with the observations of prolonged breath-holds during cold-water face immersion mentioned above are the results obtained by Sterba and Lundgren (32). Their five subjects were not trained divers but were selected on the basis of having a relatively pronounced circulatory diving response to apnea with face immersion in cold water. During maximal breath-holding efforts with the face in cold (20°C) water, their reduction in heart rate was on the average 12%, in cardiac output 6%, and in forearm blood flow 58% as compared with breath-holding with the face in thermoneutral (35°C) water. Yet, there were no

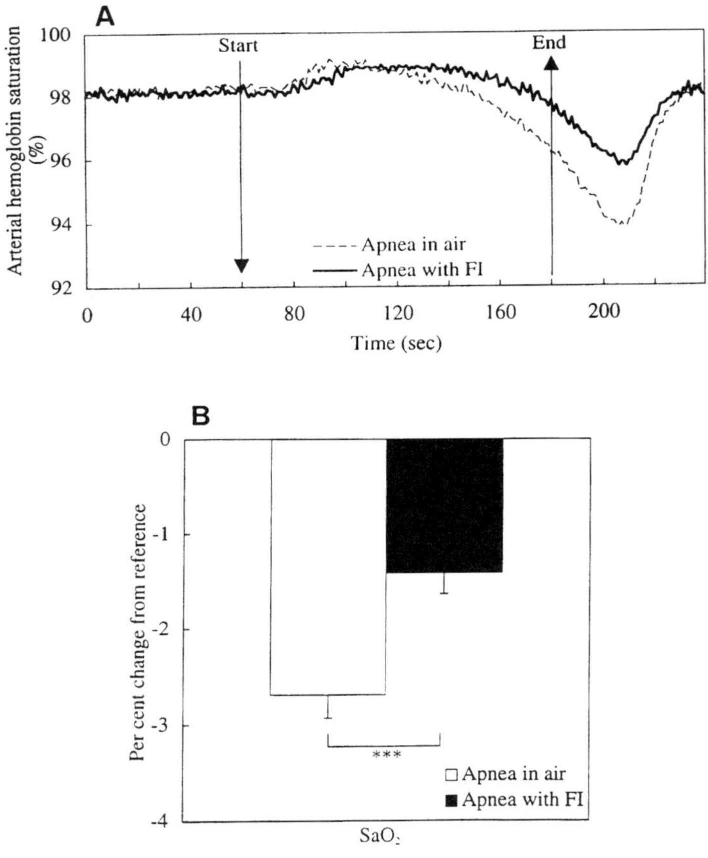

Figure 16 (A) Arterial hemoglobin oxygen saturation (pulse oximeter) versus time during a 2-min nonimmersed breath-hold (air temperature about 24°C) and a 2-min breath-hold with face immersion (FI) in cold water (about 10°C). Curves compiled from data in 16 untrained subjects. (From Ref. 95.) (B) Changes, relative to eupneic conditions, in arterial hemoglobin oxygen saturation during same conditions as in panel A. Data are mean values ± SEM. During nonimmersed breath-holding, heart rate and capillary blood flow (not shown) were reduced 7.8 ± 1.0% and 37.7 ± 3.6 (SEM)%, respectively. During face immersion, the reductions were significantly more pronounced i.e., 13.6 ± 1.0% and 55.9 ± 2.7%, respectively. (From Ref. 95.)

changes in breath-hold time, in time to first involuntary respiratory efforts (physiological breaking point), in alveolar CO_2 and O_2 tensions at the (conventional) breaking point, or in O_2 uptake from the lungs during the breath-holds. The lack of breath-hold prolongation despite a significant diving response in these subjects may perhaps, in the light of the observations of Schagatay and Andersson (52), referred to above, have been due to the fact that the subjects of Sterba and Lundgren (32) lacked specific training in breath-hold diving. According to Schagatay and Andersson (52), untrained subjects may, for psychological reasons, have a tendency to have shorter breath-holds when undergoing face immersion.

In most of the studies of the diving response and its consequences for breath-hold duration, the response has been elicited by immersion of only the face area during breath-holding. It is still uncertain whether observations under those conditions apply to actual breath-hold diving. Diving to between 40 and 70 m of depth in the ocean, three elite breath-hold divers wearing insulating wet suits exhibited elevations in blood lactate from 1.2 mmol predive up to 6.46 mmol postdive. This expression of anaerobic metabolism, which occurred at estimated power outputs of only 20 to 30% of the divers' maximal O_2 consumption, was considered a likely result of a diving response (36). The importance of this reaction pattern for performance is, however, not clear, since the dives only lasted 88 to 151 see and the same divers, when nonimmersed on a different occasion, performed breath-holds lasting up to 5 min. These prolonged breath-holds did not result in any appreciable changes in blood lactate, although they were characterized by considerable reductions in O_2 consumption as compared with the eupneic control situation (see Fig. 9) (36). In another study, in which the five subjects were thermally unprotected and underwent whole-body submersion in cold (20°C) water, apneic time was shortened by 54.9% as compared with nonsubmersed breath-holds, although the subjects exhibited an average reduction in heart rate of 25.9% (24). Two possible explanations for this paradoxical shortening of the apnea were stimulation of skin cold receptors and an increase by 256% in the metabolic rate from the cold exposure (24). Again, these observations were made in subjects who were not trained breath-hold divers. Naive subjects were also used by Hayward et al. (42), who exposed them to sudden submersion in water at temperatures from 0 to 35°C and compared heart rate and maximal breath-holding time with preimmersion control measurements. Water temperatures from 0 to 15°C reduced breath-holding time to 25 to 50% of control and heart rate to roughly half. The authors concluded that decreased breath-holding capacity, due to peripheral cold stimulation, reduces the effectiveness of the diving response and facilitates drowning (see also Sec. IV. A, "The Diving Response in Near-Drowning"). However, it is noteworthy that, when the subjects in this study were allowed a 2 min habituation period in the water and five deep breaths of hyperventilation immediately before the a second breath-hold, they were able to breath-hold twice as long as during the sudden first submersion. In fact, after habituation and when the water temperature was between 15° and 35°C, the breath-hold times exceeded the presubmersion breath-holds. The question, as of yet unanswered, is whether highly trained breath-hold divers such as the Korean and Japanese female divers, who are habituated to cool-water diving, benefit from the diving response. This question could be investigated by comparing dive performance with and without pharmacological blocking of the diving response.

III. Training and Adaptation

Some expert breath-hold divers excel in terms of the depth and duration of their dives, others in terms of the large number of dives they can do throughout a working day. The question inevitably arises whether their remarkable feats are the results of training and adaptation or genetics. It appears that there are no conclusive answers to these questions as of yet, but some observations point to the importance of training.

A. Short-Term Training

When several closely spaced maximal breath-holds are performed, there is a tendency for the second, third, and maybe fourth breath-holds to become progressively longer. This effect was noted by Israel (98) even when the recovery period between breath-holds was as short as 10 sec, but it was also present with a longer recovery of 4 min (24,99). This short-term training effect was ascribed partly to involuntary hyperventilation between breath-holds and partly to the subjects becoming inured to the unpleasant sensations of maximal breath-holds (99). The former explanation is consistent with the finding of gradual albeit small reductions in alveolar pre-breath-hold CO_2 pressures over the first few breaths while the breaking-point P_{CO_2} values were stable throughout five or six consecutive breath holds (99).

In experiments comparing the training effect of five breath-holds separated by 3-min recovery periods versus another series consisting of two breath-holds 3 min apart on each of 5 consecutive days, Hentsch and Ulmer (100) found the shorter intervals in the closely spaced breath-holds to be connected with a larger gain in breath-hold duration—i.e., 160%—while the gain in time between the first of the duplicate breath-holds increased by 60% over the 5-day period. In the series of five brief breath-holds, the onset of involuntary respiratory movements was delayed as much as 233%; the authors suggested that this may have been due to hyperventilation during the 3-min recovery periods. The corresponding delay in the 5-day series was only 14%. As pointed out by the authors (100), psychological conditioning seemed to have played an important but varied role in these experiments, which were all carried out at a depth of 1 m in a pool, since some of the 64 subjects were not comfortable with performing experiments in the water. Vasar and Kingisepp (101) suggested that an accentuated diving response observed with repeated breath-holds may be responsible for the increase in breath-holding time. However, more recently, Schagatay et al. (102) did not find diving bradycardia to be enhanced by repeated breath-holds with face immersion in cold water. Yet, breath-holding times to both physiological and conventional breaking points were increased by repeated breath-holds. Therefore, they suggested that both physiological factors associated with the accumulation of arterial CO_2 and psychological tolerance to the respiratory drive contributed to the breath-hold prolongation.

B. Long-Term Adaptation

Compared with untrained controls and older divers, young, trained breath-hold divers exhibit more pronounced diving bradycardia and peripheral vasoconstriction and longer breath-holding times (52). Adaptation to breath-holding and breath-hold diving in trained divers has also been suggested by Ferretti et al. (36), who studied three members of the same family (a father and his two daughters) who had personal depth records of 101, 80, and 70 m, respectively. As part of this study, the three elite divers and nine sex-and age-matched controls performed, at rest, a series of breath-holds of predetermined duration, increasing in 30 sec steps up to the maximum duration the subject could achieve. Each breath-hold was preceded by 1 min of hyperventilation. Samples of alveolar gas and blood samples for determination of lactic acid concentrations were obtained before and after each breath-hold. Arterial O_2 saturation was recorded continuously with an ear oximeter. The maximal duration of the breath-holds ranged between 240 and 300 sec in the divers and between 90 and 150 sec in the control group. End-tidal gas samples, obtained from the first post-breath-hold expiration, showed P_{AO_2} values as low as 28 torr in the divers, while P_{ACO_2} increased in the early stages of breath-holding, leveling off at 45 to 55 torr in both the divers and the controls (Fig. 8). The lowest arterial saturation levels recorded were 38, 63, and 78% in the divers and 83% in the controls. The changes in alveolar gas composition during breath-holding were faster in the controls than in the divers. Still, the relationship between O_2 and CO_2 pressures were the same in divers and controls (see Fig. 8). As shown in Fig. 9, the cumulative O_2 uptake in the divers during the breath holds (lasting longer than 60 sec) became increasingly lower than predicted from the eupneic $\dot{V}O_2$. Ferretti et al. (36) argued that, because lactic acid concentration did not increase at the end of the breath-holds, the missing energy must have come from high-energy phosphates and/or tissue stores in the divers. Trained divers have also been found to have a markedly different pattern of oxygen uptake than nondivers when exposed to low oxygen in the inspired air. Thus, when Schaefer's (103) subjects breathed 10.5% O_2 in nitrogen for 33 min, the divers had a consistently lower ventilation than the nondivers. Moreover, the four divers developed an O_2 debt (1033.8 ± 499 ml) three times larger than the four nondivers (347.8 ± 110.6 ml), and the authors concluded that a reduction in tissue oxidation had occurred in the divers (103). One diver, who developed an O_2 debt of 1562 ml, was studied during an ensuing recovery period of 33 min of air-breathing, at the end of which his oxygen debt still amounted to 1000 ml. This was taken to suggest that either the reduction in oxidation was still effective for a substantial period after the hypoxic exposure or that a shift to anaerobic energy production had occurred (103).

In conventional CO_2-sensitivity tests, the three earlier-mentioned expert divers had a blunted ventilatory response compared with the control subjects, whereas no difference was found in the response to hypoxia (104). The authors stated that the divers' relative insensitivity to CO_2 might be either an adaptive response or a genetic phenomenon. Similar observations of reduced CO_2 sensitivity has been demonstrated in the Korean diving women (105), in underwater hockey players (106), and in U.S. Navy breath-hold divers who also exhibited a depressed ventilatory response to hypoxia (107). In the latter, the reduced CO_2 sensitivity was clearly due to training, since it developed during a year of daily breath-hold diving to depths as deep as 90 ft. Among Japanese Ama, the Funado who make deeper and longer lasting dives exhibited low ventilatory response to CO_2 and to hypoxia, while the Kachido, who perform less strenuous dives, had no attenuation in CO_2 sensitivity but still a decreased sensitivity to hypoxia (108).

Other respiratory adaptations that may improve diving ability have also been reported. Japanese Ama (109–111) and Korean Ama (105) are able to generate a higher inspiratory pressure and have a greater vital capacity than untrained control subjects. Carey et al. (112) showed that vital capacity had increased in U.S. Navy divers after 1 year of dive training, again indicating an adaptive response. In all but one of the above studies (109), the larger VC was due to a larger inspiratory capacity. Moreover, a reduction in residual volume has been observed in swimmers after 4 months of training (113) as well as in U.S. Navy divers (112). A greater "pliability of the body wall" in Japanese Ama was described by Kobayasi et al. (114). These changes in respiratory mechanics would tend to enhance the pulmonary gas store as well as the TLC/RV relationship, which would allow dives to a greater depth without risking thoracic squeeze. The earlier-mentioned contraction of the spleen in Korean female divers, who perform very frequent breath-hold diving, has been proposed as a contributing mechanism behind the dive-related increase in hematocrit by Hurford et al. (64). The authors considered this phenomenon to be an adaptive response (see Sec. II. B. 2, "Oxygen Stores"), since it was absent in breath-hold dives performed by Japanese male scuba divers who had not routinely practiced breath-hold diving.

IV. Pathophysiology

A. The Diving Response in Near-Drowning

As already discussed, the hemodynamic changes of the diving response in humans have been found to be associated with enhanced breath-hold duration during apneic cold-water face immersion. However, the functional value of the diving response in actual breath-hold diving is not as clear cut because of the unfavorable effects of cold-water immersion on metabolism and respiratory drive (24,42). Nonetheless, the purported O_2 conserving effect of this response has been given as one explanation for the survivability of near-drowning incidents in cold water. Successful recoveries from submersions lasting as long as 38 min in an adult (115) and 65 min in a child (116) have been reported. While there is, for obvious reasons, no information about physiological reactions such as the diving response during the submersion phase in these cases, the victim is typically hypothermic when retrieved from the water. Hypothermia is not part of the diving response, but the hypothermia-induced suppression of metabolism without doubt plays a role in survival. The relative importance of the two events—i.e., the diving response and the hypothermia—depends on their temporal interplay, as pointed out in a review by Gooden (117). The following discussion of this topic is partly based on the article just mentioned.

Assuming the absence of life-threatening events, such as aspiration and its sequelae, the survival of the apneic person depends on oxygen availability and usage. As mentioned earlier, elite breath-hold divers may, under resting conditions and after 1 min of hyperventilation, even in the absence of face cooling, hold their breath for 5 min and possibly longer without suffering damage from hypoxia. It was also mentioned earlier that submersed breath-holds in trained divers were associated with a pronounced shift to anaerobic metabolism. The question is whether such changes, combined with redistribution of blood flow (which is part of the diving response), can provide enough time without hypoxic injury to allow hypothermia to develop so as to provide for long-term survival without breathing. To consider this question in a somewhat quantitative fashion, let us assume that O_2, stored in the lungs and the blood, is selectively distributed to the brain and the heart due to the dive response. This notion gets support from indications that other tissues are, to a very large extent, sustained by anaerobic metabolism, since lactic acid accumulation during breath-hold dives by a trained diver has been shown to exceed the equivalent of over 1000 ml O_2 (36). Experiments with asphyxiation of anesthetized dogs have shown that, as reflected in arterial O_2 content, more than 90% of the stored oxygen can be consumed before terminal failure of respiration and circulation (118). Based on this information, let us assume that of the total lung and blood oxygen stores in an adult of about 1250 ml, some 90%—i.e., 1125 ml—can be consumed without risk of hypoxic injury. With a reduction of the O_2 consumption of the heart to 58% of normal, due to the diving bradycardia (85)—that is, to 15 ml/min—and with a normal brain O_2 consumption of 50 ml/min for a total of 65 ml/min, 1125 ml of stored O_2 would last about 17 min. The time required to develop a degree of hypothermia sufficient to offer protection against hypoxic brain injury during apnea depends on several external factors, most notably body surface-to-mass ratio and water temperature. Amount of clothing worn and relative movement between skin and water are also important. The ideal case in terms of potential survival, as discussed by Gooden (117), is that of a small infant suddenly submersed in very cold water. In this example, the cooling rate was predicted based on data from Mohri et al. (119), indicating that in anesthetized infants, who for the purpose of surgery under hypothermia are surrounded by ice bags and ice cold water, the core temperature will fall 2.5°C in the first 10 min. Even such a modest reduction in brain temperature, if occurring while stored O_2 is available, will help to economize with the O_2. If measurements in anesthetized dogs apply, a 2°C cooling of the brain would reduce brain O_2 usage by at least 20% (120). However, in order for the brain to be cooled to a temperature that offers protection against prolonged hypoxia, the temperature must fall to 30°C (119) during the window of opportunity offered by the dive response. It is possible that the dive reflex under the conditions of a drowning incident is more effective than physiological experimentation in volunteers would indicate. As pointed out by Gooden (117), who quoted Wolf (77), anxiety and fear powerfully accentuate the diving response. It has also been suggested that the body cooling is particularly effective during a drowning incident because the victim may either inhale or swallow cold water. Based on quantitative reasoning, Gooden (117) effectively dismisses these mechanisms as unimportant.

The shortened breath-holding time in response to sudden cold-water submersion (42) was mentioned earlier. One can only surmise that, in an actual drowning situation, other important mechanisms come into play and prevent inhalation of deleterious quantities of water. For instance, respiration might in some cases be interrupted by laryngospasm as soon as a small quantity of inhaled water hits the larynx. From the foregoing, it would appear that the diving response probably plays a role in the survival from near-drowning incidents and that it may increase the likelihood that hypothermia develops to extend the tolerance to hypoxia. However, current experimental evidence does not adequately explain how nature handles the time gap between the end of the grace period offered by the dive response and the beginning of effective hypothermia.

B. Chest Squeeze

The importance of blood pooling in the chest for pressure equilibration relative to the surrounding water was discussed in Sec. II. A, "Depth." The question is: To which maximal depth will this mechanism provide adequate protection against "chest squeeze"? Neither theory, experimental evidence, nor field observations provide a conclusive answer.

Several possible mechanisms of injury can be envisioned to limit quests for deeper breath-hold dives—namely, rupture of pulmonary vessels and/or pulmonary edema, a deleterious increase in cardiac afterload, cardiac dilatation and/or serious arrhythmias, and decompression sickness. With regard to the first type of injury, it is noteworthy that West et al. (121) proposed that even a physiological act such as heavy exercise may bring the pulmonary capillaries close to stress failure, which may cause increased permeability, with protein leakage and frank hemorrhage. A case has been described by Boussuges et al. (122) in which lung injury of this nature apparently was precipitated by self-administration of aspirin before breath-hold diving. The diver dove repeatedly to 25 m over a 2-hr period, his dives lasting 2 min and alternating with recovery periods of about equal duration. At the end of the dive session, the diver developed a productive cough with hemoptysis; a chest x-ray indicated intraalveolar hemorrhage, which was verified by bronchoscopy and bronchoalveolar lavage. The patient recovered. A somewhat different chain of events, which possibly led to lung injury and the death of a breath-hold diver, has been reported by Strauss and Wright (123). The diver lost consciousness while breath-hold diving and then, supposedly after having exhaled passively to functional residual capacity, he sank to a depth where the alveolocapillary pressure gradient caused irreversible pulmonary damage. After rescue, within 3 min of the mishap, the patient's condition first improved and then progressively deteriorated. Autopsy showed extreme congestion of the lungs, edema, and interstitial and intraalveolar hemorrhage. The authors concluded that the findings were not compatible with drowning but ascribed them to thoracic squeeze.

Breath-hold diving may pose a danger to susceptible individuals by inducing cardiac arrhythmias. Apnea and face immersion in cold water not only cause diving bradycardia but may also be arrhythmogenic, as is the cardiac distention due to the redistribution of blood into the chest (124). Additionally, insults by hypoxia, acidemia, and hyperkalemia—frequent elements of the breath-hold dive—and cooling of the heart by blood returning from the periphery may be conducive to arrhythmias. Indeed, arrhythmias are frequently observed during breath-hold diving (83) and more so in cool water than in thermoneutral water (125); scuba diving, which also is likely to induce marked intrathoracic blood pooling (through the immersion effect), has been linked to arrhythmias and induced McDonough et al. (124) to propose that "cardiac arrhythmias, some of which may predispose to loss of consciousness and accidental drowning, occur during water immersion . . . such arrhythmias may be much more common than expected . . . they may comprise a significant proportion, perhaps the majority of unexplained death during water immersion."

In addition to the mechanisms just discussed, which may weaken the pumping action of the heart, another unfavorable influence may be induced by breath-hold diving. If a breath-hold dive can be made deep enough to make intrathoracic pressure lag behind the water pressure acting on the body, the cardiac afterload will increase and put further strain on the heart. However, when the maximal "safe depth" is discussed, one should remember that in terms of thoracic pressure equilibration, the addition of another 10 m from, say, 140 to 150 m, in compliance with Boyle's law, requires compression of the air in the lung by only about 6%, compared with 50% between the surface and 10 m of depth. This means that if (disregarding gas absorption in the blood) a dive starts at a lung volume of 6 L, this volume will, assuming pressure equilibrium, be compressed to 0.4 L at 140 m and the additional descent to 150 m will require an additional compression of the gas in the lung by only 25 ml, which would call for very little additional blood redistribution and/or compression of chest wall or stretching of the diaphragm.

C. Decompression Sickness

During a dive, nitrogen is taken up by the blood from the alveoli due to the increased N_2 pressure, which is caused by compression of the chest. However, Teruoka (55) speculated that during the brief dives of the Japanese Ama, not enough N_2 would dissolve in the blood to produce decompression sickness. Certainly, N_2 accumulation in the tissues can occur as a result of breath-hold diving. Using a computer model of gas exchange in the lungs, blood, and tissues, Olszowka (126) predicted a net increase of 700 ml in the amount of N_2 in the blood and tissues of a diver surfacing from a single dive to 90 m lasting 220 sec. In other words, N_2 is not unloaded to the lung as rapidly during ascent as it is taken up by the blood and tissues during descent. Nitrogen accumulation in venous blood as a result of repetitive breath-hold diving has been demonstrated in Korean female divers (127). During a 3-hr work shift, which included an average of 130 dives and 54 min under water, the venous P_{N_2} rapidly increased (half-time, 6 min) from a baseline of 584 to 640 mmHg and remained at that level until the end of the diving shift. Denitrogenation after the shift occurred much more slowly (half-time, 36 min) This amount of N_2 loading was not enough to cause decompression sickness (127), and this affliction is generally unknown among Korean and Japanese Amas. However, theoretical calculations indicate that enough N_2 could be taken up by the body to cause decompression sickness if a diver did repeated deep dives separated by short intervals at the surface (128).

The appearance of venous gas emboli, demonstrated with ultrasound Doppler technique, after repetitive breath-hold diving has been reported in a couple of studies (129, 130). However, a recent study (132) failed to detect bubbles in fishing divers who performed repetitive breath-hold dives to between 24 and 40 m, in some cases carried out with an intensity that would render them unsafe according to Lanphier (128). Yet, the authors concluded that their study was limited by too small a number of subjects and by a 3-min delay in starting the bubble monitoring after the dives. It is noteworthy that Schaefer (133), over 40 years ago, reported on observations of foam in venous and arterial blood drawn immediately after breath-hold divers surfaced from single dives to 90 ft lasting approximately 1.5 min. This phenomenon was absent in samples drawn approximately 10 sec after surfacing or 40 sec after starting ascent—i.e., at the end of the second circulation time. This foaming was considered an example of ''silent bubble formation''—i.e., symptomless bubbling (133), a condition first envisioned by Behnke et al. in 1940 (134).

Frank decompression sickness after breath-hold diving has been observed occasionally. Neurological symptoms suggestive of decompression sickness were experienced by four divers after repeated breath-hold dives to 15 to 20 m (136). In each of them, the severe neurological symptoms and signs were immediately relieved by recompression treatment. A syndrome called *taravana (tara*, to fall; *vana*, crazily) in pearl divers from the Tuamotu Archipelago has been described by Cross (3), who proposed that it may have been decompression sickness. The syndrome included nausea, vertigo, partial or complete paralysis, temporary unconsciousness, and, in some cases, death. After hyperventilation lasting 2 to 6 min, these divers descended to depths in excess of 100 fsw, staying at the bottom for 30 to 60 sec and remaining under water for about 1 ½ min. After hyperventilation, they dove again, repeating this sequence for about 6 hr per day. It is notable that another local group of diverse performing very similar dives but observing surface intervals about twice as long as the Tuamotu divers were not affected by taravana (3). Reminiscent of the taravana is the affliction of a spear fisherman described by Fanton et al. (137). This diver fell unconscious after emerging from a series of dives to 40 m consisting of 13 to 14 dives per hour for 3 hr. After 15 min of O_2 therapy at the surface, he woke up but exhibited slow mentation and temporospatial disorientation. Subsequent electroencephalography and magnetic resonance imaging investigations indicated a focal cerebral injury. The diver acknowledged several episodes of weakness in the arms after similar earlier diving activities. The account of another case suggests that even a single deep breath-hold dive can cause decompression sickness (138). The diver had made a dive (the only one that day) to about 120 m, a depth that he had reached several times earlier without problems. However, on this particular occasion he used a new assisted-ascent technique that gave him a very high rate of ascent—i.e., 4 m/sec. Shortly after reaching the surface, he experienced paresthesias in the right leg, followed within minutes by a right-sided hemiplegia. The patient was rapidly brought to recompression treatment, which was carried out according to a standard U.S. Navy table and the symptoms resolved within about 30 min. One might hypothesize that bubble formation in the arterial blood caused the symptoms in this case. Assuming a circulation time from the pulmonary capillaries to the brain of, say, 15 sec and given the very fast ascent, the blood arriving to the brain upon surfacing would have been saturated with N_2 in the lungs at a depth of about 60 m—i.e., at a pressure of 7 atm. This would have provided for a level of supersaturation in the blood, which would be highly conducive to bubbling. Indeed, if the circulation time between lungs and brain had been slowed by the diving response, the blood might have arrived at the brain with an even higher N_2 load.

D. Barotrauma During Ascent

Pulmonary barotrauma during ascent should, in theory, not be a problem for the breath-hold diver, since he or she returns to the surface with no more air in the lungs than when the dive began. Actually, allowing for gas uptake, the volume should be marginally smaller. The potential lung damage due to overdistention of the lungs during so-called free ascent from a sunken submarine or after running out of air in scuba gear is a different situation. In those cases the diver has inhaled a volume of compressed air at depth, which, during ascent, expands so as to exceed the ability of the lungs to accommodate it. This type of mishap is dealt with in Chapt. 8, ''Pulmonary Barotrauma.''

An unusual case of apparent pulmonary barotrauma and fatal air embolism in a breath-hold diver has been described by Bayne and Wurzbacher (139). The diver twice attempted to swim across a 25-yard pool at about 6 ft of depth. After the second try, he immediately suffered dizziness, headache, and ''tingling all over'' and complained ''my lungs are hurting.'' Minutes later he had a grand mal seizure and became pulseless and apneic. Advanced life support was unsuccessful. Autopsy revealed bleeding under the visceral pleura, mediastinal emphysema, and large amounts of air in the right heart and cerebral vessels; the left heart was not opened. The possibility was entertained that air was forced into the right heart from the lung circulation and that this constituted a genuine case of pulmonary barotrauma. One would then have to assume that during the dive, air shifted within the lung to a compartment that became relatively full at depth, was closed off (see Ref. 140) before ascent, and then became distended to the point of rupture during ascent to the surface. Alternatively, very forceful inhalation to total lung capacity might cause lung rupture by overdistension of a weak area in the lung, as illustrated by several case reports in Chapter 8, ''Pulmonary Barotrauma.''

E. Compressed Gas Narcosis

The narcosis experienced by air-breathing divers at depth is primarily an effect of N_2, although O_2 and CO_2 may also exert some narcotic action, as reviewed by Bennett (141). Objective and subjective manifestations of compressed-gas narcosis are usually first evident at depths of about 100 ft (30 m) and are very pronounced at 122 m (400 ft) (142,143). Since the deepest breath-hold dives performed today exceed the latter depth, the possibility of potentially incapacitating narcosis must be considered. No written accounts speak of severe narcosis during those dives. Other than a possible unwillingness of divers to share information in this regard, some other possibilities should be considered. One is that the dives typically are so brief that enough N_2 is not dissolved in the brain to exert a significant effect. Pertinent to this discussion are observations by air-breathing volunteers undergoing rapid compression and decompression in simulated individual submarine-escape procedures. Two U.S. Navy divers in a pressure chamber were compressed, while breathing air, to a pressure equivalent to 495 ft (150 m) of depth (144). Compression time was 21 sec and ascent was begun 9 sec later, at 8.65 ft (2.62 m) per sec. One diver experienced mild euphoria at maximal depth and throughout most of the ascent, which lasted 55 sec. The other diver noticed some disorientation at maximal depth, and this was manifest as a passing sense of rotation. One may conclude that N_2 narcosis was not a serious problem in these exposures, probably because the brief pressure exposure did not allow high enough N_2 concentrations to accumulate in the brain. Similarly, insufficient exposure time was thought to explain why subjects compressed to 500 ft (152 m) and decompressed 40 sec later only had a 15 to 16% increase in two choice-reaction times while at maximum depth (145). The breath-hold divers performing the extremely deep dives descend and ascend at about 2 m/sec, which means that they spend a relatively longer period of time at high pressure than did the subjects in the submarine escape simulations. For instance, F. Ferreras, in his record setting 133-m dive, would have spent about 22 sec descending from 90 to 133 m and the same amount of time ascending to 90 m, for a total of about 45 sec at depths that, in a steady state situation, would induce very pronounced narcosis. A question, not yet answered, is whether N_2 exchange between lung air and circulating blood would be hampered in lungs that are markedly compressed and engorged with blood. Another possibility to explain the lack of reports on narcosis in breath-hold divers is amnesia, which is a known effect of N_2 narcosis (141).

V. Concluding Remarks

The challenges to the respiratory function of the breath-hold diver are formidable and one has to marvel at the ability of the human body to cope with stresses that far exceed what normal terrestrial life requires. This plasticity of the system has allowed professional breath-hold divers such as the Korean and Japanese Ama to practice their vocation for centuries with remarkable safety. In order to be productive, they have limited diving depths and dive duration, so that they can tolerate daily repetitive dive schedules for years. This is contrasted with the very deep dives of, for instance, the Tuamotoan pearl divers and, in particular, those sport divers who pursue depth as an end in itself. While the diving conditions of the former have been defined by availability of shells only at great depths and an economic motive, the record breaker must push physiology to its limits. The initial predictions by scientists of the maximal ''safe'' depth were based on the ratio between the diver's total lung capacity and residual volume. Those predictions have been drastically corrected by reality. Divers have now exceeded those depths by about three fold and some interested parties have proposed, based on physiological reasoning, that the actual limit may be a good deal deeper yet. We hold that mother nature has already been sending warning signals, such as incidents of pulmonary hemorrhage and decompression sickness, as described in the foregoing. Unlike the case with most other performance sports, well-controlled experiments, close to the performance limits, cannot ethically be performed in deep breath-hold diving. However, quite a few enthusiastic divers seem determined to push the limits further, and the scientist is reduced to watching with concern and fascination. The limit may come to be defined by the unfortunate diver whose breath-hold will be of infinite duration.

Note in Proof

A potentially very dangerous trick to enhance the TLC/RV ratio known as ''buccal pumping'' or ''lung packing'' is sometimes used by breath-hold divers. After inspiring to TLC position, mouthfuls of air are repeatedly taken in and forced into the lung by keeping the glottis open while performing muscle contractions resembling swallowing. By this method, increases in VC by as much as 22–39% have been reported (151–153). The gain in lung volume is, in all likelihood, achieved partly by blood being driven out of the chest by the recoil pressures of the chest and the lungs. In a subject who increased his VC by 26% by lung packing, Örnhagen et al. (154) recorded an airway pressure, during relaxation, of 5.72 kPa versus 3.06 kPa after a normal inspiration to TLC. The authors pointed out that lung packing carries a substantial risk of lung rupture. Moreover, fainting, presumably due to a drop in venous return and hence in cardiac output, may be precipitated by lung packing. Reductions in systolic and diastolic blood pressure averaged 27% and 26%, respectively, in three subjects after lung packing (155). The potential gain in depth capacity that the breath-hold diver may achieve by lung packing may be offset by reduction in effective breath-hold endurance since the lung packing procedure is relatively time consuming (151).

References

1. Nukada M. Historical development of the Ama's diving activities. In: Rahn H, Yokoyama T, eds. Physiology of Breath-hold Diving and the Ama of Japan. Publication No. 1341. Washington, DC: National Academy of Sciences, National Research Council, 1965:25–40.
2. Schagatay E. The human diving response: effects of temperature and training. Lund, Sweden: University of Lund, Department of Animal Physiology, 1996.
3. Cross E R. Taravana: diving syndrome in the Tuamoto diver. In: Rahn H, Yokoyama T, eds. Physiology of Breath-hold Diving and the Ama of Japan. Publication No. 1341. Washington, DC: National Academy of Sciences, National Research Council, 1965:207–219.
4. Musenga G. Un pescatore di spugne (sommozzatore) che senza apparecchio si tuffa fino a 80 metri (Italian). Annali di Medicina Navale e Coloniale 1915; 163–167.
5. Maiorca E. Depth records: practical considerations. In: Lundgren CEG, Ferrigno M, eds. The Physiology of Breath-hold Diving. Undersea and Hyperbaric Medical Society Workshop. Bethesda, MD: Undersea and Hyperbaric Medical Society, 1987:291–294.
6. Rahn H. The physiologic stresses of the Ama. In: Rahn H, Yokoyama T, eds. Physiology of Breath-hold Diving and the Ama of Japan. Publication No. 1341. Washington, DC: National Academy of Sciences, National Research Council, 1965:113–137.
7. Agostoni E. Limitation to depths of diving: mechanics of chest wall. In: Rahn H, Yokoyama T, eds. Physiology of Breath-hold Diving and the Ama of Japan. Publication No. 1341, Washington, DC: National Academy of Sciences, National Research Council, 1965:139–145.
8. Ferrigno M, Warkander D E, Lundgren C E G. Unpublished observations. 1997.
9. Craig A B Jr. Depth limits of breath-hold diving (an example of Fennology). Respir Physiol 1968; 5:14–22.
10. Schaefer K E, Allison R D, Dougherty J H, Carey C R, Walker R, Yost F, Parker D. Pulmonary and circulatory adjustments determining the limits in breathhold diving. Science 1968; 162:1020–1023.
11. Warkander D E, Ferrigno M, Ferretti G, Cerretelli P, Costa M, Lundgren C E G. Unpublished observations, 1997.
12. Ferrigno M. Hickey D D, Linér M H, Lundgren C E G. Simulated breath-hold diving to 20 meters: cardiac performance in humans. J Appl Physiol 1987; 62: 2160–2167.
13. Arborelius M Jr, Balldin U I, Lilja B, Lundgren C E G. Hemodynamic changes in man during immersion with the head above water. Aerospace Med 1972; 43:592–598.

14. Kurss D I, Lundgren C E G, P°asche A J. Effect of water temperature on vital capacity in head-out immersion. In: Bachrach A J, Matzen M M, eds. Underwater Physiology VII. Bethesda MD: Undersea Medical Society 1981:297–301.
15. Dahlbäck G O, Jönsson E, Linér M H. Influence of hydrostatic compression of the chest and intrathoracic blood pooling on static lung mechanics during head-out immersion. Undersea Biomed Res 1978; 5(1):71–85.
16. Ferrigno M, Linér M H, Lundgren C E G. Cardiac performance during breath-hold diving in man: an overview. In: Lundgren C E G, Ferrigno M, eds. The Physiology of Breath-hold Diving. Bethesda, MD: Undersea and Hyperbaric Medical Society, 1987; 11:174–184.
17. Permutt S, Riley R L. Hemodynamics of collapsible vessels with tone: the vascular waterfall. J Appl Physiol 1963; 18:924–932.
18. Schaefer, K E, Allison R D, Carey C R, Strauss R. The Effects of Simulated Breat-holding Dives in the Dry and Wet Chambers on Blood Shifts into the Thorax. Report No. 729: Naval Submarine Medical Research Laboratory, October 26, 1972.
19. Rennie D, quoted in Ref 6.
20. Lin Y C, Lally D A, Moore T O, Hong S K. Physiological and conventional breath-hold breaking points. J Appl Physiol 1974; 37:291–296.
21. Whitelaw W A, McBride B, Ford G T. Effect of lung volume on breath holding. J Appl Physiol 1987; 62:1962–1969.
22. Lin Y C. Effect of O_2 and CO_2 on breath-hold breaking point. In: Lundgren CEG, Ferrigno M, eds. The Physiology of Breath-hold Diving. Bethesda, MD: Undersea and Hyperbaric Medical Society, 1987:75–87.
23. Rigg J R A, Rebuck A S, Campbell E J M. A study of factors influencing relief of discomfort in breath-holding in normal subjects. Clin Sci Mol Med 1974; 47: 193–199.
24. Sterba J A, Lundgren C E G. Diving bradycardia and breath-holding time in man. Undersea Biomed Res 1985; 12:139–150.
25. Andersson J, and Schagatay, E. Effects of lung volume and involuntary breathing movements on the human diving response. Eur J Appl Physiol 1998; 77:19–24.
26. Fowler, W S. Breaking point of breath holding. J Appl Physiol 1954; 6:539–545.
27. Whitelaw, W A, McBride, B, Amar J, Corbet, K. Respiratory neuromuscular output during breath-holding. J Appl Physiol Respir Environ Exere Physiol 1981; 50: 435–443.
28. Flume P A, Eldridge F L, Edwards L J, Houser L M. Relief of distress of breath-holding: separate effects of expiration and inspiration. Respir Physiol 1995; 101: 41–46.
29. Lanphier E H, Rahn H. Alveolar gas exchange during breathhold diving. J Appl Physiol 1963; 18:471–477.
30. Bartlett D Jr. Effects of Valsalva and Mueller maneuvers on breath-holding time. J Appl Physiol Respir Environ Exere Physiol 1977; 42:717–721.
31. Alpher V S, Nelson R B III, Blanton R L. Effects of cognitive and psychomotor tasks on breath-holding span. J Appl Physiol 1986; 61:1149–1152.
32. Sterba J A, Lundgren C E G. Breath-hold duration in man and the diving response induced by face immersion. Undersea Biomed Res 1988; 15:361–357.

33. Craig A B. Causes of loss of consciousness during underwater swimming. J Appl Physiol 1961A; 16:583–586.
34. Hong S K, Lin Y C, Lally D A, Yim B J B, Kominami N, Hong P W and Moore T O. Alveolar gas exchange and cardiovascular functions during breath holding with air. J Appl Physiol 1971; 30:540–547.
35. Chang L P, Lundgren C E G. Maximal breath-holding time and immediate tissue CO_2 storage capacity during head-out immersion in humans. Eur J Appl Physiol 1996; 73:210–218.
36. Ferretti G, Costa M, Ferrigno M, Grassi B, Marconi C, Lundgren C E G, Cerretelli P. Alveolar gas composition exchange during deep breath-hold diving and dry breath holds in elite divers. J Appl Physiol 1991; 70:794–802.
37. Craig A B Jr, Medd W L. Oxygen consumption and carbon dioxide production during breath-hold diving. J Appl Physiol 1968; 24:190–202.
38. Åstrand P. Breath holding during and after muscular exercise. J Appl Physiol 1960; 15:220–224.
39. Craig A B, Babcock S A. Alveolar CO_2 during breath holding and exercise. J Appl Physiol 1962; 17:874–876.
40. Keatinge W R, Nadel J A. Immediate respiratory response to sudden cooling of the skin. J Appl Physiol 1965; 20:65–69.
41. Cooper K E, Martin S, Riben P. Respiratory and other responses in subjects immersed in cold water. J Appl Physiol 1976; 40:903–910.
42. Hayward J S, Hay C, Matthews B R, Overweel C H, Radford D D. Temperature effect on the human diving response in relation to cold water near-drowning. J Appl Physiol Respir Environ Exerc Physiol 1984; 56:202–206.
43. Alvis H J. Breath-holding breakpoint at various increased pressures. MRL Report No. 177. 1951; 10:110–120.
44. Hesser C M. The role of nitrogen in breath holding at increased pressures. In: Schaefer K E, ed. Man's Dependence on the Earthly Atmosphere. New York: Macmillan, 1962:327–334.
45. Klocke F J, Rahn H. Breath holding after breathing of oxygen. J Appl Physiol 1959; 14:689–693.
46. Hesser C M, Beskow D, Holmgren B. Unpublished observations (1964) quoted in Ref. 47.
47. Hesser C M. Breath holding under high pressure. In: Rahn H, Yokoyama T, eds. Physiology of Breath-hold Diving and the Ama of Japan, Publication No. 1341. Washington, National Academy of Sciences, National Research Council, DC: 1965:165–181.
48. Hill L, Flack M. The influence of oxygen inhalations on muscular work. J Physiol (Lond) 1910; 40:347–372.
49. Pollok N W, Corkey W B, Natoli M J, Vann R D, Thalmann E D, Lundgren C E G. Oxygen-enhanced breath-hold (abstr). Undersea Hyper Med 1998; 25 (suppl), Abstract 69, 27.
50. Rahn H. Oxygen stores of man. In: Dickens F, Neil E, eds. Oxygen in the Animal Organism. Pergamon/Macmillan, 1964:609–618.
51. Mithoefer J C. Mechanism of pulmonary gas exchange and CO_2 transport during breath holding. J Appl Physiol 1959; 14:706–710.

52. Schagatay E, Andersson J. Diving response and apneic time in humans. Undersea Hyper Med 1998; 25(1):13–19.
53. Mithoefer J C, Stevens C D, Ryder H W, McGuire J. Lung volume restriction: hypoxia and hypercapnia as inter-related respiratory stimuli in normal man. J Appl Physiol 1953; 5:797–802.
54. Landsberg P G. Hyperventilation: an unpredictable danger to the sports diver. In: Lundgren C E G, Ferrigno M, eds. The Physiology of Breath-hold Diving. Bethesda, M D: Undersea and Hyperbaric Medical Society, 1987:256–265.
55. Teruoka G. Die Ama und Ihre Arbeit. Arbeitsphysiologie 1932; 5:239–251.
56. Lanphier E H, Rahn H. Alveolar gas exchange during breath holding with air. J Appl Physiol 1963; 18:478–482.
57. Linér M H, Ferrigno M, Lundgren C E G. Alveolar gas exchange during simulated breath-hold diving to 20 m. Undersea Hyper Med 1993; 20(1):27–38.
58. Ferrigno M, Hickey D D, Linér M H, Lundgren C E G. Cardiac performance in humans during breath holding. J Appl Physiol 1986; 60:1871–1877.
59. Schaefer K E, Carey C R. Alveolar pathways during 90-foot breath-hold dives. Science 1962; 137:1051–1052.
60. Hong S K, Rahn H, Kang D H, Song S H, Kang B S. Diving patterns, lung volumes and alveolar gas of the Korean diving women (AMA). J Appl Physiol 1963; 18:457–465.
61. Craig A B Jr, Harley A D. Alveolar gas exchange during breath-hold dives. J Appl Physiol 1968; 24:182–189.
62. Qvist J, Hurford W E, Park Y S, Radermacher P, Falke K J, Ahn D W, Gruyton J P, Stanek K S, Hong S K, Weber R E and Zapol W M. Arterial blood gas tensions during breath-hold diving in the Korean Ama. J Appl Physiol 1993; 75:285–293.
63. Stanek K S, Guyton J P, Hurford W E, Park Y S, Ohn D W, Qvist J, Falke K J, Hong S K, Kobayashi K, Kobayashi H, Zapol W M. Continuous pulse oximetry in breath-hold diving women of Korea and Japan. Undersea Hyper Med 1993; 20: 297–307.
64. Hurford W E, Hong S K, Park Y S, Ahn D W, Shiraki K, Mohri M, Zapol W M. Splenic contraction during breath-hold diving in the Korean Ama. J Appl Physiol 1990; 69:932–936.
65. Linér M H, Linnarsson D. Tissue oxygen and carbon dioxide stores and breath-hold diving in humans. J Appl Physiol 1994; 77:542–547.
66. Olszowka A J, Rahn H. Breath-hold diving. In: Sutton J R, Houston C S, Coates G, eds. Hypoxia and Cold. New York: Praeger. 1987:417–428.
67. Cherniack N S, Longobardo G S. Oxygen and carbon dioxide gas stores of the body. Physiol Rev 1970; 50:196–243.
68. Farhi L E, Rahn H. Dynamics of changes in carbon dioxide stores. Anesthesiology 1960; 21:604–614.
69. Corkey W B, Pollock N W, Natoli M J, Vann R D, Thalmann E D, Lundgren C E G. Unpublished observation, 1998.
70. Craig A B. Underwater swimming and loss of consciousness. JAMA 1961; 176: 255–258.
71. Craig A B. Summary of 58 cases of loss of consciousness during underwater swimming and diving. Med Sci Sports 1976; 8(3):171–175.

72. Norfleet T, Bradley C L. Can eucapnic hyperventilation prolong a subsequent breath-hold? Respir Physiol 1987; 70:369–376.
73. Farhi L E. Gas stores of the body. In: Fenn W O and Rahn H, eds. Handbook of Physiology; Respiration Vol 1. Baltimore, MD: Williams & Wilkins, 1964:873–885.
74. Paulev P-E, Neraa N. Hypoxia and carbon dioxide retention following breath-hold diving. J Appl Physiol 1976; 22:436–440.
75. Linér M H, Linnarsson D. Intrapulmonary distribution of alveolar gas exchange during breath-hold diving in humans. J Appl Physiol 1995; 78:410–416.
76. Arborelius M Jr, Balldin U I, Lilja B, Lundgren C E G. Regional lung function in man during immersion with the head above water Aerospace Med 1972; 43: 701–707.
77. Wolf S. Psychophysiological influences on the dive reflex in man. In: Neural Mechanisms in Cardiac Arrhythmias. New York: Raven Press, 1978:237–250.
78. Muktar M R, Patrick J M. Bronchoconstriction: a component of the ''diving response'' in man. Eur J Appl Physiol 1984; 53:155–158.
79. Lin, Y C. Physiological limitations of humans as breath-hold divers. In: Lin Y C, Shida K K, eds., Man in the Sea, Honolulu, HI: University of Hawaii Press, 1990, II:33–56.
80. Kawakami Y, Natelson B H, DuBois A B. Cardiovascular effects of face immersion and factors affecting diving reflex in man. J Appl Physiol 1967; 23: 964–970.
81. Schagatay E, Holm B. Effect of water and ambient air temperatures on human diving bradycardia. Eur J Appl Physiol 1996; 73:1–6.
82. Hong S K Breath-hold bradycardia in man: an overview. In: Lundgren C E G, Ferrigno M, eds. The Physiology of Breath-hold Diving. Bethesda, M D: Undersea and Hyperbaric Medical Society, 1987:158–167.
83. Scholander P F, Hammel H T, LeMessurier H, Hemmingsen E, Garey W. Circulatory adjustments in pearl divers. J Appl Physiol 1962; 17: 184–190.
84. Elsner R W, Garey W F, Scholander P F. Selective ischemia in diving man. Am Heart J 1963; 65:571–573.
85. Bjertnaes L, Hauge A, Kjekshus J, Soyland E. Cardiovascular responses to face immersion and apnea during steady state muscle exercise: a heart catheterization study on humans. Acta Physiol Scand 1984; 120:605–612.
86. Song S H, Lee W K, Chung Y A, Hong S K. Mechanisms of apneic bradycardia in man. J Appl Physiol 1969; 27:323–327.
87. Angeleone A, Coulter N A Jr. Heart rate response to held lung volume. J Appl Physiol 1965; 20:464–468.
88. Asmussen E, Kristiansson N G. The ''diving bradycardia'' in exercising man. Acta Physiol Scand 1968; 73:139–150.
89. Craig A B Jr. Effects of submersion and pulmonary mechanics on cardiovascular function in man. In: Rahn H, Yokoyama T, eds. Physiology of Breath-hold Diving and the Ama of Japan. Publication 1341, Washington, DC: National Academy of Sciences, National Research Council, 1965:295–302.
90. Lin, Y C, Shida K K, Hong S K. Effect of hypercapnia, hypoxia, and rebreathing

on heart rate response to apnea. J Appl Physiol Respir Environ Exerc Physiol 1983; 54:166–171.

91. Moore T O, Elsner R, Lin Y C, Lally D A, Hong S K. Effects of Alveolar PO_2 and PCO_2 on apneic bradycardia in man. J Appl Physiol 1973; 34: 795–798.
92. Elsner R W, Gooden B A, Robinson S M. Arterial blood-gas changes and the diving response in man. Aust J Exp Biol Med Sci 1971; 49:435–444.
93. Elsner R, Gooden B. Diving and Asphyxia. Monographs of the Physiological Society. New York: Cambridge University Press, 1983.
94. Wolf S, Schneider R A, Groover M E. Further studies on the circulatory and metabolic alterations of the oxygen-conserving (diving) reflex in man. Trans Assoc Am Phy 1965; 78:242–254.
95. Andersson J, Schagatay, E. Arterial oxygen desaturation during apnea in humans. Undersea Hyper Med 1998; 25(1):21–25.
96. Mukhtar M R, Patrick J M. Ventilatory drive during face immersion in man. J Physiol (Lond) 1986; 370:13–24.
97. Mukhtar M R, Patrick J M. Face immersion prolongs maximal breath-holding in man. J Physiol (Lond) 1985; 361:67P.
98. Israel S. Neue Gesichtspunkte zum Atemanhalteversuch in Klinik und sportärztlicher Praxis. *Zeitschr Inn* Med 1957; 12:1048–1052.
99. Heath J R, Irwin C H. An increase in breath-hold time appearing after breath-holding. Respir Physiol 1968; 4:73–77.
100. Hentsch U, Ulmer H-V. Trainability of underwater breath-holding time. Int J Sports Med 1984; 5:343–347.
101. Vasar E, Kingisepp P H. Physiological characteristics of repeated breath-holding. Adv Physiol Sci 1984; 10:639–646.
102. Schagatay E K, Van Kampen M, Andersson J. The effect of repeated diving apnea on apneic time and diving response in humans. Personal communication, 1998.
103. Schaefer, K E. Adaptation to breath-hold diving. In: Rahn H, Yokoyama T, eds. Physiology of Breath-hold Diving and the Ama of Japan. Publication No. 1341. Washington, DC: National Academy of Sciences, National Research Council, 1965:237–252.
104. Grassi B, Ferretti G, Costa M, Ferrigno M, Panzacchi A, Lundgren C E G, Marconi C, Cerretelli P. Ventilatory responses to hypercapnia and hypoxia in elite breath-hold divers. Respir Physiol 1994; 97:323–332.
105. Song, S H, Kang, D H, Kang B S, Hong S K. Lung volumes and ventilatory responses to high CO_2 and low O_2 in the Ama. J Appl Physiol 1963; 18:466–470.
106. Davis F M, Graves M P, Gey H J B, Prisk G K, Tanner T E. Carbon dioxide response and breath-hold times in underwater hockey players. Undersea Biomed Res 1987; 14:527–534.
107. Schaefer K E, Cornish E R, Lukas C A, Carey C R. Respiration and circulation during and after inhalation of various concentrations of carbon dioxide. MRL Report No. 189, XI, No. 6, 1952, quoted by Schaefer KE (Ref. 133).
108. Honda Y, Masuda Y, Hayashi F, Yoshida A. Differences in ventilatory responses to hypoxia and hypercapnia between assisted (funado) and non-assisted (cachido)

breath-hold divers. In: Shiraki K, Matsuoka S, eds. Hyperbaric Medicine and Underwater Physiology. Kitakyushu Japan: University of Occupational and Environmental Health, 1983:45–58.

109. Shiraki, K, Konda, N, Sagawa, S, Park Y S, Komatsu T, and Hong, S K. Diving pattern of Tsushima male breath-hold divers (Katsugi). Undersea Biomed Res 1985; 12:439–452.
110. Tatai, K, Tatai K. Anthropometric studies on the Japanese Ama. In: Rahn H, Yokoyamat. eds. Physiology of Breath-hold Diving and the Ama of Japan Publication No. 1341. Washington, DC: National Academy of Sciences, National Research Council 1965:71–83.
111. Tatai K. Comparisons of ventilatory capacities among fishing divers, nurses and telephone operators in Japanese females. Jpn Physiol 1957;7:37–41.
112. Carey C R, Schaefer K E, Alvis H. Effect of skin diving on lung volumes. J Appl Physiol 1956;8:519–523.
113. Bachman, J C, Horvath S M. Pulmonary function changes which accompany athletic conditioning program. Res Q 1969;30:235–239.
114. Kobayashi S, Ogawa T, Adachi C, Ishikawa F, Takahashi K. Maximal respiratory pressure and pliability of the body wall of the Japanese Ama. Acta Med Biol 1971;18:249–260.
115. Nemiroff, M J, Saltz G R, Weg J G. Survival after cold-water near-drowning: the protective effect of the diving reflex. Am Rev Respir Dis 1977;115:145.
116. Antretter H, Müller L C, Cottogni M, Dapunt O E. Erfolgreiche Reanimation bei ausgeprägter Hypothermie nach Beinahe-Ertrinken. Dtsch Med Wochenschr 1994; 119:837–840.
117. Gooden B A. Why some people do not drown: hypothermia versus the diving response. Med J Austr 1992; 157:629–632.
118. Herbert F J. Metabolic changes of blood and tissues during asphyxia. Am J Physiol 1948;152:687–695.
119. Mohri H, Dillard D H, Crawford E W, Martin W E, Merendino K A. Method of surface-induced deep hypothermia for open-heart surgery in infants. J Thorac Cardiovasc Surg 1969;58:262–270.
120. Steen P A, Newberg L, Milde J H, Michenfelder J D. Hypothermia and barbiturates: individual and combined effects on canine cerebral oxygen consumption. Anesthesiology 1983;58:527–532.
121. West J B. Tsukimoto K, Mathien-Costello, O, Prediletto, R. Stress failure in pulmonary capillaries. J Appl Physiol 1991;70: 1731–1742.
122. Boussuges A, Succo E, Bergmann E, Sainty J M. Hémorragie intra-alvéolaire: un accident inhabituel chez un plongeur en apnée. Presse Med 1995;24:1169–1170.
123. Strauss M B, Wright P W. Thoracic squeeze diving casualty. Clin Aviat Aerosp Med 1971; 42:673–675.
124. McDonough J R, Barutt J P, Saffron J C. Cardiac arrhythmias as a precursor to drowning accidents. In: Lundgren C E G, Ferrigno M, eds. The Physiology of Breath-hold Diving. Undersea and Hyperbaric Medical Society Workshop. Bethesda, M D: Undersea and Hyperbaric Medical Society, 1987:212–226.
125. Ferrigno M, Ferretti G, Ellis A, Warkander D, Costa M, Cerretelli P, Lundgren

C E G. Cardiovascular changes during deep breath-hold dives in a pressure chamber. J Appl Physiol 1997;83:1282–1290.

126. Olszowka A. Depth and time in relation to gas exchange. In: Lundgren C E G, Ferrigno M, eds. The Physiology of Breath-hold Diving. Undersea and Hyperbaric Medical Society Workshop. Bethesda, MD: Undersea and Hyperbaric Medical Society, 1987:12–31.
127. Radermacher P, Falke K J, Park Y S, Ahn D W, Hong S K, Qvist J, Zapol W M. Nitrogen tensions in brachial vein blood of Korean Ama divers. J Appl Physiol 1992;73:2592–2595.
128. Lanphier E H. Application of Decompression Tables to Repeated Breath-Hold Dives. In: Rahn H, Yokoyama T, eds. Physiology of Breath-hold Diving and The Ama of Japan. Publication No. 1341. Washington DC: National Academy of Sciences, National Research Council, 1965:227–236.
129. Spencer M P and Okino H. Venous gas emboli following repeated breath-hold dives (abstr). Fed Proc 1972; 31:355.
130. Nashimoto I. Intravascular bubbles following repeated breath-hold dives (in Japanese). Jpn J Hyg 1976; 31:439.
131. Lin Y C and Hong S K. Hyperbaria: breath-hold diving. In: Fregly M J, Blatteis C M, eds. Handbook of Physiology, Environmental Physiology. Vol II. New York: Oxford University Press, 1996:979–995.
132. Boussuges A, Abdellaqui S, Gardette B, Sainty J M. Circulating bubbles and breath-hold underwater fishing divers: a two-dimensional echocardiography and continuous wave Doppler study. Undersea Hyper Med 1997;24:309–314.
133. Schaefer K E. The role of carbon dioxide in the physiology of human diving. In: Grolf L G, ed. Underwater Physiology Symposium. Publication No. 377. Washington, DC: National Academy of Sciences, National Research Council, 1955: 131–141.
134. Behnke A R, Feen B G, Willmon T L. Preliminary report on aero-embolism and equipment for oxygen inhalation US NRC, CAM Report No. 3. Washington, DC: Experimental Diving Unit, US Navy Yard, December 1940.
135. Bateman J B. Preoxygenation and nitrogen elimination. In: Fulton J F, ed. Decompression Sickness. Philadelphia: Saunders, 1951:242–277.
136. Paulev P. Decompression sickness following repeated breath-hold dives. J Appl Physiol 1965;20:1028–1031.
137. Fanton Y, Grandjean B, Sobrepere G. Accident de decompression en apnée. Presse Med 1994; 23:1094.
138. Ferrigno M, Lundgren C E G. Unpublished information provided by the diver. 1998.
139. Bayne C G, Wurzbacher T. Can pulmonary barotrauma cause cerebral air embolism in a non-diver? Chest 1982;81:648–650.
140. Dahlbäck G O, Lundgren C E G. Pulmonary air-trapping induced by water immersion. Aerospace Med 1972; 434:768–774.
141. Bennett P B. Inert gas narcosis. In: Bennett P B, Elliott D H, eds. The Physiology and Medicine of Diving. London: Saunders, 1993:170–193.
142. Adolfson J. Deterioration of mental and motor functions in hyperbaric air. Scand J Psychol 1965;6:26–31.

143. Adolfson, J, Muren A. Airbreathing at 13 atmospheres: psychological and physiological observations. Swed J Def Med (Försvarsmedicin) 1965; 1:31–37.
144. Summitt J K, Herron J M, Flynn E T, Hall D A. Research Report 4–69, AD #694–937. Washington, DC: US Navy Experimental Diving Unit, May 9, 1969.
145. Bennett P B, Dossett A N, Ray P. Nitrogen narcosis in subjects compressed very rapidly with air to 400 and 500 feet. Report, Medical Research Council, R N Personnel Research Committee UPS 239, London, 1964. Quoted in Ref 141.
146. Sterba J A. Influence of the Diving Response and Submersion on the Breath-holding Time in Man. PhD thesis. Department of Physiology, School of Medicine, State University of New York at Buffalo, 1981.
147. Rahn H, Fenn W O. A graphical analysis of the respiratory gas exchange: the O_2–CO_2 diagram. Washington, DC: American Physiological Society, 1955.
148. Otis A, Rahn H, Fenn W O. Alveolar gas changes during breath holding. Am J Physiol 1948; 152:674–686.
149. Otis W O, Rahn H, Epstein M A, Fenn W O. Performance as related to composition of alveolar air. Am J Physiol 1946; 146:207–221.
150. Rahn H, Otis A B, Hodgeand M, Epstein M A, Hunter S W, Fenn W O. The effects of hypocapnia on performance. J Aviat Med 1946;17:374–380.
151. Hamilton R W, Olstad C S, Petersen, R E. Spurious increase in vital capacity by lung ''packing''. Undersea and Hyperbaric Med 1993; 20(suppl):66.
152. Vann R D. Pressure-volume characteristics of ''lung-packing.'' Undersea and Hyperbaric Med 1994; 21(suppl):42.
153. Chaduteau P, Friemel F. Etude d'une manoeuvre pour améliorer la performance en apnée profonde. Colloque International de Medecine de Plonger, Paris Dec 1996. FFDESSM et Societe de Physiologie et de Medecine Subaquatiques et Hyperbares de Langue Francaise (1996) quoted by Örnhagen et al., Ref. 154.
154. Örnhagen H, Schagatay E, Andersson J, Bergsten E, Gustafsson, P Sandström S. Mechanisms of ''buccal-pumping'' (''lung packing'') and its pulmonary effects. Diving and Hyperbaric Medicine: Collection of manuscripts for the XXIV Annual Scientific Meeting of the European Underwater and Baromedical Society, Stockholm, Sweden, FOA Report: FOA-B-98-00342-721-SE, 1998:80–83.
155. Andersson J, Schagatay E, Gustafsson P, Örnhagen H. Cardiovascular effects of ''buccal pumping'' in breath-hold divers. Diving and Hyperbaric Medicine: Collection of manuscripts for the XXIV Annual Scientific Meeting of the European Underwater and Baromedical Society, Stockholm, Sweden, National Defence Research Establishment, Sweden, 1998:103–106.

14

Diving Animals

GERALD L. KOOYMAN, PAUL J. PONGANIS, and ROBERT S. HOWARD

Scripps Institution of Oceanography
University of California, San Diego
La Jolla, California

I. Introduction

Most physiology texts that explain and discuss the physiology of diving seldom mention the diversity of vertebrate divers. In terms of the total number of species in a taxon, they are few, especially those that have invaded the marine environment. The limited diversity exists partly because it takes special and hard won adaptations for vertebrates to deal with limitations of access to one of the most critical of life-sustaining resources—oxygen. Nevertheless, although few in number of species, vertebrate divers have made up for this limited species radiation in abundance and biomass. Many were and some still are the most plentiful, widely distributed, and physically largest of all vertebrates that exist now or ever have existed. Few animals also have as remarkable a lifestyle as this polyglot group of vertebrates. In no context is this more obvious than when their physiology or behavior is discussed. To gain a better perspective of these animals, the following pages describe briefly the various major marine groups, give some detail of select species, and then discuss diving physiology, especially the lung at depth, in a few species representing the major groups of reptiles, birds, and mammals. The chapter is limited to marine species because few of the freshwater species are "real" divers in the strict sense; many are very good breath-holders, but they are adapted to subsurface swimming and not to descending to depth—e.g., freshwater turtles, many ducks, muskrats, and humans. This becomes clear from a comparison of the routine feats described in this chapter and the almost superhuman efforts reported for some champion human divers described in Chap. 13.

There are two major and two minor groups of marine species in the taxonomic class Reptilia. Out of a total number of 46 families, 2 families, turtles and snakes, have had major species radiation. There are eight species of sea turtle. In former times all were extremely abundant, but now all are listed as endangered species. Some species are restricted to the tropics or subtropics of either the Atlantic or Pacific Ocean, but one, the leatherback sea turtle (*Dermochelys coriacea*), occurs in all oceans and ranges as far north as subpolar waters. It also has the largest body mass of any extant reptile.

What sea snakes lack in individual body mass relative to sea turtles they make up in diversity. There are over fifty species. Most are found in the near shore waters of southeast Asia, but one, the yellow-bellied sea snake (*Pelamis platurus*), is found throughout the Indo-Pacific tropical waters from near Acapulco to Zanzibar.

A few crocodile species occur in coastal waters of some tropical regions, such as the American crocodile of the Everglades. They probably do very little if any diving to depth. Even more restrictive is the distribution of the only marine lizard, and that is the Galapagos marine iguana (*Amblyrhynchus cristatus*). It is a vegetarian that feeds on marine algae in or near the surf zone, and only the adult animals dive. Although totally dependent on sustenance from the sea, it has no distinct aquatic adaptations (1).

Out of 163 families and about 8600 species of bird, only 5 families are completely or partially marine divers. They represent 76 species. In the family of penguins (Spheniscidae), the most aquatic of all birds, there are only 17 species, and all occur in the southern hemisphere, give or take a degree or two of latitude for the rare Galapagos penguin (*Spheniscus mendiculus*). The penguin of the north, the flightless great auk (*Alea impennis*), was eliminated in the 1840s as a result of one of the saddest tales of human greed in an era of many sorry stories.

In the southern hemisphere, in addition to the familiar penguins, there are 14 species of diminutive diving petrels. Another extremely specialized group of divers are the loons and grebes, in which the legs are so modified for aquatic propulsion that these birds cannot walk on land. Cormorants and shags, of which there are 28 species occurring in almost every sea and lake of the world, are well known to any fisherman or any seaside or lake shore visitor. Within the alcids (puffins, auks, auklets, and murres) there are 22 species, many of which are unknown to the casual observer of sea birds. Within this group, the murres are the most penguin-like of any flying bird in body shape and perhaps diving ability as well. Ducks are the most diverse of all families of aquatic birds. They range from freshwater rivers to marine seas. Some ducks only dabble just barely below the surface, while others dive to at least 60 or 70 m. Not surprisingly, the domestic duck was the first subject of physiological studies of the response to breath-holding by Bert (2). Since then, a host of other investigators continue to study the domestic duck as well as a few other species. However, our discussion below focuses on penguins, which are the only group that have been studied in regard to the lung at depth.

Whales and dolphins, which are the most aquatic and diverse of all marine mammals, are represented by 10 species of baleen whale—e.g., blue whale (*Balaenoptera musculus*)—and 67 species of toothed whale, including the largest predator of warm-blooded prey that has probably ever existed. Because of their extreme specialization to the marine environment, physiological studies of this group have been limited, as will be our reference to them in the following discussions about the lung at depth.

The sea cows, which include four species of tropical-dwelling coastal, riverine, and estuarine mammals, are the only herbivorous marine mammal. Most if not all of their life is spent in shallow waters and little is known about their diving habits. Equally uncharacteristic of marine mammals are the sea otters. These relatively small marine predators from the weasel family are coastal species. Few people except locals know of or have seen the marine otter (*Lutra felina*) of South America. Little is known about its habits. In contrast, many people have heard about the widely distributed and high-profile California and Alaskan sea otters (*Enhydra lutra*). Their diving physiology is unstudied. Some aspects of sea otter biology would be especially interesting to the pulmonary physiologist because of this animal's unusually large lung—proportionately the largest of any mammal (3).

Of the 12 species of sea lion and 18 species of seal, one form or more occurs on every cold temperate or polar coast and a few tropical coasts of the world. These creatures range in body mass from the 25-kg female Galapagos fur seal to the 3000-kg male southern elephant seal. Their amphibious traits as well as their widespread distribution has made them readily available to zoos and laboratories. In regard to the physiology of breath-holding, they are the most studied group next to the domestic duck. Much attention in this chapter is given to some species in this group.

Because our emphasis is on the lung at depth, we present data and discuss results for only a chosen few diving vertebrates. The reasons are twofold: (1) data are available in regard to the effects of pressure on only a few species of divers. It should be kept in mind that all divers are not built alike and there have always been a few surprises with each new species investigated. (2) The species of most interest are those that dive to depth—that is, the mesopelagic predators. These species dive daily and routinely from a few to several hundred meters below the surface. This is not true of the neritic feeders, which comprise most of the sea snakes, many birds, and sea otters. Because of the unique physiological studies on the yellow-bellied (*Pelamis platurus*) and blue-banded (*Hydrophis belcheri*) sea snakes, they are reviewed along with the behavioral traits of the leatherback sea turtle and physiological studies of the green sea turtle (*Chelonia mydas*). Some aspects of the behavior and physiology of fur seals and sea lions are presented as a collage to develop a picture of how these animals might cope with pressure. Most emphasis on what we know will come from work on the well-studied Weddell (*Leptonychotes weddellii*) and northern elephant (*Mirounga angustirostris*) seals, with supportive evidence from the southern elephant (*Mirounga leonina*) and grey (*Halichoerus grypus*) seals.

Finally, and not the least, we conclude with one of the biggest puzzles in diving physiology and especially in the physiology of the lung at depth—that is, how birds survive diving to depth, especially to the extreme depths reached by emperor (*Aptenodytes forsteri*) and king (*Aptenodytes patagonicus*) penguins. In the lesson from the birds, we may take comfort in the expression "It is a wise ignorance that knows itself" (Pascal).

In order to develop a comprehensive framework of the conditions to which divers must have adapted, we present a few highlights of the diving characteristics of the species whose physiology is discussed. Then we present four major topics: (1) gas stores and the importance of the lung as an O_2 store as well as an N_2 store; (2) the general cardiovascular responses that are germane to how the vascular and lung O_2 and N_2 stores are distributed in the body while diving; (3) the effects of compression that relate to decompression sickness; and (4) the aerobic limits of the diver.

II. Behavior

The behavioral information discussed below is gleaned from an active field in which the amount of ecological data related to diving has expanded explosively. It is nothing short of phenomenal and has not really received its due recognition in the biological sciences. We are unraveling mysteries about animals dwelling in a habitat that is totally alien to us. Importantly, it is setting the boundaries within which our concepts about physiology must work. Despite the ever more elegant techniques and powerful measuring devices available to physiologists, they have been unable to keep pace with the behaviorists and ecologists. More functional questions are being asked than we can answer.

We have chosen to discuss one or two species from the major groups of sea turtles, penguins, and seals. The emphasis is on common foraging patterns and routine diving depths. To put this in the perspective of what the divers can do, the maximum diving depths for a variety of divers are presented in Table 1.

Table 1 Maximum Depths of Marine Divers

Species[a]	Maximum depth (m)	Method[b]	Source
Ridley sea turtle (*Lepidochelys olivacea*)	300	O	Landis, 1965 (4)
Leatherback sea turtle (*Dermochelys coriacea*)	>1000	R	Eckert et al., 1989 (5)
Cassin's auklet (*Ptychoramphus aleuticus*)	43	R	Burger and Powell, 1990 (6)
Common diving petrel (*Pelecanoides urinatrix*)	64	R	Chastel, 1994 (7)
Blue-eyed shag (*Phalacrocorax atriceps*)	116	R	Croxall et al., 1991 (8)
Common loon (*Gavia immer*)	60	N	Schorger, 1947 (9)
Thick-billed murre (*Uria lomvia*)	210	R	Croll et al., 1992 (10)
Atlantic puffin (*Fratercula arctica*)	60	N	Piatt and Nettleship, 1985 (11)
Chinstrap penguin (*Pygoscelis antarctica*)	70	R	Lishman and Croxall, 1983 (12)
Gentoo penguin (*Pygoscelis papua*)	156	R	Williams et al., 1992 (13)
Macaroni penguin (*Eudyptes chrysolophus*)	115	R	Croxall, 1993 (14)
King penguin (*Aptenodytes patagonicus*)	304	R	Kooyman et al., 1992 (15)
Emperor penguin (*Aptenodytes forsteri*)	534	R	Kooyman and Kooyman, 1995 (16)
Northern fur seal (*Callorhinus ursinus*)	256	R	Ponganis et al., 1992 (17)
Crabeater seal (*Lobodon carcinophagus*)	528	R	Nordoy et al., 1995 (18)
Weddell seal (*Leptonychotes weddellii*)	626	R	Castellini et al., 1992 (19)
Northern elephant seal (*Mirounga angustirostris*)	1581	R	Stewart and DeLong, 1994 (20)
Southern elephant seal (*Mirounga leonina*)	1430	R	Slip et al., 1994 (21)
Common porpoise (*Delphinus delphis*)	260	R	Evans, 1971 (22)
White sided dolphin (*Lagenorhynchus obliquidens*)	215	T	Hall, 1970 (23)

Table 1 Continued

Species[a]	Maximum depth (m)	Method[b]	Source
Bottle-nose dolphin (*Tursiops truncatus*)	535	T	Ridgway, 1986 (24)
Pilot whale (*Globicephala melaena*)	610	T	Bowers and Henderson, 1972 (25)
Beluga whale (*Delphinapteras leucas*)	650	T	Ridgway et al., 1984 (26)
Killer whale (*Orcinus orca*)	260	T	Bowers and Henderson, 1972 (25)
Sperm whale (*Physeter catodon*)	2035	S	Watkins et al., 1993 (27)
Fin whale (*Balaenoptera physalus*)	350	H	Scholander, 1940 (28)

[a] Additional fur seal and sea lion data in Table 2.
[b] E = echosounder; H = harpooned; N = net, trap, or cable; O = direct observation; R = attached recorder; S = sonar transponder; T = trained.

Note that the deepest measured dives of a whale, seal, bird, and turtle are 2035, 1581, 534, and >1000 m, respectively (5,16,20,27).

Leatherback sea turtles exhibit a trait that may be common among pelagic deep or mesopelagic foragers in ice-free zones. They dive continuously with few extended surface intervals, and >90% of their time is spent submerged, usually at depths greater than 100 m. Animals that exhibit this kind of behavior are more aptly called *surfacers* than *divers* (29). Such behavior has especially important implications for considering the lung at depth. The subject is dealt with in more detail below.

The continuous diving activity of the leatherback is best discussed in light of Fig. 1a. As noted below, despite the fact that they are reptiles, this behavior of routinely diving between 100 to 300 m for about 10 to 15 min is similar to that of a large seal rather than what might be expected of a sea turtle. The extremely deep and long dives that occur uncommonly may be made for predator avoidance. The only refuge for a large, slow-swimming animal that may be harassed by other air-breathing divers such as killer whales (*Orcinus orca*) may be simply to outdive them.

Both elephant seals and Weddell seals exhibit similar diving patterns (Fig. 1B and C) to those of the leatherback sea turtle. One of the major differences between elephant seals and Weddell seals is that the Weddell spends long intervals on the surface, when it rests in ice holes or on sea ice. It is not a continuous diver and therefore would fit the classification of a diver rather than

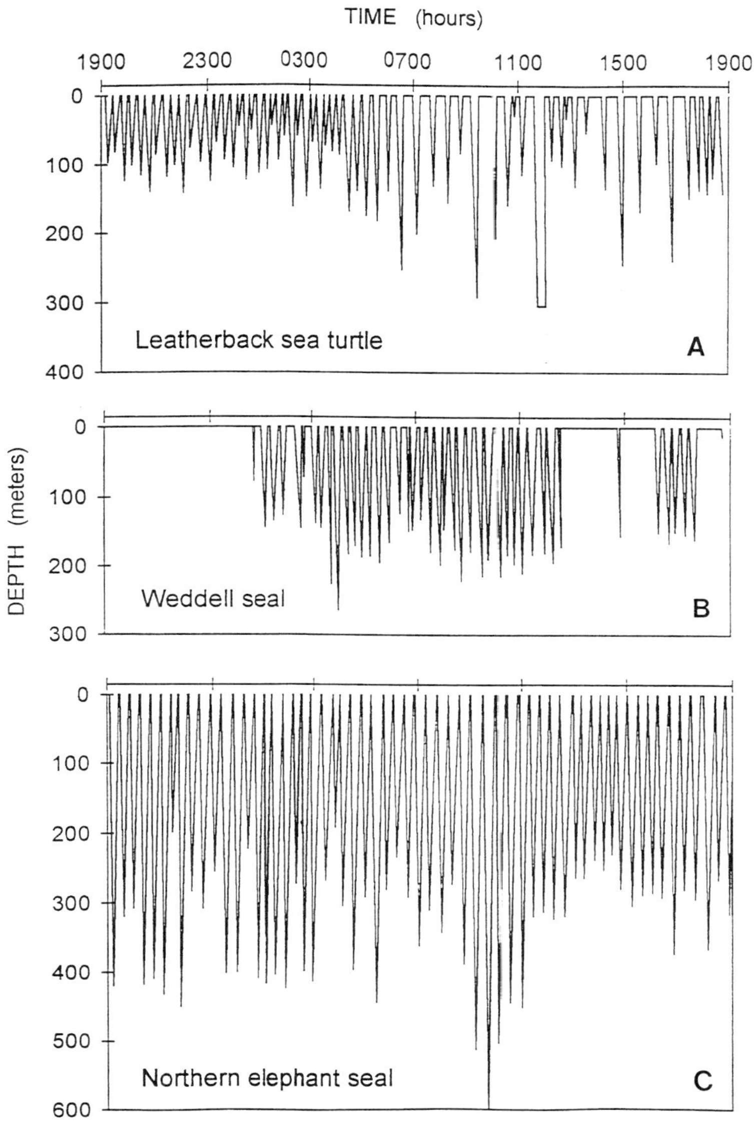

Figure 1 Twenty-four hour dive profiles of (A) leatherback sea turtle, (B) Weddell seal, and (C) elephant seal. The continuous diving of leatherback sea turtles and elephant seals classify these animals as "surfacers," whereas the intermittent dives of the Weddell seal characterize it as a "diver." (Unpublished data, G. L. Kooyman, 1986.)

Table 2 Fur Seal and Sea Lion Dive Characteristics

Species	Dive duration (min)		Dive depth (m)		Percent time diving[a]
	Mean	Max	Mean	Max	
Northern fur seal (*Callorhinus ursinus*)	2.2	7.6	68	256	26
Antarctic fur seal (*Arctocephalus gazella*)	<2.0	4.9	30	101	35
South African fur seal (*Arctocephalus pusillus*)	2.1	7.5	45	204	—
South American fur seal (*Arctocephalus australis*)	2.5	7.1	34	170	24
Galapagos fur seal (*Arctocephalus galapagoensis*)	<2.0	5.0	26	115	24
Galapagos sea lion (*Zalophus californianus wollebaeki*)	<2.0	6.0	37	186	64
California sea lion (*Zalophus californianus*)	2.1	9.9	62	274	33

[a] Percent time diving refers to percentage of time diving during a foraging trip to sea.
Sources: All data are from Gentry and Kooyman (30) except California sea lion data, which are from Feldkamp et al. (31), and maximum (max) dive depth of northern fur seal from Ponganis et al. (17).

a surfacer. The Weddell seal dives routinely for about 15 min to depths of 200 to 400 m (19). However, there are many shallow dives of less than 50 m. This is in striking contrast to the elephant seal, a surfacer, that seldom dives to depths of less than 200 m. They also dive longer and deeper, averaging depths of about 400 to 500 m and durations of 20 to 25 min (20). Noteworthy is that the female elephant seal, Weddell seal, and the female leatherback all have similar body mass.

The traditional order of comparative reports where birds are usually presented before mammals is reversed for the rest of this chapter in order to place more emphasis on what we do not know than what we do. This becomes more apparent in later sections of this chapter. Prior to 1989 little was known about diving depth, duration, or patterns in penguins or any other bird. Some of us assumed that the diving characteristics exhibited by penguins would be similar to those of fur seals, which at that time had been studied more broadly than those of any other diver (30). It was assumed that female fur seals would be the most similar comparative model because they are small (25 to 70 kg), rely on pelage for insulation, occur in cold water, and their locomotion is by forelimbs; their body O_2 store distribution and size were considered to be similar to those of penguins. The salient features of fur seal diving are presented in Table 2. This summary shows that dives >200 m are rare, average dive times are short (<2 min), and maximum durations are about 7 min. However, even prior to 1989, there were some troubling data on penguins suggesting that there might be some major differences between penguins and fur seals. Maximum dives for some species of penguin were deep compared to those of fur seals. For example, king and emperor penguins were both known even then to dive deeper than 240 m (32,33).

More recent studies have revealed that king and emperor penguins dive considerably deeper and longer than fur seals (15,16). We present one part of a dive record to show what a premier diver the emperor penguin is (Fig. 2). Similar results are available for king penguins except that the foraging and maximum depths are about half as great (15). The record highlighted is one of many obtained from birds nurturing chicks at penguin colonies on the edge of the western Ross Sea.

During the first few days no dive exceeded 298 m. On day 8, the bird began a remarkable deep-diving episode that lasted nearly 3 days (Fig. 2). During this period, a depth-frequency analysis of only deep dives (>350 m) shows that nearly 45% were between 400 to 425 m (Fig. 3). Over 40% of the diving durations were between 8.5 to 9.0 min. The average diving depth was 416 ± 18.9 m, $n=69$, range $(R)=364$ to 464 m. The average dive time was 8.8 ± 0.52 min,

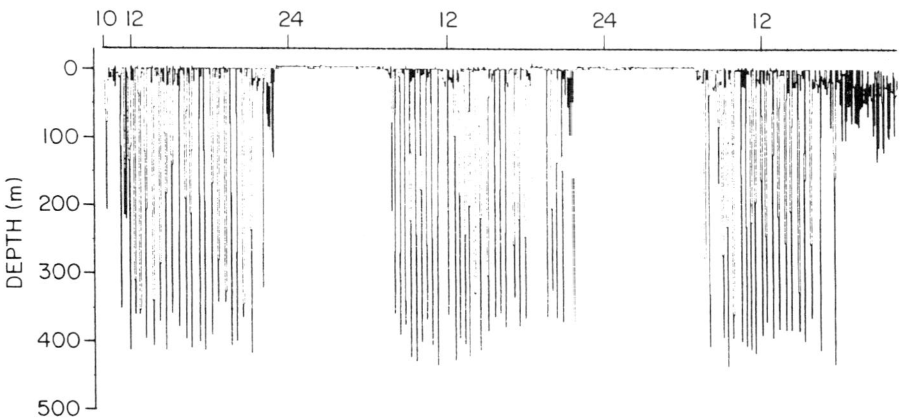

Figure 2 Deep diving episode of an emperor penguin that was away from the colony for 13 days. The abscissa is hour of the day in local time. (Unpublished data, G. L. Kooyman, 1995.)

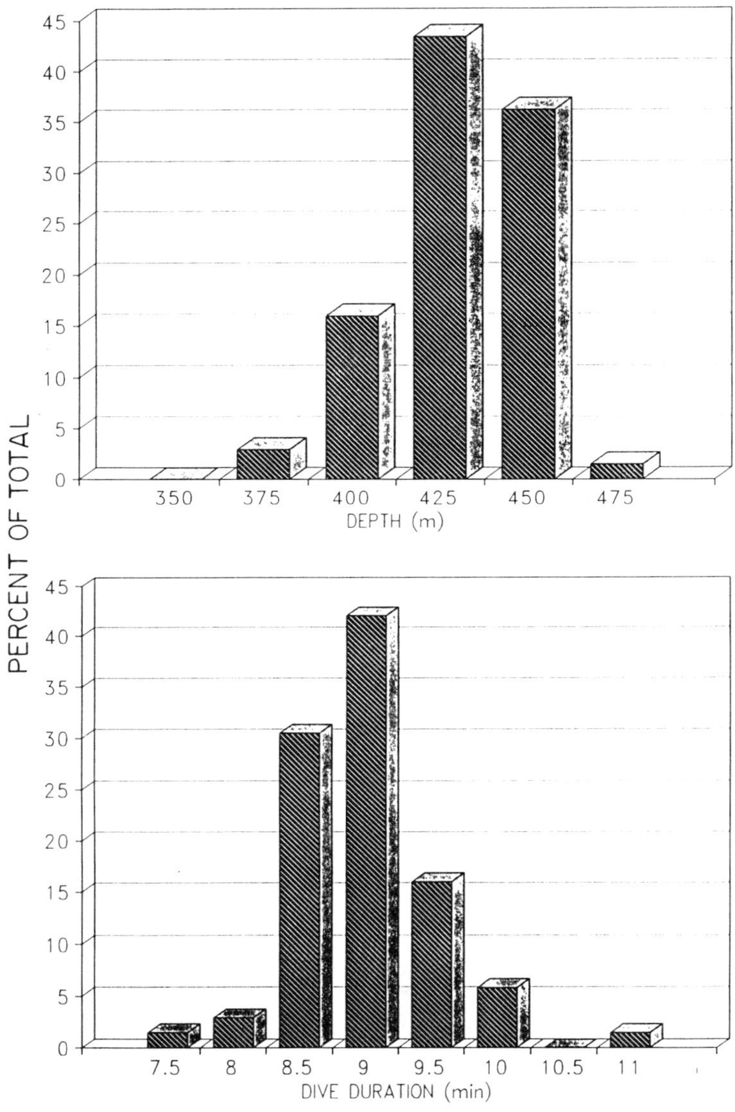

Figure 3 Histogram of the 69 deep dives >364 m that occurred during the three deep diving bouts. Top, the dive depth histogram; bottom, the dive duration histogram.

R=7.5 to 10.8 min. Deep dives greater than 375 m occurred at a rate of two to three per hour, with an average ''surface'' interval of 18.6 min ± 10.1 (R=45.9 to 1.2). The surface interval includes shallow dives of less than 60 m and diving durations of <4.7 min.

Several dives over 500 m have been recorded; the deepest was 534 m (15). To our knowledge, 534 m is the deepest dive ever recorded for a bird and it doubles the previous depth report for an emperor penguin of 265 m (33). Another emperor penguin has dived to over 450 m in the Australian sector of the antarctic as well (34). It is therefore important to note that these may not be rare events, nor may they represent the maximum ability of the birds; rather, they may be almost routine in a special diving mode where presumably deep-dwelling prey are being hunted.

III. Physiology

A. Oxygen Stores

The respiratory, blood, and muscle O_2 stores within a diver are determined by multiple factors (Table 3). Although assumptions as to the extent of O_2 depletion during routine dives as well as the arteriovenous blood volume distribution require further research, the calculations in Table 4 provide our current best estimates of total O_2 stores and their distribution in four long-duration, deep-diving species (leatherback sea turtles, Weddell seals, elephant seals, and emperor penguins). Comparison of the distribution of O_2 within the three storage compart-

Table 3 O_2 Store Determinants

Species	Diving lung volume ($ml \cdot kg^{-1}$)	Hb (g%)	Blood volume ($ml\ kg^{-1}$)	Mb (g%)	Muscle mass (% BM)
Leatherback sea turtle	38 (35,36)	15.6 (37)	77 (35)	0.5 (37)	30[A]
Weddell seal	27 (38)	26.0 (39)	210 (39)	5.4 (39)	35 (40)
Elephant seal	27 (38)	25.0 (41)	250 (41)	6.5 (42)	28 (43)
Emperor penguin	165 (44)	16.8 (45)	60 (46)	6.4/2.1*	29/8 (47)**

Abbreviations: Hb = hemoglobin; Mb = myoglobin; BM = body mass; A = assumed, * = pectoral and leg Mb concentrations (Ponganis and Kooyman, unpublished data), ** = pectoral and leg muscle masses. Reference numbers in parentheses.

Assumptions: 12.5% O_2 available in lung in turtle, 15% in seals and penguins; 0.33 blood volume is arterial, 0.67 is venous; initial arterial Hb saturation is 95%, final is 20%; initial venous O_2 content is 5 vol% less than initial arterial value, all of venous O_2 store is consumed; initial Mb saturation is 100%, Mb concentration is uniform except as indicated in emperor penguin, all of muscle O_2 is consumed.

Table 4 Oxygen Stores

Species	Mass (kg)	O_2 store ($ml\ O_2 \cdot kg^{-1}$)	O_2 store distribution (%)		
			Respiratory	Blood	Muscle
Leatherback sea turtle	300	18	26	63	11
Weddell seal	400	87	5	66	29
Elephant seal	400	97	4	71	25
Emperor penguin	25	62	40	16	44

ments is potentially valuable in understanding diving physiology and O_2-store management adaptations among these species. Direct interspecies comparisons of the magnitudes of O_2 stores is limited, however, because of the differences in body mass, body temperature, and probable metabolic rate of these four species.

It is notable that the total O_2 stores of the two pinnipeds are about one-third greater than estimated values in past studies and reviews (48–50). This is secondary to higher myoglobin (Mb) concentrations (39,42) and to higher blood volume (BV) estimates. We have selected the highest BV measurements available for these species (41,39), since splanchnic or splenic sequestration of red blood cells potentially complicates blood volume measurements in seals and may lead to underestimation of blood volume in animals with large spleens (51). In pregnant elephant seals, BV and its O_2 store may be even greater, since BV increases during pregnancy [by as much as 50% absolute volume in humans (52)]; this may contribute to the exceptional diving capacity (28 min mean dive duration, 1- to 2-hr maximum dive durations) of these animals (48,49).

In the seals and leatherback sea turtle, the blood O_2 store is about two-thirds of the total O_2 store, while in the penguin, it represents less than one-fifth of the total store (Table 4). This is the result of relatively high hemoglobin (Hb) concentrations and BVs in the seals and turtle. In contrast, these factors in emperors and other penguins (45) are only in the upper range of most avian values.

Penguins, on the other hand, do have a very large respiratory O_2 store as a result of a large air sac–lung volume (44). The magnitude of the respiratory air volume is not different from that of other birds. However, this differs markedly from the seals, in which the lung O_2 store is almost insignificant (Table 4). The respiratory O_2 store of the leatherback sea turtle is intermediate in value between the seals and penguins. This is secondary to its total lung capacity, which is less than those of shallow-diving turtles (35,53,54).

Muscle O_2 stores are elevated in all marine diving species because of high Mb concentrations. The relative magnitude of this store ranges from 11% in the leatherback sea turtle to 44% in the emperor penguin. It is notable that, in the latter, 40% of the total O_2 store is located within the locomotory muscle complex because of both the mass and Mb concentration of the pectoral and supracoracoideus muscles.

These varied O_2-store distributions may reflect different O_2-store management adaptations and indirectly have different physiological implications. The two seal species are characterized by a large, mobile O_2 store in the circulatory system and a significant muscle O_2 store. Since the lungs are not a large component of the O_2 store, lung collapse during diving minimizes the risks of N_2 narcosis and decompression sickness without significantly decreasing the amount of O_2 available to the seal during a dive (see Sec. IV, ''Effects of Compression,'' below). The muscle O_2 store in seals should also enhance ischemic tolerance and decrease muscle O_2 transport requirements during diving. In the leatherback sea turtle, a significant quantity of O_2 is within the respiratory system; continued gas exchange at depth may be a significant risk for decompression sickness, as discussed below (36). The penguins contrast with these previous species in that they have large O_2 stores in the respiratory system and in muscle. The exceptionally large locomotory muscle O_2 store of emperors should make this tissue more tolerant of ischemia than even seal muscle. Reduced muscle blood flow, however, in combination with dependence of central-organ oxygenation on continued lung perfusion and blood oxygen uptake, should predispose the emperor to elevated tissue P_{N_2} and its associated risks (55).

Although the question of lung collapse during deep dives of penguins and turtles remains open, it is generally accepted that alveolar compression and lung collapse occur in deep-diving phocid seals (38,56) (see Sec. IV, below). This may prevent buildup of excessive tissue P_{N_2}, but the effect of such collapse on pulmonary vascular resistance and the pulmonary circulation is unknown. In addition, hypoxemia, hypercarbia, acidosis, and hypoxic pulmonary vasoconstriction should also contribute to an elevated pulmonary vascular resistance by the end of a long dive. It should be noted that, as in other mammals, the foramen ovale and ductus arteriosus close at an early age in seals (57) and therefore do not serve as a low-resistance pulmonary shunt. Drabek has suggested that the long, narrow shape of the right ventricle of phocid seals is an adaptation for such elevated pulmonary pressures (58). During compression chamber dives to 800-kPa pulmonary artery pressures of harbor seals ranged from 40/30 to 24/12 torr (59). The mechanisms by which the pulmonary circulation is managed during the continuous, long, deep diving of elephant seals require further investigation and may be relevant to clinical situations associated with elevated pulmonary vascular resistance and right heart failure (60).

In summary, although O_2 stores are increased among all these divers, different patterns of O_2-store distribution among the respiratory, blood, and muscle compartments suggest different O_2-store management patterns. Whether O_2

is stored in a mobile circulatory compartment or in relatively fixed respiratory or muscle compartments has implications for diving cardiovascular adaptations as well as for the risks of N_2 narcosis and decompression sickness.

B. Cardiovascular Responses

The bradycardia, peripheral vasoconstriction, and blood flow redistribution associated with forced submersions have been extensively studied in turtles, birds, and pinnipeds (28,61–64). Forced submersions differ from diving in the following ways: (1) the apnea is involuntary, (2) the subject is restrained and immobile (though not necessarily ''at rest''), (3) the subject has no idea how long the submersion will be, and (4) unless the subject is in a compression chamber, there are usually no pressure changes. Although forced submersion experiments have provided much information on the nature of these cardiovascular responses, physiological differences between forced submersions and diving do exist. For example, in adult Weddell seals, postsubmersion increases in blood lactate always occur after forced submersions regardless of duration (64,65). Such increases generally occur only after voluntary dives of about 19 min duration in adult seals (66,67).

The heart rate reductions during diving and rest apneas of Weddell seals are not as great as during forced submersions (64,68,69). This is also true of heart rate reductions during spontaneous apneas in elephant seals (70), turtles (71), and penguins (72). In addition, repetitive exposure of harbor seals (*Phoca vitulina*) to a forced submersion protocol (P. Jobsis, personal communication) results in adaptation of the forced submersion response. With training, heart rate and muscle blood flow are greater during the submersion, and postsubmersion blood lactates and catecholamines are lower.

Heart rate responses during diving or spontaneous apneas have been examined in three of the four species selected for this review. Diving heart rates among leatherback sea turtles have not been recorded. The extensive heart rate data available for Weddell seals (68,69,73) indicate that (1) mean diving heart rates are about equivalent to sleep apneic heart rates, (2) such diving heart rates are about half the eupneic value, and (3) diving heart rates can be variable at times. The sleep apneic heart rates of northern elephant seals are also about half the eupneic value and are equivalent to the heart rate during the slow phase of the seal's ventilatory sinus arrhythmia (70). Similar responses have been reported during the diving of harbor seals (74), northern elephant seals (75), and sleep apnea of leopard seals (*Hydrurga leptonyx*) (76). Extremely low heart rates, however, may occur; heart rates as low as those recorded during forced submersions have been recorded during some dives of ringed seals (*Phoca hispida*) (77) and gray seals (*Halichoerus grypus*) (78). In emperor and Adelie

(*Pygoscelis adeliae*) penguins, diving heart rates are at or below resting values and are less than half of surface swimming values (72,79,80).

C. Blood Flow Distribution

The significant blood flow reductions to muscle, kidneys, and splanchnic organs during the severe bradycardias of forced submersions have been well documented in birds and pinnipeds (28,62–64,81,82). Studies during free diving are few and limited primarily to the Weddell seal. No data are available for turtles. In immature Weddell seals, during routine foraging dives, inulin and indocyanine green clearance rates were similar to those at rest and considered consistent with maintained renal and hepatic blood flow during such dives (83). Since decreased clearance rates had been observed in isolated short dives and in dives of long duration—i.e., greater than 20 min (83,84)—it would appear that splanchnic and renal blood flow can be variable during dives regardless of duration. However, at least in routine dives of foraging bouts of Weddell seals, it appears that such blood flows are maintained. This is consonant with the above clearance rates, the development of lipemic serum in such dive bouts (83), and the previous discussion of heart rates.

During dives, muscle blood flow may trickle (85), pulse (67), or even cease completely as in forced submersions (62,64). Indirect evidence for some flow to muscle in dives includes an elevated blood lactate concentration late in a long dive of a Weddell seal (84) and the maintenance of a constant and occasionally decreased locomotory muscle temperature (86). An ''extramuscular throttle'' may make muscle blood flow regulation during diving independent of local vasodilatory effects (85). In Adelie penguins, femoral blood flow during diving decreased to about one-half resting values; this decrease contrasted with the increase in flow measured during surface swimming (72). In contrast to diminished flow during diving in seals and penguins, locomotory muscle blood flow in the tufted duck (*Aythya fuligula*) is maintained during diving (87). However, diving heart rate and cardiac output during the 14-sec dives of tufted ducks are 30% greater than resting values. This contrasts to the situation in emperor penguins and phocid seals, in which diving heart rate is at or below resting levels. In addition, the much greater Mb concentrations in these species than in tufted ducks (88) suggests a greater tolerance to ischemia.

In summary, blood flow distribution during diving appears variable and dependent on the nature of the dive. At least during the foraging dives of Weddell seals, hepatic and renal blood flows appear to be maintained. Muscle blood flow patterns are unknown, but flow has been postulated to trickle, pulse, or entirely cease. The Mb-O_2 store in muscle presumably allows prolonged aerobic metabolism during diving without a significant increase in muscle blood flow.

D. Blood Chemistry

Intramuscular O_2 depletion and lactate formation during forced submersions and the subsequent postsubmersion lactate washout were observed in seals and penguins by Scholander and coworkers (28,82). Similar postsubmersion increases in blood lactate have also been measured after forced submersions in numerous other species, including Weddell seals (64), green sea turtles (61), and painted turtles (*Chrysemys picta*) (89). However, during voluntary diving of Weddell seals, postdive lactate levels were rarely elevated and led to the concept that most voluntary dives were aerobic (66,84,90,91). Postdive blood lactate levels began to rise above 2 mM after dives with durations greater than 19 to 20 min in adult Weddell seals. In the extreme condition after a 61-min dive, blood lactate peaked at 27 mM (66). It is notable that resting blood lactate levels are not required before a seal will dive and that elevated blood lactate levels can decrease during diving (50,90).

Other blood metabolites have been examined during voluntary diving. Blood glucose remained relatively constant between 3 and 6 mM during diving bout surface periods of Weddell seals (90). The glucose concentration was lower during diving of Weddell seals (83), did not change more than 1 mM during dives (84) and increased after diving to predive or greater than predive levels (66,84). Plasma free fatty acid concentrations and whole-blood free amino acid concentrations did not change significantly during diving and recovery (84).

Arterial blood gas determinations during and immediately after voluntary diving have been limited again to the Weddell seal. The highest Pa_{CO_2} values are from 50 to 60 torr (66,92); Pa_{CO_2} after a 42-min dive returned to 40 torr within 6 min of surface time (66). An arterial P_{O_2} of 18 torr (28% Hb saturation) has been measured at 1 min prior to the end of a 37-min dive (92). End-tidal P_{O_2} values ranged between 23 and 50 torr after 5- to 20-min dives and from 13 to 23 torr after dives $>$20 min (39). Such values support the 20% end-of-dive arterial saturation in calculation of usable O_2 stores. The time required for arterial or end-tidal P_{O_2} to increase above 60 torr (assumed 90% Hb saturation) was less than 2 min in these studies. Pulmonary gas exchange at the surface appears to be efficient. Rapid expansion of previously atelectatic alveoli presumably occurs during ascent and/or the first breath. Surfactant properties and the mechanism of such routine alveolar reexpansion may have relevant clinical implications.

IV. Effects of Compression

Every type of diver must deal with some of the same problems when diving to depth: (1) major compressive forces, which have significant mechanical effects on the body; (2) a precipitous decline in ambient light; (3) for dives occurring in temperate and tropical seas, a great decrease in water temperature with depth; and (4) the long distance they must travel from their most precious resource—oxygen. How the reptiles, birds, and mammals have dealt with some of these common liabilities is discussed below. It is an eclectic presentation because so few experiments have addressed this aspect of diving. Also, the body structures of those various groups require different solutions. For example, most of the gas volume in birds resides in air sacs external to the lung, whereas most of the respiratory gas volume in mammals is contained within the lung. Air spaces of any sort are a liability, and the cranial sinuses present in all terrestrial mammals are absent from marine mammals. In brief, the questions and the experimental results described below reflect some of these anatomical differences in marine reptiles, birds, and mammals.

A. Reptiles

The effects of pressure have been studied on both sea snakes and sea turtles. Seymour performed a series of elegant studies on sea snakes (93). In a completely aquatic species, *Hydrophis belcheri*, he showed that 76% of the total systemic flow bypasses the lung. With such a large shunt at the surface, the species is preadapted to avoid high arterial P_{N_2}. At a 40-m submersion depth, the shunt fraction was 83% and the calculated P_{N_2} was always below the level required for gas liberation on return to the surface. Nearly as large a shunt of 60% occurs in the yellow-bellied sea snake when it is exposed to elevated hydrostatic pressure (50). In addition to this shunt, there is at least 12% cutaneous respiration (94). A consequence of these responses is that high Pa_{N_2} does not occur in sea snakes while they are at depth.

The only studies on sea turtles have been the experiments carried out by Berkson (36). Unfortunately, he selected the only species, the green sea turtle, that is generally herbivorous and therefore may seldom dive deeply. In addition to the artificiality of forced submersions, he kept the turtles submerged an excessive duration and decompressed them much more rapidly than their normal ascent rate would require. With these procedures, he induced the only recorded case of decompression sickness in a diving animal. However, as Fig. 4 shows, there are many uncertainties about the result. For example, Pa_{N_2} rose slowly when the turtle was compressed to an equivalent of 177 m. The maximum Pa_{N_2}, 800 kPa, was obtained about 30 min after compression. There were no intermediate samples. This result is inconclusive in regard to the hazards of deep diving for sea turtles, but it did show that Pa_{N_2} could rise much higher than that observed in sea snakes or marine mammals.

No experiments similar to those done on the green sea turtle have been carried out on more pelagic species. Of course, the species of most interest

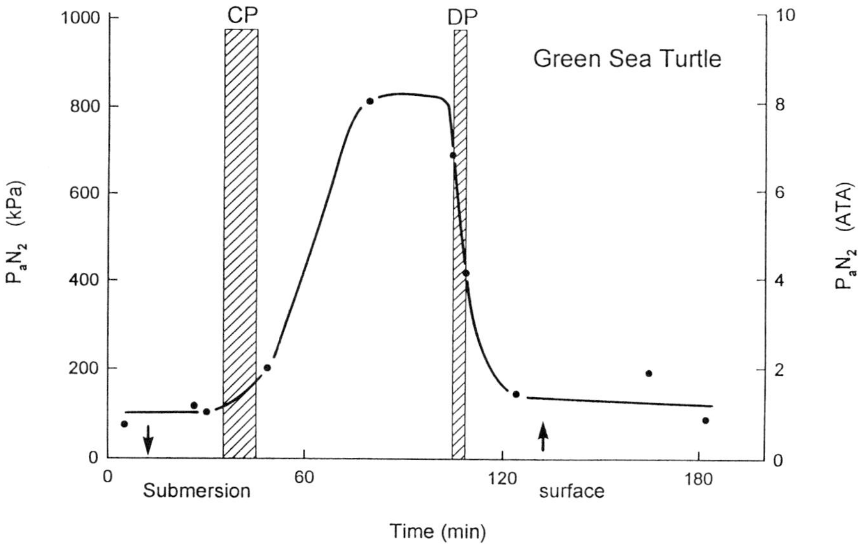

Figure 4 Pa_{N_2} profile of a green sea turtle during a forced compression to 1990 kPa. CP = compression; DP = decompression. (Adapted from Ref. 36.)

would be the leatherback sea turtle. They routinely dive to depth and because of this behavior they must have some protection against pulmonary N_2 uptake. Possible adaptations are their small lungs compared to other species (35) and a well-developed pulmonary artery sphincter (95), which may induce a large pulmonary shunt any time the turtle dives to depth.

B. Marine Mammals

The lungs of marine mammals are the most structurally modified of any mammalian group (96). Among marine mammals, the toothed whales, especially small dolphins, are the most extreme in their reinforcement of peripheral airways, the loss of respiratory bronchioles, and the presence of a series of bronchial sphincters (97) (Fig. 5).

Like dolphins, sea lions have robust cartilaginous airway reinforcement extending to the alveolar sac. In seals, the terminal airway is reinforced by connective tissue and smooth muscle but not cartilage. It has been proposed that the pinniped and cetacean type of lung makes it possible for a graded collapse to occur and that most of the lung air is forced into the upper airways during a dive to depth (28,96). Radiographic evidence in Weddell seals during compression to 300 m supports this model (98).

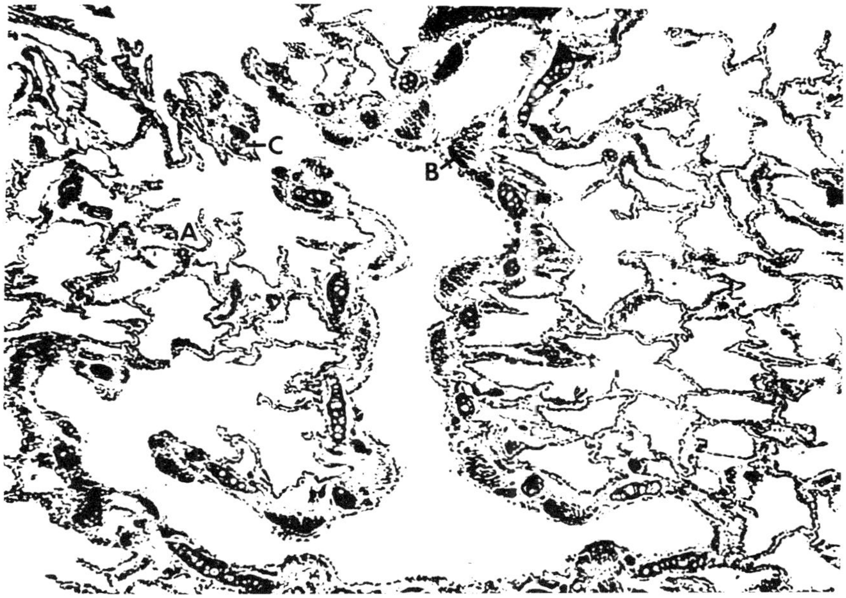

Figure 5 Histological section of spinner dolphin lung, *Stenella longirostris*. A, alveolus; B, bronchial sphincter; C, bronchial cartilage. (Unpublished data, G. L. Kooyman, 1979.)

These airway structures are not the only unusual feature about marine mammals that suggest an adaptation to pressure. Volume-pressure curves of the chest wall and lung of seals show that both are nearly limitless in the degree of compression collapse that they can tolerate (Fig. 6).

From Table 3 it is clear that at least pinnipeds do not dive with a large lung volume. Nevertheless, given the depth and duration of dives, blood and tissue P_{N_2} could rise substantially if there were no structural adaptations, as mentioned earlier. Just how high P_{N_2} may go has been shown in a few experiments.

Bottlenose dolphins were trained to dive serially to a depth of 100 m. After some of these dives, the muscle tissue was sampled with a mass spectrometer probe inserted into the dorsal musculature. Indirect evidence from these measurements indicated that tissue P_{N_2} never rose above about 213 kPa and that lung collapse probably occurred at a depth of about 70 m (100).

In more direct estimates of pulmonary shunts, it was found that the degree of shunt in a California sea lion is dependent on the depth of dive to about 170 m, where lung collapse is complete (101). Few dives of sea lions are to such a

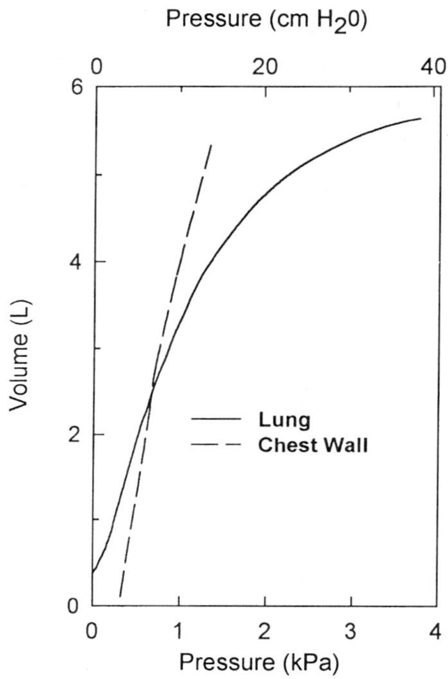

Figure 6 Chest wall and lung compliance of a 55-kg ribbon seal, *Phoca fasciata*. (Adapted from Ref. 99.)

depth, and this indicates that for most of their dives there would be gas exchange in the lungs. Exposure to high pressure would be brief because of the shortness of the dive, but the lung could continue to function as an O_2 reservoir. This reservoir function could be important, because the lung O_2 is 13% of the total body O_2 store in sea lions (50). This is not the case in the seal.

In two independent studies it has been shown that blood P_{N_2} in seals rises only slightly no matter how deep the dive. In the first example, the conditions were the most extreme because the seals were forcibly submerged in a compression chamber. Since N_2 tension in blood and tissue are dependent upon the distribution of the circulating blood in addition to the depth and duration of the dive, the forced submersion should raise the Pa_{N_2} to the highest possible level. This would be so because peripheral blood flow during a forced submersion is most restricted, as discussed above; therefore much less tissue would be exposed to the blood-borne N_2. Under these conditions, the Pa_{N_2} of the elephant seal peaked at 300 kPa and equilibrated to 200 kPa, where it was approximately the same as venous P_{N_2} (38) (Fig. 7). This was independent of the ambient pressure from 37 to 138 m (1480 kPa). Similar values were obtained for Weddell seals diving voluntarily to depths as great as 230 m (2400 kPa) (56) (Fig. 7). The Pa_{N_2} never exceeded 323 kPa. These modest increases in Pa_{N_2} indicate that lung collapse in both species occurred between 20 and 50 m. The early occurrence of lung collapse in seals makes the lung almost useless as an O_2 store, but it limits N_2 absorption during the dive. All of the reported N_2 values in diving seals are below the minimum P_{N_2} of 330 kPa found to be necessary for bubble formation in cats (102). These N_2 values in seals are greater than the 135-kPa steady-state pressure exposure, which resulted in a 50% incidence of venous gas emboli in humans on decompression (103). However, none of the subjects in that Doppler ultrasound study exhibited signs or symptoms of decompression sickness. Whether such asymptomatic bubble formation occurs in seals is unknown. Doppler ultrasound methodology may be a valuable technique for the further investigation of pressure effects in seals.

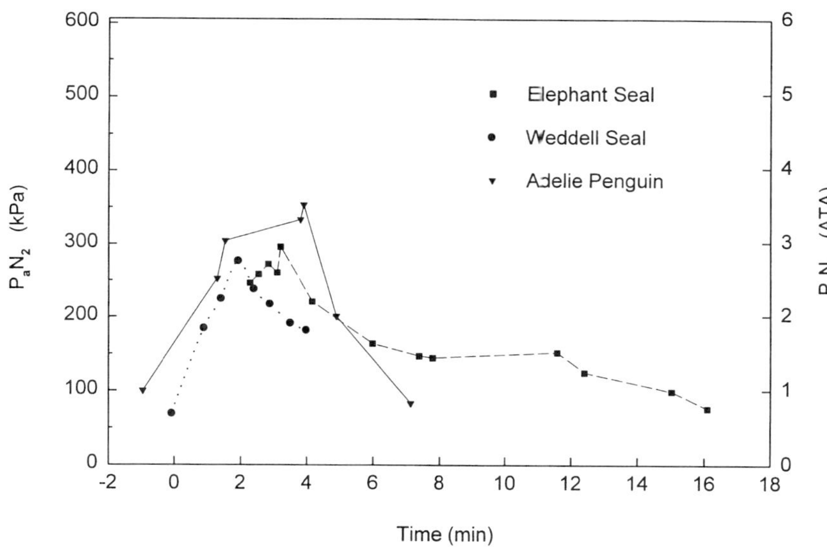

Figure 7 Arterial P_{N_2} profiles of a Weddell seal, elephant seal, and Adelie penguin. The Weddell seal data are from an 8-min free dive to 89 m; no data were collected after 4 min (56). The elephant seal profile is pooled data from simulated dives to 30–272 m (400–2820 kPa). Peak values during dives did not change with depth (38); decompression occurred at 9 min. Adelie penguin P_aN_2 during a simulated dive to 68 m (780 kPa); decompression occurred at 3.5 min (44).

C. Birds

The recent observations on the deep diving behavior of king and emperor penguins have raised some difficult physiological questions about how birds respond to pressure. The problem with birds is that they dive with such a large gas volume that it represents not only a proportionally important O_2 store for the bird, but it is also a large reservoir of N_2. Consequently, if much of the N_2 in the respiratory system is absorbed, blood and tissue PN_2's could rise to high levels.

Penguins dive with a large gas store that, in relation to body mass, is five to six times that of a diving seal (44) (Table 3). During simulated dives to 68 m (44), blood N_2 tensions in Adelie penguins were slightly higher than those measured in elephant seals (Fig. 7). None of these levels are dangerously high, and natural diving durations are shorter than were those experimental dives. Therefore, the shortness and shallowness of the diving patterns in this species are adequate protection against high blood P_{N_2} (44).

During routine deep dives of emperors (Fig. 2), pressures are well over 4000 kPa. The total time below 100 m was 8.5 min in the 464-m dive discussed and illustrated earlier. This seriously weakens the premise, at least for king and emperor penguins, that the main protection of diving birds is short, shallow dives (44). The ascent rates from deep dives may also be too rapid to allow for adequate N_2 elimination. During the 464-m dive, the bird ascended at a rate of more than 100 m/min.

If tissue nitrogen uptake remains simply driven by the differential between ambient and tissue partial pressures, it is possible to use traditional decompression theory to calculate the resulting nitrogen tension for any given half-time tissue (104). For a tissue with half-time $t_{1/2}$, the tissue pressure Pt_{N_2} is calculated by integrating

$$dPt_{N_2}/dt = (\ln 2/t_{1/2}) \times (PA_{N_2} - Pt_{N_2}) \tag{1}$$

where PA_{N_2}= ambient driving pressure, here set to 80 kPa during surface intervals (i.e., an air mixture with about 80% N_2) and to 80 kPa times an assumed parabolic-shaped depth profile during dives. The tissue N_2 levels predicted just after final ascent from a bout of 30 parabolic dives to 400 m, each lasting 9 min and separated by surface intervals of 20 min., are shown in Fig. 8. Just how the emperor penguin avoids the decompression risks of such extreme nitrogen values predicted by traditional theory is unknown. Intervening shallow dives might act as "decompression stops," and brief surface intervals might reduce the decompression risk so long as the tissue N_2 remains in solution (105,106). The long recoveries are more likely driven by a metabolic acidosis resulting from a substantial O_2 debt. If only the potential deleterious effects of

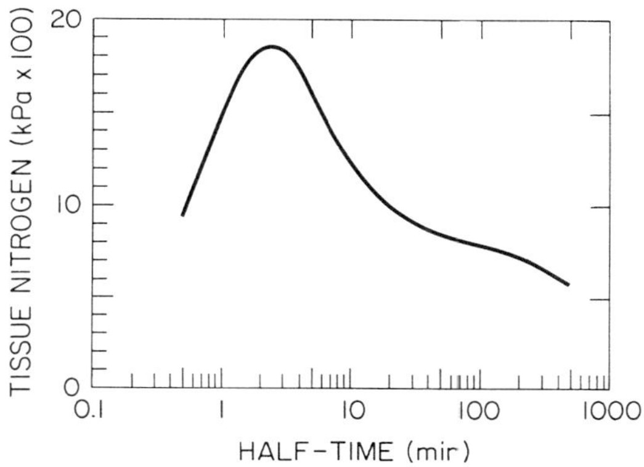

Figure 8 Theoretical tissue nitrogen pressure vs. tissue half-times following a deep diving bout of an emperor penguin, similar to Fig. 2. There is free gas exchange between the lung, blood, and tissue at all depths (see text for details of the dive bout). For example, if the penguin has a tissue that half saturates in 10 min ($t_{1/2}$ = 10 min), we predict the tissue P_{N_2} equals approximately 1200 kPa immediately after the animal surfaces from the last dive of the bout.

high blood and tissue P_{N_2} are considered, further physiological studies of birds are clearly needed in order to develop suitable gas-exchange models.

Relative to mammals, the avian lung is a small portion of the respiratory system and about 90% of the respiratory air volume resides in the air sacs (107). The lung is bonded to the dorsal surface of the thoracic cavity, including the ribs, and there is, relative to mammals, little ability to expand and contract. Instead, this semirigid structure is made up of a series of parallel parabronchial tubes that have perpendicular side branches of air capillaries where gas exchange occurs. There is unidirectional flow through the parabronchial tubes during both inspiration and expiration (108). Gas transport into the small air capillaries is by diffusion. The radius of curvature of these air capillaries is so small that reexpansion pressure would be very high; consequently, it would take very large pressures to reopen them after collapse (107). In brief, the mechanics of compression collapse and reinflation would not be the same as in mammals. However, there must be a way of reducing gas exchange.

If we assume that a shunt mechanism limits the Pa_{N_2} to remain at or below 400 kPa (about the level measured in shallower diving penguins) (44), then this would initially require about a 90% blood flow bypass or shunt that must increase as systemic venous blood $P\bar{v}_{N_2}$ rises. With pulmonary end-capillary Pc_{N_2} presumed equal to air sac gas partial pressure (about 0.8×4000 kPa for a dive to 400 m), application of the shunt equation can provide a lower limit for the effective shunt by setting mixed venous $P\bar{v}_{N_2}$ to its smallest initial value of 80 kPa:

$$\frac{\dot{Q}S}{\dot{Q}T} = \frac{Pc_{N_2} - Pa_{N_2}}{Pc_{N_2} - P\bar{v}_{N_2}} = \frac{3200 - 400}{3200 - 80} = 90\% \tag{2}$$

where $\dot{Q}T$ is the cardiac output, and $\dot{Q}S$ is shunt flow. With such a large, effective shunt, the arterial Pa_{O_2} must then be only slightly higher than the $P\bar{v}_{O_2}$ since for a 90% shunt, Ca_{O_2} (arterial O_2 content) $= 0.9\ C\bar{v}_{O_2} + 0.1\ Cc_{O_2}$ (109). At or below this N_2 tension (400 kPa), bubble formation is unlikely even if the bird ascends so rapidly from depth that no reduction in tissue P_{N_2} occurs before reaching the surface. However, at this level of shunt, Pa_{O_2} would be essentially equal to $P\bar{v}_{O_2}$.

Such a low Pa_{O_2} might seem to put the bird on the border of brain hypoxia when it reaches the bottom of its dive. However, this level of hypoxia is not so remarkable in light of what we know about birds flying at high altitudes. It is about the same as what the Pa_{O_2} must be of birds flying high enough to cross the Himalayas, as is done by bar-headed geese (*Anser indicus*) (110). Also, as the penguin ascends and the gas-exchanging surfaces expand, the Pa_{O_2} may stabilize or even rise. So how might this reduction in gas-exchange surface area occur in penguins?

In a recent study of the lung of the Humboldt penguin, *Spheniscus humboldti*, it was found that there is a thick blood-gas barrier and small gas-exchange area as compared with other birds (111). In addition, pulmonary capillary blood volume is almost twice that of other birds (111). We speculate that this extra blood volume, if present in the emperor penguin, may reflect a potential for further expanding into the parabronchial air space as the bird dives to depth. The reduction in the parabronchial space to compensate for the effect of increased ambient pressure may cause a reduction in the gas-exchange surface area. If so, then a major reduction in gas exchange might occur.

This very preliminary and simple model tells us that at least a major reduction in blood/gas exchange within the lung must occur in order for these birds to tolerate dives to such great depths. How it is accomplished is conjecture that illustrates what little we know about how pressure affects deep diving in birds. The emperor is an enigma.

V. Aerobic Diving Limits

An additional puzzle, especially in birds, is the management of O_2 stores in such a way that they remain within an aerobic diving limit (ADL). This was defined in 1985 by Kooyman based on some combined physiological and behavioral measurements made on Weddell seals (67). That definition "the maximum breath-hold that is possible without any increase in blood lactate concentration during or after the dive'' emphasized that, somewhere in the body, oxygen was depleted enough that lactate production became dominant and that lactate was produced in excess of what was consumed either locally or in other parts of the body. So far the only measurements of a lactate endurance curve (Fig. 9) have been for the Weddell seal (66,84,91). It was also found that this measured ADL was equal to the ADL calculated on the basis of O_2 stores and metabolic rate (66,91). Most dives of the Weddell seal appeared to be aerobic since only about 5% of all dives exceeded the ADL (66).

The fact that the measured ADL equals the calculated ADL in Weddell seals does not necessarily mean that the entire O_2 store is consumed in that time period. The Weddell seal can dive at least four times longer than the ADL.

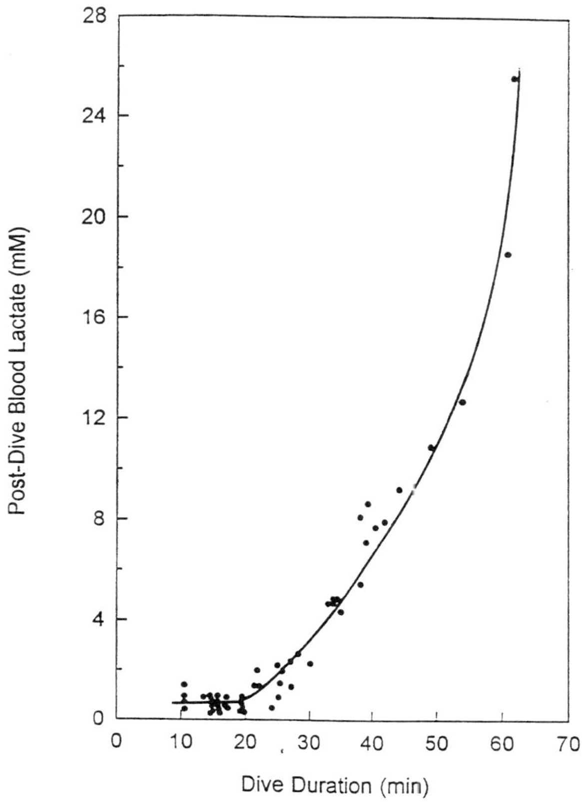

Figure 9 Postdive blood lactate concentrations and diving durations of adult Weddell seals. The inflection point at 19 min is the aerobic diving limit (ADL). (Modified from Ref. 66.)

Table 5 Myoglobin Concentrations in Marine Divers

Species	Myoglobin (g 100 g^{-1})	Source
Loggerhead sea turtle (*Caretta caretta*)	0.29	Lutz and Bentley, 1985 (53)
Leatherback sea turtle (*Dermochelys coriacea*)	0.49	Lutcavage et al., 1990 (37)
Thick-billed murre (*Uria lomvia*)	1.9	Croll et al., 1992 (10)
Common murre (*Uria aalge*)	1.4	Davis and Guderley, 1987 (112)
Atlantic puffin (*Fratercula arctica*)	1.3	Davis and Guderley, 1987 (112)
Adelie penguin (*Pygoscelis adeliae*)	3.0	Weber et al., 1974 (113)
Gentoo penguin (*Pygoscelis papua*)	4.4	Weber et al., 1974 (113)
Little blue penguin (*Eudyptula minor*)	2.8	Mill and Baldwin, 1983 (114)
King penguin (*Aptenodytes patagonicus*)	4.3	Baldwin et al., 1984 (115)
Emperor penguin (*Aptenodytes forsteri*)	6.4	Ponganis and Kooyman (unpublished data)
Manatee (*Trichechus manutus*)	1.5	Blessing, 1972 (116)
Sea otter (*Enhydra lutris*)	3.1	Castellini and Somero, 1981 (117)
Walrus (*Odobenus rosmarus*)	3.0	Lenfant et al., 1970 (118)
California sea lion (*Zalophus californianus*)	3.2	Lenfant et al., 1970 (118)
Northern fur seal (*Callorhinus ursinus*)	3.5	Lenfant et al., 1970 (118)
Antarctic fur seal (*Arctocephalus gazella*)	3.1	Reed et al., 1994 (119)
Harbor seal (*Phoca vitulina*)	5.5 4.4	Lenfant et al., 1970 (118) Castellini and Somero, 1981 (117)
Ribbon seal (*Phoca fasciata*)	8.1	Lenfant et al., 1970 (118)
Ringed seal (*Phoca hispida*)	4.1	Lydersen et al., 1992 (120)
Grey seal (*Halichoerus grypus*)	5.4	Reed et al., 1994 (119)

Table 5 Continued

Species	Myoglobin ($g\ 100\ g^{-1}$)	Source
Weddell seal (*Leptonychotes weddellii*)	5.4	Ponganis et al., 1993 (39)
Northern elephant seal (*Mirounga angustirostris*)	6.5	Thorson, 1993 (42)
Bottle-nose dolphin (*Tursiops truncatus*)	3.3	Blessing and Hartschen-Niemeyer, 1969 (121)
Harbor porpoise (*Phocoena phocoena*)	3.0	Blessing, 1972 (116)
Sperm whale (*Physeter catodon*)	5.0	Hapner et al., 1968 (122)

Sufficient O_2 must be available during such a dive to protect the central nervous system from anoxia. During prolonged dives, heart rate and peripheral vasoconstriction responses presumably decrease the depletion rate of the central (lung and blood) O_2 store with perfusion-related decreases in splanchnic and renal O_2 consumption and with isolation of muscle O_2 demand from the circulation. The latter probably accounts for the elevated myoglobin concentrations found in diving species (Table 5).

As discussed previously, the distribution of O_2 stores in seals (Table 4) minimizes the contribution of the lung to the total O_2 store. The duration of the ADL will not be greatly affected if lung collapse occurs in seals at depth. This is not the case, however, in deep-diving turtles and penguins, in which 30 to 70% of the "nonmuscle" central O_2 store is located in the respiratory system. How deep-diving turtles and penguins maximize O_2 utilization yet minimize P_{N_2} elevation remains a mystery of the lung at depth.

VI. Concluding Remarks

1. With the advent of microprocessor-based dive recorders, our knowledge of diving ecology and behavior has eclipsed that of diving physiology.
2. Our understanding of the lung at depth in seals and probably other marine mammals is well supported by experimental data on seals—the lung does not function in gas exchange.

3. Novel structures in cetaceans—i.e., thoracic retes (123) and bronchial sphincters—are possible adaptations to pressure, but their function is unknown.
4. Although large gas stores exist in sea turtle lungs, a pulmonary artery sphincter, at least in the leatherback sea turtle, probably contracts during dives, directing blood flow to the systemic circulation and causing a pulmonary bypass.
5. Lung function and management of the large gas stores of air sacs in deep-diving birds remain puzzles.
6. Inert gas narcosis (124), high-pressure nervous syndrome (125), and surfactant function during lung collapse and reinflation have not been addressed in deep-diving animals and await future investigations.

Acknowledgments

Preparation of this review was supported by NSF OPP-9219872 and NIH HL 17731-20.

References

1. Dawson WR, Bartholomew GA, Bennett AF. A reappraisal of the aquatic specializations of the Galapagos marine iguana (*Amblyrhynchus cristatus*). Evolution 1977; 31:891–897.
2. Bert P. Sur les differences dans la resistance a l'asphyxie que presentent divers animaux. Paris: Societe de Biologie, Paris comptes rendus hebonda daires des seances et memoires, 1869:186–189.
3. Kooyman GL. Respiratory adaptations in marine mammals. Am Zool 1973; 13: 457–478.
4. Landis AT. New high pressure research animal? Nav Undersea Ctr Tech Paper 1965; 6:21.
5. Eckert SA, Eckert KL, Ponganis PJ, Kooyman GL. Diving and foraging behavior of leatherback sea turtles (*Dermochelys coriacea*). Can J Zool 1989; 67:2834–2840.
6. Burger AE, Powell DW. Diving depths and diet of Cassin's Auklet at Reef Island, British Columbia. Can J Zool 1990; 68:1572–1577.
7. Chastel O. Maximum diving depths of common diving petrels, *Pelecanoides urinatrix*, at Kerguelen Islands. Polar Biol 1994; 14:211–213.
8. Croxall JP, Naito Y, Kato A, et al. Diving patterns and performance in the antarctic blue-eyed shag *Phalacrocorax atriceps*. J Zool (Lond) 1991; 225:177–199.
9. Schorger AW. The deep diving of the Loon and the Old Squaw and its mechanism. Wilson Bull 1947; 59:151–159.
10. Croll DA, Gaston AJ, Berger AE, Konoff D. Foraging behavior and physiological adaptations for diving in Thick-billed Murres. Ecology 1992; 73:344–356.

11. Piatt JF, Nettleship DN. Diving depths of four alcids. The Auk 1985; 102:293–297.
12. Lishman GS, Croxall JP. Diving depths of the Chinstrap penguin, *Pygoscelis antarctica*. Br Antarct Bull 1983; 61:21–25.
13. Williams TD, Briggs DR, Croxall JP, et al. Diving pattern and performance in relation to foraging ecology in the gentoo penguin, *Pygoscelis papua*. J Zool (Lond) 1992; 227:211–230.
14. Croxall, JP. Diving pattern and performance in the macaroni penguin *(Eupdyptes chrysolophus*). J Zool 1993; 230:31–47.
15. Kooyman GL, Cherel Y, Le Maho Y, et al. Diving behavior and energetics during foraging cycles in king penguins. Ecol Monogr 1992; 62:143–163.
16. Kooyman GL, Kooyman TG. Diving behavior of emperor penguins nurturing chicks at Coulman Island, Antarctica. Condor 1995; 97:536–549.
17. Ponganis PJ, Gentry RL, Ponganis EP, Ponganis KV. Analysis of swim velocities during deep and shallow dives of two northern fur seals, *Callorhinus ursinus*. Mar Mamm Sci 1992; 8:69–75.
18. Nordoy ES, Folkow L, Blix AS. Distribution and diving behaviour of crabeater seals (*Lobodon carcinophagus*) off Queen Maud land. Polar Biol 1995; 15:261–268.
19. Castellini MA, Davis RW, Kooyman GL. Annual cycles of diving behavior and ecology of the Weddell seal. Bulletin of the Scripps Institution of Oceanography, Vol. 28, University of California, San Diego. Berkeley, CA: University of California Press, 1992:1–54.
20. Stewart BS, DeLong RL. Postbreeding foraging migrations of northern elephant seals. In: Le Boeuf BJ, Laws RM, eds. Elephant Seals: Population Ecology, Behavior, and Physiology. Berkeley, CA: University of California Press, 1994:290–309.
21. Slip DJ, Hindell MA, Burton HR. Diving behavior of southern elephant seals from Macquarie Island: An overview. In: Le Boeuf BJ, Laws RM, eds. Elephant Seals: Population, Ecology, Behavior, and Physiology, Berkeley, CA: University of California Press, 1994:253–270.
22. Evans WE. Orientation behavior of delphinids: Radio telemetric studies. Ann NY Acad Sci 1971; 188:142–160.
23. Hall JD. Conditioning Pacific white striped dolphin, *Lagenorhynchus obliquidens*, for open ocean release. Nav Undersea Ctr Tech Paper 1970; 200:1–16.
24. Ridgway SH. Diving by cetaceans. In: Brabakk AO, Kanwisher JW, Sundnes G, eds. Diving in Animals and Man. Trondheim, Norway: Royal Norwegian Society of Science and Letters, 1986:33–62.
25. Bowers CA, Henderson RS. Project Deep OPS: Deep object recovery with pilot and killer whales. Nav Undersea Ctr Tech Pub 1972; 306:1–86.
26. Ridgway SH, Bowers CA, Miller D, et al. Diving and blood oxygen in the white whale. Can J Zool 1984; 62:2349–2351.
27. Watkins WA, Daher MA, Fristrup KM, Howald TJ. Sperm whales tagged with transponders and tracked underwater by sonar. Mar Mam Sci 1993; 9:55–67.
28. Scholander PF. Experimental investigations on the respiratory function in diving

mammals and birds. Hvalradets Skrifter Norske Videnskaps: Akad Oslo 1940; 22: 1–131.

29. Kramer DL. The behavioral ecology of air breathing by aquatic animals. Can J Zool 1988; 66:89–94.
30. Gentry RL, Kooyman GL, eds. Fur Seals: Maternal Strategies on Land and at Sea. Princeton, NJ: Princeton University Press, 1986.
31. Feldkamp S, DeLong RL, Antonelis CA. Diving patterns of California sea lions, *Zalophus californianus*. Can J Zool 1989; 67:872–883.
32. Kooyman GL, Davis RW, Croxall JP, Costa DP. Diving depths and energy requirements of king penguins. Science 1982; 217:726–727.
33. Kooyman GL, Drabek CM, Elsner R, Campbell WB. Diving behavior of the emperor penguin, *Aptenodytes forsteri*. Auk 1971; 88:775–795.
34. Robertson GG. The foraging ecology of emperor penguins (*Aptenodytes forsteri*) at two Mawson Coast colonies, Antarctica. ANARE Reports 138 Antarctic Division, Department of the Environment, Sport, and Territories, Australia, 1995.
35. Lutcavage M. Bushnell P, Jones DR. Oxygen stores and aerobic metabolism in the leather back sea turtle. Can J Zool 1992; 70:348–351.
36. Berkson H. Physiological adjustments to deep diving in the Pacific green turtle (*Chelonia mydas*). Comp Biochem Physiol 1967; 21:507–524.
37. Lutcavage ME, Bushnell PG, Jones DR. Oxygen transport in the leatherback sea turtle *Dermochelys coriacea*. Phys Zool 1990; 63:1012–1024.
38. Kooyman GL, Schroeder JP, Denison DM, et al. Blood N2 tensions of seals during simulated deep dives. Am J Physiol 1972; 223:1016–1020.
39. Ponganis PJ, Kooyman GL, Castellini MA. Determinants of the aerobic dive limit of Weddell seals: Analysis of diving metabolic rates, post-dive and tidal P_{O_2}'s and blood and muscle oxygen stores. Physiol Zool 1993; 66:732–749.
40. Fujise Y, Hidake H, Tatsukawa R, Miyazaki N. External measurements and organ weights of five Weddell seals (*Leptonychotes weddelli*) caught near Syowa Station. Antarctic Record (Tokyo) 1985; 85:96–101.
41. Simpson JG, Gilmartin WG, Ridgway SH. Blood volume and other hematologic values in young elephant seals (*Mirounga angustirostris*). Am J Vet Res 1970; 31: 1449–1452.
42. Thorson PH. Development of diving in the northern elephant seal. Doctoral thesis. University of California, Santa Cruz, 1993.
43. Bryden MM. Body size and composition of elephant seals (*Mirounga leonina*): Absolute measurements and estimates from bone dimensions. J Zool (Lond) 1972; 167:265–276.
44. Kooyman GL, Schroeder JP, Greene DG, Smith VA. Gas exchange in penguins during simulated dives to 30 and 68 m. Am J Physiol 1973; 225:1467–1471.
45. Lenfant C, Kooyman GL, Elsner R, Drabek CM. Respiratory function of the blood of the Adelie penguin (*Pygoscelis adeliae*). Am J Physiol 1969; 216:1598–1600.
46. Groscolas R. Effet d'une exposition a la chaleur sur la temperature corporelle et quelques parametres hematologiques du manchot empereur (*Aptenodytes forsteri*). Comp Biochem Physiol 1975; 50A:533–543.
47. Cherel Y, Charassin JB, Handrich Y. Comparison of body reserve buildup in pre-

fasting chicks and adults of king penguins (*Aptenodytes patagonicus*). Physiol Zool 1993; 66:750–770.

48. Le Boeuf BJ, Costa DP, Huntley AC, Feldkamp SD. Continuous deep diving in female northern elephant seals, *Mirounga angustirostris*. Can J Zool 1988; 66:446–458.
49. Hindell MA, Slip DJ, Burton HR, Bryden MM. Physiological implications of continuous, prolonged, and deep dives of the southern elephant seal (*Mirounga leonina*). Can J Zool 1992; 70:370–379.
50. Kooyman GL. In: Johansen K, Farner DS, eds. Diverse Divers: Physiology and Behavior. Zoophysiol Series, Vol 23. New York: Springer-Verlag, 1989.
51. Persson SGB, Ekman L, Lyden G, Tufvesson G. Circulation effects of splenectomy in the horse I-IV. II. Effect on plasma volume and total and circulating red cell volume. Zentralbl Veterinaermed 1973; 20:456–468.
52. Danforth DN. Obstetrics and Gynecology. Hagerstown, MD: Harper & Row, 1977.
53. Lutz PL, Bentley TB. Respiratory physiology of diving in the sea turtle. Copeia 1985; 1985:671–679.
54. Tenney SM, Tenney JB. Quantitative morphology of cold-blooded lungs: Amphibia and reptilia. Respir Physiol 1970; 9:197–215.
55. Kooyman GL, Ponganis PJ. Behavior and physiology of diving in emperor and king penguins. In: Davis LS, Darby J, eds. Penguin Biology. New York: Academic Press, 1990:231–244.
56. Falke KJ, Hill RD, Qvist J, et al. Seal lungs collapse during free diving: Evidence from arterial nitrogen tensions. Science 1985; 229:556–558.
57. van Nie CJ, van der Kamp JS. The closure of the foramen ovale and the ductus arteriosus in the common seal (*Phoca vitulina*, L. 1758). A morphological approach. Aquat Mam 1988; 14:82–85.
58. Drabek CM. Some anatomical aspects of the cardiovascular system of antarctic seals and their possible functional significance in diving. J Morphol 1975; 145:85–106.
59. Sinnett EE, Kooyman GL, Wahrenbrock EA. Pulmonary circulation of the harbor seal. J Appl Physiol 1978; 45:718–727.
60. Calvin JE Jr. Acute right heart failure: pathophysiology, recognition and pharmacological management. J Cardiothorac Vasc Anesthesiol 1991; 5:507–513.
61. Berkson H. Physiological adjustments to prolonged diving in the Pacific green turtle (*Chelonia mydas agassizii*). Comp Biochem Physiol 1966; 18:101–119.
62. Blix AS, Elsner RW, Kjekshus JK. Cardiac output and its distribution through capillaries and A-V shunts in diving seals. Acta Physiol Scand 1983; 118:109–116.
63. Jones DR, Bryan RM Jr, West NH, et al. Regional distribution of blood flow during diving in the duck (*Anas platyrhynchos*). Can J Zool 1979; 57:995–1002.
64. Zapol WM, Liggins GC, Schneider RC, et al. Regional blood flow during simulated diving in the conscious Weddell seal. J Appl Physiol 1979; 47:968–973.
65. Murphy B, Zapol WM, Hochachka PW. Metabolic activities of heart, lung, and brain during diving and recovery in the Weddell seal. J Appl Physiol 1980; 48: 596–605.
66. Kooyman GL, Wahrenbrock EA, Castellini MA, et al. Aerobic and anaerobic metab-

olism during diving in the Weddell seals: Evidence of preferred pathways from blood chemistry and behavior. J Comp Physiol 1980; 138:335–346.

67. Kooyman GL. Physiology without restraint in diving mammals. Mar Mamm Sci 1985; 1:166–178.
68. Kooyman GL, Campbell WB. Heart rate in freely diving Weddell seals (*Leptonychotes weddelli*). Comp Biochem Physiol 1973; 43:31–6.
69. Hill RD, Schneider RC, Liggins GC, et al. Heart rate and body temperature during free diving of Weddell seals. Am J Physiol 1987; 253:R344–R351.
70. Castellini MA, Milsom WK, Berger RJ, et al. Patterns of respiration and heart rate during wakefulness and sleep in elephant seal pups. Am J Physiol 1994; 266:R863–R869.
71. Belkin DA. Variation in heart rate during voluntary diving in the turtle, *Pseudemys concinna*. Copeia 1964; 1964:321–330.
72. Millard RW, Johansen K, Milson WK. Radiotelemetry of cardiovascular responses to exercise and diving in penguins. Comp Biochem Physiol 1973; 46:227–240.
73. Kooyman GL. An analysis of some behavioral and physiological characteristics related to diving in the Weddell seal. Antarct Biol Ser 1968; 11:227–261.
74. Fedak MA, Pullen MR, Kanwisher J. Circulatory responses of seals to periodic breathing: Heart rate and breathing during exercise and diving in the laboratory and open sea. Can J Zool 1988; 66:53–60.
75. Andrews RD, Williams JD, Jones DR. Heart rate responses to apnea on land and at sea in northern elephant seals (*Mirounga angustirostris*). Am Zool 1992; 32: 31A.
76. Williams R, Bryden MM. Observations of blood values, heart rate and respiratory rate of leopard seals (*Hydrurga leptonyx*) (Carnivora: Phocidae). Aust J Zool 1993; 41:433–439.
77. Elsner R, Wartzok D, Sonafrank NB, Kelly BP. Behavioral and physiological reactions of arctic seals during under-ice pilotage. Can J Zool 1989; 67:2506–2513.
78. Thompson D, Fedak MA. Cardiac responses of grey seals during diving at sea. J Exp Biol 1993; 174:139–164.
79. Kooyman GL, Ponganis PJ, Castellini MA, et al. Heart rates and swim speeds of emperor penguins diving under sea ice. J Exp Biol 1992; 165:161–180.
80. Kooyman GL, Ponganis PJ. Emperor penguin oxygen consumption, heart rate and plasma lactate levels during graded swimming exercise. J Exp Biol 1994; 195:199–209.
81. Elsner R, Franklin DL, Van Citters RL, Kenney DW. Cardiovascular defense against asphyxia. Science 1966; 153:941–949.
82. Scholander PF, Irving L, Grinnell SW. Aerobic and anaerobic changes in seal muscle during diving. J Biol Chem 1942; 142:431–440.
83. Davis RW, Castellini MA, Kooyman GL, Maui R. Renal GFR and hepatic blood flow during voluntary diving in Weddell seals. Am J Physiol 1983; 245:743–748.
84. Guppy M, Hill RD, Schneider RC, et al. Microcomputer-assisted metabolic studies of voluntary diving of Weddell seals. Am J Physiol 1986; 250:175–187.
85. Gooden BA, Elsner R. What diving mammals might tell us about blood flow regulation. Perspect Biol Med 1985; 28:463–474.

86. Ponganis PJ, Kooyman GL, Castellini MA, et al. Muscle temperature and swim velocity profiles during diving in a Weddell seal, *Leptonychotes weddellii*. J Exp Biol 1993; 183:341–348.
87. Bevan RM, Butler PJ. Cardiac output and blood flow distribution during swimming and voluntary diving of the tufted duck (*Aythya fuligula*). J Exp Biol 1992; 168:199–277.
88. Stephenson R, Turner DL, Butler PJ. The relationship between diving activity and oxygen storage capacity in the tufted duck I (*Aythya fuligula*). J Exp Biol 1989: 141:265–275.
89. Gatten RE Jr. Anaerobic metabolism in freely diving painted turtles (*Chrysemys picta*). J Exp Biol 1981; 216:377–385.
90. Castellini MA, Davis RW, Kooyman GL. Blood chemistry during repetitive diving in Weddell seals. Physiol Zool 1988; 61:379–386.
91. Kooyman GL, Castellini MA, Davis RW, Maue RA. Aerobic dive limits in immature Weddell seals. J Comp Physiol 1983; 151:171–174.
92. Qvist J, Hill RD, Schneider RC, et al. Hemoglobin concentrations and blood gas tensions of free-diving Weddell seals. J Appl Physiol 1986; 61:1560–1569.
93. Seymour RS. Gas tensions and blood distribution in sea snakes at surface pressure and at simulated depth. Physiol Zool 1978; 51:388–407.
94. Graham JB. Aquatic respiration in the sea snake. Respir Physiol 1974; 21:1–7.
95. Dunlap CE. Notes on the visceral anatomy of the giant leatherback sea turtle, *Dermochelys coriacea*. Bull Tulane Med Fac 1955; 14:55–69.
96. Denison DM, Kooyman GL. The structure and function of the small airways in pinniped and sea otter lungs. Respir Physiol 1973; 17:1–10.
97. Kooyman GL, Sinnett EE. Mechanical properties of the harbor porpoise lung. Respir Physiol 1979; 36:287–300.
98. Kooyman GL, Hammond DD, Schroeder JP. Bronchograms and tracheograms of seals under pressure. Science 1970; 169:82–84.
99. Leith D. Comparative mammalian respiratory mechanics. Physiologist 1976; 19: 485–510.
100. Ridgway SH, Howard R. Dolphin lung collapse and intramuscular circulation during free diving: Evidence from nitrogen washout. Science 1979; 206:1182–1183.
101. Kooyman GL, Sinnett EE. Pulmonary shunts in harbor seals and sea lions during simulated dives to depth. Physiol Zool 1982; 55:105–111.
102. Harvey EN, McElroy WD, Whiteley AH, et al. Bubble formation in animals: III. An analysis of gas tension and hydrostatic pressure in cats. J Cell Comp Physiol 1944; 24:117–132.
103. Eckenhoff RC, Olstad CS, Carrod G. Human dose-response relationship for decompression and endogenous bubble formation. J Appl Physiol 1990; 69:914–918.
104. Workman R. Calculation of decompression schedules for nitrogen-oxygen and helium-oxygen dives. Report 6-65. Washington, DC: U.S. Navy Experimental Diving Unit, 1965.
105. Hills BA. Relevant phase conditions for predicting occurrence of decompression sickness. J Appl Physiol 1968; 25:310–315.

106. Griffiths HB. On the role of separated gas in decompression procedures. Proc R Soc Lond B 1971; 178:389–406.
107. Duncker H-R. Structure of the avian respiratory tract. Respir Physiol 1974; 22:1–19.
108. Scheid P. Mechanisms of gas exchange in bird lungs. Rev Physiol Biochem 1979; 86:138–186.
109. McIlroy MB. Pulmonary shunts. In: Handbook of Physiology. Sec 3, Vol 2. Washington, D.C.: American Physiological Society, 1965:1519–1529.
110. Swan LW. Goose of the Himalayas. Nat Hist 1970; 79:68–75.
111. Maina JN, King AS. A morphometric study of the lung of a Humboldt penguin (*Spheniscus humboldti*). Anat Histol Embryol 1987; 16:293–297.
112. Davis MB, Guderley H. Energy metabolism in the locomotor muscles of the Common Murre (*Uria aalge*) and the Atlantic Puffin (*Fratercula arctica*). Auk 1987; 104:733–739.
113. Weber RE, Hemmingsen EA, Johansen K. Functional and biochemical studies of penguin myoglobins. Comp Biochem Physiol 1974; 49:197–214.
114. Mill GK, Baldwin J. Biochemical correlates of swimming and diving behavior in the little penguin, Eudyptula minor. Physiol. Zool 1983; 56:242–254.
115. Baldwin J, Hardel J-P, Montague T, Tomkin R. Energy metabolism in penguin swimming muscles. Molec Physiol 1984; 6:33–42.
116. Blessing MH. Studies on the concentration of myoglobin in the sea-cow and porpoise. Comp Biochem Physiol 1972; 41A:475–480.
117. Castellini MA, Somero GN. Buffering capacity of vertebrate muscle: Correlations with potentials for anaerobic function. J Comp Physiol 1981; 143:191–198.
118. Lenfant C, Johansen K, Torrance JD. Gas transport and oxygen storage capacity in some pinnipeds and the sea otter. Respir Physiol 1970; 9:277–286.
119. Reed JZ, Butler PJ, Fedak MA. The metabolic characteristics of the locomotory muscles of grey seals (*Halichoerus grypus*), harbour seals (*Phoca vitulina*) and antarctic fur seals (*Arctocephalus gazella*). J Exp Biol 1994; 194:33–46.
120. Lydersen C, Ryg MS. Oxygen stores and aerobic dive limit of ringed seals (*Phoca hispida*). Can J Zool 1992; 70:458–461.
121. Blessing MH, Hartschen-Niemeyer E. Uber den Myoglobingehalt der Herz und Skelettmuskulatur insbesondere einiger mariner Sauger. 1969; 116:302–313.
122. Hapner KD, Bradshaw RA, Hartzell CR, Gurd FRN. Comparison of myoglobins from harbor seal, porpoise, and sperm whale. J Biol Chem 1968; 243:683–689.
123. McFarland WL, Jacobs MS, Morgane PJ. Blood supply to the brain of the dolphin, *Tursiops truncatus*, with comparative observations on special aspects of the cerebrovascular supply of other vertebrates. Neurosci Biobehav Res 1979; 3(suppl 1):193.
124. Bennett PB. Inert gas narcosis. In: Bennett PB, Elliott DH, eds. The Physiology and Medicine of Diving and Compressed Air Work. Baltimore: Williams & Wilkins, 1975:207–229.
125. Brauer PB. The high pressure nervous syndrome: Animals. In: Bennett PB, Elliott DH, eds. The Physiology and Medicine of Diving and Compressed Air Work. Baltimore: Williams & Wilkins, 1975:231–247.

AUTHOR INDEX

Italicized numbers give the page on which the complete reference is listed.

A

B

C

E

F

G

H

I

J

K

L

M

N

O

P

S

T

U

V

W

Y

Z

SUBJECT INDEX

A

B

C

D

E

G

O

P

R

T

U

W